NUTRITION FOR SPORT, EXERCISE, AND HEALTH

Marie A. Spano, MS, RD, CSCS, CSSD
Spano Sports Nutrition Consulting, LLC

Laura J. Kruskall, PhD, RDN, CSSD, LD, FACSM, FAND
University of Nevada, Las Vegas

D. Travis Thomas, PhD, RDN, CSSD, LD, FAND
University of Kentucky

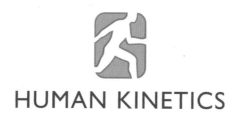

HUMAN KINETICS

Library of Congress Cataloging-in-Publication Data

Names: Spano, Marie A., 1972- author. | Kruskall, Laura J., 1967- author. |
  Thomas, D. Travis, 1977- author.
Title: Nutrition for sport, exercise, and health / Marie A. Spano, Laura J.
  Kruskall, and D. Travis Thomas.
Description: Champaign, IL : Human Kinetics, [2017] | Includes
  bibliographical references and index.
Identifiers: LCCN 2016025648| ISBN 9781450414876 (print) | ISBN 9781492546108 (e-book)
Subjects: | MESH: Sports Nutritional Physiological Phenomena | Physical
  Fitness--physiology
Classification: LCC RA784 | NLM QT 263 | DDC 613.7--dc23
LC record available at https://lccn.loc.gov/2016025648

ISBN: 978-1-4504-1487-6 (print)

Senior Acquisitions Editor: Amy N. Tocco; **Developmental Editor:** Melissa J. Zavala; **Managing Editor:** Anna Lan Seaman; **Copyeditor:** John Wentworth; **Indexer:** Nancy Ball; **Permissions Manager:** Dalene Reeder; **Senior Graphic Designer:** Joe Buck; **Cover Designer:** Keith Blomberg; **Photograph (cover):** lzf/iStockphoto/Getty Images; **Photo Asset Manager:** Laura Fitch; **Photo Production Manager:** Jason Allen; **Senior Art Manager:** Kelly Hendren; **Art Style Development:** Joanne Brummett; **Illustrations:** © Human Kinetics, unless otherwise noted; **Printer:** Walsworth

Printed in the United States of America   10 9 8 7 6 5 4 3 2 1

The paper in this book is certified under a sustainable forestry program.

Human Kinetics
Website: www.HumanKinetics.com

United States: Human Kinetics
P.O. Box 5076
Champaign, IL 61825-5076
800-747-4457
e-mail: info@hkusa.com

Canada: Human Kinetics
475 Devonshire Road Unit 100
Windsor, ON N8Y 2L5
800-465-7301 (in Canada only)
e-mail: info@hkcanada.com

Europe: Human Kinetics
107 Bradford Road
Stanningley
Leeds LS28 6AT, United Kingdom
+44 (0) 113 255 5665
e-mail: hk@hkeurope.com

For information about Human Kinetics' coverage in other areas of the world, please visit our website: www.HumanKinetics.com

PART IV APPLICATION OF NUTRITION FOR SPORT, EXERCISE, AND HEALTH 253

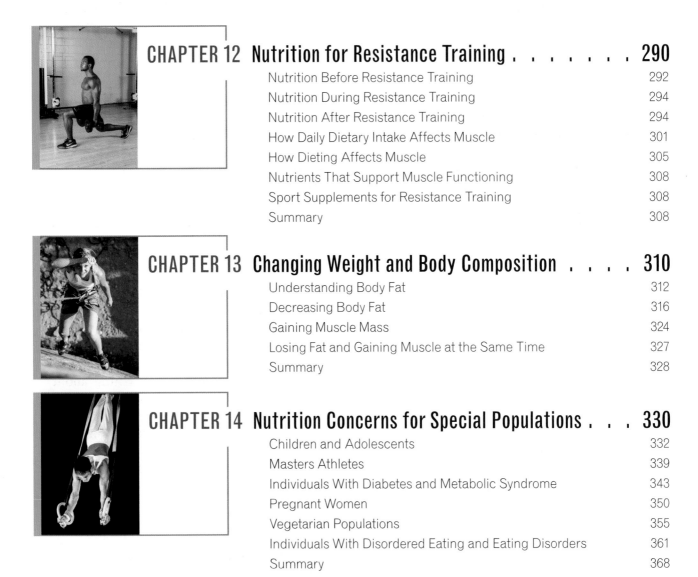

Nutrition affects overall health and exercise performance in myriad ways. In *Nutrition for Sport, Exercise, and Health* our goal is to provide readers with practical information they can use to enhance their everyday lives as well as the sports and physical activities that are part of their lives. For the student with an interest in working in the field of sport nutrition, sports medicine, or another related field, our goal is to supply in a single text the foundation of knowledge you will need to get the best start on your career path.

Given the plethora of nutrition misinformation consumers are hearing and reading from television, the Internet, magazines, coaches, trainers, parents, and their peers, this comprehensive textbook will help readers distinguish between nutrition recommendations that are based on quality scientific research and those that are not backed by science and have no foothold in basic biochemistry or physiology.

eBook available at your campus bookstore or HumanKinetics.com

WHO NEEDS THIS BOOK

We have written *Nutrition for Sport, Exercise, and Health* for students studying fitness, exercise science, health, nutrition, physical therapy, and closely related majors. This text is also an excellent reference for athletic trainers, strength coaches, wellness professionals, health coaches, health and physical education teachers, coaches, fitness instructors, athletic directors, exercise physiologists, registered dietitians, military personnel, and government employees working in health and human performance.

TOPICS COVERED

Our text covers the basics of nutrition for health, including the functions and daily allowances for the energy-yielding macronutrients—carbohydrate, protein, and fat—and micronutrients; nutrition in health and disease prevention; population-based nutrition considerations for training and sports; and practical information on measuring and altering body composition.

The text is organized in a logical sequence, with each chapter building on what was learned in the previous chapter. In part I, we provide an overview of the role nutrition plays in overall well-being throughout the life span. Energy metabolism is discussed, including the roles of macronutrients and micronutrients and how exercise affects nutrient needs. The three chapters in part II focus on each energy-yielding macronutrient, its role in health and disease, and dietary recommendations that support health and an active lifestyle. After learning about macronutrients, readers are introduced in part III to the roles of micronutrients in health and performance. Chapters on vitamins and minerals cover population-specific intake recommendations, consequences of excess intake or dietary shortfalls, and supplemental intake. This part of the book covers water and electrolytes as well as nutrition supplements and drugs. The role of fluid in health and human performance is discussed, and fluid and electrolyte guidelines are recommended. The chapter on nutrition supplements and drugs covers popular dietary supplements, supplement claims, third-party testing, drugs in sports, and the untoward effects of alcohol on sports performance. In part IV we provide information on the application of nutrition to health and fitness. Ideal body weight and body composition is discussed, including how to measure body composition and achieve optimal body composition and weight; nutrition recommendations are provided for aerobic endurance and resistance training. In the final chapter we discuss nutrition concerns and recommendations for special populations and individuals at distinct life stages, including children, adolescents, masters athletes, diabetics, vegetarians, pregnant women, and individuals with eating disorders or disordered eating.

UNIQUE FEATURES THAT ENHANCE LEARNING

The book includes a number of features that help highlight key concepts and provide practical examples to enhance understanding. Each chapter includes the following elements:

> Chapter objectives

  Included at the start of each chapter, these give you an overview of what lies ahead.

> "Putting It Into Perspective" sidebars

  These elements help engage college readers by providing information that is relevant to them, including practical case studies; tips on improving health, enhancing sports performance, or achieving a desired physique; and other helpful material that can be applied in everyday living.

> "Do You Know?" sidebars

  These brief information nuggets provide key insights, little-known details, and evidence-based facts that might surprise you.

> "Reflection Time" sidebars

  These elements prompt readers to dig deeper and consider how certain concepts presented in the book relate to their everyday lives.

> "Nutrition Tip" sidebars

  Intriguing, real-world tips related to nutrition for the college student.

> Review questions

  Questions to evoke further thought and ensure that readers have digested the key points in each chapter.

> Glossary

  A handy listing of key terms to help you fill your memory bank—or for your future reference.

INSTRUCTOR RESOURCES

Instructor ancillaries include an instructor guide, presentation package, test package, and chapter quizzes. The instructor guide includes chapter outlines and chapter summaries, objectives, and review questions from the book. The presentation package includes PowerPoint slides and an image bank of most of the art and tables from the book that instructors may use to create customized lecture presentations. The test package and chapter quizzes provide questions in various formats that can be used to create customized tests. Ancillary products supporting this textbook are available at www.HumanKinetics.com/NutritionForSportExerciseAndHealth.

PART I

THE BIG PICTURE

Nutrition is a complex and vast science that covers the role of food, supplementation, and hydration for growth and development, metabolism, health, disease prevention, and sports performance. Looking at the big picture, nutrition needs change throughout the lifecycle. A nutrient-rich diet supplies the body with the macronutrients and micronutrients needed for optimal growth and development, health, and well-being throughout the lifecycle. Medical nutrition therapy, a subdiscipline within the field of nutrition, covers the nutrition needs for specific disease states and health conditions. Chapter 1 provides an overview of nutrition for health throughout the lifecycle, for disease states, and for athletic performance. In addition, food guidance systems intended for the general public are covered, as well as information on the research process and reliable sources of nutrition information.

Following an overview of nutrition for health and well-being, chapter 2 explores energy metabolism. Before delving into the specific role of nutrition in exercise and athletic performance, you'll learn about the different energy systems the body can use to generate fuel during various types of exercise at both high and low intensity.

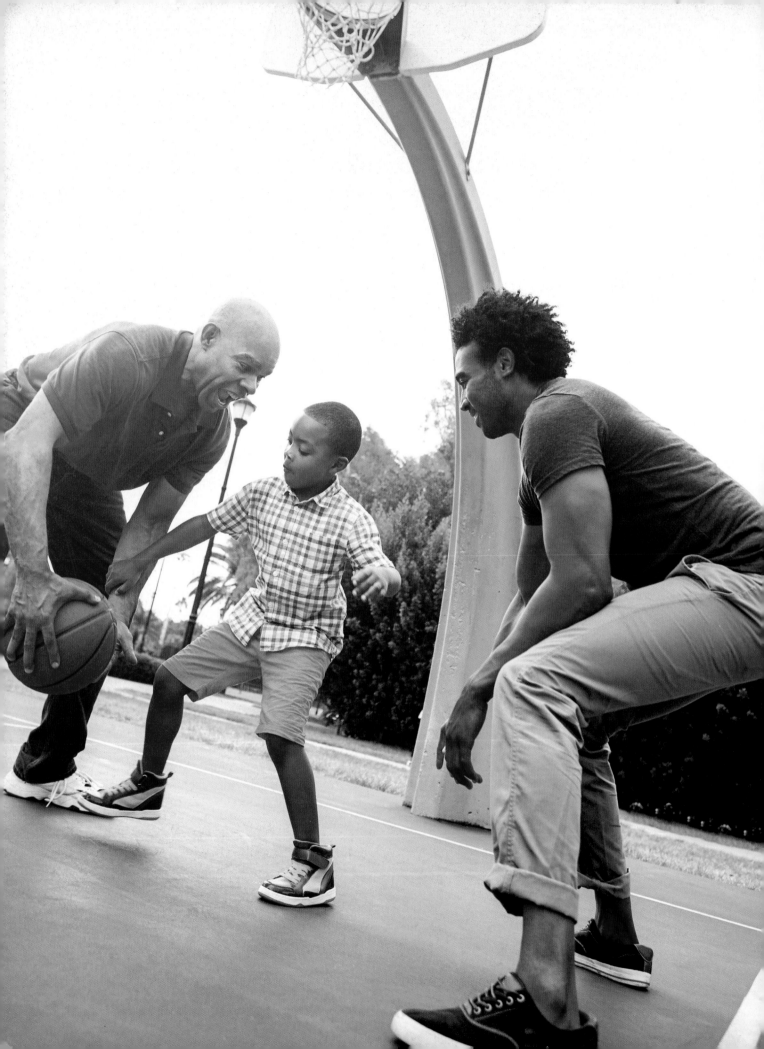

CHAPTER 1

Optimizing Health and Well-Being Throughout the Lifespan

> **CHAPTER OBJECTIVES**
>
> After completing this chapter, you will be able to do the following:
>
> - Explain functions of nutrients and their roles in health.
> - Describe the differences between macronutrients and micronutrients.
> - Explain the difference between general nutrition information and medical nutrition therapy.
> - Identify and understand the major food guidance systems in the United States (Dietary Guidelines, Food Labels, Dietary Reference Intakes, and MyPlate).
> - Describe the basic principles of exercise and training.
> - Discuss the role of nutrition in optimizing athletic performance.
> - Summarize the scientific research process and types of research designs, as well as how to evaluate reputable sources for sport nutrition information.
> - Understand credentials available in exercise science and the scope of practice between nutrition and exercise professionals.

Nutrition, as a scientific discipline, is the study of how food and its components affect growth and development, metabolism, health, and disease as well as mental and physical performance. **Food** refers to anything people eat or drink that supports life and growth. **Nutrients** are substances that elicit a biochemical or physiological function in the body. The science of nutrition involves the processes of consumption or ingestion, digestion, absorption, metabolism, transport, storage, and elimination. In addition to the science behind it, nutrition is an extremely broad field that encompasses everything from the food supply and food safety to eating behavior and nutrient recommendations for optimal health (44, 58). **Sport nutrition** is a specialty discipline that merges nutrition and sports science research, resulting in nutrition guidelines for optimal training, performance, and recovery from exercise.

NUTRIENTS

There are six groups of nutrients: carbohydrate, lipids, protein, vitamins, minerals, and water. Alcohol is not a nutrient, but it does contain energy (calories). Carbohydrates, fats (including fatty acids and cholesterol), protein (including amino acids), fiber, and water are **macronutrients**, which are required in the diet in larger amounts. Carbohydrates, fats, and proteins are also referred to as **energy-yielding macronutrients** because they supply the body with energy. Vitamins and minerals are **micronutrients**, which are required in the body in smaller amounts in comparison to macronutrients. A common misconception is that vitamins and minerals are energy nutrients. These do not contain energy, though they play essential roles in the production of energy. Deficiencies of certain vitamins and minerals can lead to fatigue. Macronutrients and micronutrients work together for optimal physiological function (44, 58). The unit of energy in food is called a **kilocalorie**, commonly referred to as a calorie or kcal. A kilocalorie is the amount of heat it takes to raise the temperature of one kilogram of water by one degree Celsius. A person's energy requirements refer to the number of kilocalories needed each day. Food labels list calories per serving of the item. Both carbohydrate and protein contain 4 calories per gram, while lipids provide 9 calories per gram, making lipids more energy dense—that is, they contain more calories per mass or volume than do carbohydrate or protein (44, 58).

Dietary Reference Intakes

The Institute of Medicine (IOM) of the United States Department of Agriculture (USDA) developed the Dietary Reference Intakes (DRIs), a set of recommendations based on the latest "scientific knowledge of the nutrient needs of healthy populations" (46) (figure 1.1). The DRIs include:

> **Estimated Average Requirement (EAR).** The EAR is the estimated mean daily requirement for a nutrient as determined to meet the requirements of 50 percent of healthy people in each life stage and gender group (different amounts are provided based on age ranges and life stages, such as pregnancy and lactation). The EAR is based on the reduction of disease and other health parameters. It does not reflect the daily needs of individuals but is used to set the RDA and for research purposes.

> **Recommended Dietary Allowance (RDA).** The RDA is set to meet the needs of nearly all (97–98%) healthy people in each gender and life stage. This is the amount that should be consumed on a daily basis. The RDA is two standard

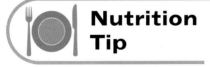

Nutrition Tip

Counting your carbs? Note that while all vegetables contain primarily carbohydrate, their content per serving is not the same. Vegetables can be categorized as starchy or nonstarchy. Starchy vegetables, such as potatoes, corn, and peas, contain approximately 15 grams of carbohydrate in a half-cup serving. Nonstarchy vegetables, such as broccoli, beets, and asparagus, contain considerably less carbohydrate—about 5 grams per half-cup serving. So if you want to reduce your intake of carbohydrate, choose nonstarchy vegetables.

deviations above the EAR based on variability in requirements, or if the standard deviation is not known, the RDA is 1.2 times the EAR.

> **Adequate Intake (AI).** The AI is the recommended average daily nutrient level assumed to be adequate for all healthy people. The AI is based on estimates—observed or experimentally determined approximations—and used when the RDA cannot be established because of insufficient data (46).

> **Tolerable Upper Intake Level (UL).** The UL is the highest average daily intake considered safe for almost all individuals. The UL represents average daily intake from all sources, including food, water, and supplements. Lack of a published UL does not indicate that high levels of the nutrient are safe. Instead, it means there isn't enough research available at this time to establish a UL (46).

> **Acceptable Macronutrient Distribution Range (AMDR).** The AMDR is a range given as a percentage of total calorie intake—including carbohydrate, protein, and fat—and is associated with a reduced risk of chronic disease and adequate intake of essential nutrients (18).

> **Estimated Energy Requirement (EER).** The EER is the average daily energy intake that should maintain energy balance in a healthy person. Factors such as gender, age, height, weight, and activity level are all considerations when calculating this value (46).

Energy-Yielding Macronutrients

The primary function of carbohydrate is to provide energy. Carbohydrate becomes increasingly important when exercising at a high intensity. High-intensity exercise increases energy (calorie) demands, and carbohydrate is a fast source of energy—the body can quickly access it—whereas fat, another source of energy, is much slower in meeting the body's demand for energy during high-intensity exercise. Carbohydrate can be stored, to an extent, in the human body as an energy reserve in the form of glycogen in the liver and muscle. The AMDR for carbohydrate is 45 to 65 percent of kilocalories for both males and females ages 19 and older (18). Common sources of carbohydrate are rice, pasta, wheat products, and grains such as corn, beans, legumes, fruits, vegetables, and milk. Some carbohydrates are considered nutrient-dense because they contain nutrients important for good health, including vitamins, minerals, and dietary fiber. A type of carbohydrate, fiber is discussed in detail in chapter 3.

Dietary fats and oils are examples of lipids. Dietary fats and oils provide energy and aid in the absorption of fat-soluble vitamins and food components. Fat can be stored in limitless quantities in the body, serving as an energy reserve (18). Fat can be an important energy source during long-duration activities, such as an ultra-endurance race. The AMDR for fat is 20

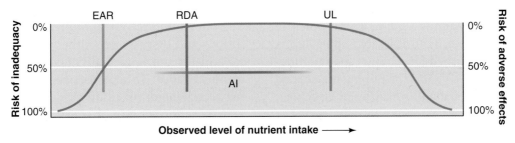

EAR is inadequate for 50% of the population.

RDA is inadequate for 2 to 3% of the population.

AI is the recommended average daily intake assumed to be adequate for all healthy people. AI is used when a RDA cannot be established.

UL is the maximum safe level above which risk for adverse effects increases.

Figure 1.1 Dietary Reference Intakes. The AI or RDA describes the recommended daily amount of a nutrient, while the UL describes the amount not to exceed. Too little or too much of a nutrient can increase the risk of undesirable effects.

to 35 percent for both males and females ages 19 years and older (18). Common sources of fats include meat, nuts, seeds, oils, dairy products, and vegetable spreads (47).

Protein can be used for energy, but its primary function is to support cell and tissue growth, maintenance, and repair. Unlike carbohydrate and lipids, the primary purpose of protein is not to supply energy, so it is important to get an adequate amount on a regular basis (18). The RDA for protein is 56 grams per day for males aged 19 and over, and 46 grams per day for females aged 14 and over. The RDA for pregnant and lactating women of all ages is 71 grams per day (18). Despite these recommendations, considerable evidence suggests that the RDA for protein is too low to support muscle growth and maintenance, particularly for athletes and older adults (32, 34, 35). The AMDR for protein is 10 to 35 percent of calories for both males and females ages 19 and older (18). Common sources of protein include poultry, beef, fish, eggs, dairy foods, and some plant foods, particularly soy foods, nuts, and seeds (44, 47, 58).

Micronutrients

Vitamins are essential nutrients, necessary for releasing and using energy in the metabolism of carbohydrates, lipids, and proteins. Vitamins also support proper growth and development, vision, organ and immune functioning, muscle contraction and relaxation, oxygen transport, building and maintaining bone and cartilage, building and repairing muscle tissue, and protecting the body's cells from damage. Vitamins are classified as fat-soluble or water-soluble depending on how they are absorbed, transported, and stored in the body. Most water-soluble vitamins (e.g., some B vitamins, vitamin C) are not stored in the body, and any excess is excreted in urine; fat-soluble vitamins (e.g., vitamins A, D, E, K) are stored in adipose (fat) tissue (18). Tolerable upper limits have been established for many of the micronutrients (46). Daily vitamin requirements depend on many factors, including health status, gender, life stage, and age (27). Vitamin deficiencies or insufficiencies may negatively impact training gains and athletic performance, though there is no evidence to suggest those who exercise or train

for competition need greater intakes beyond their requirements for general health (24, 44, 58).

Minerals are structural components of many body tissues, including bones, nails, and teeth. They also help regulate fluid balance, muscle pH, muscle contraction (including heartbeat), nerve impulses, oxygen transport, immune functioning, and muscle building and repair and are part of enzymes that facilitate several metabolic functions (15, 44, 58).

Macrominerals are required in higher amounts (i.e., grams and milligrams) than are trace minerals (i.e., micrograms). Mineral deficiencies can impair health as well as exercise and athletic performance, though research does not indicate that excess intake, beyond the DRIs, will improve results from an exercise program or improve athletic performance (24, 44, 58).

Water

Water plays a role in nutrient transport, waste removal, biochemical reactions, blood pressure, and regulation of body temperature. Water needs depend on many factors, including age, body size, health status, medication use, environment (heat), altitude, and physical activity, particularly sweat losses. Daily water requirements can be met through a combination of fluids and the water found in food (28). In particular, soups, fruits, and vegetables contain a considerable amount of water (38, 44, 58).

GENERAL NUTRITION GUIDELINES

Nutrition plays a significant role in health **wellness**. Nutrition guidelines exist for healthy persons as well as those with specific diseases or conditions. Medical nutrition therapy includes diet interventions to treat or prevent health conditions and diseases (2). Other guidelines exist for athletes and active individuals specific to the activity or sport. In some aspects, there is overlap between general nutrition guidelines for health and those for activity or sports. It is important to have an understanding of both in order to differentiate when general versus sport-specific guidelines should be considered.

PUTTING IT INTO PERSPECTIVE

GENERAL NUTRITION INFORMATION VERSUS MEDICAL NUTRITION THERAPY

General, nonmedical nutrition information is designed to provide healthy individuals with food and nutrition guidelines for health promotion and disease prevention. Many of these guidelines come from government agencies, including the United States Department of Agriculture (USDA). If a person has a health condition or disease for which food and nutrition plays a role in the prevention or management, this is called **medical nutrition therapy (MNT)**. MNT is most often provided by a Registered Dietitian Nutritionist (RD or RDN), and in many states providing MNT is limited to practitioners who hold a license.

Dietary Guidelines

While the rate of many infectious diseases has dropped over the years, largely because of immunizations (6), an increase has occurred in chronic diseases and conditions related to poor nutrition habits and physical inactivity (59). Examples include cardiovascular disease, high blood pressure, type 2 diabetes, some types of cancer, and osteoporosis (14). In addition, more than two-thirds of adults and almost one-third of children and adolescents are overweight or obese (31). The *2015–2020 Dietary Guidelines for Americans* includes evidence-based recommendations and guidelines designed for professionals to help guide Americans toward healthier eating patterns and **physical activity levels (PALs)** to improve and maintain good health and reduce risk of chronic disease (48).

The *Dietary Guidelines* are used to develop federal food, nutrition, and health policies and programs. The *Dietary Guidelines* are evidence-based and intended for policymakers and nutrition and health professionals, not the general public. Educational materials and programs are developed based on the *Dietary Guidelines* and for the public. The current *Dietary Guidelines* translates nutrition science and physical activity research into food-based guidance as well as physical activity recommendations that individuals can use to choose foods and incorporate physical activity patterns into their lives to promote optimal health and reduce risk of chronic disease (49). The guidelines are too extensive to fully discuss in this text, but they can be obtained free of charge by visiting the USDA website. Resources and toolkits for both health professionals and consumers are also being developed from the *Guidelines* (48, 49).

Food Labels

The **United States Food and Drug Administration (FDA)** requires nutrition labeling on most foods; and any nutrient content claims and health messages comply with agency regulations. Some foods are exempt from nutrition labeling. For example, foods that do not provide significant nutrition value, including coffee and most spices, are exempt. Fresh produce is also exempt (57). For those foods requiring a label, five key components must be listed (57):

1. Name of the product or something to identify what it is
2. The net weight, volume, or numerical count of the package contents
3. Ingredients by common name and in descending order by weight
4. The name and address of the manufacturer, packer, or distributor
5. The Nutrition Facts Panel (figure 1.2)

Fortunately, government agencies help make the process of translating nutrition requirements into food choices a fairly simple process. The FDA regulates the contents of most food labels affixed to packaged products in the United States, whereas meat and poultry product labels are governed by the United States Department of Agriculture (USDA) Food Safety and Inspection Service

Nutrition Facts (a)

Nutrition Facts	
Serving Size 2/3 cup (55g)	
Servings Per Container about 8	

Amount Per Serving

Calories 230	Calories from Fat 40

	% Daily Value*
Total Fat 8g	**12%**
Saturated Fat 1g	**5%**
Trans Fat 0g	
Cholesterol 0mg	**0%**
Sodium 160mg	**7%**
Total Carbohydrate 37g	**12%**
Dietary Fiber 4g	**16%**
Sugars 1g	
Protein 3g	

Vitamin A 10%	Calcium 20%
Vitamin C 8%	Iron 45%

*Percent Daily Values are based on a 2,000 calorie diet. Your daily values may be higher or lower depending on your calorie needs:

	Calories	2,000	2,500
Total Fat	Less Than	65g	80g
Saturated Fat	Less Than	20g	25g
Cholesterol	Less Than	300mg	300mg
Sodium	Less Than	2,400mg	2,400mg
Total Carbohydrate		300g	375g
Dietary Fiber		25g	30g

Nutrition Facts (b)

Nutrition Facts	
8 servings per container	
Serving size	**2/3 cup (55g)**

Amount per 2/3 cup

Calories	**230**

	% Daily Value*
Total Fat 8g	**12%**
Saturated Fat 1g	**5%**
Trans Fat 0g	
Cholesterol 0mg	**0%**
Sodium 160mg	**7%**
Total Carbohydrate 37g	**12%**
Dietary Fiber 4g	**14%**
Total Sugars 1g	
Added Sugars 0g	
Protein 3g	

Vitamin D 2mcg	10%
Calcium 260mg	20%
Iron 8mg	45%
Potassium 235mg	6%

* The % Daily Value (DV) tells you how much a nutrient in a serving of food contributes to a daily diet. 2,000 calories a day is used for general nutrition advice.

Figure 1.2 The Nutrition Facts Panel has been updated for easy understanding of the information provided. *(a)* This label is what you have been seeing for several years. *(b)* This updated label will be widely used by July 26, 2018, but food manufacturers with annual food sales of less than $10 million may take up to one more year to comply with the new FDA regulations (52).

(FSIS). Food labels display, among other nutrients, the amount of carbohydrate, fiber, fat, and protein included in each serving of the product. Serving sizes are somewhat standardized among products but, more importantly, are in familiar household measurements such as cups, tablespoons, and whole units (pieces).

DO YOU KNOW ?

Vitamin D, calcium, iron, and potassium are listed on the Nutrition Facts Panel because many Americans are not meeting recommendations for these nutrients (52).

Serving size is an important consideration. For example, a sports drink may have three servings per bottle, yet the nutrition information is listed per serving—that is, for one third of the bottle. Servings must be listed in common household measures as well as in the metric unit of grams. The quantity of energy-yielding nutrients—carbohydrate, fat, and protein—content are provided in grams, which can be useful for nutrition guidelines presented in grams per day or grams per kilograms of body weight, as commonly used in sports nutrition guidelines. Macronutrients and micronutrients

are also expressed in terms of percent of **daily value (DV)**. DV is an indicator of how much of one serving of a food item contributes to a person's nutrition needs, based on a 2,000-calorie diet. The percent DV (%DV) puts nutrition information in context of overall daily diet. Less than 5 percent of the DV is low for a nutrient; greater than 20 percent is high (55). Finally, a footnote at the bottom of the Nutrition Facts Panel describes %DV: "The % Daily Value tells you how much a nutrient in a serving of food contributes to a daily diet. 2,000 calories a day is used for general nutrition advice" (52).

Food products and dietary supplements are allowed to make **nutrient content claims** and **health claims**, as regulated by the FDA. Nutrient content claims describe the level of a nutrient or ingredient in a food product. For instance, a claim may say "high in oat bran," "fat free," or "light cheesecake." Examples of terms defined by the FDA include "light," "lite," "sodium free," "trivial source of sodium," "reduced," "less," "low-fat," "sugar free," "low calorie," "good source," "high," "more," and "high potency." Some of the terms compare the level of the nutrient in a product to the DV for that nutrient (e.g., "excellent source"), whereas others compare one product to a reference food. A reference food is defined as a food within the same category (potato chips and pretzels, for instance) or similar food (comparing two brands of potato chips, for example). Detailed descriptions of FDA-approved nutrient content claims can be found on the FDA's website (30, 51, 53).

Health claims can be used on food as well as dietary supplements to describe a relationship between a substance and a health-related condition or disease. There are several requirements that must be met prior to FDA approval of a health claim, including significant scientific agreement supporting the proposed claim. Only a limited number of health claims have been approved for use; the complete list can be found on the FDA's website (54, 56).

MyPlate

MyPlate is a visual reminder that "all food and beverage choices matter." MyPlate outlines healthy dietary patterns based on the *Dietary Guidelines* and focuses on variety, amount, and nutrition. More nutritious food choices are encouraged from the five food groups: fruits, vegetables, grains, protein, and dairy. For example, whole grains are a better choice than refined white bread or pasta. See figure 1.3 for more details. MyPlate also encourages staying within one's daily calorie limits (45).

The website for MyPlate is: www .choosemyplate.gov. Once a person establishes a profile by entering sex, age, current activity level, and weight goals, the system creates a meal plan with the number of servings recommended from each of the five food groups. The user can explore each food group in great detail to determine the healthiest choices and the guidelines for serving sizes. The website can also track daily dietary

intake and physical activity and include details about nutrient intake and patterns of energy balance. Though other, more sophisticated, programs are on the market for diet and physical activity tracking, www.choosemyplate.gov is free of charge (45). When assessing any diet analysis program, accuracy and ease of use are both important. Accurate programs use the USDA database for the calorie and nutrient content of foods in addition to information from food labels on packaged foods.

MyPlate can teach athletes about portion sizes and accompanying nutrient content. For example, a half-cup of cooked rice is a serving size of grains

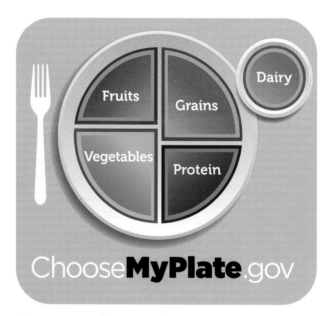

Figure 1.3 MyPlate is easily identifiable. It provides a simple reminder that all food groups are important. Half of the plate should be filled with fruits and vegetables, one quarter with lean protein, and one quarter with quality grain. Dairy is represented as a side dish or a beverage, as commonly consumed.

USDA's Center for Nutrition Policy and Promotion.

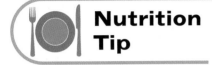

Nutrition Tip

The terms "light" or "lite" can have several meanings when used on a food product. These terms are regulated by the FDA yet remain confusing to consumers. When one of these terms is used it can mean the product contains one-third fewer calories, or no more than half the fat of the original version of the product. It can also refer to sodium, meaning that the food has no more than half the sodium compared to the comparable product. Examples include "light" salad dressing, referring to calories and fat; and light soy sauce, meaning the product has half the sodium of a typical soy sauce. Here is the tricky part: These terms can also refer to color and texture, and in such cases the terms have no relation to nutrition value. For example, "light" brown sugar is a description of the color and something described as "light and fluffy" refers to food texture.

and provides about 15 grams of carbohydrate. However, MyPlate and educational materials based on MyPlate provide calorie guidelines and portions for individuals who get less than 30 minutes of moderate physical activity most days of the week, so their guidelines need to be adjusted when used by athletes.

Guidelines for Athletes

The DRIs do not take exercise into account. Although athletes might benefit from greater intake of certain micronutrients to keep levels in the body within normal limits, many can meet these needs with a well-planned diet that meets their caloric demands. Greater calorie intake provides the opportunity to consume more food and therefore more nutrients. Micronutrients of greater concern for athletes are discussed in chapters 6 and 7. The AMDRs are generally not used for athletes, and specific guidelines for carbohydrates, lipids, and proteins are expressed in grams or as grams per kilogram of body weight. These are discussed in detail in chapters 3, 4, and 5. The ULs apply to athletes and

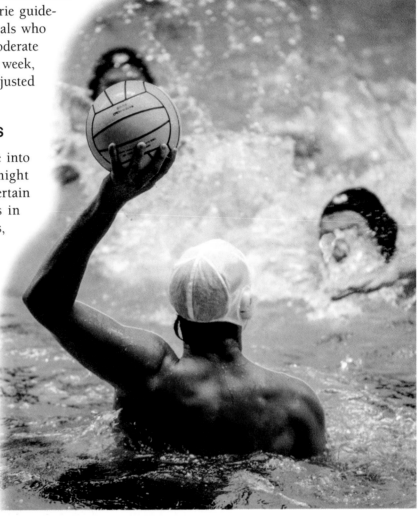

Nutritional requirements for athletes may vary by sport. Water polo, for example, is a high-intensity activity. If you are an athlete, consider what aspects of your sport may require specialized nutrition to replenish your body and improve performance.

active individuals. When considering the UL for vitamins and minerals, one must take into account total intake of nutrients from all sources, including food, sports nutrition products (e.g., bars, protein powders), and supplements.

Learning to read food labels can help athletes plan their diets. Most energy-yielding macronutrient guidelines for athletes are expressed in grams, as listed on food labels. Grams per serving for carbohydrate, fat, and protein are clearly listed on the Nutrition Facts Panel.

EXERCISE

Exercise is considered a type of physical activity that is planned and repetitive. Exercise is important throughout one's life, as it can help prevent or delay the development of many diseases and health conditions, including certain types of cancer, cardiovascular disease, osteoporosis, and sarcopenia (age-related loss of muscle mass). Sport-specific training results in physiological adaptations to improve performance.

Health Benefits of Exercise

The *Physical Activity Guidelines for Americans* (50) is a public document that summarizes the research findings on the health benefits of physical activity. Some of the major findings include:

> - All adults should avoid physical inactivity; some physical activity is better than none; regular physical activity reduces the risk of many adverse health outcomes.
> - For most health outcomes, there is a dose-response relationship. As the amount of physical activity increases through higher intensity, greater frequency, or longer duration, many health outcomes improve.
> - Most health benefits occur with at least 150 minutes (2 hours and 30 minutes) a week of moderate-intensity **aerobic physical activity** or 75 minutes (1 hour and 15 minutes) a week of vigorous-intensity aerobic physical activity, or an equivalent combination of the two intensities.
> - For additional and more extensive health benefits, adults should aim to achieve 300

minutes (5 hours) a week of moderate-intensity aerobic physical activity, or 150 minutes a week of vigorous-intensity aerobic physical activity, or an equivalent combination of the two intensities. Additional health benefits may be gained by engaging in physical activity beyond this amount.

> - Both endurance (aerobic) and resistance training are beneficial. Resistance training should be moderate or high intensity and involve all major muscle groups 2 or more days per week.

DO YOU KNOW ?

Some people think they are too old to reap the benefits of exercise. In reality, it is never too late. Though muscle mass declines with age, older adults can improve strength through resistance training. This can lead to improved health and enhanced mobility and daily functioning (7, 22)

> - Health benefits occur for children and adolescents, young and middle-aged adults, older adults, those in every studied racial and ethnic group, and for people with disabilities.
> - The benefits of physical activity far outweigh the possibility of adverse outcomes.

Many competitive athletes far exceed these general recommendations for health.

Components of Fitness

Physical fitness involves many systems of the body working together to produce a desired outcome. The key components of fitness include cardiovascular or cardiorespiratory endurance, muscular strength and endurance, flexibility, and body composition. Aerobic power (aerobic capacity) is dependent on a continuous supply of oxygen and is determined by measuring maximal oxygen uptake (also referred to as maximal oxygen consumption; $\dot{V}O_2max$). $\dot{V}O_2max$ measures the maximum volume ($\dot{V}$) of oxygen (O_2) taken in, transported, and used by muscles to produce energy. $\dot{V}O_2max$ is measured using an incremental (increases in speed, incline, or both) exercise test on a cycle ergometer or treadmill (36) A higher

$\dot{V}O_2$max means the athlete can consume more oxygen and deliver it to hard-working muscles. $\dot{V}O_2$max declines with age (10), yet aerobic training can increase $\dot{V}O_2$max in people of all ages, including older adults (12, 33). High-intensity, low-duration training and low-intensity, high-duration training increase $\dot{V}O_2$max to a similar extent (42).

Anaerobic means literally *without oxygen*. **Anaerobic activity** is intense activity performed without sufficient oxygen over a short period of time (figure 1.4). Sprinting is an example. Increasing anaerobic power or capacity depends on the anaerobic energy systems, the adenosine triphosphate-phosphocreatine system (ATP-PC), and anaerobic glycolysis (see chapter 2 for more details). Optimizing anaerobic power means the body has trained these systems to maximally produce ATP, a high-energy molecule used in all cells of the body and during exercise (20).

Muscular strength is the maximal force that a skeletal muscle or group of muscles can produce, whereas **muscular power** is the rate at which the work (contraction) is performed. Muscular power is the product of strength and velocity or speed of the contraction. **Muscular endurance** is the ability to perform repeated skeletal muscle contractions or to hold a contraction over a period of time. Both skeletal muscle strength and endurance can be increased with training. **Muscular flexibility** is the ability to move through a joints' range of motion. Like other components of fitness, flexibility can be improved through exercise (20).

Body composition describes the makeup of tissues in the body. Percent body fat is the percentage of body weight that is fat, rather than fat-free mass such as muscle, organs, water, connective tissue, and bone (20). Ranges of body fat associated with both health and athletic performance are discussed in later chapters of this book. While excess body fat is a risk factor for developing

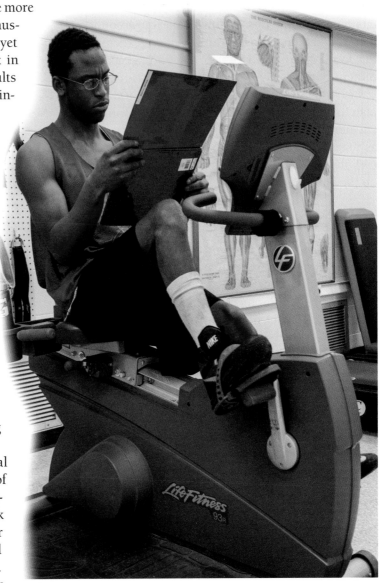

Exercise improves attention span, increases learning retention, and decreases stress. Instead of skipping a workout when you're busy prepping for final exams, take your studying to the gym.

several chronic diseases, too little body fat is also detrimental to health. In some sports, athletes require a high level of muscle mass and strength, while other sports require leanness and optimal muscle endurance. More details on body composition are provided in chapters 10 and 13.

Both genetics and environmental factors, including physical activity, activities of daily living, and nutrition, influence body composition (5, 9, 11, 60). Though genetics can influence tendency for overweight and obesity,

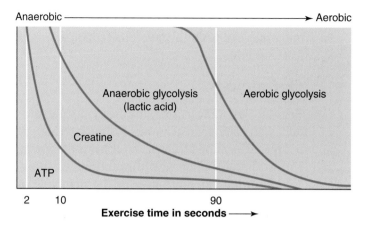

Figure 1.4 Anaerobic activities do not require oxygen for ATP generation. Training results in optimization of this system for enhanced ATP production and greater performance.

Based on Rick University, WebMed. Available: http://www.rice.edu/~jenky/images/creatine_reviewPCT11.JPG

as well as where fat is deposited on the body (hips, buttocks, breasts, etc.), many people with obesity genes never become overweight or obese (16). Environment plays a tremendous role, and there is also a link between genetics and the environment (61). Making good nutrition choices, decreasing calories to lose weight or consuming enough calories to maintain yet not gain weight, and physical activity all have profound influence on genetic predisposition to overweight or obesity (4, 37, 39, 40).

Principles of Exercise Training

Exercise training describes the body's response to consistent exercise, resulting in desired physiological adaptations (20). A well-designed training program combined with proper nutrition and adequate sleep and recovery generally leads to performance improvements, while overtraining or undertraining can result in a performance decrement.

Specificity

The **principle of specificity** dictates that training adaptations and performance improvements are specific to the type, intensity, and duration of training. Training must induce a physical stress specific to the system needed for performance enhancements. For example, a triathlete must perform endurance activities that are long in duration and that include the activities in competition: swimming, cycling, and running. Weightlifting promotes increased muscle strength and hypertrophy (growth), which are beneficial adaptations for power lifters. Endurance training alone will not promote the increased muscular strength and hypertrophy necessary for power lifting. In simplest terms, for the principle to apply, the training program must be specific to the sport or activity and support the physiological adaptations needed to succeed at the desired sport or activity (20, 50).

Overload

In order to see improvements in performance, it is necessary to **overload** the system (e.g., cardiovascular, muscular) being trained with a greater load than normal. For example, you bench press 150 lbs. for a maximum of 8 repetitions at which time your muscles becomes fatigued, and you cannot lift one more repetition. This 150 lbs. is called your 8 repetition max, or 8RM. With regular training over time, you will be able to lift the same 150 lbs. more than 8 times before your muscles fatigue and you must stop. If you wish to become stronger, you must add more weight to your press in order to establish a new 8RM or experience complete muscle fatigue after 8 repetitions. As resistance training continues, weight needs to be added until fatigue sets in after six to eight repetitions. Adjusting weight and number of repetitions while focusing on **eccentric contractions** can improve muscle hypertrophy and strength. For endurance performance improvement, you must increase total training volume via intensity or duration or a combination of the two (20, 50).

DO YOU KNOW ?

Though less time in between sets will increase muscular fatigue, longer rest periods between sets—3 minutes instead of 1 minute, for instance—can improve hypertrophy and strength gains in resistance-trained individuals (41).

Periodization

The **principle of periodization** schedules training for a particular sport or event into smaller blocks of time (figure 1.5). Proper periodization allows for the intensity of training required for the desired performance outcome while also allowing adequate rest and recovery. Traditional periodization plans are usually mapped over a long duration, such as a year to four years. Within that timeframe are various cycles of months (macrocycles), weeks (mesocycles), days (microcycles), and individual training sessions. Such a plan might work well for individuals training for a single competition like a marathon, in which the focus is on one system (the cardiovascular system). Training blocks can also be customized to a particular sport or activity to emphasize a smaller number of performance outcomes at once or to design a smaller number of blocks at one time. These blocks might be a shorter duration than in single-sport training

(e.g., a few weeks). The number, sequence, and outcomes can be highly customized for the sport or event (19).

Detraining

Regular resistance or endurance training produces physiological training responses that are beneficial for both athletes and other individuals. Unfortunately, when you discontinue training, your training gains are lost, or the **principle of detraining**. Maintenance-level training programs are needed to prevent physiological declines from the trained state. Physiological reductions with detraining can be partial or full, and cardiorespiratory endurance decrements appear to be greater than loss of muscular strength and power. Data vary regarding muscle strength, power, and endurance, but some research suggests that just two weeks of inactivity can lead to declines in muscular endurance. Fortunately, resuming training can result in restoration of both cardiorespiratory endurance and skeletal muscle performance (8, 23, 29).

Overtraining

It is fairly well established that appropriate training and adequate recovery and rest leads to enhanced performance, but unfortunately, many athletes believe that more is better and that there is no limit to performance enhancement. Exces-

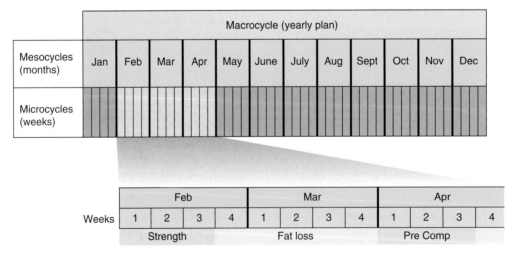

Figure 1.5 Periodization is a concept that simplifies training regimens and goals into smaller blocks of time. Intensity and duration of training may vary depending on the desired performance outcome. The actual length of time in each block or period will depend on the sport or activity.

PUTTING IT INTO PERSPECTIVE

YOU CAN COME BACK FROM DETRAINING

Have you ever worked hard in an exercise program and then, for whatever reason, taken an unexpected long break? Though your body will become detrained during your down time, you can bounce back. For most people, once exercise resumes, physiological gains occur faster than initial changes.

sive training usually results in a performance decrement, often followed by the compensatory behavior of even more physical effort. The American College of Sports Medicine and the European College of Sports Science have a Joint Consensus Statement on this topic (26). The two terms to describe the condition of excessive training are overreaching and overtraining. **Overreaching** describes excessive exercise volume that results in short-term performance decrement and usually occurs during periods of competition. These can be reversed in several days to several weeks through proper training, nutrition intervention,

and rest. Key nutrients include adequate fluid to restore hydration, carbohydrate to replenish glycogen stores, and protein to optimize protein synthesis (particularly in muscle) and healing. The symptoms accompanying overreaching include overall fatigue, muscular fatigue, chronic muscle tenderness and soreness, lack of concentration, and disrupted eating habits or loss of interest in food. **Overtraining** results in a compendium of symptoms referred to as the overtraining syndrome (OTS) (figure 1.6). This condition is more serious than overreaching, often causing long-term performance impairment that can take

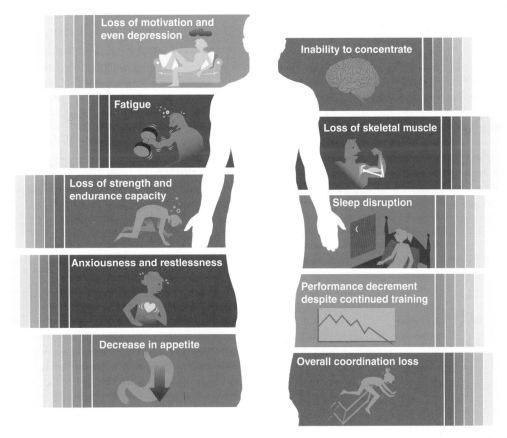

Figure 1.6   Common signs and symptoms characteristic of overtraining syndrome (OTS).

several weeks or months to recover from. OTS is complex because there are both physiological abnormalities and often psychological challenges stemming from the stress of competition, family and social relationships, and other life demands. There are no set diagnostic criteria for OTS, as symptoms vary from athlete to athlete and are highly individualized. Athletes with suspected OTS should seek medical attention to rule out other confounding conditions and to develop a sound plan for recovery (26).

SPORT NUTRITION

Exercise physiology is the study of the body's response to exercise, from acute bouts to chronic adaptations with repeated activity and long-term training (20). Nutrition includes the science of the ingestion, digestion, absorption, and metabolism of nutrients and the accompanying physiological and biochemical functions of those nutrients (18). Sport nutrition integrates exercise physiology and nutrition. Athletes and active individuals should adhere to the principles of sound nutrition for optimal health but also need to address the appropriate nutrition intake to support training, performance, and recovery from exercise. Nutrition guidelines have been established to support the unique needs of various sports and physical activities.

General Principles

The ultimate goal for most athletes is to optimize performance in their sport or activity. Training is required for the metabolic adaptations leading to improved performance, while nutrition strategies are important to providing adequate fuel and nutrients to support that training. Sports nutrition strategies encompass food intake and **nutrient absorption** and utilization on a regular or daily basis, and then specifically before, during, and after competition or activity. Nutrition goals need to be individualized for each athlete within and between sports. For example, while general carbohydrate guidelines exist for the endurance athlete, the actual amounts that should be consumed are far different for a small female athlete versus a large male athlete. In addition, endurance athletes have different carbohydrate and protein needs than strength athletes. Individualization should also take into account food preferences, food intolerances or allergies, and any other special needs that help the athlete maintain compliance.

In addition to individualized needs from person to person, sports nutrition guidelines are dynamic and change depending on exercise training cycles. In **nutrition periodization**, nutrition guidelines are adjusted depending on the cycle of training or individual training sessions. For example, nutrition needs will differ depending on whether an individual is in training, precompetition, competition, or the off-season. There are many protocols for nutrition periodization that can be individualized to meet the needs of any athlete. A common periodization program is broken into the same cycles as exercise training: macrocycles, mesocycles, and microcycles. During the off-season, if athletes are not in training, their nutrient needs will reduce significantly. Optimal body composition for performance is a goal for many athletes. If an athlete wishes to lose body weight or fat, this is usually recommended during the off-season, or very early in training, to avoid any performance declines caused by an energy deficit (43).

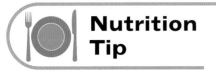

Nutrition Tip

Since nutrition guidelines exist for many sports and training regimens, you might think that athletes must be extremely rigid to achieve success. While it is important to have adequate fuel and nutrients to support training and recovery from exercise, eating with extreme rigidity can lead to the development of compulsive behaviors or disordered eating patterns, such as binge eating, which, like other eating disorders, is a psychological condition. Varying your food choices and eating patterns, within the nutrition guidelines you are following, should provide a good balance (25).

Evidence-Based Practice

Most reputable professional organizations related to health care have a code of ethics. While codes of ethics vary across disciplines, a common element is evidence-based practice. Generally speaking, evidence-based practice requires the use of a systematic process for identifying, assessing, analyzing, and synthesizing the available evidence; using the best evidence in making recommendations; and promoting the use of professional expertise when evidence is weak or lacking (13). All evidence-based practice is founded on well-established, scientific guidelines and never relies on anecdotal information.

Scientific Evidence

In large part because of the media, conflicting information regarding nutrition abounds. When trying to determine if information is accurate and complete, one method to employ is the scientific method (figure 1.7). The scientific method is a standardized process used by scientists and other professionals to answer research questions. The process begins with an observation of a relation between two or more elements. The scientist (or other professional) then develops a hypothesis, or educated guess, regarding the basis for the observation. The hypothesis is also considered

the research question. For instance, hypotheses may be developed based on the effect of a dietary intervention on performance, the effect of a sports supplement on body composition, or a relation between two variables (e.g., Is vitamin D deficiency related to bone fracture risk?). Once a hypothesis is established, the scientist develops a study design that includes an appropriate number of subjects, methodology, and statistical control. Data are then collected and analyzed, and decisions, and sometimes conclusions, are made from the experiment. The study design and statistical analyses must be appropriate to answer the research question(s), and the experiment must be repeatable to other scientists to see if they obtain similar results. After many repeated experiments demonstrate similar results, a theory can be proposed.

Reputable Sources of Nutrition Information

In the nutrition world, there is a lot of **quackery**—misleading, unproven, or unsupported information—driven by marketing rather than science and often promoted for the purpose of financial gain. Thus, it may be difficult to distinguish misinformation from sound scientific evidence. Several factors should be considered when evaluating a nutrition or dietary supplement claim:

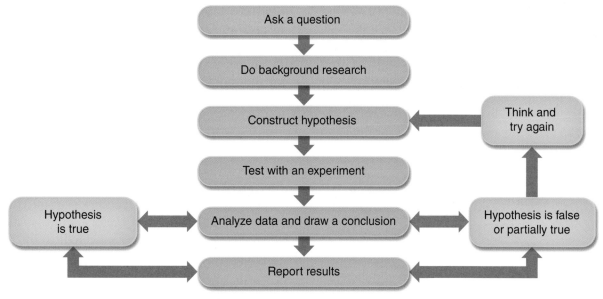

Figure 1.7 The scientific method is a way of ensuring a standardized process is used when examining scientific evidence and evaluating claims.

> Who is making the claim or report? What are their training and credentials? Anyone can claim to be an expert in a subject and publish in popular print or on the Internet (and even credentialed persons can misinterpret scientific research).

> Where is the information published? While quality information can be published in popular outlets, it is not guaranteed to be correct and not to mislead. Scientific evidence is published in peer-reviewed journals in which the research or review information is critiqued by other experts in the field.

> Is the report based on credible research? Has the research been interpreted correctly? In an effort to convince consumers, some websites for dietary supplements cite research that wasn't conducted on their product or stretch the truth regarding the research on their product.

> Is the report founded on personal observation, testimony or small, unpublished research findings?

> Are there claims being made that are too good to be true? Does the report criticize the scientific community? Companies who manufacture "breakthrough" products sometimes criticize scientific experts.

Because of the abundance of available nutrition information, it is important to ensure sound scientific principles are being considered. Some research studies are difficult to fully understand, and access to some studies may be limited. Though it is easy to type questions into a search engine or skim through popular magazines or websites, it is worth taking the time to critically evaluate nutrition claims and information before considering a dietary supplement or diet change.

CREDENTIALS AND SCOPE OF PRACTICE

Credentials and certifications vary tremendously among the professions of nutrition and dietetics and exercise sciences. Nutrition and dietetics have one uniform credential that is recognized by all 50 states in the United States, while this is not the case for exercise professionals. Dietitians of Canada is an organization that issues and regulates the profession of nutrition and dietetics in Canada. The credentials may vary slightly by province but most use the credential Registered Dietitian (RD). Both professions require education and skills in order to provide proper care for members of the public.

Exercise Science and Fitness Certifications

There is no single accrediting body governing academic programs in the exercise sciences that leads to a nationally recognized practice credential. Titles for exercise professionals—personal trainer, fitness professional, exercise physiologist, etc.—can be used by anyone. Further, the term "certified" can be meaningless, depending on where the certification came from. Some certifications come from reputable exercise and fitness professional organizations; others can be obtained over the Internet with a credit card. This makes it confusing for the public when seeking professional exercise advice. Making matters more confusing, many people who call themselves nutrition experts may have taken a weekend nutrition or nutrition and fitness certification class but have no formal training or education in nutrition. Further, some exercise science degree programs may require one or two nutrition courses, while others may have no requirement for nutrition classes. Limited nutrition education does not provide the training and skills necessary to perform an individualized nutrition assessment and intervention, especially for those who have health conditions or diseases.

Because of these concerns, the American College of Sports Medicine (ACSM), the National Strength and Conditioning Association (NSCA), the American Council on Exercise (ACE), and other professional organizations suggest that the general public seek an exercise professional who holds a certification that is accredited by the National Commission for Certifying Agencies (NCCA). The NCCA provides a standardized, independent, and objective third-party evaluation of the certification programs and subsequent examinations (17).

EVALUATING WEBSITES

The Internet is loaded with nutrition misinformation. Here are some tips to help find credible websites:

> Who is sponsoring the site? Individual people, private companies, nonprofit organizations, or government agencies all create websites. Look for the credentials and training of individuals who contribute to the content of the site as well as who is sponsoring it. If a food or supplement manufacturer or trade organization is sponsoring the site, the information may be credible but biased. Be sure to evaluate the content carefully.

> When was the website last updated? The nutrition field is constantly developing, so information should be current.

> Check the three letters following the "dot" in the web address. Dot gov (.gov) is for a government website, dot edu (.edu) is an educational institution, dot org (.org) is for nonprofit or professional organizations, and dot com (.com) is for commercial and business sites. The first two are usually reputable (though some dot-edu sites are the personal websites of faculty members, who might have their own agenda or post their own opinions to sound like facts). Dot org may or may not be credible, as organizations often have sponsors they must please or promote.

> Does the site distrust credible organizations? Does there appear to be financial gain for the authors of the site?

Credentials in Nutrition and Dietetics

The Academy of Nutrition and Dietetics (known simply as the Academy) governs the practice credential **Registered Dietitian Nutritionist (RD or RDN**, which are interchangeable; we will use RDN in this text). This credential is granted and maintained by the Commission on Dietetic Registration (CDR) of the Academy (1). To be eligible to take the National Registration Examination for Dietitians in order to obtain the RDN credential, one must (1) obtain a bachelor's degree, (2) complete a program in nutrition and dietetics (DPND) accredited by the Accreditation Council for Education in Nutrition and Dietetics (ACEND) of the Academy, and (3) complete an ACEND-accredited dietetic internship program that provides at least 1,200 hours of supervised practice experience (or a combination of the IOC diploma in sports nutrition plus 700 hours of supervised practice experience). There are additional board certifications beyond the RDN credential, including the Certified Specialist in Sports Dietetics (CSSD) (3). The person holding the CSSD credential has specialized experience in sports dietetics. The CSSD translates that information to specific dietary guidance when working with athletes of all levels participating in different sports and activities. The CSSD conducts an appropriate nutrition assessment and uses the data to provide safe and effective nutrition interventions aimed at promoting health and optimizing performance (21, 43).

Currently, 46 states, the District of Columbia, and Puerto Rico have enacted statutory provisions regulating the practice of nutrition and dietetics either through state licensure or statutory certification. Many states require RDNs be licensed to practice nutrition and dietetics. In these cases, breaking the state licensure law is a criminal offense, subject to misdemeanor or felony penalties ranging from a cease-and-desist order to fines and imprisonment. Statutory certification limits the use of particular titles (e.g., certified dietitian, certified nutritionist) to individuals meeting the state's credentialing criteria. Approximately 10 states have statutory certification or title protection for nutrition and dietetics professionals. Specific title protection for "RDN" (or "RD") means that only those with the credential may use the title (21).

REPUTABLE SPORTS NUTRITION ORGANIZATIONS

REFLECTION TIME

You might consider spending some time learning about the following organizations to see which ones interest you most.

> Sports, Cardiovascular, and Wellness Nutrition (SCAN) (www.scandpg.org). SCAN is a dietetic practice group of the Academy of Nutrition and Dietetics. It is a sound source of sports nutrition information and can be used to find a Certified Specialist in Sports Dietetics (CSSD). While this organization reserves most of its resources for members, there are links to some publicly available position papers, sports nutrition fact sheets for consumers, and useful websites with sports nutrition–related information. Other resources are available for purchase. SCAN holds an annual symposium, where current sports nutrition–related information is presented to attendees.

> Professionals in Nutrition for Exercise and Sport (PINES) (www.pinesnutrition.org). PINES is an international organization that promotes sports nutrition practice and research. Associate membership is available to those who hold current employment in a health sciences field that requires ongoing continuing education. Students enrolled in a sport nutrition, sport science, or sport medicine program are also eligible for membership. PINES provides a variety of sports nutrition resources and links to other organizations and documents related to the field.

> American College of Sports Medicine (ACSM) (www.acsm.org). ACSM is a resource for the exercise sciences as well as sports nutrition. There is a nutrition interest group within ACSM. ACSM offers several levels of membership, from student members to degreed professionals. The organization provides access to information related to sports medicine, position papers, and, for members, journals. ACSM also provides numerous exercise-related certifications.

> National Strength and Conditioning Association (NSCA) (www.nsca.com). The NSCA is a professional membership organization for thousands of elite strength coaches, personal trainers, and dedicated individuals conducting research and providing education. There are different levels of membership for students, non-NSCA-certified individuals, and NSCA-certified professionals. Members gain access to various educational materials, events, and career services.

Some individuals might hold a master's or doctoral degree in nutrition but might not hold the credential RDN. Depending on the state, these individuals may not be able to practice dietetics (e.g., complete a nutrition assessment, an intervention, or a provision of medical nutrition therapy). However, these individuals may have extensive training in nutrition sciences and can be a reliable resource for sound nutrition information (21).

Scope of Practice

State licensure supersedes both registration and certification. Thus, in states with licensure, only those with a license can practice nutrition and dietetics. Does this mean that only RDNs can provide education? The answer is no. Other health professionals may discuss nutrition as long as it is general, nonmedical nutrition information. For instance, these individuals may state "dietary fiber is important for gut health and preventing constipation." This is an example of general nutrition information. Education should be limited to healthy individuals and based on sound scientific nutrition principles. Conducting a nutrition assessment and providing a nutrition intervention is considered dietetics, and licensure is required for this in certain states. Further, if working with a person with a disease or health-related condition, the assessment of nutrition status and nutrition intervention is considered medical nutrition therapy and should be reserved for the RDN.

General, nonmedical nutrition therapy includes any public guidance systems such as the *2015–2020 Dietary Guidelines*, reading food labels as guided by the FDA, the DRIs, and interactive systems such as MyPlate. Topics may also include the functions of nutrients in the body and principles of healthy food preparation. For a more detailed list, please refer to table 1.1. Providing nutrition education within one's scope of practice and taking actions one can take as defined by their professional license are encouraged and beneficial to the public. It is critical to understand the laws where you live and to understand your own level of nutrition knowledge and skills before communicating information to the public (21).

Table 1.1 Samples of General, Nonmedical Nutrition Information

Nutrition principle	Example application of the principle
Principles of healthy food preparation	Baking fish or chicken is healthier than batter dipping and deep frying.
Foods to be included in the normal daily diet of healthy individuals	Fruits, vegetables, quality grains, lean proteins, low-fat dairy, and healthy fats are all part of a healthy, balanced diet.
The functions of nutrients on the body	Carbohydrate is a fuel source for skeletal muscle and organs; iron is a component of hemoglobin.
Recommended amounts of the essential nutrients (DRIs) for HEALTHY individuals	Share the USDA DRI tables.
The effects of deficiencies or excesses of nutrients	Excess energy leads to obesity; iron deficiency leads to the medical condition iron-deficiency anemia.
Food sources of essential nutrients	Orange juice is an excellent source of vitamin C; whole grains contain dietary fiber.
Providing information about food guidance systems (e.g., *Dietary Guidelines*, food labels, and Choose MyPlate)	Showing the actual food label or MyPlate system.
The basic roles of carbohydrates, proteins, fats, vitamins, minerals, water	Protein is important for tissue growth and repair; calcium is an important mineral for bone health; water plays an important role in body temperature regulation.
Giving statistical information about the relationship between chronic disease and the excesses or deficiencies of certain nutrients	Obesity is a leading cause of type 2 diabetes mellitus.
Proper hydration in HEALTHY individuals	Use the current position stand on this topic (43).

NUTRITION PROFESSIONALS WHO WORK WITH ATHLETES

Are you interested in a profession working with athletes? A Certified Specialist in Sports Dietetics (CSSD) is a specialty credential that can be earned by RDNs. Individuals holding the CSSD credential have specialized knowledge in performance nutrition. In addition to providing general sports nutrition guidelines, the CSSD can provide individualized nutrition plans for optimizing performance and, as an RDN, can work with athletes who have (or might have) a disease or nutrition-related condition. This credential can be earned after an RDN has at least 1,500 practice hours in sports dietetics. For more information on earning this credential, visit this website: www.scandpg.org (3).

SUMMARY

Nutrition is a scientific discipline that examines the role of food and its nutrients on physiological function and health. The science of nutrition is rapidly evolving, with new information published regularly. These scientific findings are translated to the nutrition guidelines that are used to determine which foods and nutrients to consume. The energy-yielding macronutrients—carbohydrate, fat, and protein—play a significant role in fueling, and in the case of protein, repairing the body. The micronutrients—vitamins and minerals—have numerous roles in physiological functions within the body. Water is an essential macronutrient for survival and is critical for several physiological processes, including regulation of body temperature. The nutrients work together to keep the body systems running smoothly.

Look for evidence-based nutrition guidelines; these have been compiled and designed to translate the science into food and nutrient choices for all individuals. Food labels, Dietary Reference Intakes, and MyPlate are some of the food guidance systems that can be used for healthy individuals of all ages. While these systems and tools are not specifically designed for athletes, they can be useful when making food choices based on a desired nutrient content.

There is a strong relationship between physical activity and health. Athletes usually exceed the general physical activity guidelines, as training is essential for performance in their activity or sport. Athletes must understand the basic principles of training that can lead to the physical gains they need for effective performance in their sport. While adequate training is required for sports performance, overtraining can disrupt normal physiological function and impair performance.

Sports nutrition is a relatively young subdiscipline that integrates the disciplines of nutrition sciences and exercise physiology. It is a dynamic field with new research chronically evolving. Many of the principles of nutrition for health promotion and disease prevention apply to all athletes and active individuals. There are, however, defined guidelines set for various nutrients that are sport- and activity-specific. Nutrition and sports nutrition are areas that are rich in misinformation and quackery, so it is critical to seek sound scientific information before decisions are made and implemented. Nutrition and dietetics are regulated in many states; those who provide nutrition education must take care to do so within their scope of practice.

■ FOR REVIEW ▶

1. What is the percent of daily value, and why is it used?
2. Explain the difference between a nutrient content claim and health claim.
3. What are the general physical activity guidelines for adults for both aerobic training and resistance training?
4. List the factors that influence body composition.
5. Describe the differences between overreaching and overtraining.
6. How do you go about finding accurate nutrition information?
7. Should athletes follow the DRIs and MyPlate? Why or why not?
8. List the benefits associated with regular exercise.

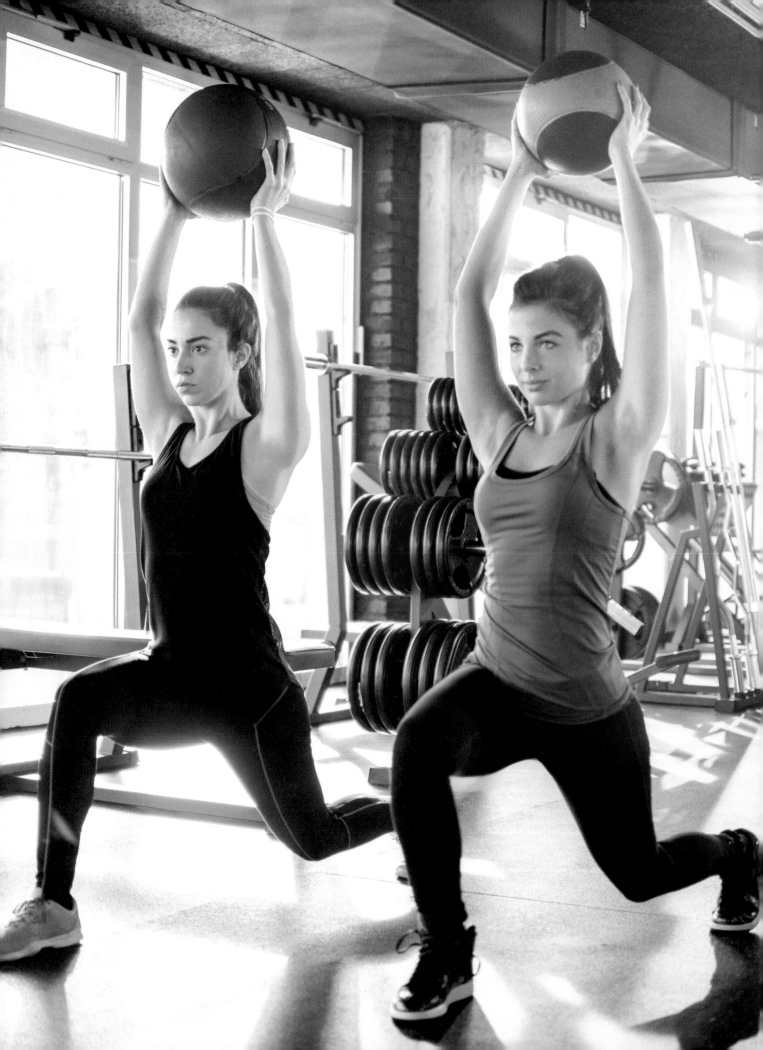

CHAPTER 2

Energy Metabolism

▶ CHAPTER OBJECTIVES

After completing this chapter, you will be able to do the following:

- Summarize the principles of energy metabolism and the production of ATP.
- Describe how energy expenditure is measured and estimated.
- Identify the energy systems.
- Explain which fuels are used in the different energy systems.
- Explain why the fuels used in energy metabolism are used during different exercise intensities.
- Discuss other systems that enhance performance: gluconeogenesis, Cori cycle, glucose-alanine cycle.
- Describe how energy content of food is measured.

Appropriate energy intake is the cornerstone of the athlete's diet. Proper energy intake supports optimal body function, determines the capacity for intake of macro- and micronutrients, and assists in manipulating body composition. Fortunately, the human body works hard as an efficient factory by transferring the chemical energy derived from food via digestion, absorption, and metabolism to generate power that fuels muscle contraction. The body can also use this chemical energy to synthesize new products in the body, such as chemical messengers or structural proteins, direct some energy for storage in glycogen and fat tissue, and help discard waste. A significant site of the body's energy factory is muscle tissue. The metabolic factory analogy of energy metabolism in active muscle tissue includes the cellular enzymes, organelles, and many metabolic pathways responsible for converting and using chemical energy to support muscle contraction. The muscle metabolic factory is on at all times, always responding when chemical energy from food is either scarce or plentiful.

HOW ENERGY FUELS THE BODY

Collectively, the use of energy for bodily processes, including all chemical changes, is known as **metabolism**. Metabolic processes involving thousands of chemical reactions can be further categorized as anabolism and catabolism. **Anabolism**, sometimes referred to as "growth," involves metabolic processes that use energy to synthesize building blocks to produce new molecules. **Catabolism** is characterized by the breakdown of molecules to generate useable energy.

The phrase "metabolic pathway" describes a series of chemical reactions that can result in catabolic or anabolic outcomes. These metabolic pathways are never completely inactive and constantly adapt to external stimuli that the body experiences

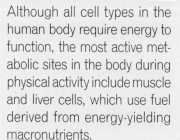

DO YOU KNOW ?

Although all cell types in the human body require energy to function, the most active metabolic sites in the body during physical activity include muscle and liver cells, which use fuel derived from energy-yielding macronutrients.

(figure 2.1). For example, let's say someone schedules a challenging workout with friends before afternoon classes. On these days, the carbohydrate consumed for lunch is broken down into glucose units. The muscle cells can further catabolize (break down) these glucose units in metabolic pathways occurring in the **cytosol** and mitochondria of the cell to produce **adenosine triphosphate (ATP)** to fuel muscle contraction. Once the workout is over and the group is sitting in class eating a banana as a recovery snack, their bodies take the carbohydrate consumed and the subsequent glucose units to assemble, via anabolism, glycogen.

The law of energy conservation states that energy can be neither created nor destroyed; rather, it transforms from one form to another. The total amount of "energy" in the universe is constant. While it can change from one form to another and can move from one location to another, the system never gains or loses energy. The conservation of energy law is a principle component of the first law of thermodynamics. So how does this apply to the human body? Where does the energy come from to power the body? While there are several forms of energy in the universe, including heat, mechanical, and electrical, it is the **chemical energy** derived from food that fuels our body. This form of energy is essential to human life and is responsible for much more than muscle work. Chemical energy provides energy needs for many processes, including breathing, pumping blood, maintaining body temperature, delivering oxygen to tissues, removing waste products, synthesizing new tissue for growth or adaptation to exercise and stress, and repairing damaged or worn-out tissues. Energy demands never cease but continue even when you are sleeping. When awake, the body needs not only energy to support the aforementioned processes but also additional energy to support physical movement as well as digestion and absorption of foods.

Chemical energy is derived from the molecular bonds that make up carbohydrate, fat, and protein that are consumed or broken down (catabolized) from stored forms of these nutrients in our body (glycogen, fat tissue, and skeletal muscle, though skeletal muscle is dense with protein, as mentioned in chapter 1—it isn't intended to serve as a backup source of amino acids). As discussed in a future chapter, energy can also be derived from the break-

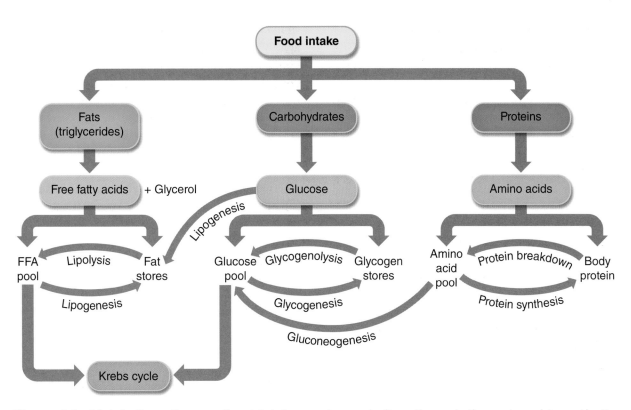

Figure 2.1   Metabolic pathways. Food intake sparks anabolism through the various biosynthetic pathways.

Reprinted, by permission, from L.W. Kenney, J.H. Wilmore, and D.L. Costill, 2015, *Physiology of sport and exercise*, 6th ed. (Champaign, IL: Human Kinetics), 51.

down of alcohol. The next step in the process is for our bodies to harness and transfer this energy from food into cellular energy to perform physiological tasks. We extract energy from food in three stages. Stage 1 is digestion, absorption, and transportation of energy-yielding nutrients. These are simple sugars from carbohydrate, amino acids from protein, **fatty acids** from lipids, and alcohol. Stage 2 consists of a more in-depth breakdown of small food-derived molecules to key energy-producing metabolites. For example, the simple sugar glucose derived from carbohydrate foods can be converted to the metabolite pyruvate. Two three-carbon pyruvate metabolites are formed from the breakdown of one six-carbon glucose molecule. These important molecules serve as metabolic intermediates. This process of breaking down glucose to pyruvate releases useable energy for the body to harness but, more important, serves as a precursor for the final stage. During stage 3, the body's cells can use energy-producing metabolites (such as acetyl-CoA derived from pyruvate) to completely break down ("burn") these compounds to a converted

form of energy the body can use. While it is true this process releases some energy as heat, unfortunately, the human body is not good at using heat to power cellular functions. Instead, cells transfer this energy into ATP as the form of chemical energy the body can use. This transfer of energy is not entirely efficient, and a significant portion of the food energy consumed is lost as heat (30). However, the energy we do use from the food we consume and the energy we store in glycogen and fat tissue allows the continuous synthesis of ATP from energy stores that are comparable to an energy "bank account," where energy consumed from food can be used as needed and the leftover excess can be "saved" for future use.

DO YOU KNOW ?

In survival situations, such as when stranded, food consumption, particularly protein, helps the body stay warm because of the metabolic production of heat. During digestion, protein produces more heat than either carbohydrate or fat.

HUMAN ENERGY METABOLISM

To fully comprehend and appreciate how our bodies use and transfer energy into ATP, we need to understand the centers within the cells that do the work. Although the body is made up of many types of cells, the cells share many of the same basic structures to facilitate metabolism. The two major compartments of the cell are its **cytoplasm** and **nucleus**. The cytoplasm is enclosed within the cell membrane and consists of a semi-fluid called cytosol. This cytosol is the site of a catabolic process known as **glycolysis** and anabolic processes such as fatty acid synthesis and glycogen synthesis. Also found within the cytoplasm are tiny, specialized factories known as **organelles**, which have unique metabolic functions. When discussing energy, arguably the most important organelle is known as the **mitochondria**, the powerhouse of the cell (figure 2.2). Liver, brain, kidney, and muscle cells all have similar organelle structure and multiple mitochondria. This is because several metabolic pathways exist in this organelle, and it is the final stop in the energy-transfer journey, where in the presence of oxygen, metabolites originating from carbohydrate, protein, fat, and alcohol produce ATP, carbon dioxide, and small amounts of water. The structure of the mitochondrion consists of two highly specialized membranes: an outer membrane and a highly folded inner membrane that surrounds the mitochondrial matrix. In conjunction with important metabolic processes that occur in the cytoplasm, key metabolic pathways occur in specific locations within the mitochondrion. In the matrix, the **tricarboxylic acid (TCA) cycle**, also known as the Krebs cycle, can accept various metabolites that enter from the cytosol as pyruvate, fatty acids, and amino acids following oxidation to form **acetyl-CoA**. This process is illustrated in figure 2.3. The catabolism of acetyl-CoA in the TCA cycle breaks carbon bonds through a process known as **oxidative decarboxylation** and produces free electrons that bind with coenzymes, which carry the electrons to the **electron transport chain (ETC)**. The ETC is made up of a series of complex protein channels that accept the electrons from the coenzymes. This process harnesses energy to fuel the final step in ATP formation, known as **oxidative phosphorylation (OP)**. ATP is often called the molecular unit of currency for our bodies to perform work. ATP is the fundamental energy molecule to power cellular functions. In order to make ATP, catalytic enzymes play key roles in the cell by speeding up chemical reactions in the ATP biosynthesis pathway. These enzymes bind with smaller, vitamin-derived molecules called coenzymes. The coenzyme molecules nicotinamide adenine dinucleotide (**NADH**) and flavin adenine dinucleotide (**FADH$_2$**), serve as important couriers that carry liberated electrons as a form of energy from fuel catabolism to the ETC for the synthesis of ATP. When breaking down energy-producing nutrients, carbohydrate, fat, and protein, the carbon chains are broken by catabolic enzymes. This process frees high-energy electrons that must be harnessed to reach the site of ATP production, the ETC. In order to do this, these electrons ride on special electron acceptor molecules NAD^+ and FAD. These molecules are derivatives of the B-vitamins niacin and riboflavin, respectively, and have several energy-transfer points where NAD^+ and FAD accept two high-energy electrons and two protons ($2H^+$) to form the reduced coenzymes NADH and FADH$_2$.

PUTTING IT INTO PERSPECTIVE

LEO THE LION SAYS "GER"

During the synthesis of ATP, electrons are transferred when carbon-carbon bonds are split during the formation of pyruvate, acetyl-CoA, and metabolites found within the TCA cycle. A helpful mnemonic can help you remember the process of electron movement and molecule charge. When a molecule Loses an Electron, the molecule is Oxidized (LEO); when a molecule Gains an Electron, the molecule is Reduced (GER).

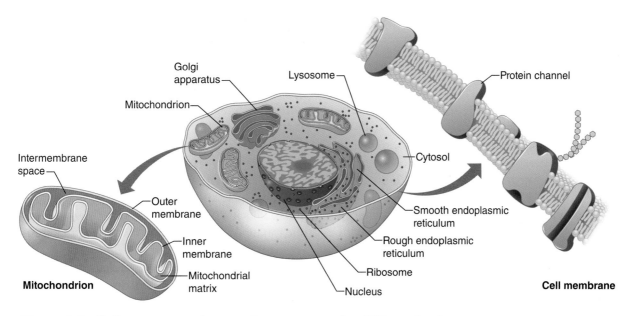

Figure 2.2 Cell structure and organelles necessary for ATP production.

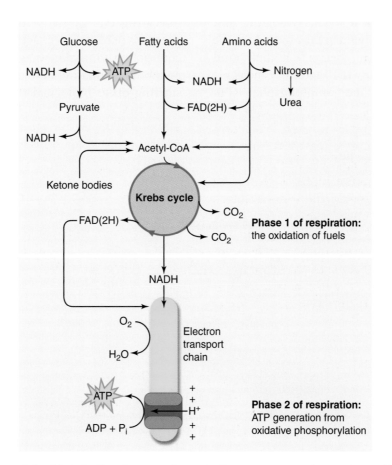

Figure 2.3 Metabolic phases of respiration necessary to produce ATP.

Transforming Energy to a Useable Form in the Body

The use of ATP in the body is constant and never-ending—it exists as long as life exists. ATP is the kick-start that initiates the complete breakdown and oxidation of glucose and fatty acids. It also powers energy-consuming processes, such as making new glucose for the body when a meal is missed. ATP's role in biosynthesis is synonymous with building construction. In order to make larger molecules from smaller molecules, energy is required to form the chemical bonds as well as the physical structure, just as construction workers are necessary to lay the bricks of a new building foundation.

The production of ATP is the fundamental goal of energy-producing pathways in metabolism. The ATP molecule has three phosphate groups attached to the organic molecule adenosine. When the phosphate bonds break, a tremendous amount of energy is released, and cells can use this to power biological work. When the first phosphate-adenosine bond breaks from ATP, the reaction leaves the still energy-rich compound **adenosine diphosphate (ADP)** and a free molecule of **pyrophosphate**, or inorganic phosphate (Pi).

Breaking the remaining phosphate bond releases a lesser amount of energy and breaks down ADP to **adenosine monophosphate (AMP)** and P_i. Under normal conditions, concentrations of AMP are very low in the cell, as ADP is constantly re-phosphorylated into ATP. However, as energy demands rise, physiological processes increasingly rely on conversion from ADP to AMP, although this is less energy efficient. As seen in figure 2.4, AMP is interconvertible with both ADP and ATP, and because it contains only one phosphate it does not contain any high-energy phosphate to phosphate bonds. These reactions are considered interconvertible because P_i can break free from adenosine to release energy or can be bound to adenosine from the extraction of energy from carbohydrate, protein, and fat. This most commonly occurs with ADP binding with P_i, forming a phosphate bond and capturing energy in a new ATP molecule. As energy is required, the reaction then goes in the opposite direction, breaking the phosphate bond and liberating energy while reforming ADP. This energy is used to power activities such as muscle contraction, transporting substances across cell membranes, making new molecules, and jump-starting other biological pathways. ATP is not

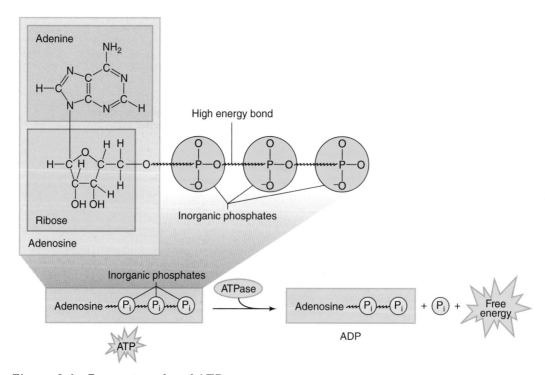

Figure 2.4   Energy transfer of ATP.

considered an energy-storage molecule; in fact, the body's pool of ATP is a very small (~100 g), immediately accessible energy reservoir capable of providing energy for only several seconds. ATP production rate is directly related to muscle mass and the changing energy demands of the body. For example, at rest, the body uses approximately 90 pounds (40 kg) of ATP over 24 hours. At the immediate onset of strenuous exercise or physical activity, it is possible to rapidly break down over a pound (.45 kg) of ATP per minute, while the production of ATP skyrockets to keep up with the energy demand of quickly contracting muscles.

Energy Systems Used By the Human Body

Before discussing the specifics of ATP production and how each energy-yielding macronutrient is used to generate ATP using both unique and commonly used metabolic pathways, it is helpful to categorize ATP production from a systems approach. This approach not only aids in understanding the integrated nature of ATP production, but also helps with real-life application of how different systems are used to meet our ever-changing ATP demand. As discussed earlier, the body readily uses carbohydrate and fat from the diet or from body stores to make ATP. Protein also contributes but at a much lower relative percentage. In energy metabolism, carbohydrate, fat, and protein are all considered biological substrates. A substrate is a molecule upon which an enzyme acts to create different metabolite products along its journey to make ATP. While carbohydrate, fat, and protein are the three major fuel substrates, there is a fourth that originates from **phosphocreatine (PCr)**. You may

have heard of this compound in the gym, where it is a popular dietary supplement (much more on supplements in chapter 9).

In muscle tissue, phosphocreatine can be split into a creatine component and a phosphate (P_i) component. It is the presence of this additional P_i from the phosphocreatine compound that can be used to resynthesize ADP into ATP. This general process describes the phosphagen system (ATP-PC system). This system uses exclusively phosphocreatine to regenerate ATP in muscle tissue. In addition to the phosphagen system, the body has two other energy systems that use energy-yielding macronutrients to make ATP. These energy systems are known as the **anaerobic system** and the **aerobic system**. Each of these energy systems can be described by the complexity of their metabolic pathways, rate or speed of ATP production, capacity to produce ATP, and the lag time required to contribute significant amounts of ATP when ATP is in demand. The relative contribution of each energy system to ATP production in different sporting activities is described in table 2.1. In brief, the phosphagen system uses small stores of ATP and PC to support short bursts of energy, the anaerobic system burns carbohydrate and produces lactic acid for bouts of exercise up to a couple minutes, and the aerobic system uses a variety of substrates in conjunction with oxygen to support exercise lasting tens of minutes to many hours. At any given point in time, ATP is being produced by these energy systems to some degree, even if only in a minute amount. No energy system is *ever* turned off. Figure 2.5 illustrates the constant change in the relative proportion of ATP produced from different body tissues at any one point in time.

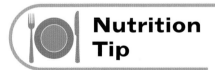 **Nutrition Tip**

About half of the creatine in our bodies is from the consumption of meat and fish. The other half is made from amino acids in the liver, kidney, and pancreas. Taken together, depending on how much meat is consumed, these processes can account for roughly 1 to 3 grams of creatine per day that can be converted into phosphocreatine to store in our muscle to help with ATP generation. Vegetarians, including vegans, who do not consume creatine phosphate supplements have been shown to have lower muscle stores of phosphocreatine than their meat-eating or supplementing peers (5) and may have a compromised ability to generate ATP with this energy system when high-intensity, short-duration efforts are important for competition.

In the world of exercise and sport, we think about how these energy systems are integrated in muscle tissue to produce ATP along a wide spectrum of intensity, ranging from sleep, to playing sedentary video games, to steady-state exercise, to high-intensity, stop-and-go sports.

Before exploring each energy system in detail, let's review the chemical energy sources that can be used by the three energy systems to produce ATP. As mentioned, phosphocreatine is specific to the phosphagen system. The carbohydrate family contributes serum glucose, also known as blood sugar, liver glycogen, and muscle glycogen. Fat contributes serum-free fatty acids (FFAs), serum triglycerides (TG), muscle TG, and adipose TG. Finally, protein contributes muscle protein, mostly in small amounts. If we think about each of these sources of stored energy as total kilocalories available to the body to burn, stored adipose TG have the highest caloric value, theoretically

providing tens of thousands of kilocalories, followed by muscle protein at no more than half of the kilocalories that could potentially be supplied by **adipose tissue** (fat tissue). We certainly do not want to make a habit of digging into our muscle tissue to supply our energy needs, as this can decrease muscle mass and strength. Fortunately, stored fat tissue and any available carbohydrate help to meet the body's energy demands.

Although it might sound as if we have near endless amounts of stored energy in our body to use for exercise and sport, several variables come into play that limit our ability to access this energy. Some barriers relate to the practical aspects of exercise, where the onset of fatigue limits the ability to continue exercise, which, in turn, limits the ability to maximally use stored energy. Other variables involve limitations of the energy systems to produce ATP because they have reached their capacity to make ATP. With regards to stored

Table 2.1 Relative Contribution of Each Energy System to ATP Production

	Phosphagen	Anaerobic	Aerobic
Neighborhood walk	Tertiary	Secondary	Primary
100-yard sprint	Primary	Secondary	Tertiary
Soccer game	Tertiary	Primary	Primary
Marathon	Tertiary	Secondary	Primary

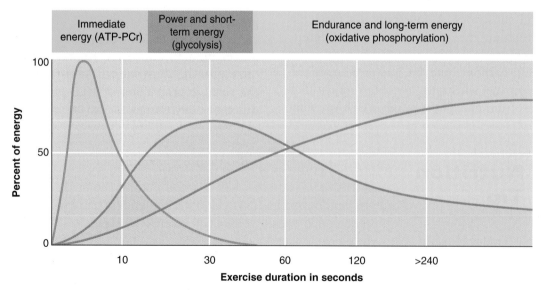

Figure 2.5 The three systems of energy transfer, and the percentage contribution to total energy output during all-out exercise of different durations.

lipid in the body, the amount of energy derived from fat stores to support exercise or training is a small fraction of the thousands of kilocalories of stored energy in adipose, making it evident that we cannot completely exhaust this stored fuel source. Further, of the described energy-yielding macronutrients found in the body that are fed into the energy systems for ATP production, a key point is that only carbohydrate can be used by the anaerobic system. In contrast, the aerobic system can use and completely break down all energy-yielding macronutrient fuel sources. While on the surface it seems that the aerobic system should pick up the slack to maximally tap into our stored fuel sources, it is not that simple. Consistent with all energy systems, the aerobic system also faces barriers to produce ATP, with the most significant of these barriers being oxygen availability. Without adequate oxygen delivery to the muscle, ATP production through the aerobic system is severely compromised. Other energy systems must step up to meet ATP needs, or exercise cannot continue.

Phosphagen System

The phosphagen system relies only on the P_i that is liberated from phosphocreatine to produce ATP, so by nature it is not a highly complex energy system (figure 2.6). The minimal lag time and rate of ATP production are this system's most impressive attributes. The rate or speed of ATP generation is the fastest of all energy systems. Because it is such a simple chemical reaction (not defined as a metabolic pathway), there is no

lag time to produce ATP, which occurs virtually instantaneously. Despite these impressive characteristics, this system's capacity to produce ATP is severely limited by the amount of phosphocreatine substrate found in muscle tissue. This limits the utility of this energy system to produce significant amounts of ATP for longer than a few seconds.

Precisely how many seconds depends on phosphocreatine concentrations in the muscle tissue and the intensity of the physical movement or exercise required that will have a direct impact on ATP demand to complete the activity. Maximal physical efforts tap into this energy system, immediately stimulating the simple metabolic reaction to occur continuously until phosphocreatine substrate is depleted in the engaged muscle groups. The best examples of this energy system at play are when you must move your body or another heavy object quickly. "Heavy" implies a certain level of elevated intensity that produces an immediate, exponential increase in ATP demand that can be met with the phosphagen system. These examples are clearly different from, say, moving your hand quickly from the keyboard to the computer mouse, an exertion for which very little ATP is required. In athletes, heavy weightlifting and sprinting are examples of activities requiring an increase in rate of ATP production. While it is certainly true that the phosphagen system in these examples can affect performance, in reality, any athlete who must give an all-out effort by intensely moving an object or their body relies on the phosphagen system until phosphocreatine is depleted. This can be for the duration of the event (if only seconds in duration) or, if

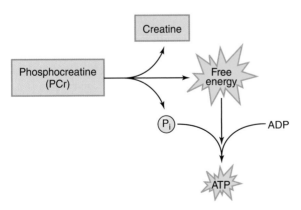

Figure 2.6 The phosphagen system.

intensity decreases, can serve as a bridge until other energy systems can help out and pick up the slack.

Anaerobic System

The anaerobic system contributes to ATP generation and is much more complex than the phosphagen system. This system features a 12-step process known as glycolysis. The rate of ATP production in the anaerobic system is fast and runs a close second to the phosphagen system. The speed of the anaerobic system allows it to be ready to receive the handoff from the phosphagen system as the primary ATP producer when all-out exercise efforts continue beyond 10 seconds. A great example of this occurs in the 200-meter sprint. Within seconds of exploding off the starting block, phosphocreatine stores rapidly plummet in the leg muscles, while the anaerobic system begins to skyrocket its ATP production. While the lag time for ATP production in the anaerobic system is seconds behind the phosphagen system, the capacity of this system to make ATP is significantly greater because more substrate, in the form of carbohydrate, is available. Still, in this aspect, the anaerobic system is limited when compared to the aerobic system.

Glycolysis, a key metabolic pathway, occurs in the cytoplasm of the cell and is associated with both the anaerobic and aerobic energy systems.

REFLECTION TIME

CREATINE SUPPLEMENTATION: POINTS TO PONDER

Many athletes consume a dietary supplement containing phosphocreatine in an effort to gain strength and muscle mass. This can be an effective strategy for some, combined with a well-rounded diet and exercise plan. Creatine supplementation effectiveness is related to many mechanisms (9) including the bolstering of phosphocreatine concentrations in muscle that create a larger P_i pool, which takes a longer time to be depleted in short-lived, high-intensity efforts. Supplementation of phosphocreatine (usually 5 to 20 g per day) is three to four times higher than what is naturally synthesized by the body and consumed in the diet. For many people in an exercise program that engages the phosphagen system, creatine supplementation can augment this system to allow athletes to lift slightly heavier weights and complete more repetitions of an exercise. This process helps to create more contractile protein breakdown to stimulate the muscle to grow larger and become stronger. Although this sounds great and in many cases is effective to help athletes meet strength goals, there are caveats. For instance, not everyone responds to creatine supplements, and dietary supplement manufacturers are not required to prove safety to the U.S. Food and Drug Administration (FDA), meaning there is no 100 percent guarantee that the product is safe and free from banned substances. However, many dietary supplement companies claim to ensure a greater level of safety through third-party testing. Despite anecdotal reports and some remaining controversy about long-term safety, most available evidence suggests that creatine consumption is safe. In fact, many studies are currently being conducted to examine the health benefits of creatine supplementation in cardiovascular disease, Parkinson's disease, and in patients who experienced mild traumatic brain injury (concussion). Although interest in creatine use and its growing safety profile is expanding, we should all stay up to date on studies on creatine safety, particularly its use long term (over years), its use by adult athletes with disease processes or conditions in which creatine may be contraindicated, and its use by young adults and preadolescents. Though creatine use in young athletes remains controversial (9), the International Society of Sports Nutrition provides prudent guidelines for adolescent use (4). For further discussion of creatine, see chapter 9.

Glycolysis takes a six-carbon molecule of glucose and breaks it down into two three-carbon molecules of pyruvate along with electron carriers NADH and FADH$_2$. Glycolysis ends with the synthesis of pyruvate and the production of a minimal amount of ATP. The key distinction between glycolysis that occurs in the anaerobic system and that which occurs in the aerobic system is that anaerobic glycolysis takes place without adequate oxygen delivery to the mitochondria, which results in a large portion of pyruvate being converted to **lactic acid**, also known as **lactate** (the chemical suffix "–ate" means acid). Alternatively, if oxygen is present, pyruvate is metabolized in other metabolic pathways involving the aerobic energy system in the mitochondria to produce more ATP.

In the anaerobic system (figure 2.7), two molecules of lactic acid form from the oxidation (donating electrons) of pyruvate. The basic reason for this is that, in an anaerobic environment, the participation of mitochondria in ATP production is drastically reduced, so calling exercise "anaerobic" or "without oxygen" is about the same as saying "without mitochondria." In this example, then, anaerobic glycolysis is the only efficient way to make ATP to fuel intense muscle contractions, and in order for this energy system to be self-functioning, it must also produce lactic acid from pyruvate via the acceptance of hydrogen ions (H$^+$). The NADH that is also produced from glycolysis (a carrier of H$^+$) is oxidized and recycled to NAD$^+$ via the enzyme **lactate dehydrogenase**

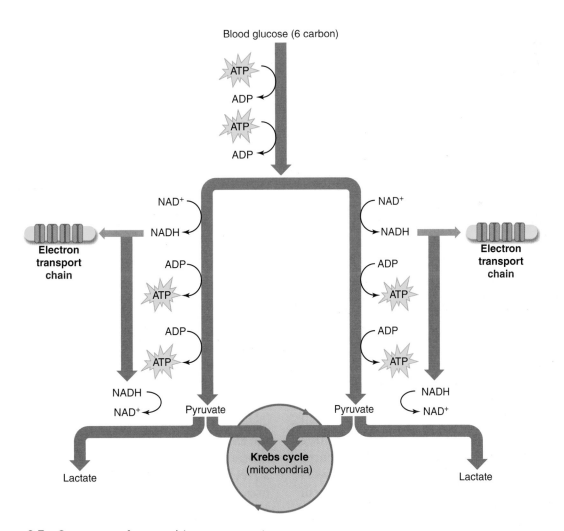

Figure 2.7 Summary of anaerobic energy system.

Reprinted, by permission, from NSCA, 2015, Bioenergetics of exercise and training, T.J. Herda and J.T. Cramer. In *Essentials of strength training and conditioning*, 4th ed. edited by G.G. Haff and N.T. Briplett (Champaign, IL: Human Kinetics), 47.

(LDH). This allows for the continuous glucose breakdown to pyruvate to make ATP.

LDH accomplishes this process by recycling NAD^+ from NADH to allow the anaerobic system to continue. At high concentrations of lactate (the conjugate base of lactic acid after the H+ is donated), LDH exhibits **feedback inhibition**, and the rate of conversion of pyruvate to lactic acid is decreased. The eventual fate of cytosolic NADH that has not yet donated its H+ ultimately depends on mitochondrial oxygen availability. If oxygen is limited, NADH is oxidized by LDH, and LDH then reduces (donates electrons) to pyruvate to form lactic acid. If mitochondrial oxygen is adequate, NADH is able to be shuttled to the ETC within the mitochondria for the aerobic energy system to proceed. See figure 2.7 for a summary of the basic processes of the anaerobic energy system.

The muscle oxygen deficit associated with the anaerobic energy system that leads to this cascade of events does not imply that someone is holding their breath to limit oxygen consumption. Instead, it means that oxygen *delivery* to the active muscle cell with high ATP demands is compromised to some degree. In the highly trained sprint athlete, this occurs in a 100-meter or 200-meter running event. The ATP demand at maximal physical exertion is so great to move the body at competitive speeds; it is not physiologically possible to deliver enough oxygen by increasing respiration rate. As oxygen is consumed through inhalation, it still must be processed by the lungs and delivered to the active muscle cell by the end of the race. This is not feasible, so the anaerobic system is in place to meet ATP needs where the phosphagen system left off. For a sedentary individual just starting a running program, the anaerobic energy system is also very important because oxygen insufficiency in untrained muscle is much more prevalent, even during low-intensity exercise, than in a trained athlete. As the sedentary person begins running the first mile on the first training day, the phosphagen system is immediately activated. This is quickly followed by the anaerobic energy system or, to some degree, the aerobic system, depending on oxygen availability of the mitochondria. If this formerly sedentary individual continues to push to maintain a running pace faster than they are used to, they will have to significantly rely on the anaerobic system. While the anaerobic energy system is extremely important for supporting the energy needs of high-intensity efforts, it is limited by the hydrogen ions it produces that lowers the pH, increasing the acidity of the muscle tissue. This is a contributing factor to muscular fatigue. The anaerobic energy system is also limited by substrate availability, as carbohydrate is the only substrate that can be used in this system. Over time, with repeated training, muscles can make physiological adaptations to muscle tissue acidity by improving buffering mechanisms that can limit the drop in tissue pH caused by hydrogen ions. Other physiological adaptations include improved muscle handling of lactate, improvements in the capacity of the phosphagen system, and many mechanisms associated with improved oxygen delivery to working muscle. Arguably the most important physiological adaptation resulting from intense anaerobic training is the increased capacity for the muscle to store and use carbohydrate in the anaerobic energy system. Since carbohydrate is the only fuel source that can be used when training and competing at the highest intensity (90–100% of $\dot{V}O_2$ max) (resulting in an anaerobic muscle environment), adequate carbohydrate consumption is vital to optimal high-intensity performance. If a suboptimal amount of carbohydrate is consumed, carbohydrate becomes a limited fuel, and the intensity of the exercise effort will inevitably decrease.

Aerobic System

The aerobic energy system is the most complex of the three energy systems. As illustrated in figure 2.8, this system incorporates many pathways to process each energy-yielding macronutrient for ATP production. These pathways include beta-oxidation (fat), glycolysis (carbohydrate), deamination (protein), and the TCA cycle and the ETC (all energy-yielding macronutrients). In contrast, the phosphagen system does not use a metabolic pathway, and the anaerobic system uses only glycolysis. The aerobic energy system requires adequate oxygen availability for the mitochondria. The available oxygen is used in the final set of metabolic reactions that occur in the ETC, where oxygen serves as the final electron acceptor.

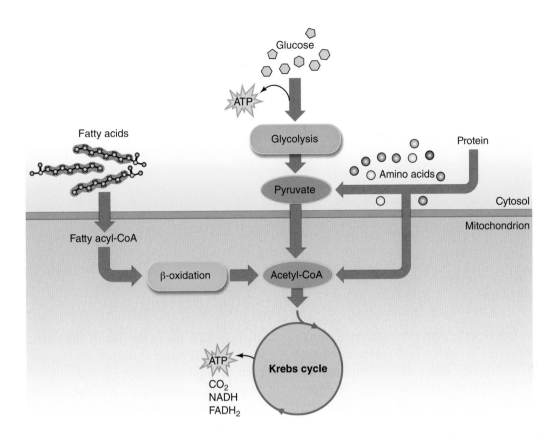

Figure 2.8 The aerobic energy system allows entry points of fat, carbohydrate, and protein in the oxidative pathway.

Reprinted, by permission, from A. Jeukendrup and M. Gleeson, 2010, Fuel sources for muscle and exercise metabolism. In *Sport nutrition* (Champaign, IL: Human Kinetics), 52.

Because of the aerobic energy system's requirement for oxygen, the maximal rate of ATP production is considered relatively slow in comparison to the phosphagen and anaerobic system. This is because of the time it takes to deliver oxygen from the air we breathe to the mitochondrial matrix. This also contributes to the longest lag time to increase ATP production of any energy system. While the phosphagen and anaerobic systems are activated either immediately or over the course of a few seconds, the aerobic energy system can take minutes to produce enough ATP to fuel a physical workload that is within an individual's **aerobic capacity**. The aerobic capacity is the maximal amount of oxygen (measured in milliliters) that an athlete can use in 1 minute per kilogram of body weight ($ml \cdot kg^{-1} \cdot min^{-1}$). For the purposes of fuel metabolism to produce ATP via the aerobic system, this is used to estimate the maximal

amount of oxygen the muscle can use aerobically and is tightly connected to aerobic fitness and how long an individual can rely on the aerobic system as exercise intensity increases (figure 2.9). The term aerobic capacity is also used alongside $\dot{V}O_2max$, the maximal amount of oxygen someone can use. As exercise intensity increases, everyone has a $\dot{V}O_2max$ that they are approaching. Once the maximum peak of oxygen consumption (by the muscle) is met, any additional intensity that requires additional ATP must be met by the anaerobic system. With repeated aerobic training that tests the limits of the $\dot{V}O_2max$, an individual can increase their $\dot{V}O_2max$, within their genetic potential, to improve the ability of the muscle to make ATP from all energy-yielding macronutrient substrates aerobically.

This reference to aerobic capacity is different from the aerobic system's capacity to make ATP.

PUTTING IT INTO PERSPECTIVE

TRAINING AT HIGH ALTITUDES

We have all heard of athletes who travel to high-altitude locations (greater than 2,000 meters, or 6,600 feet) to train and prepare for future competition. They do so in an effort to produce metabolic changes to adapt to breathing air that contains less oxygen. While there are several metabolic reasons why this can be advantageous to the athlete, one of the fundamental concerns that athletes should be aware of is how limited oxygen availability affects the ability to oxidize metabolic fuels. Limited oxygen availability will limit the aerobic system's ability to perform. While over time, as athletes train in this environment, their bodies will begin to make metabolic adaptations to improve aerobic system efficiency; their immediate concern is ensuring their anaerobic system has the energy substrate it needs to pick up the slack in ATP production. Since oxygen is already limited in the air, mitochondrial oxygen deficits will occur much sooner as exercise intensity increases. Adequate carbohydrate ingestion during the acute 3- to 6-week adaptation phase is critical because it is the only fuel that can be used anaerobically.

In theory, the aerobic system's capacity to make ATP is practically unlimited when adequate oxygen is available, which is why the aerobic system is the ATP production system of choice when the body is at rest, when it can easily tap into carbohydrate and access seemingly unlimited fat stores to meet the body's chemical energy needs. For the well-trained athlete who has benefitted from cardiovascular, muscle, and metabolic adaptations that allow more efficient oxygen uptake and delivery to muscle tissue, the use of the aerobic system is much more robust than what is observed in a sedentary, untrained individual. The trained athlete is capable of tapping into their aerobic system for meeting a significant portion of their ATP needs earlier in the exercise bout, for a much greater duration during the exercise bout, and at higher exercise intensities than their untrained counterparts. Ultimately, their capacity to make ATP aerobically is hindered only by having some carbohydrate available for the TCA cycle to run smoothly and any muscle fatigue they encounter that may eventually stop the exercise or competitive session. This means that some elite endurance athletes, such as triathletes and ultramarathoners, can maintain aerobic exercise for more than 8 hours on end!

In summary, the three energy systems the body uses are tightly integrated to make ATP based on the intensity of the exercise, which dictates ATP

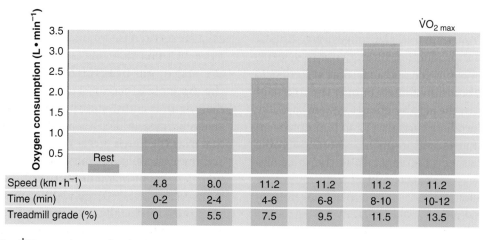

Speed (km·h⁻¹)		4.8	8.0	11.2	11.2	11.2	11.2
Time (min)		0-2	2-4	4-6	6-8	8-10	10-12
Treadmill grade (%)		0	5.5	7.5	9.5	11.5	13.5

Figure 2.9 $\dot{V}O_2$max is reached when oxygen consumption fails to increase the expected amount or decreases slightly with increased exercise intensity.

demand to fuel muscle contraction and oxygen availability. In the aerobic and anaerobic systems, the glycolysis pathway does not change; only the fate of pyruvate is different. For energy-yielding macronutrient oxidation to make ATP aerobically, each macronutrient starts the breakdown process with a metabolic pathway specific to that nutrient. Carbohydrate participates in glycolysis, protein in deamination, and fat in beta-oxidation. Once this initial catabolic process is complete, metabolites from each individual breakdown source enter the TCA cycle at different entry points to yield high-energy electrons from oxidative decarboxylation and complete the ATP production cycle in the ETC.

Breakdown and Release of Energy

During the first steps of the complete breakdown of carbohydrate, fat, and protein, several metabolic pathways are involved. However, as breakdown of each energy-yielding macronutrient proceeds, all eventually converge along two shared metabolic pathways: the TCA cycle and the ETC. In this section we will start with an overview of carbohydrate breakdown, and then discuss the steps involved in protein and fat breakdown.

Chemical Energy Derived From Carbohydrate

Most of the cells in the body extract energy from carbohydrate via four metabolic processes: glycolysis, pyruvate to acetyl-CoA, the TCA cycle, and the ETC. For each of the metabolic pathways glucose is involved in, a different amount of ATP is produced. For instance, glycolysis produces only a small amount of ATP (+ 2ATP) per each glucose molecule, but the complete aerobic breakdown of glucose that ends at the ETC produces roughly 16 times the amount of ATP that is produced from the anaerobic breakdown of glucose (+ 30–32ATP).

Glycolysis occurs in the cytosol of the cell and does not require oxygen to proceed. The sequence of reactions involves splitting a six-carbon glucose molecule into *two* three-carbon pyruvate molecules. This catabolic process requires 2ATP per glucose molecule and yields a gain of 4ATP for a net gain of 2ATP + 2NADH + 2Pyruvates. The ATP required for this reaction serves to "prime the pump" to get the series of enzymatic reactions started.

In the muscle cell, glucose is the only simple sugar carbohydrate that can be absorbed, and once absorbed the muscle will not let it go. The muscle does this by adding a phosphorous group to glucose, turning it into glucose-6-phosphate (G-6-P). The structure of G-6-P will not allow it to leave the muscle cell and seals glucose's fate to either participate in the catabolic pathway (when energy is needed) of glycolysis or the anabolic process of **glycogenesis** (when energy demands are low) to store carbohydrate as a future energy source in the form of glycogen. What about the other simple sugars, fructose and galactose? These sugars from our diet are absorbed by the liver for further metabolic processing to glucose that can be stored as liver glycogen or released into the bloodstream as glucose.

The next step in the aerobic energy system process is to convert pyruvate into acetyl-CoA. This is a highly regulated process that takes into account the cell's energy demands (i.e., how much ATP is needed to maintain muscle work) and oxygen availability within the cell. The **pyruvate dehydrogenase complex (PDC)**, which converts pyruvate from glycolysis into acetyl-CoA for the TCA cycle, helps regulate this step by receiving feedback from the cell from the available concentrations of ADP versus ATP as well as the availability of NAD⁺ and FAD to accept electrons and protons for energy transfer. For example, high levels of ATP within the cell suggests energy adequacy that will slow down additional conversion of pyruvate to acetyl-CoA. Conversely, high ADP concentrations suggest an energy deficit and the need to speed up the rate in which pyruvate is converted to acetyl-CoA. The most important factor that affects this conversion pathway is the availability of oxygen. When a cell

DO YOU KNOW ?

Muscle is the primary disposal organ of glucose. This is a fundamental reason why exercise is important for diabetes prevention and treatment. Exercise uses glucose for muscle contraction, which helps decrease the amount of glucose in the blood. If you have a genetic history for diabetes, you have all the more reason to maintain fitness through exercise. With regular exercise, your chances of getting diabetes are significantly reduced.

requires energy, and oxygen is readily available, aerobic reactions in the mitochondria convert each pyruvate molecule to an acetyl-CoA molecule. This reaction produces a pair of electrons to form NADH while also producing carbon dioxide. The NADH will then shuttle the electrons to the ETC. The phrase "oxygen availability" is best conceptualized when thinking about the pyruvate to acetyl-CoA pathway in muscle cells. At rest, in healthy individuals, it is not very difficult for the body to deliver inhaled oxygen to muscle cells. This gets tricky when someone begins to exercise. How well oxygen remains available to exercising muscle depends on two things: an individual's aerobic fitness and the relative intensity of the exercise session. Oxygen will become less available sooner in an unfit individual as exercise intensity increases. Fit individuals have created physiological adaptations to deliver oxygen much more efficiently in exercising muscle and can maintain "oxygen availability" at high intensities. From a metabolic perspective, everyone has an intensity limit, even fit athletes, at which oxygen becomes unavailable, and it is at this time the conversion of pyruvate to acetyl-CoA ceases.

While many metabolic pathways can proceed either forward or backward, the formation of acetyl-CoA is an irreversible process once it is initiated in the presence of adequate oxygen. To form acetyl-CoA, metabolic reactions remove one carbon from the three-carbon pyruvate and add the **coenzyme A** that is derived from the B vitamin, pantothenic acid. After combining with oxygen, the carbon is released as part of carbon dioxide. The end products from this process that started with two pyruvate molecules are now two NADH and two acetyl-CoA molecules. The acetyl-CoA molecules produced from pyruvate are trapped inside the mitochondria and ready to enter the TCA cycle.

The oxygen-dependent reactions of the TCA cycle and the ETC liberate large amounts of energy in the form of ATP. The TCA cycle—also known as the citric acid cycle or the Krebs cycle—occurs in the mitochondria and serves to take the acetyl portion (CH_3COO-) of acetyl-CoA through oxidative processes (i.e., breaking carbon-carbon bonds to liberate electrons) to yield three molecules of NADH, two molecules of carbon dioxide, and one

molecule each of $FADH_2$ and GTP (guanosine triphosphate, an energy carrier similar to ATP). The TCA process begins with acetyl-CoA combining with **oxaloacetate**, freeing coenzyme A and yielding a six-carbon compound called citrate. The coenzyme A can then be recycled to form another acetyl-CoA by binding with a new pyruvate molecule. Subsequent reactions in the TCA cycle convert citrate into a series of intermediate compounds, removing two additional carbons (freeing high-energy electrons) and releasing two molecules of carbon dioxide. The final step in the TCA cycle regenerates oxaloacetate (figure 2.10), which in turn reacts with pyruvate to create citric acid and start the cycle anew. The primary purpose of the TCA cycle for energy-generation purposes is to extract most of the energy from oxidative decarboxylation to harness high-energy electrons and protons to be shuttled to the ETC. For each acetyl-CoA entering the cycle, one complete cycle or "turn" produces one GTP and transfers pairs of high-energy electrons to three NADH and one $FADH_2$. Recall that the anaerobic breakdown of one glucose molecule yields two molecules of acetyl-CoA and that the TCA cycle "turns" or cycles with each acetyl-CoA molecule provided. This produces twice the amount of high-energy electron carriers (i.e., six NADH, two $FADH_2$, and two GTP). In addition to providing electron substrate for coenzyme energy transfer to the ETC, the TCA cycle is also an important source of building blocks for the biosynthesis of amino acids and fatty acids. When there is plenty of ATP to meet the energy demand of the cell, the TCA cycle's intermediate molecules can leave the cycle and join biosynthetic metabolic pathways. For example, during times of energy excess (i.e., consuming more calories than are burned with activity), citrate can leave the cycle to provide substrate for fatty acid synthesis and subsequent fat storage.

The ETC produces most of the ATP available from glucose and serves as the final step in glucose oxidation by accepting the high-energy electrons from the TCA cycle. The ETC consists of a sequence of linked reactions that take place on what visually appears to be a chain of linked protein channels found on the inner mitochondrial membrane (figure 2.11). Most ATP

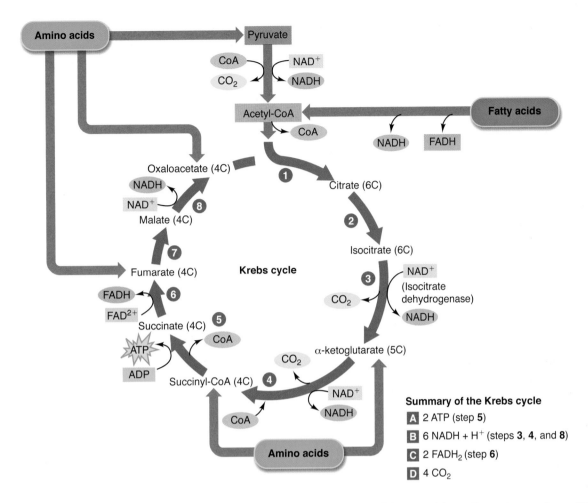

Summary of the Krebs cycle

A 2 ATP (step **5**)

B 6 NADH + H$^+$ (steps **3**, **4**, and **8**)

C 2 FADH$_2$ (step **6**)

D 4 CO$_2$

Figure 2.10 The TCA cycle is a metabolic pathway that is part of the aerobic pathway to produce ATP.

is produced here, and as long as mitochondrial oxygen supply is adequate, it can maintain ATP production to fuel exercise for hours. The site of the ETC is where NADH and FADH$_2$ deliver its pair of high-energy electrons to the beginning of the chain. In the inner mitochondrial membrane, these electrons are passed along a chain of linked reactions, giving up energy along the way to power the final production of ATP. At the end of the ETC, oxygen accepts the energy-depleted electrons and reacts with hydrogen to form water (this is where most of the oxygen we breathe goes!). This series of oxidation-reduction reactions (i.e., losing and gaining electrons) is known as oxidative phosphorylation and is characterized by the flow of electrons down the chain and the phosphorylation of ADP to form significant amounts of ATP.

As electrons are donated and passed down the ETC, they create an electrochemical gradient that

causes a pressure change between the inner mitochondrial space and the mitochondrial matrix. This creates a phenomenon known as **proton motive force** that forces protons (H$^+$) through the ETC proton channels from the matrix into the inner mitochondrial space. The pressure that starts to build in the inner mitochondrial space provides the force to push hydrogen ions back through to the matrix through a complex protein channel called **ATP synthase**. This protein complex has been described as an energy turbine that turns and manufactures ATP by serving as the physical tool that binds P$_i$ to ADP. This process is analogous to blowing up a balloon—the opening of the balloon serves as the pressure release valve that drives the ATP synthase machinery to form ATP. Collectively, this entire process has been termed the **chemiosmotic coupling** and is illustrated in figure 2.12. The difference in NADH and

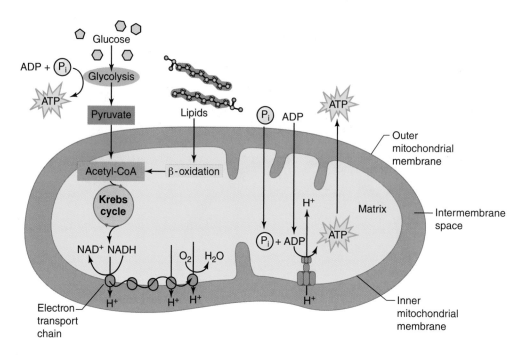

Figure 2.11 Mitochondrial matrix. The ETC and beta-oxidation occur in the mitochondria, the powerhouse of the cell.

$FADH_2$ contribution to ATP production is where on the ETC they donate their electrons. NADH donates electrons at the beginning of the chain, whereas $FADH_2$ electrons enter the ETC at a later point. Because they travel through fewer reactions, the electrons from $FADH_2$ generate fewer ATP molecules from less proton motive force. As illustrated in table 2.2, the total amount of ATP molecules produced from one glucose molecule is currently estimated at 30 to 32 ATP (8).

Chemical Energy Derived From Fat

To generate chemical energy from fat, the body must first break down triglycerides into their component glycerol and fatty acids. Different hormones and metabolic processes are involved to take on this task from both fats (technically termed triglycerides) derived from the diet and those stored in fat cells. Glycerol, a small three-carbon molecule, carries a small amount of energy within its carbon-carbon bonds and the liver readily accepts it to convert it to pyruvate or glucose. The fatty acids derived from triglycerides provide nearly all of the energy found in this compound. All fatty acid breakdown and oxidation occurs within the mitochondria. However, before

a fatty acid can cross into mitochondria, it must be linked to coenzyme A. This is the activation step of fatty acid delivery into the mitochondria and requires one molecule of ATP to launch the process. Figure 2.13 provides an overview of how fat is transported and used for ATP production.

The next step of fatty acid delivery into the mitochondria involves activated fatty acid interaction with the **carnitine shuttle**. Carnitine is a compound formed from the amino acid lysine and has the unique task of shepherding the activated fatty acid across the outer mitochondrial membrane from the cytosol to the mitochondrion matrix.

Once fatty acids enter the mitochondria, a process known as beta-oxidation breaks the fatty acids down into multiple molecules of acetyl-CoA for entry into the TCA cycle. Once fatty acids become individual acetyl-CoA units, the remaining metabolic pathways to make ATP are the same as glucose and involve both the TCA cycle and the ETC, as previously described. Beta-oxidation involves disassembling long fatty acid chains. Beta-oxidation of fatty acids takes place primarily in the mitochondrial matrix. However, fatty acids must be activated for degradation by coenzyme A by forming a fatty acyl-CoA bond. Starting from

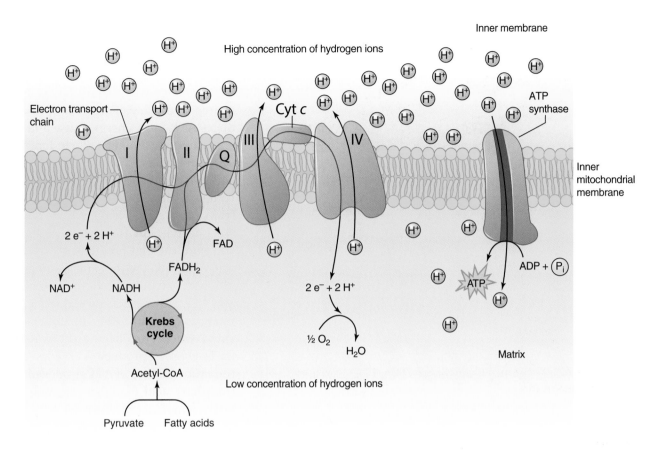

Figure 2.12 Chemiosmotic coupling. An electrochemical gradient is formed from electrons passing through the electron transport chain, causing hydrogen ions (protons) to move across from the mitochondrial matrix, producing proton motive force that activates the protein complex ATP synthase to regenerate ATP.

the second carbon from the acidic end of the fatty acid chain, called the beta carbon, fat enzymes will clip a two-carbon "link" off the end of the chain. Every time this happens, other reactions take place to convert this link to one acetyl-CoA, while also transferring one pair of electrons to $FADH_2$ and another pair to NADH. This process always occurs in a stepwise fashion, where only two carbons are clipped at a time to generate a molecule of acetyl-CoA until only one two-carbon

Table 2.2 Net ATP From the Complete Aerobic Oxidation of One Molecule of Glucose

Step	Coenzyme electron carriers	ATP yield
Glycolysis		2
TCA	GTP	2
Oxidative phosphorylation	2 NADH × 1.5 (G-3PO)	3
	2 NADH (oxidative decarboxylation of pyruvate) × 2.5	5
	2 FADH (TCA) × 1.5	3
	6 NADH (TCA) × 2.5	15
	Total yield	**30 (32) ATP**

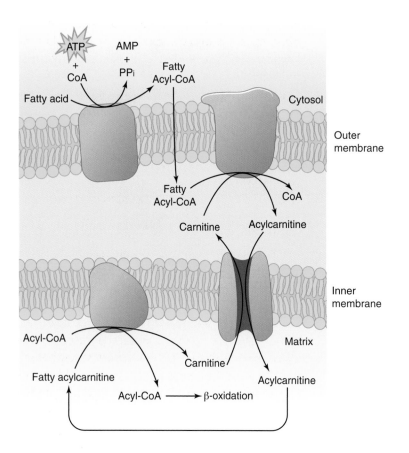

Figure 2.13 Fat used in ATP production. These steps are essential for fatty acids to be oxidized in the mitochondria.

segment remains. The final acetyl-CoA formed does not produce an FADH$_2$ or NADH, because the final step does not generate high-energy electrons without additional carbon-carbon bonds being split.

Almost all fatty acids that originate from food have an even number of carbons and vary in length from 4 to 26 carbons. Although most fatty acids are 16 to 18 carbons long, if the mitochondrion encounters an odd-numbered fatty acid, it will break down the chain in the same way until it reaches a final three-carbon link. Instead of continued breakdown, the final three-carbon molecule will join with coenzyme A and enter the TCA cycle as one of the downstream intermediates (i.e., not as acetyl-CoA). Because this process skips some of the early TCA reactions, it has a shorter journey than acetyl-CoA and produces fewer high-energy electrons and thus fewer NADH molecules.

Because beta-oxidation produces many acetyl-CoA molecules from just one fatty acid (figure 2.14), it is easy to see why dietary fat, as a source of dietary energy that produces ATP, is so energy dense and contributes a higher calorie load for our bodies. The ETC within the matrix of the mitochondria complete the extraction of energy from fatty acids, just as they do with acetyl-CoA from glucose. In addition, the end products of fatty acid oxidation are the same as with glucose: carbon dioxide, water, and ATP. However, a few metabolic nuances are important to understand when considering the way fat is used to produce ATP. First, the exact amount of ATP produced from fatty acid oxidation depends on the length of the fatty acid chain. Longer chains have more carbon bonds and hence will produce more chemical energy in the form of ATP. The complete breakdown of an 18-carbon fatty acid produces 120 ATP. This is substantially more ATP than is produced from one molecule of glucose. To take this a step further, most of the fat we consume in our diet is in the form of triglycerides. A *single* triglyceride with three 18-carbon fatty acids that are completely oxidized will produce 360 ATP, a value more than 10 times the ATP produced from the complete oxidation of a single glucose molecule.

Another metabolic consideration important to understand is that fat metabolism is tightly synchronized with carbohydrate metabolism and, unlike carbohydrate breakdown, requires oxygen. Acetyl-CoA from beta-oxidation can enter the TCA cycle only when fat and carbohydrate occur in concert. When carbohydrate availability to normal human metabolism is low, such as with very low-carbohydrate diets or during starvation, the TCA intermediate oxaloacetate readily leaves the TCA cycle to travel to the liver and help the body make more blood glucose to prevent hypoglycemia. This metabolic pathway

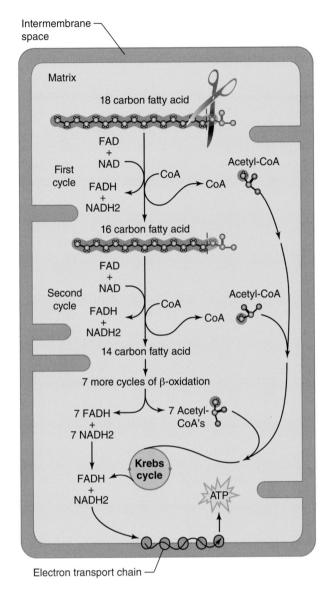

Figure 2.14 Beta-oxidation is specific to fat metabolism and provides substrate to the aerobic energy system.

ered products of incomplete fat oxidation. The body makes and uses small amounts of ketone bodies at all times, and they serve as a readily oxidized fuel source for ATP production by the heart and kidneys. For acetyl-CoA derived from the oxidation of fatty acids to enter the TCA cycle, fat and carbohydrate metabolism must be synchronized. When acetyl-CoA cannot enter the TCA cycle, it is shunted to form ketone bodies.

Similar to the aerobic oxidation of glucose, the mitochondria must also have adequate oxygen availability in order to completely oxidize fatty acids. Unlike carbohydrate, fatty acids cannot produce ATP anaerobically and must follow mitochondrial pathways leading up to the ETC with oxygen serving as the final electron acceptor. Take, for example, a foot race between a trained athlete versus an unfit couch potato. Just as there are differences in carbohydrate metabolism between the two race participants, differences also exist in the ability to use fat as a fuel source to generate ATP. At rest, both the athlete and couch potato have no problems burning fat as a fuel source. ATP demand is low, and oxygen is available to all mitochondria. This drastically changes at the onset of exercise. Athletes have adapted to be able to deliver more oxygen to working muscles and can do so at higher exercise intensities than the untrained. The couch potato will experience an oxygen deficit much sooner as intensity increases. This will put the brakes on fat oxidation, as ATP will be generated with anaerobic glycolysis (relying on the breakdown of carbohydrate) with much less capacity than with fat oxidation.

Chemical Energy Derived From Protein

As previously discussed, the human body's preference is to use protein in structural and functional roles, such as warming the body and remodeling muscle tissue, so protein is not considered a major resource for ATP production. That said, recall that no metabolic pathway involving carbohydrate, fat, or protein is ever "turned off." Some tissues will always be using protein as an ATP source, but its contribution is relatively small compared

takes precedence under these circumstances because we cannot function properly or, in some cases, even survive if our blood glucose gets too low. Because of this metabolic shift, oxaloacetate is much less available to combine with acetyl-CoA, from beta-oxidation, to form citrate and continue the TCA process. Instead, acetyl-CoAs are blocked from entry into the TCA cycle and rerouted to form a family of compounds called ketone bodies. These ketone bodies are consid-

to that of carbohydrate and fat to meet chemical energy needs. However, if for some reason our energy production falters, such as in starvation or when inadequate amounts of calories are available, energy production from body protein stores will increase. During starvation, when energy needs and blood glucose is vital to sustaining life, the body will break down protein and use amino acids.

To make ATP from protein, amino acids must first be stripped of their nitrogen component ($-NH_2$) in a process called deamination. The remaining carbon structure, often referred to as the "carbon skeleton," can be used by the TCA cycle, whereas the nitrogen component is converted to ammonia and then to urea (essentially, a waste product) by the liver. The carbon skeletons from amino acid catabolism can enter the breakdown pathways of the TCA cycle at many different points. This is a key distinction from carbohydrate and fat breakdown that must enter the TCA cycle as acetyl-CoA (see figure 2.10). The carbon skeleton from each amino acid has a unique structure and number of carbon atoms. These differences determine the carbon skeleton's fate. Some skeletons take the form of pyruvate (alanine) or enter the TCA as acetyl-CoA (leucine), while others can enter as one of the many intermediates of the TCA cycle (asparagine, tyrosine, methionine, glutamate). The complete breakdown of an amino acid yields urea, carbon dioxide, water, and ATP. How much ATP the amino acid produces depends on where the carbon skeleton enters the TCA cycle. For example, alanine enters the TCA cycle early and can produce 12.5 ATP. In contrast, methionine enters the TCA cycle following deamination approximately halfway through the cycle, producing only five ATPs. When compared to carbohydrate and fat fuel sources, amino acids produce relatively low amounts of ATP.

Chemical Energy Derived From Alcohol

Alcohol in human nutrition usually refers to beer, wine, and distilled spirits. The technical name for alcohol is ethanol and, when consumed, the energy value is 7 kilocalories per gram (kcal/g), providing a chemical energy source the body can use to make ATP. Since alcohol provides an energy source, it has been classified as a food; however, alcohol performs no essential functions in the body and is therefore not a nutrient.

The body works extremely hard to get rid of alcohol in order to prevent it from accumulating and destroying cells and organs. For example, the liver will selectively metabolize alcohol before other compounds and can use alternative metabolic pathways in the liver in an effort to handle and clear excessive (i.e., binge) consumption. Generally, when small to moderate amounts of alcohol is consumed it is first converted to acetaldehyde and rapidly converted to acetate and then acetyl-CoA (figure 2.15). Generally, very little acetyl-CoA enters the TCA cycle and, instead, is shuttled to anabolic pathways to form fat. This occurs because the metabolic reactions that convert alcohol to acetate rapidly consume the available NAD^+ that is normally available to receive high-energy electrons from the oxidation of carbohydrate and fat. The limited availability of NAD^+ restricts the speed of the TCA cycle. Since alcohol detoxification is the body's priority, accumulating acetyl-CoAs are rerouted to fatty acid synthesis. Fat accumulation in the liver can be seen after a single bout of heavy drinking. This fatty acid synthesis adapts and accelerates with chronic heavy alcohol consumption, leading to a fatty liver—the first stage of liver destruction that occurs with chronic alcohol abuse.

DO YOU KNOW?

Although some supplement manufacturers claim the supplement carnitine can enhance "fat burning," the bulk of the scientific literature remains equivocal (25, 32). Despite these findings, carnitine research continues to grow, with new research questions addressing dose efficacy, exercise performance, and recovery. However, some of this movement has been dampened by data that suggest that carnitine supplementation may be harmful by potentially increasing the risk of cardiovascular disease (17). The highly respected Australian Institute of Sports has classified carnitine as a Group B supplement that is "deserving of further research and could be considered for provision to athletes under a research protocol or case-managed monitoring situation."

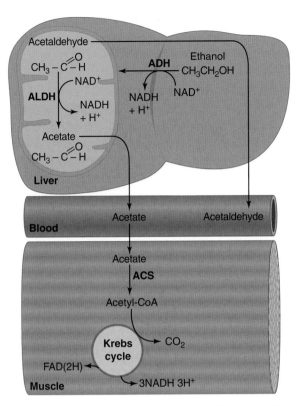

Figure 2.15 The process of ethanol metabolism.

ent (32). In the postexercise phase, alcohol may interfere with recovery by impairing glycogen resynthesis and storage (6). Alcohol consumption postexercise can also slow rates of rehydration via its suppressive effect on antidiuretic hormone (14) and impair the muscle protein synthesis response that is desired for muscle adaptation and repair (7, 24). For some athletes, other effects on body function are likely, such as mild disturbances in acid-base balance, increased inflammation, and compromised glucose metabolism and cardiovascular function (34). Finally, binge drinking can indirectly affect athlete recovery goals through inattention to following proper guidelines for training recovery, such as dealing with a hangover, missing meals, overeating, and excessive sleep. In general, athletes are advised to consider both public health guidelines and team rules regarding use of alcohol and are encouraged to minimize or avoid alcohol consumption in the postexercise period when issues of recovery and injury repair are a priority (32). Further discussion of the effects of alcohol on athletic performance appears in chapter 9.

BENEFITS OF TRAINING ON HEALTH AND ATHLETIC PERFORMANCE

Whether you train to increase strength or endurance, your body will adapt in order to accommodate or get used to the repeated stimulus, which ultimately will improve performance. The concept of training to improve performance encompasses the three key principles outlined in chapter 1. Although the magnitude and **specificity** of these changes will depend on the individual and the characteristics of the training program, any program that improves aerobic capacity will have a significant effect on fuel utilization and the energy systems. Since many athletes adopt a training regimen that promotes improvements in strength, power, and endurance, metabolic adaptations geared toward improving mitochondrial oxygen availability are prominent.

Figure 2.16 describes some key metabolic adaptations. Structural and biochemical adaptations to endurance training include increased

For athletes and others who want to maintain a high level of exercise and performance, misuse of alcohol can interfere with athletic goals in a variety of ways related to the negative effects of acute intake of alcohol on the performance of, or recovery from, exercise (32). Negative effects of chronic binge drinking can also manifest as poor health and difficult management of body composition (higher body fat) (20). Besides the calorie load of alcohol, alcohol suppresses fat oxidation, increases the likelihood of unplanned food consumption, and might compromise the achievement of a lean body composition (32).

The available evidence warns against intake of significant amounts of alcohol in the preexercise period and during training because of the direct negative effects of alcohol on exercise metabolism, thermoregulation, physical skills, and concentration (2). Any negative effects of alcohol on strength and performance may persist for several hours, even after signs and symptoms of intoxication or hangover are no longer pres-

mitochondrial number and size and increased concentration of oxidative enzymes involved in beta-oxidation, the TCA cycle, and the ETC. These changes improve the muscle environment and efficiency of the aerobic energy system. The NADH shuttling system and a change in LDH protein structure is also observed. These adaptations improve electron delivery to the ETC and increase the ability of the muscle to oxidize lactate. A host of cardiovascular changes also take place to support adaptation. The most significant changes are related to improvements in the heart's **stroke volume** and **angiogenesis**, which creates improved capillary density and capacity to transport fatty acids from the plasma to the muscle cell. Again, these are key adaptations that promote aerobic system efficiency, and in this case improve oxygen delivery to working muscle. Unfortunately, the principle of **reversibility** still holds true when training ceases. Most of these adaptations are lost after approximately 5 weeks of detraining, and about half of the increase in muscle mitochondrial content is lost after just 1 week of detraining. It is even more troubling to consider that it takes about 4 weeks of retraining to regain the adaptations lost in the first week of detraining. This is one of the fundamental reasons why exercise is recommended as part of a healthy lifestyle that is done daily, in some form, as a key strategy to promote health, longevity, and chronic disease prevention.

There is no doubt that the training stimulus is instrumental in promoting a multitude of cardiovascular system, muscle tissue, and cellular changes to improve energy system efficiency. While these adaptations have a clear benefit on metabolic health that should not be understated, other outcomes are related to fuel substrate utilization that offer key benefits for the competitive athlete and anyone else starting an exercise program to improve health. These benefits are best described by understanding the **crossover concept** of carbohydrate and fat utilization during exercise. By definition, the "crossover" is the point on the graph at which the body starts using more carbohydrate than fat as its energy source (for more on the crossover concept, see figure 11.1). Recall that exercise intensity is directly proportional to carbohydrate use because of the anaerobic environment that increasing intensity

creates. Also recall that an individual's ability to oxidize fat during exercise with increasing intensity will depend on their aerobic capacity. This means that if someone were to draw a simple figure to represent the crossover concept for a sedentary friend and compare it to an athlete friend, the figure, especially where the crossover occurs on the percent $\dot{V}O_2$max axis, would look very different. Consistent with the cardiovascular, muscle tissue, and cellular changes that occur with training, the crossover point also shifts to the right with training. This phenomenon has huge metabolic significance, both for individuals trying to become healthier through exercise and for athletes. For those starting an exercise program, the shift to the right that occurs with chronic training adaption means they will be able to work out longer and harder using a more efficient aerobic energy system to primarily oxidize fatty acids. While this finding may be initially interpreted as a direct strategy to lose body fat by directly oxidizing fat, this is not the key outcome of this adaptation and is not the key player that promotes body fat loss. The key benefit is that this adaptation allows for higher-intensity exercise capacity, an acquired advantage to training that is of primary importance for promoting weight loss and weight maintenance. Think of trading in your four-cylinder car for a car with a V-8 engine. While in the car world, this trade is clearly not good for fuel economy, the shift in the crossover with training allows you to aerobically burn fuels more efficiently and burn more calories using large muscle groups with a reduced reliance on the lactate-producing anaerobic system. By continuing to push yourself with repeated training, you can further augment this adaption and increase muscle mass that can burn more fuel (calories) at rest. Consider how long it takes someone to run a mile before training compared to how long it takes after training. Regardless of the time difference in running the mile, the amount of calories burned will be similar. The major difference is the energy-yielding macronutrient distribution of fuels oxidized, the energy systems used, and the calories burned divided by the amount of time to run the mile. The trained individual will oxidize more fat, feel better during the run because of less lactate production, and burn more calories per

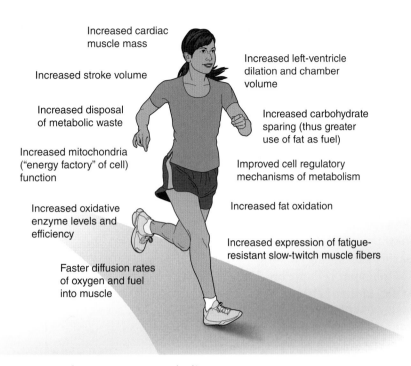

Increased cardiac muscle mass

Increased stroke volume

Increased disposal of metabolic waste

Increased mitochondria ("energy factory" of cell) function

Increased oxidative enzyme levels and efficiency

Faster diffusion rates of oxygen and fuel into muscle

Increased left-ventricle dilation and chamber volume

Increased carbohydrate sparing (thus greater use of fat as fuel)

Improved cell regulatory mechanisms of metabolism

Increased fat oxidation

Increased expression of fatigue-resistant slow-twitch muscle fibers

Figure 2.16 Advantages of training on metabolism.

unit of time. This usually results in an enjoyable experience during which mileage and calorie expenditure is increased, improving metabolic health and maintaining a healthy body weight.

When continued training promotes metabolic adaptation that shifts the crossover point to the right, the athlete benefits from the same metabolic advantages as the nonathlete but to a greater degree. These adaptations support the athlete's high-intensity efforts and allow for fat, as an endless fuel source, to be used earlier in the activity and at much greater intensities and power outputs than in the nonathlete. However, the most important metabolic benefit of this crossover adaptation is not weight and body composition management—the most important benefit is the ability to preserve and protect limited carbohydrate stores until the highest-intensity effort is required to compete in an athletic event. Since carbohydrate stores in the body are limited in muscle tissue, and a relatively small amount in the liver, the preservation of this fuel source for anaerobic system activity to fuel ATP generation is imperative to high-intensity performance. Think of a trained distance runner metabolically capable of tapping primarily into fat stores to fuel much of the ATP demand for most of a race. When it is

important for the runner to overtake other runners in the final portion of the race, the increased intensity (and increased ATP demand) will need to be met anaerobically with the only fuel the anaerobic system can use—carbohydrate. If this runner did not adequately prepare for the race by consuming enough carbohydrate leading up to the race, their capacity to produce ATP anaerobically will be compromised and produce a negative effect on performance.

BIOSYNTHESIS AND STORAGE PATHWAYS IN METABOLISM

From an evolutionary perspective, the human body does not like to get rid of unexpended energy; and referring back to the first law of thermodynamics, recall that energy cannot be destroyed. So what happens in our bodies when we have excess energy remaining from the food we consume? Consider how your clothes fit after visiting home for the holidays—a little tighter than before, right? Although your biosynthetic metabolic pathways work hard to capture excess energy to create heat and store ATP for future energy needs, and though some of the excess energy can be used to synthesize new proteins or to store glycogen, a significant portion of the excess goes to fat storage—which is why after the holidays many of us must loosen our belts.

Now fast-forward to the New Year, when waist-line growth and resolutions often result in new gym memberships. After several workouts, the cumulative result of increased energy expend-iture and reduced calorie intake creates weight loss—and the observation that your clothes are fitting different because of muscle gain. A differ-ent biosynthetic pathway is now working hard to assemble new proteins. Other pathways are at work synthesizing and storing carbohydrate, pro-tein, and fat. While some cells are breaking down carbohydrate, fat, and protein to extract energy, other cells are busy building glucose, fatty acids, and amino acids. Depending on the energy needs of the body and the amount of energy available, either breakdown pathways or biosynthetic path-ways will dominate.

Gluconeogenesis

Gluconeogenesis (figure 2.17) is a biosynthetic pathway that creates glucose for the body from noncarbohydrate precursors, such as amino acids, lactic acid, and glycerol (12). Note, how-ever, that fatty acids *cannot* be converted to glucose, and that gluconeogenesis is not simply the reverse of glycolysis. Along with amino acid involvement in the gluconeogenic pathway, the other gluconeogenic precursors are pyruvate, lactic acid, and glycerol. When someone is not taking in enough carbohydrate, the body can make glucose from pyruvate in the gluconeogenic pathway. About 90 percent of this pathway takes place in the liver, and the kidneys pick up the rest (37). The liver and kidney cells make glucose from pyruvate by way of oxaloacetate by detour-ing around some of the irreversible metabolic steps found in glycolysis. These detours require the use of some ATP to bypass the glycolysis pathways that are flowing in the opposite direc-tion. In times of glucose need, some glucose can be synthesized from lactate. While some lactate is continuously formed and degraded, lactate generation accelerates in exercising muscle dic-tated by the anaerobic condition of the muscle. Circulating lactate can be absorbed by the liver,

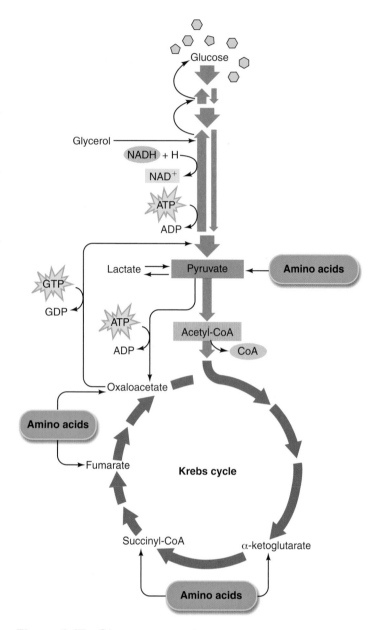

Figure 2.17 Gluconeogenesis.

where gluconeogenesis converts some of the lactate back to glucose via the **Cori cycle** (figure 2.18). In this metabolic pathway, the enzyme LDH catalyzes the conversion of lactic acid to pyruvic acid (pyruvate).

Glycogenesis

Glycogenesis is a biosynthetic pathway that assembles glucose molecules into branched chains for storage as glycogen. Glycogen is a

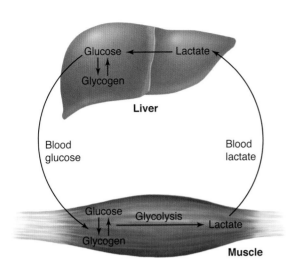

Figure 2.18 The Cori cycle.

branched-chain **polysaccharide** made of glucose units (3). Liver glycogen serves as a glucose reserve for the blood, and muscle glycogen provides a glucose reserve for exercising muscle tissue. As discussed earlier, glycogen stores are limited and can be depleted after an overnight fast (in the liver) or after repeated high-intensity exercise bouts (in the muscle). When glucose is needed, a breakdown reaction called **glycogenolysis** liberates glucose molecules from glycogen chains. In the liver, this process produces glucose that can freely enter the blood stream. In the muscle, glucose is trapped and is often shuttled to glycolysis for the production of ATP.

Lipogenesis

The biosynthetic pathway involving **lipogenesis** is accelerated during times of excess calorie consumption and often leads to the gain of fat tissue. When ATP supply exceeds the body's energy demand excess, acetyl-CoA is available to make long-chain fatty acids. Accumulating acetyl Co-A

molecules are assembled within this biosynthetic pathway as links to form fatty acid chains in the cytosol. Fatty acid synthesis via the lipogenesis pathway also requires energy in the form of nicotinamide adenine dinucleotide phosphate (**NADPH**) to drive the synthetic reaction (note that NADH and NADPH, although similar molecules, have very different biological roles) (31). As the final step, the **endoplasmic reticulum** will then take the surplus of fatty acids formed and combine them with glycerol to form triglycerides, the body's primary storage form of fat.

Since only acetyl-CoA molecules feed the lipogenesis synthetic pathway, note that any precursor substrates involved in acetyl-CoA synthesis can feed fatty acid synthesis. This is an important concept to grasp because carbohydrates, many amino acids, alcohol, and fatty acids can all contribute to acetyl-CoA production. Therefore, when energy intake exceeds ATP demands, additional intake from any of these precursor sources may efficiently activate lipogenesis to store additional body fat. From a practical standpoint, excess energy consumption in any form—sugar-sweetened beverages, meat, protein supplements, fat, alcohol—can contribute to fat storage. The key point here is that overeating, usually a result of a lack of self-awareness and self-monitoring is the primary driving force behind increasing body fat storage.

HORMONAL CONTROL OF METABOLISM

So how are these breakdown and synthetic biological pathways regulated? What triggers the shift in the dominant pathway from one to the other after consuming food (fed state) or after a night of sleeping (fasted state)? The answer is hormonal control of metabolism. The body can

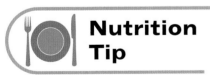

Nutrition Tip Need an energy boost? You won't find it in your coffee cup. You might feel as if coffee, or a caffeinated alternative, increases your energy, but based on the first law of thermodynamics, this makes no sense. Caffeine is not an energy source; it is a central nervous system stimulant. For an energy boost, try eating food rich in nutrients.

tightly regulate and control the reactions of metabolic pathways. In many ways, hormones that circulate through the body act as traffic police, ensuring that each metabolic pathway proceeds at just the right speed. While it is true that the body has many strategies to help control metabolism simultaneously, hormones serve as the master regulators, and the key players are illustrated in figure 2.19.

MEASURING ENERGY INTAKE AND EXPENDITURE

By definition, energy is the capacity to do work. Without energy, our bodies cannot function. The energy in the food we eat is considered chemical energy, which our bodies convert from potential energy to mechanical, electrical, or heat energy. For an energy boost, we must eat nutrient-rich food, which is then converted to ATP via the process described earlier. Every muscle movement, every nerve impulse, every cellular reaction requires ATP, and carbohydrate, triglycerides, and proteins are the vehicles through which this energy is supplied.

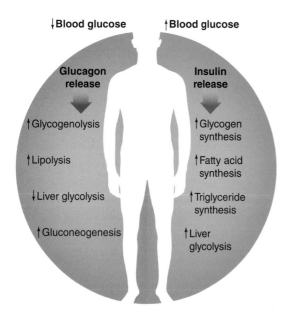

Figure 2.19 Glucagon and insulin are major players in the metabolic pathway control.

Based on Lieberman 2012.

Estimating Energy Content of Food

In the field of nutrition science, we discuss the potential energy in food, or the body's use of energy (i.e., using ATP), in units of heat called kilocalories (or simply calories). One kilocalorie (kcal) is the amount of energy (in the form of heat) required to raise the temperature of 1 kilogram (kg) of water by 1 degree Celsius. While this might sound like an abstract concept, it makes more sense when thinking about how a bomb calorimeter (i.e., a meter for calorie measure) works to liberate chemical energy from food that is placed in it to heat energy. As shown in figure 2.20, food is placed within a sealed chamber, and the food is completely burned while sensors placed outside of the chamber in a water bath measure the amount of heat produced by combustion within the inner chamber. The difference in water temperature from the heat energy produced is a measure of the sample's energy output and provides an accurate assessment of the total energy content of the particular food. Because this method is a direct method of measuring heat production, the use of the bomb calorimeter is often categorized as direct calorimetry. While the human body is not as efficient as the bomb calorimeter in energy transfer from one form to another, following a few metabolic adjustments, the same basic principle applies and can be used to determine the amount of food energy we consume from our diet. Thus, the number of calories from complete combustion in a bomb calorimeter is adjusted downward:

> 4 kilocalories per gram pure carbohydrate
> 4 kilocalories per gram pure protein
> 9 kilocalories per gram pure fat
> 7 kilocalories per gram of pure alcohol

So, the number of kilocalories derived from the complete combustion of these energy-yielding macronutrients and alcohol in a bomb calorimeter is slightly higher than what is listed here. This is primarily because the human body does not completely digest all food and, as discussed earlier, nitrogen from protein foods cannot be oxidized to

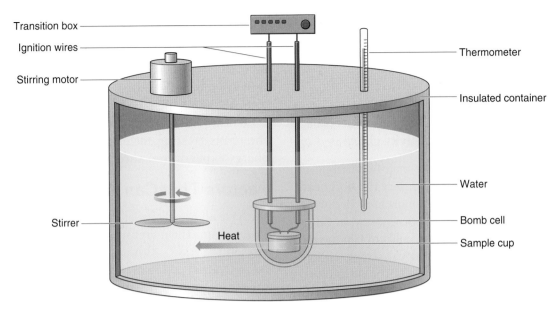

Figure 2.20 A bomb calorimeter determines the total energy content of food.

Assessing an Athlete's Energy Intake

produce ATP. Because of these adjustments that led to knowing the kilocalorie content of each energy-producing food component we consume, we can use these numbers to estimate its calorie content, as long as we know the weight of each component.

Athletes must have an idea of how much energy they consume at different stages of their training regimen, both to support athletic performance and to promote health and injury prevention. Since an athlete's energy requirements vary from day to day throughout the yearly training plan, relative to changes in training volume and intensity, reliable estimates of energy intake can be helpful in developing an individualized nutrition plan. An athlete's energy intake from food, fluids, and supplements can be estimated from measured food records, a multi-pass 24-hour dietary recall, or from food frequency questionnaires (11). For athletes and nonathletes alike, it is important to understand that there are limitations with all of these methods, with a bias to the underreporting of intakes (32). Extensive education regarding the purpose and protocols of documenting calorie intake may assist with compliance to the measurement techniques and enhance the accuracy and validity of self-reported information.

Factors that can increase energy intake needs in athletes (22)

> Exposure to cold or heat
> Fear
> Stress
> High altitude
> Some physical injuries, wound healing
> Stimulant drugs (caffeine, nicotine)
> Increases in **fat-free mass (FFM)**

Factors that can decrease energy intake needs in athletes (28)

> Aging
> Decreases in FFM
> Sedentary behavior between training sessions

Estimating Energy Expenditure

Energy expenditure (EE), or the amount of calories burned by the body, can be measured and estimated using several different methods.

The body uses energy (expends calories) for three primary reasons.

1. To maintain basic physiological function, such as pumping blood and breathing
2. To process the food we eat
3. To power muscles for all movements—called the **thermic effect of activity (TEA)**

These are examples of the major contributors to energy expenditure, but in fact the body can also use additional fuel to support growth during childhood, adolescence, and pregnancy. In times of stress, such as exposure to cold environments, fever, trauma, and psychological stress, energy expenditure is also increased. The sum of all energy expended over a set period of time (usually 24 hours) is called the **total energy expenditure (TEE)**. The TEE calculation has several energy expenditure variables that we can measure independently and account for to estimate TEE.

Energy Expenditure During Rest

People who are not normally physically active and consider themselves sedentary expend most of their energy at rest to maintain the basic body functions to sustain life. This type of energy expenditure is called **resting energy expenditure (REE)** and is required to maintain body temperature, heartbeat, and other functions. Just like TEE, REE is an absolute measure over a period of time, such as a day. When REE measures are expressed as a rate, or as the number of kilocalories expended per hour, energy expenditure is measured as either the **basal metabolic rate (BMR)** or the **resting metabolic rate (RMR)**. RMR may account for up to 60 to 80 percent of TEE (32).

In research, measuring RMR and BMR involves different procedures that produce slightly different values. The measurement of BMR is more stringent and requires the subject to be lying at rest for an extended period of time or to have just woken up from a normal overnight sleep and remaining in bed. BMR measures also require a 10- to 12-hour fast and no physical activity for at least 12 hours. Since these ideal conditions are difficult to meet when studying large groups of human subjects, the RMR measure is often

preferred. In measuring RMR, the subject must be in a resting position for several minutes and be 3 to 4 hours removed from a meal or strenuous activity. Because of the differences in the protocols for these measures, RMR values tend to be slightly higher, but most researchers prefer measuring RMR for its practicality. We will use the terms "resting metabolic rate" and "resting energy expenditure" throughout this book.

Factors That Can Alter RMR

We have all heard that exercise can increase your metabolism. The increase is a direct effect of exercise on the RMR. Although the absolute change an individual can experience in their RMR is at the most around 5 percent, these changes can be meaningful to long-term health. When examining large groups of people, variations in RMR can be as much as 25 percent. This is largely because of large differences in muscle and organ mass, which helps explain why muscle-building exercise can have a meaningful impact on RMR. Resting muscle tissue and organ tissue make up most of the contribution to RMR because of their higher fuel needs to support metabolic activities. These two tissue compartments, along with the bone tissue and fluids that make up the human body, are collectively known as **lean body mass (LBM)**. Differences in LBM explain 60 to 80 percent of the variation that is seen in RMR kcal values among individuals (21).

Several other factors can also create small but meaningful changes in RMR values. First of all, anything that can change LBM will affect RMR. Age, sex, exercise, and body size are primary influences on LBM. Increasing body size and regular exercise increases or maintains LBM. Males typically have more LBM per pound of body weight than females, and LBM steadily falls with increasing age. As we age, RMR is reduced by

DO YOU KNOW ?

Two individuals of approximately the same body weight can have far-different RMR values. An individual with more LBM will have a significantly higher RMR than someone with lower LBM and higher fat mass.

about 2 to 3 percent per decade (29). Most of this is attributed to declining LBM, but declining organ function might also contribute. Regular exercise becomes even more valuable as we age because it is a strong stimulus to slow the loss of LBM, while discouraging the gain of fat mass. Body size has a strong influence on metabolic rate because it takes more energy to move a larger mass. A large person will expend more energy (calories) per unit of time doing the same activity as a smaller person. Fitness level and sport experience is another factor that influences energy expenditure. Athletes tend to have stronger muscles with greater endurance that are trained for the competitive task, making them more efficient with energy utilization and conservation than those who are untrained and attempting to complete similar tasks.

Thermic Effect of Activity

The energy expenditure required to move our bodies is broadly defined as any movement—not only exercise and sport but also everyday activities and movements required at work. Along with **nonexercise activity thermogenesis (NEAT)**, any type of activity, even fidgeting, is included in this category. Energy expenditure in this category typically accounts for about 15 to 30 percent of TEE (35) but can vary significantly based on duration, mode (walking, running, eating, dancing, etc.), and intensity. This is why elite athletes who are committed to training several hours a day can have a thermic effect of activity (TEA) that easily exceeds 50 percent of the TEE for a given day. As a component of TEA, energy expenditure from exercise (EEE) can be estimated in several ways, including activity logs (1–7 days duration), using subjective estimates of exercise intensity; activity codes; and metabolic equivalents (MET) (1, 13, 33). While RMR represents 60 to 80 percent of TEE for most individuals, it may be as little as 38 to 47 percent of TEE for elite endurance athletes, who might have a TEA as high as 50 percent of TEE (22).

Energy Expenditure to Process the Food We Consume

Energy expenditure is also required to digest, absorb, and metabolize the food we eat. The met-

abolic processes involved generate heat, and the energy output is collectively called the **thermic effect of food (TEF)**. This phenomenon generally peaks about 1 hour after the consumption of food and usually dissipates within 4 to 5 hours after eating, depending on the amount and composition of the meal. TEF values vary for each of the energy-yielding macronutrients and are highest for protein and lowest for fat. This means the body is more efficient at storing excess dietary fat as body fat than at converting excess protein and carbohydrate to fat stores. TEF typically accounts for approximately 10 percent of total energy expenditure (15). Although changes in energy-yielding macronutrient distribution of the diet can alter TEF's contribution to total energy expenditure, the changes are considered to have marginal impact.

Measuring Energy Expenditure

The general measurement of energy expenditure is referred to as **calorimetry** and is further broken down by methodological differences as **direct calorimetry** (mentioned earlier in the chapter) and **indirect calorimetry**. These measurements can be used by health care professionals and nutrition and exercise scientists to examine individual differences in energy expenditure and to help understand the effects of age, gender, and exercise on total energy expenditure (table 2.3). However, despite improvements in technology, measuring energy expenditure is generally not practical. As a result, many energy expenditure equations have been developed and are commonly used for making predictions.

Direct Calorimetry

As you recall from our earlier example of the bomb calorimeter, direct calorimetry measures heat production by the body. When the body breaks down food, it captures some of the energy in ATP production, while losing the rest as heat. When this heat loss is measured, the measure is proportional to the body's total energy expenditure and can be measured directly within a sealed chamber (figure 2.21). With this method, a research subject is typically asked to stay in the chamber for 24 hours. The chambers are typically furnished with a bed

Table 2.3 Percentage of Energy Expended to Process Food Intake

Energy-yielding macronutrient	% of calories used for processing
Protein	20–25
Carbohydrate	5–15
Fat	0–5

and a television and in some cases equipment for exercising. While the individual is in the chamber, changes in temperature and oxygen and carbon dioxide gas exchange can be measured to calculate the total calories expended. Though highly accurate, this method is not considered practical for most research studies. The equipment is complex, expensive, and takes up a lot of space. Plus, the chamber must comfortably accommodate people of various sizes while maintaining the precision to measure small changes in temperature. Given the alternative methods available to estimate energy expenditure, direct calorimetry is used primarily in large research universities and institutions with a heavy interest in human research studies investigating changes in metabolism.

Indirect Calorimetry

Indirect calorimetry is a method to determine energy expenditure without directly measuring the production of heat. Methods include measuring oxygen consumption and carbon dioxide production, collectively referred to as gas exchange, and the doubly labeled water technique. Overall, indirect techniques are less expensive than direct calorimetry. These methods are defined as "indirect" because energy expenditure as heat is not measured. The gas exchange method is based on the principle that our metabolized fuels (i.e., carbohydrate, protein, fat) require oxygen to be completely burned (oxidized). One of the by-products of burning these fuels is carbon dioxide. What is fascinating is that the consumed oxygen and carbon dioxide release is in direct proportion to the amount of fuel burned and the amount of energy (measured as calories) released. During the process, a technician can collect respiratory gases from a volunteer during rest or short bouts of exercise. This is accomplished by attaching a face mask, using a mouthpiece with the nose closed shut, or by using a canopy system. While these methods are commonly used in research settings, they are still considered cumbersome by many researchers and research volunteers and thus carry limitations on how the methods can be used effectively in different living situations (figure 2.22).

The doubly labeled water technique is highly effective at measuring daily energy expenditure over extended time periods while subjects are living in their usual environment. This method relies on measuring the stable **isotopes** of hydrogen and oxygen in excreted water and carbon dioxide. Isotopes are defined as different forms

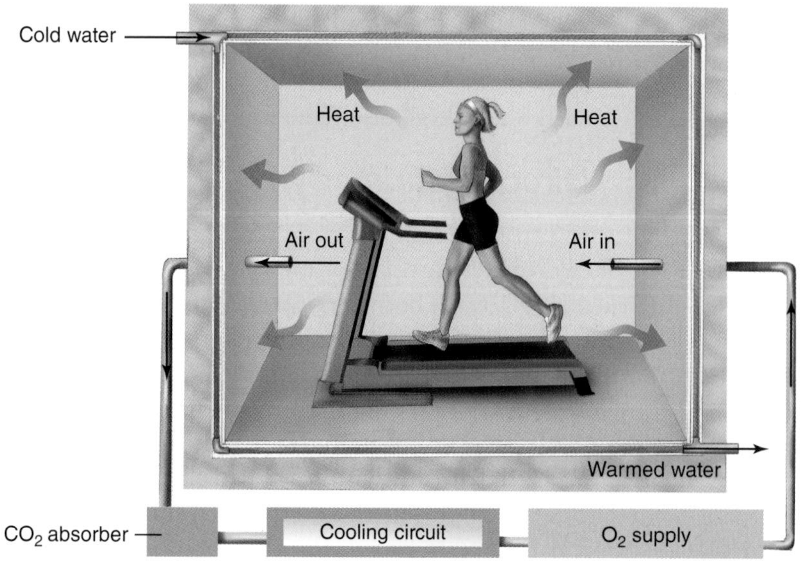

Cold water

Heat — Heat

Air out — Air in

Warmed water

CO_2 absorber — Cooling circuit — O_2 supply

Figure 2.21 Direct calorimeter.

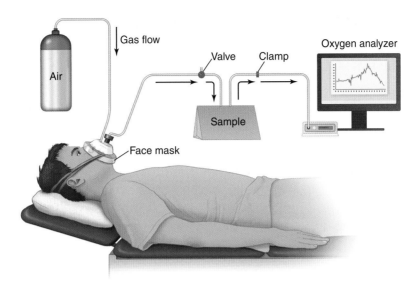

Figure 2.22   Indirect calorimeter.

of an element in which the atoms have the same number of protons but different number of neutrons. These isotopes are nonradioactive and safe for human consumption and retain the same characteristics of the usual element, with the only difference being a higher than usual atomic mass. Small amounts of water that are isotopically labeled with deuterium and oxygen-18 (^2H_2O and $H_2{}^{18}O$) are ingested, while the difference between the rates at which the body loses each isotope can be measured to determine energy expenditure. This method is unique and very practical because it avoids the need to measure heat and gas exchange.

PUTTING IT INTO PERSPECTIVE

ESTIMATING TOTAL ENERGY EXPENDITURE

Estimate of the total energy expenditure of an 18-year-old college freshman with a height of 183 centimeters and a weight of 73 kilograms.

$$TEE = BMR + TEF + TEA$$

BMR can be estimated using the Harris-Benedict equation.

For men, the equation looks like this:

$$BMR = 66.4730 + (13.7516 \times \text{weight in kg}) + (5.0033 \times \text{height in cm}) - (6.7550 \times \text{age in yr})$$

Therefore, BMR for this individual

$$= 66.4730 + (13.7516 \times 73 \text{ kg}) + (5.0033 \times 183 \text{ cm}) - (6.7550 \times 18 \text{ yr})$$

$$= 66.4730 + (1003.8668) + (915.6039) - (121.59)$$

$$= 1,864.35$$

$$\sim 1,850-1,900 \text{ kcal}$$

TEF = thermic effect of food; TEA = planned exercise expenditure + spontaneous physical activity + nonexercise activity thermogenesis

PUTTING IT INTO PERSPECTIVE

USING THE CUNNINGHAM EQUATION TO ESTIMATE RMR

RMR = 500 + 22 (fat-free mass in kg)

A 22-year-old collegiate female swimmer is 5 feet 10 inches and weighs 160 pounds. At 20 percent body fat, she has approximately 58 kilograms of fat-free mass (160 lb. × 0.2 = 32 lb.; 160 lb. − 32 lb. = 128 lb.; 128 lb./2.2 lb./kg = 58.2 kg)

RMR = 500 + 22(58.2 kg)

RMR = 500 + 1,280

RMR = 1,780 kcal/d

Two types of water are consumed, one with the hydrogen isotope deuterium and the other with an isotope of oxygen. Following consumption, researchers can measure isotope appearance in excreted urine (as ^2H_2O) and examine the difference between the rate of deuterium loss and ^{18}O loss to calculate the output of carbon dioxide and determine TEE. The doubly labeled water method is often considered the gold standard for determining energy expenditure and has been used alongside measuring weight change and diet assessment methods to help determine the validity of energy intake assessment techniques. This method is noninvasive and unobtrusive and allows subjects to act normally in their typical environment. On the other hand, testing protocols are recommended to last at least 14 days for the best accuracy, the technique is not widely available, and it is expensive. Isotopes and equipment to analyze isotope appearance in urine can cost thousands of dollars and are often too costly for many research budgets. Further, this technique is best at giving a summary of energy expenditure over the 14-day protocol period and cannot give information about individual days or day-to-day variability.

Estimating TEE With Prediction Equations

Because the direct measurement of a person's TEE requires costly equipment and training that is not easily accessible outside of research settings, energy expenditure is widely estimated by nutrition professionals through the use of a range of equations. Calculated estimates use many variables that are known to have a strong influence on energy expenditure, such as age, height, weight, gender, and fat-free mass. In order to use various equations effectively, it is important to understand their limitations, the population they are intended for, what the calculated calorie values mean (i.e., BMR vs. RMR vs. TEE), and most important, remembering that these values are indeed estimates. When equations provide an RMR or BMR value, in order to determine TEE, energy for physical activity and the TEF must be included. When energy is expended from physical activity and exercise can be accounted for by using a multiple of the REE based on the level of activity intensity and duration. For example, the activity level for most of the U.S. population is considered light or moderate, and the TEF is about 10 percent of the sum of REE plus the energy expenditure of physical activity. The sum of these three components provides the estimated TEE.

Techniques used to measure or estimate components of TEE in sedentary and moderately active populations can also be applied to athletes. However, there are some limitations to this approach, particularly in highly competitive athletes (32). As previously discussed, it is more practical to measure resting metabolic rate (RMR),

PUTTING IT INTO PERSPECTIVE

WEARABLE ACTIVITY MONITORS AND DEVICES

If you observe exercisers in a gym, you will see that many are wearing a kind of physical activity tracker or exercise monitor. These accelerometry-based devices allow us to estimate physical activity and energy expenditure (EE), as well as track data over time via the Internet or on a cell phone. Improvements in technology and reduced costs have resulted in a flood of various brands of physical activity monitors, making these devices highly accessible (36). The monitors are valuable in that they can provide a stimulus to promote behavioral change to increase physical activity and manage energy intake, leading to long-term metabolic health and reduced risk for diabetes, cardiovascular disease, and other conditions.

Do you question the accuracy of these devices? Their limitations? The wide variety of brands available suggests a wide range in quality. Some devices are more accurate than others. Accelerometer-based devices provide measures of body movement with validity derived from studies using doubly labeled water. Generally speaking, many commercially available monitors score lower in measures of step count and energy expenditure accuracy than more sophisticated activity monitors used for health research. A recent study examined the validity of eight different consumer-based, activity-monitoring technologies with estimates of EE from a portable metabolic analyzer as a comparison. Absolute percent error ranged from approximately 9 to 23.5 percent. Overall, the performance and overall accuracy of these monitors is impressive.

The most important feature of these devices is that they promote increased physical activity (27). Meanwhile, companies are trying to entice more consumers by making monitors that provide goal-setting features, tracking tools, and social networking links, which could have implications for behaviorally focused research applications (18).

but a reasonable estimate of BMR can be obtained using either the Cunningham (10) or the Harris-Benedict (26) equations, with an appropriate activity factor being applied to estimate TEE.

Note that the perfect energy expenditure prediction equation does not currently exist. Practitioners often use a combination of methods when working with athletes and refine their intervention over time based on new data becoming available, such as changes in weight, a new body composition assessment, changing training volume, and so on. It is also important to use caution in the application of these methods since RMR may over- or underestimate requirements by 10 to 20 percent. Remember that RMR is only one factor that accounts for TEE and should not be overemphasized without careful consideration of the other variables that make up TEE.

AN EMERGING TOPIC OF INTEREST FOR ATHLETES
Energy Availability in Sport

Energy availability (EA) is a relatively new topic in the field of sports nutrition. EA extends beyond the study of energy balance (EB) by considering the energy requirements needed to promote optimal health and function during periods of high EEE. Energy availability is defined as dietary intake minus exercise energy expenditure normalized to FFM. The resulting number from this calculation is the amount of energy available to the body to perform all other functions after the cost of exercise is subtracted (19).

The concept of EA emerged from the study of the **female athlete triad (triad)**, which started as a recognition of the interrelatedness of clinical issues with disordered eating, menstrual

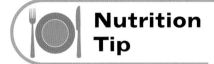

dysfunction, and low bone mineral density in female athletes (19). The concept then evolved into a broader understanding of the concerns associated with any movement along the spectra away from optimal energy availability, menstrual status, and bone health (16). Low EA can occur from insufficient energy intake, high TEE, or a combination of the two. It might also be associated with disordered eating, a misguided or excessively rapid program for loss of body mass, or inadvertent failure to meet energy requirements during a period of high-volume training or competition (19). It is now thought that additional physiological consequences may occur beyond that of what is found in the female athlete triad and is also thought to affect male athletes. Potential complications are thought to contribute to endocrine, gastrointestinal, renal, neuro-psychiatric, musculoskeletal, and cardiovascular dysfunction (16).

In order to capture the negative effects of low EA in both male and female athletes, an extension of the Triad has been proposed, called **relative energy deficiency in sport (RED-S)**. RED-S is as an inclusive description of the entire cluster of physiological complications observed in male and female athletes who consume energy intakes that are insufficient to meet the needs for optimal body function once the energy cost of exercise has been removed (23). Regardless of the terminology used to describe low EA, this phenomenon may compromise athletic performance in the short and long term for both male and female athletes. Screening and treatment guidelines have been established for management of low EA (16, 23).

Potential performance effects of RED-S might include decreased endurance, increased injury risk, decreased training response, impaired judgment, decreased coordination, decreased concentration, irritability, depression, decreased glycogen stores, and decreased muscle strength (23). In terms of health, RED-S can negatively affect menstrual function, bone health, endocrine, metabolic, hematological, growth and development, psychological, cardiovascular, gastrointestinal, and immunological systems (32). It is now recognized that impairments of health and function occur across the continuum of reductions in EA, rather than occurring uniformly at an EA threshold, and require further research (23).

SUMMARY

The understanding of energy metabolism is essential to lay a solid foundation for understanding the nutrition needs to support all forms of physical activity and exercise. Energy from the foods we consume is converted into a useable chemical form of energy our bodies can use (ATP). ATP is generated by three distinct energy systems that work together in concert using several metabolic pathways to fuel muscle contraction. Several substrates are used by the energy systems to meet our ATP demands, including phosphocreatine, carbohydrate, protein, fat, and alcohol. We use kilocalories (calories) as our universal energy currency to estimate the amount of energy we consume and expend. Several methods are available to measure both energy intake and expenditure that vary in their practicality, accuracy, time commitment, and cost. Collectively, these methods provide a mechanism to assess important aspects of energy metabolism in athletes, including energy balance and energy availability.

■ FOR REVIEW ▶

1. What is energy and the various forms of energy? Which form of energy is most important to human physiology?

2. List the energy systems used by the body to make ATP. How do they differ in complexity, lag time, and capacity to make ATP?

3. Describe the crossover concept, and explain the most important physiological adaptations that occur as a result of training.

4. Describe the fuel substrates the body uses to make ATP. What is the only substrate that can be used to make ATP anaerobically?

5. Differentiate between BMR, RMR, TEA, TEE, and TEF, as defined in this chapter.

6. Several metabolic pathways were described in this chapter. List the metabolic pathways used by each energy system and where in the cell these pathways occur.

7. From the food that we eat, describe some of the metabolic fates of glucose, lipid, and amino acids that are digested and absorbed.

8. Explain how the mitochondria generate ATP aerobically. How is oxygen used? How are hydrogen ions and electrons delivered to the mitochondria?

PART II

ROLE OF ENERGY-YIELDING MACRONUTRIENTS

Energy-yielding macronutrients are covered in chapters 3, 4, and 5. Foods providing carbohydrate, protein, and fat supply a different array of vitamins, minerals and, in the case of plant-based foods, plant compounds that support good health. Therefore, carbohydrate, protein, and fat can have different effects on long-term health and disease risk factors.

A slower digesting carbohydrate, high-fiber food, is beneficial for health and reducing chronic disease risk. A faster-digesting carbohydrate, low-fiber food, is helpful before, during, and after exercise because it is a quick, easy-to-digest source of energy. Protein varies based on the speed of digestion and amino acid profile and helps make up structures in the body. Dietary fat is energy dense, has many metabolic roles, and affects disease risk factors. Within the body, fat also has essential roles in structure and function.

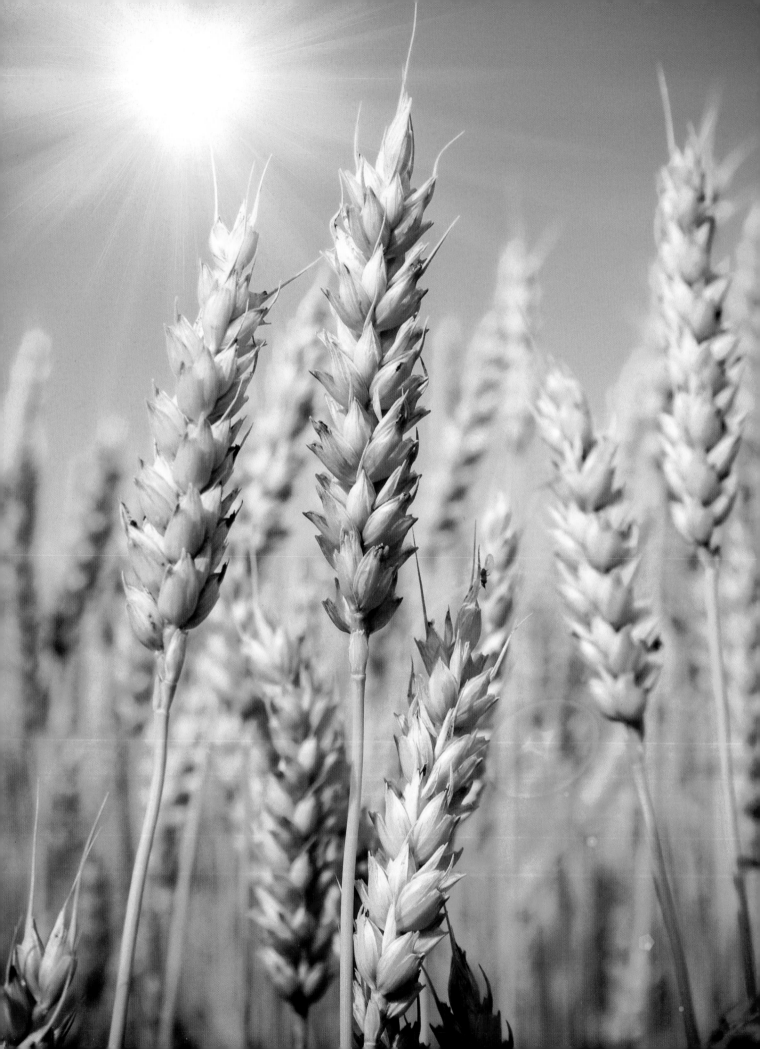

CHAPTER 3

Carbohydrate

▶ **CHAPTER OBJECTIVES**

After completing this chapter, you will be able to do the following:

> Identify the classification of carbohydrate.

> Describe the digestion and absorption of carbohydrate.

> Discuss the metabolic fates of glucose once inside the body.

> Describe how glucose is regulated in the body.

> Explain the relationship between carbohydrate and exercise performance.

> Discuss the role of carbohydrate in fatigue during exercise.

> Identify carbohydrate recommendations for the general population, active individuals, and athletes.

> Explain where to find the carbohydrate content of foods.

> Discuss the role of carbohydrate in health.

Carbohydrate is an organic compound derived from plants and contains the elements carbon, hydrogen, and oxygen. Through **photosynthesis** (figure 3.1), plants use energy from the sun interacts with water and minerals in the soil and carbon dioxide in the air to produce glucose, the simplest form of carbohydrate. The primary purpose of carbohydrate in the human body, both at rest and during physical activity, is as a fuel source (40). Carbohydrate is an energy source for most cells in the body, a preferred fuel source for nerve and brain cells, and the required fuel for red blood cells. During physical activity, the biologically usable form of energy for the skeletal muscle, ATP, can be generated from both dietary and stored carbohydrate. The amount and source of carbohydrate the skeletal muscle uses depends on the length and intensity of exercise and the amount of carbohydrate available (26). In this chapter we provide an overview of the types of carbohydrate and how they are digested, absorbed, metabolized, and stored in the human body during rest and exercise. Dietary recommendations, food sources, and the role of carbohydrate in health and disease will also be discussed.

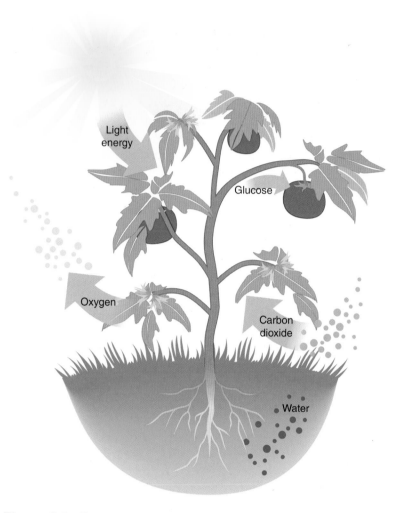

Figure 3.1 During photosynthesis, plants use energy from the sun to synthesize glucose.

CLASSIFICATION OF CARBOHYDRATE

Carbohydrate is often classified into one of two primary classes that describe the physical structure of the nutrient: **simple carbohydrates** are relatively small compounds comprised of either one or two sugar molecules, whereas **complex carbohydrates** are larger compounds that contain more than three sugar molecules joined together (40).

Simple Carbohydrates

Monosaccharides and disaccharides are commonly referred to as simple carbohydrates, or **simple sugars**. The simplest unit of a carbohydrate is a monosaccharide—*mono* meaning one and *saccharide* meaning sugar (figure 3.2). Three common monosaccharides are present in the human diet: glucose, fructose, and galactose. All contain the elements carbon, hydrogen, and oxygen, but they differ slightly in their structure and in their level of sweetness. **Glucose** is an abundant sugar molecule in the human diet. **Fructose** is the sweetest of the monosaccharides and sometimes referred to as fruit sugar. While fructose is naturally found in fruits, it can also be found in processed foods, most commonly in the form of high-fructose corn syrup or sucrose. **Galactose** is not usually found alone in foods; rather, it is most commonly bound to glucose to form the disaccharide lactose (35).

Two monosaccharides joined together are called **disaccharides**—*di* meaning two (figure 3.3). The chemical bond holding these together can be broken (digested) by the action of enzymes in the human digestive tract, thereby releasing the component monosaccharides from one another. The common natural disaccharides in the human diet are sucrose, lactose, and maltose. **Sucrose** is the sweetest and most common of the disaccharides and is composed of one glucose molecule and one fructose molecule. Sucrose can be found naturally in sugar cane, sugar beets, honey, and to some extent fruits and vegetables, but it is more commonly processed into "table sugar" and added to a variety of foods during processing. **Lactose** is comprised of one glucose molecule and one galactose molecule and is called "milk sugar" because it is found naturally in dairy products. **Maltose** is composed of two glucose molecules joined together. It is not commonly found in foods but rather as a by-product of the breakdown of larger carbohydrate compounds, such as starch. Maltose also forms as a result of the fermentation process during production of some alcoholic beverages. However, the complete fermentation reaction results in a final low maltose concentration, so these alcoholic beverages are not a good source of dietary carbohydrate (22, 40).

Complex Carbohydrates

Complex carbohydrates are assemblies of at least three and as many as thousands of monosaccha-

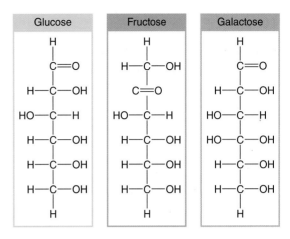

Figure 3.2 Monosaccharides.

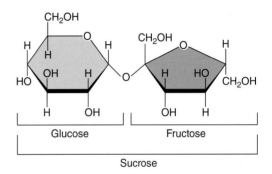

Figure 3.3 Disaccharide.

ride molecules. The term "complex carbohydrate" was once used to describe a slower digestive process compared to sugars, but now the term refers only to the chemical structure of the molecule, not digestive speed. Relatively shorter assemblies of only 3 to 10 monosaccharides are referred to as **oligosaccharides**, and larger assemblies are called

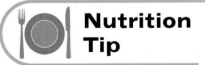

Nutrition Tip

Glucose is the form of fuel the brain depends on for functioning. Research studies have demonstrated that reduced glucose availability can negatively alter attention, memory, and learning in individuals who regularly consume carbohydrate in their diet (as opposed to those who have adapted to a lower carbohydrate diet). Consuming adequate dietary carbohydrate throughout the day can reverse these dips in glucose levels. The brain also has increased glucose demands as mental tasks become more challenging. Studying for exams and completing assignments require higher cognitive function, so a steady glucose supply to the brain is critical. Do not skip meals and snacks during times of mental stress, when cognition is important for success (35).

polysaccharides. Oligosaccharides are commonly found in beans, legumes, some cruciferous vegetables, whole grains, and some manufactured products such as sports drinks. These usually appear on a food label as fructooligosaccharides, maltodextrins, or polydextrose. **Polysaccharides** have more than ten monosaccharides and are primarily in the form of starch and fiber. **Starch** is the primary form of carbohydrate polysaccharide found in plants and consists of simple chains of glucose molecules joined together by **alpha bonds**, which are breakable by human digestive enzymes. The most common forms of starch are **amylose**, which is a straight chain of glucose molecules, and **amylopectin**, which is a branched chain of the same molecules. Once consumed and digested into its component monosaccharides, the glucose molecules from starch are absorbed into the bloodstream and become indistinguishable from all other glucose molecules in the body (22, 40).

Fiber is another type of carbohydrate polysaccharide found in plants. It is similar to starch; both contain long chains of glucose molecules joined by bonds, except that the bonds in fiber are **beta bonds** that cannot be broken by human enzymes. Thus fiber is not digested, absorbed, and metabolized in the human body. Nonetheless, fiber does possess health benefits, which are discussed later in this chapter. From a structural standpoint, fiber can be classified as soluble or insoluble. **Soluble fibers** are generally found in and around plant tissue cells, are dissolvable in water, have a gel-like consistency when wet, and are digested by gut bacteria (**fermentation**). Common sources include citrus fruit, berries, oats, and beans. **Insoluble fibers** are the structural component of plant cell walls, are not dissolvable in water, and are usually not fermentable. They are commonly found in the outer husks of whole grains, fruits, vegetables, and legumes. The structural classification of fiber does not adequately describe how

insoluble and soluble fibers behave once inside the human body, so another way of viewing fiber is from the standpoint of how it affects physiological processes. For example, different fibers have varying impacts on gastric emptying, post-meal blood glucose levels, and the absorption of dietary fat and cholesterol from the gut. In other words, some fibers are better than others at improving **satiety**, making one feel fuller for a longer period of time, blunting the rise in blood sugar after eating, and improving serum lipid levels (total and LDL cholesterol). The Institute of Medicine uses the terms "dietary fiber" and "functional fiber" for those isolated, nondigestible food or commercially produced carbohydrates (36) to describe the different effects that fibers have on physiological processes within the human body.

The third category of carbohydrate polysaccharide is called **glycogen**. Glycogen is the storage form of carbohydrates (glucose) in humans and animals, where it is stored primarily in the liver and skeletal muscle. Glycogen and starch are similar in that they are chains of glucose molecules; they differ in that glycogen is much more highly branched and contains greater surface area for enzymatic action (figure 3.4) (22, 40). In addition, glycogen stored in the liver and muscle in its hydrated form contains three to four parts water (27). Approximately three quarters of the glycogen in the body is stored in skeletal muscle; the remaining quarter is stored in the liver (9, 23).

Starch (amylose)

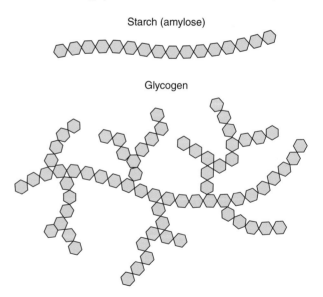

Glycogen

Figure 3.4 Structure of starch and glycogen.

Complex carbohydrates vary extensively in quality from the standpoint of the level of processing they undergo from farm to table. Some carbohydrates have been minimally processed and are made of **whole grains**. Refined grains have been extensively processed, to the point that some components of the whole grain have been removed or added back in order to make the product more palatable. Whole grains contain all of the nutrients and fiber that nature intended, but processed grains have much less fiber and fewer naturally occurring vitamins and minerals (though some vitamins and minerals are added back through a process called **enrichment**). Enriched products may have lower or higher levels of some nutrients than their whole-product counterparts (35, 40, 50).

DIGESTION AND ABSORPTION

The **digestive tract** is essentially a long tube within the body that extends from the **mouth** to the anus and whose purpose is to facilitate the digestion of food and subsequent absorption of nutrients into the body. Any food contained in the digestive tract is not considered to be part of the body until it is broken down into smaller components (**digestion**) and moved across the wall of the digestive tract into the bloodstream (absorption). A critical feature of digestion is excretion of undesirable or indigestible material from the diet (elimination). The digestive tract contains multiple segments, each of which contributes to breaking food down into smaller components that can move across the wall of the digestive tract and into the body. The primary segments of the digestive tract where carbohydrate digestion and absorption occur are the mouth and the small intestine (figure 3.5) (35, 40).

Carbohydrate in the diet is in the form of sugars, starches, and fibers, most of which are too large to be absorbed in their consumed form and must be

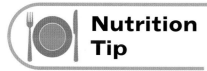

Nutrition Tip

When choosing food products, high-quality carbohydrates are those made from whole-grain flour and usually have the term "whole grain" on the label. A Whole Grain Stamp has been introduced in an attempt to simplify the shopping process for consumers. There are two varieties of the Whole Grain Stamp: the "basic stamp" and the "100% stamp." If a product displays the "100% stamp," all of its grain ingredients are whole grains and contain a minimum of 16 grams (a full serving) of whole grain. A product with the "basic stamp" has a minimum of 8 grams of whole grain but may also contain some refined grain. The stamps can be helpful but might also be misleading because not all products that display the stamps are the best choices for health. This is especially true in the cereal aisle, where products may contain whole grains but also have significant levels of added sugars. When checking food labels, beware of terms such as "wheat" and "wheat flour" (rather than "whole wheat") because these indicate that parts of the grain, along with the vitamins and minerals within the grain, are likely missing. The term "whole grain" usually indicates the product contains at least one type of whole grain; "whole wheat" indicates the specific type of grain used. Either term may identify a food rich in fiber, vitamins, and minerals. Many nutrition professionals recommend looking for a "whole food" label in addition to the term "whole grain." A "**rule of five**" can be used to find whole-grain products that are generally better for health. A good choice will have 5 grams or more of fiber per serving of the food and less than 5 grams of sugar per serving (46).

broken down along the digestive tract. Digestion of carbohydrate begins in the mouth. Chewing food causes **mechanical digestion**, as chewing physically breaks large polysaccharides into smaller ones, and the salivary glands in the mouth secrete an enzyme called **salivary amylase** that begins the **chemical digestion** of polysaccharides. Digestion of carbohydrate in the mouth is not complete; the broken-down polysaccharides are still not small enough to cross the walls of the digestive tract. The amount of digestion occurring in the mouth depends primarily on the extent of chewing and the length of time food stays in the mouth prior to swallowing. Once swallowed, the carbohydrate exits the mouth and does not receive further *significant* digestion until it reaches the **small intestine**, which is the segment of the digestive tract where the vast majority of carbohydrate digestion and absorption occurs (figure 3.6). The intestinal wall is comprised of numerous folds called **villi** that increase the surface area for absorption. The villi contain an abundance of absorptive cells called **enterocytes**, each of which has brush-like projections called **microvilli** that further increase the surface area for absorption (35, 40).

The primary forms of carbohydrate upon entering the small intestine are oligosaccharides, polysaccharides, and some disaccharides but very few monosaccharides. Since only monosaccharides can be absorbed into the bloodstream, there still exists the need for a great deal of processing to convert carbohydrates into monosaccharides in the small intestine. Unlike in the mouth, where mechanical digestion via chewing was significant, no such events occur in the small intestine. In fact, virtually all carbohydrate digestion in the small intestine is chemical digestion involving several enzymes released by the pancreas. The **pancreas** is an accessory organ that helps facilitate digestion by secreting many enzymes into the small intestine. One such enzyme is called **pancreatic amylase**, which

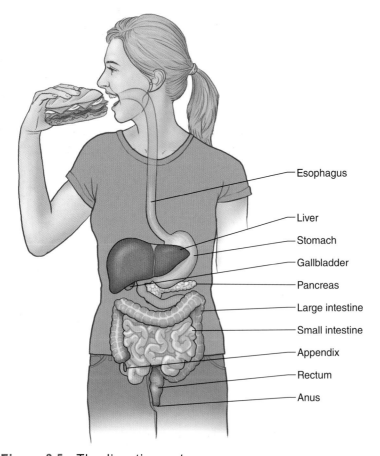

Esophagus

Liver

Stomach

Gallbladder

Pancreas

Large intestine

Small intestine

Appendix

Rectum

Anus

Figure 3.5 The digestive system.

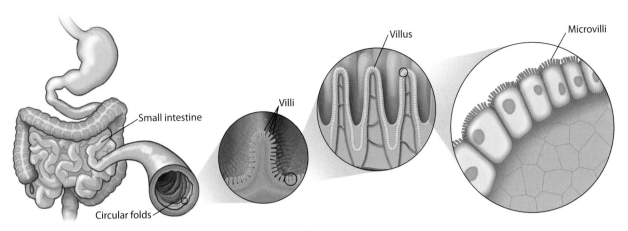

Figure 3.6 Villi and microvilli of the small intestine.

helps further break down polysaccharides into disaccharides, primarily maltose. Additional enzymes, namely, **maltase**, **sucrase**, and **lactase**, are secreted by cells in the intestinal wall to aid in the terminal digestion of disaccharides into their component monosaccharides (table 3.1) (35, 40).

The monosaccharides can then cross the intestinal wall and be absorbed into the body. Monosaccharides in the small intestine enter the enterocytes and move into the bloodstream via capillaries adjacent to the villi on enterocytes. Both glucose and galactose are absorbed by an active transport process requiring ATP, but fructose relies on a more passive diffusion process that doesn't require ATP. This difference in the manner in which the monosaccharides are absorbed results in a slower absorption of fructose than that of glucose and galactose, which means fructose tends to remain in the small intestine longer (35, 40).

METABOLISM OF CARBOHYDRATE

Once the monosaccharides are absorbed by the small intestine and enter the bloodstream, they are transported to the **liver**, where they undergo significant transformations. The vast majority of fructose and galactose monosaccharides are converted to glucose in the liver, although there are other relatively insignificant fates for these monosaccharides. The key point here is that glucose is the primary usable form of carbohydrate in the body, and virtually all ingested carbohydrates are ultimately converted to glucose for use or storage.

DO YOU KNOW ?

Virtually all chemical carbohydrate digestion ceases in the stomach because of the stomach's extremely acidic environment, which destroys salivary amylase. However, some digestion of carbohydrate does continue, particularly mechanical digestion via the churning of the stomach.

Table 3.1 Enzymes Involved in the Digestion of Carbohydrates

Organ	Enzyme	Action
Mouth	Salivary amylase	Breaks down starch in the mouth
Pancreas	Pancreatic amylase	Breaks down starch in the small intestine
Small intestine	Maltase	Breaks down maltose to the monosaccharide glucose
Small intestine	Sucrase	Breaks down sucrose to the monosaccharides glucose and fructose
Small intestine	Lactase	Breaks down lactose to glucose and galactose

Assuming glucose as the definitive starting point, there are several *metabolic fates* for glucose, depending primarily on the energy needs of the body cells (figure 3.7). If cells of the body need energy, they use glucose to generate ATP; otherwise, glucose is stored in a different form (primarily glycogen in the liver and muscle) for later use as a reserve or is converted to fatty acids and stored in adipose tissue (35, 40).

Glycogen storage is favored after an energy-depleting workout and when glucose and the hormone insulin are present after the consumption or ingestion of carbohydrate. For an average person, the liver can store approximately 70 to 110 grams of glycogen (280 to 440 kcal) and the skeletal muscle 120 to 500 grams (480 to 2,000 kcal) (table 3.2). These values can vary greatly depending on habitual dietary intake, dietary manipulation for training and competition, muscle mass, and physiological adaptations to training (23-26, 40).

Since the liver and skeletal muscle have a limited storage capacity for glycogen, excess glucose is typically metabolized into an alternate form of energy storage that is virtually limitless—that is, adipose tissue. Liver cells, and to a lesser extent fat cells (**adipocytes**), can convert glucose into fatty acids via a process called lipogenesis. Fatty acids combine with glycerol to form triglycerides and are stored in adipose tissue. Note that this process occurs only when carbohydrate is chronically consumed in *excess of need* or amount expended during physical activity. If an excessive amount of blood glucose is not being metabolized properly or quickly enough, the glucose can be excreted in the urine. This is most commonly seen in a person with uncontrolled diabetes mellitus (35, 40).

REGULATION OF GLUCOSE METABOLISM

Because glucose is such an important biological substrate required by almost every cell in the body, the process of managing the various fates of glucose is tightly controlled to ensure sufficient glucose availability and delivery to cells that need it. The term "glucose metabolism" encompasses all the activities that, among other functions, regulate the amount of glucose (a) circulating in blood; (b) used to produce ATP by cells; (c) stored as glycogen in skeletal muscle and the liver; (d) converted to fatty acids and stored in adipose tissue; and (e) synthesized from noncarbohydrate precursors to glucose whenever glucose is in short supply in the body.

Blood glucose is normally maintained within the range of 70 to 100 mg/dl under fasting conditions. This range of blood glucose concentrate under normal conditions in a healthy person is widely accepted to be sufficient to provide nourishment to the body's cells under normal resting conditions. Blood glucose values below this range are considered hypoglycemic, within the range **euglycemia**, and above the range

DO YOU KNOW ?

The amount of glucose circulating in your blood is very small and, unless replenished by reserves in your liver and can provide only enough energy for you to walk about one mile (35, 40).

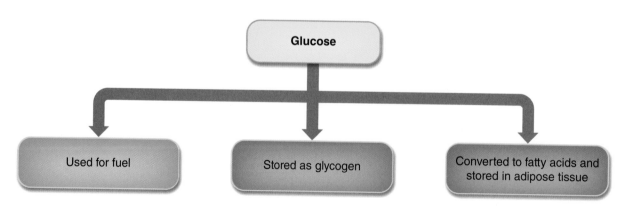

Figure 3.7 Metabolic fates of glucose.

Glucose

Used for fuel

Stored as glycogen

Converted to fatty acids and stored in adipose tissue

Table 3.2 Glucose and Glycogen Content in the Human Body

Source	Amount (g)	Amount (kcal)
Blood glucose	5–25	20–100
Liver glycogen	70–110	280–440
Muscle glycogen	120–500	480–2,000

Based on Ivy 1991; Jensen et al. 2011; Karpinski and Rosenbloom 2017; Kenney, Wilmore, and Costill 2015; Thompson, Manore, and Vaughan 2017.

hyperglycemia (see chapter 14). It is normal to have acute fluctuations after and between carbohydrate-containing meals, but depending on the amount of carbohydrate consumed, blood glucose levels usually return to resting levels between 30 minutes and 2 hours after eating. An individual who has chronic hypoglycemia (low blood sugar) or hyperglycemia (high blood sugar) may have a condition such as diabetes mellitus or impaired carbohydrate metabolism. Diabetes mellitus is characterized by chronic hyperglycemia caused by the cells' inability to sufficiently uptake glucose and metabolize it for fuel. Diabetes mellitus is a potentially devastating medical condition, often suspected when fasting blood glucose levels exceed 126 mg/dl; however, looming dangers are associated with fasting blood glucose levels that are only moderately elevated (between 100 and 125 mg/dl), as these levels might indicate impaired glucose tolerance, a type of prediabetes (35, 40).

What causes fasting blood glucose levels to rise in individuals with impaired glucose metabolism? The answer lies in the inability of body cells to import glucose into the cell. In order for cells to use glucose for energy or storage, the glucose molecules must first enter the cell by crossing its **cell membrane** (figure 3.8).

Glucose molecules are too large to cross cell membranes and usually require assistance from transport proteins located in the cell membrane, which physically move glucose from the space outside the cell into the cell's cytoplasm. These transport proteins tend to remain inside the cytoplasm and move to the cell membrane only when needed to carry glucose into the cell. How does the cell know that glucose needs to be transported? In most cells, the hormone **insulin**, which is secreted into the bloodstream by the **beta cells** of the pancreas in response to elevated blood glucose, binds to receptors on the cell membranes and triggers the glucose transport proteins (primarily **GLUT4**) to move from the cytoplasm to the

DO YOU KNOW ❓

Although fasting blood glucose levels may indicate diabetes mellitus, many physicians won't diagnose this disease unless a patient fails an **oral glucose tolerance test (OGTT)**. During this test the patient consumes 75 grams of glucose, and blood samples are drawn every 30 to 60 minutes over the next 3 hours. At the end of the test period, blood glucose values between 140 and 200 mg/dl indicate impaired glucose tolerance, and a value of 200 mg/dl or higher suggests diabetes (33, 34).

PUTTING IT INTO PERSPECTIVE

GLYCOGEN STORAGE IS LIMITED

While dietary strategies are used to maximize the amount of glycogen stored in the liver and skeletal muscle, the amount is limited because of the size of the liver and muscles. You cannot simply grow new muscle tissue in response to excess dietary carbohydrate. If that were true, you would not need to resistance train to increase muscle mass. Instead you could eat an abundant amount of carbohydrate without exercise, and your skeletal muscle would expand to accommodate (35, 40).

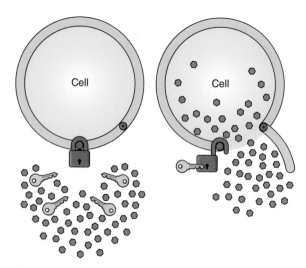

Figure 3.8 Glucose transport into a cell. Insulin is like a key that opens the lock on a door, allowing glucose to enter the cell.

cell membrane and begin shuttling glucose across the cell membrane back into the cytoplasm. This process is known as **insulin-dependent glucose transport (IDGT)** and is often described as a lock-and-key mechanism where insulin is the key that unlocks the membrane and allows glucose to enter. When IDGT fails to work properly, glucose does not enter the cell and tends to build up outside the cell and in the blood, resulting in elevated blood glucose levels. IDGT may fail because the pancreas cannot produce insulin, so there is no insulin available to trigger glucose uptake. This is the cause of type 1 diabetes mellitus. IDGT may also fail because the cell becomes insensitive to insulin, and even though insulin is available, it does not have the normal effect of signaling glucose transport proteins to the cell membrane, which is what causes type 2 diabetes mellitus. Not all glucose import into a cell requires an insulin trigger. In fact, all brain cells and some liver cells use an insulin-independent process, and exercising skeletal muscle can also take up glucose without requiring insulin when glucose demand is high in order to generate ATP for that activity, a situation that can be quite opportune (35, 40).

What happens when blood glucose levels temporarily drop, such as in cases when carbohydrate is not eaten for a period of time? Transient hypoglycemia triggers the pancreas to secrete the hormone **glucagon**, which has an action opposite of insulin. Whereas insulin is released as blood glucose concentration decreases, glucagon is secreted during hypoglycemia. This dual function underscores how important the pancreas is in the regulation of glucose homeostasis in the body. Glucagon stimulates the liver to convert stored glycogen to glucose (glycogenolysis), which is then released into the bloodstream. In addition, glucagon also stimulates the intrinsic (naturally occurring within the body) synthesis of glucose from noncarbohydrate precursors (gluconeogenesis). Two gluconeogenic pathways commonly convert different noncarbohydrate precursors to glucose—namely, the glucose-alanine cycle (amino acids) and the Cori cycle (lactate). The combined effect of the two glucagon-stimulated processes, glycogenolysis and gluconeogenesis, is to increase the quantity of glucose circulating in blood (figure 3.9) (26, 35, 40).

In addition to insulin and glucagon, other hormones contribute to the regulation of blood glucose levels, especially during periods of increased physical activity (table 3.3). Epinephrine and norepinephrine released into the bloodstream increase significantly with the onset of exercise and work together to stimulate glycogenolysis to make glucose readily available to working skeletal muscle. Cortisol also plays a role in raising blood glucose during exercise via its stimulatory effects on gluconeogenesis (26, 35, 40).

Preventing hypoglycemia during physical activity is a unique challenge for the body that differs from when at rest. Exercise creates an internal body environment that allows skeletal muscles to uptake glucose from blood via noninsulin-dependent glucose transport. As glucose is taken up by the muscle, blood glucose concentrations fall, and glucagon rises and stimulates both glycogenolysis and gluconeogenesis to help restore blood glucose levels to normal. It appears that exercising muscle prefers stored glycogen as its carbohydrate source; gluconeogenesis is a secondary system, providing a small amount of glucose to muscle in the later stages of prolonged exercise but ultimately cannot keep up with the energy demands. It should be noted that this is a finite process, as eventually the glucose production via these mechanisms cannot keep up with the utilization (26, 35, 40).

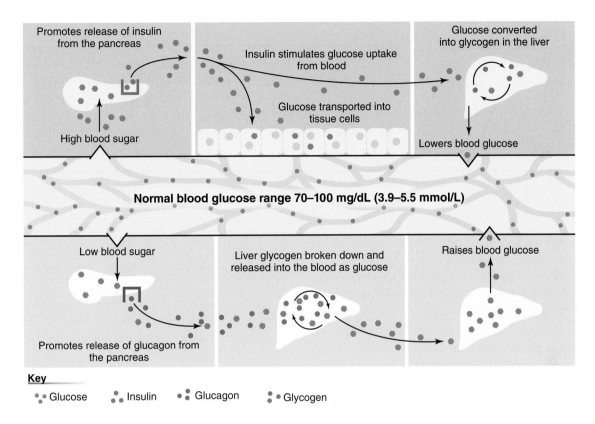

Figure 3.9 Regulation of blood glucose.

GLYCEMIC RESPONSE

It is well established that eating carbohydrates causes insulin and blood glucose levels to rise for a period of time after consumption before returning to baseline values; however, the rapidity, magnitude, and duration of this rise, better known as the **glycemic response**, is not easily predicted because many variables influence it. For many years, it was assumed that simple sugars caused a greater glycemic response than complex carbohydrates, but this theory was overly simplistic and has been summarily discarded. The chemical classification of carbohydrates does not fully describe the effects on digestion and metabolism. Newer theories based on the glycemic index and glycemic load of foods more accurately explain the glycemic response observed after consuming various foods (32, 35).

Table 3.3 Hormones Involved in Blood Glucose Regulation

Hormone	Secreting organ	Action
Epinephrine	Adrenal gland	Activates glycogenolysis
Norepinephrine	Adrenal gland	Activates glycogenolysis
Cortisol	Adrenal gland	Activates gluconeogenesis
Glucagon	Pancreas	Activates gluconeogenesis and glycogenolysis
Insulin	Pancreas	Activates glycogen synthesis Decreases gluconeogenesis

Data from Ross et al. 2014; Thompson, Manore, and Vaughan 2017.

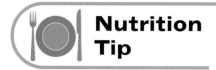

Nutrition Tip

Many people choose foods low in glycemic index (GI) to help them lose weight; however, the research studies are mixed, and some report no significant differences in energy intake or body weight as a result of eating a low GI diet. One study did report that a low GI diet in combination with high protein enhanced weight loss and prevented weight regain (3). Until more research is available to support the use of low GI diets for weight loss, a combination of an overall healthy, energy-restricted diet and regular exercise remains the most common recommendation for losing weight.

Glycemic Index

Glycemic index, a concept first introduced in 1981, continues to be employed today. The glycemic index is a qualitative method of ranking foods based on the relative blood glucose response observed after ingesting them. The glycemic index of a specific food is determined by measuring blood glucose levels for two hours following consumption of a fixed amount of available carbohydrate (e.g., 50 g) and then comparing these results to the blood glucose response observed following consumption of the same amount of a reference food, such as pure glucose. Foods that cause a large blood glucose response compared to the reference food has a high glycemic index, and foods causing a relatively low blood glucose response has a low glycemic index. The reference food is usually assumed to have a glycemic index of 100, meaning that all foods causing a lower blood glucose response than the reference food will have a glycemic index below 100 and vice versa. This system has a few limitations. Pub-lished glycemic index values of the same foods may vary considerably because of differences in ingredients used, ripeness, method of food processing, cooking methods, and food storage (10, 11, 19).

Also, people rarely consume a single food item in isolation, and addition of other foods to a carbohydrate-containing food will affect the glycemic index. For example, a potato might have a high glycemic index in isolation, but when consumed with protein and fat, it causes a much slower rise in blood glucose than would be expected based solely on glycemic index (10, 14, 32).

Glycemic Load

In 1997 the concept of **glycemic load** was introduced in attempt to quantify the overall glycemic response of a portion of food, not just the amount of available carbohydrate. The glycemic load is an indicator of the blood glucose response that results from total carbohydrate ingestion. The formula for determining glycemic load is:

PUTTING IT INTO PERSPECTIVE

GLYCEMIC INDEX IS A TOOL, NOT A RULE

Glycemic index is an empirical measurement that can never truly be duplicated because it is impossible to repeat the test on exactly the same person under the exact same conditions (i.e., time of day) and using the *exact* same food (i.e., same cooking time, same cooking method, same maturation or ripening, etc.). Moreover, the glycemic response to a specific food in one individual can be quite different from that observed in another. Furthermore, glycemic index is based on a set amount of carbohydrate, not necessarily a typical portion of the food. For example, carrots might have a high glycemic index, but a large portion is needed for a significant blood glucose response. All considered, it is most practical to think of glycemic index as simply an indicator of how high and how fast blood glucose *tends* to rise after eating the food, but it should never be used to predict the magnitude of the glycemic response to food with great accuracy.

Glycemic load = glycemic index of the food × g CHO per portion ÷ 100

It is possible for a food to have a high glycemic index and low glycemic load if consumed in a small quantity, and vice versa when a larger portion size is consumed. Glycemic index should never be the sole factor considered when consuming carbohydrates. Factors such as energy density, other macronutrients, micronutrients, and phytochemicals should also be considered (6, 32).

Table 3.4 includes some examples of the glycemic index and glycemic load of common foods. The scientific literature offers more comprehensive tables on glycemic index and glycemic load on a wide variety of foods (4, 17).

Glycemic Index and Glycemic Load in Sport and Exercise

Athletes need to use caution when selecting foods based solely on glycemic index or glycemic load.

Table 3.4 Glycemic Index and Load of Common Foods

Food	Serving size	Serving size (g)	Glycemic index	Available carbohydrates and serving (g)	Glycemic load
Wheat bread	1 slice	30	53	20	11
Oatmeal	2/3 cup	50	69	35	24
English muffin	1 half	30	77	14	11
White bagel	Diameter 3 in.	70	72	35	25
White rice	1 cup	150	51	42	21
Brown rice	3/4 cup	150	50	33	16
Cheese pizza	1 slice	100	36	24	9
Mashed potatoes	3/4 cup	150	74	20	18
Baked potato	5.3 oz.	150	60	30	18
Corn	3/4 cup	150	53	32	17
Kidney beans	0.5 cup	150	52	17	9
Apple	Diameter 2-3/4 in.	120	38	15	6
Apple juice	8 fl. oz.	250 ml	40	29	12
Soda	8.5 fl. oz.	250 ml	53	26	14
Chocolate milk	1 cup	50	43	28	12
Low-fat yogurt	7 oz.	200	31	30	9
Chocolate pudding	3.5 oz.	100	47	16	7
Chocolate ice cream	3/4 cup	50	87	13	8
Angel food cake	2 oz.	50	67	29	19
Vanilla wafers	4 cookies	25	77	18	14
Ripe banana	7 in.	120	51	25	13
Grapes	25	120	46	18	8
Strawberries	3/4 cup	120	40	3	1
Raisins	2 oz.	60	64	44	28

Adapted from K. Foster-Powell, S.H. Holt, and J.C. Brand-Miller, 2002, "International table of glycemic index and glycemic load values: 2002," *American Journal of Clinical Nutrition* 76: 5-56.

Simply choosing or avoiding a food classified as low, medium, or high glycemic index or load is not always warranted. For example, some athletes experience **reactive hypoglycemia**, or **postprandial hypoglycemia**, a condition in which blood sugar drops below normal after consuming certain foods. This can be problematic if the drop occurs at the start of a race. Experimentation with prerace foods would be beneficial to see if this is a potential concern. Otherwise, research to suggest that high- or low-glycemic foods are more advantageous prior to exercise is insufficient (5, 37). Though carbohydrates that rapidly increase insulin, such as glucose, will lead to an initial drop in blood sugar at the beginning of exercise, blood sugar levels typically return to normal within approximately 20 minutes, and the initial drop has no negative effect on performance (28).

DO YOU KNOW ?

The average male marathon runner stores 400 to 500 grams of skeletal muscle glycogen, which is long enough to run for 80 minutes at his normal running pace, assuming no other substrate is used to make ATP (23-26, 40).

CARBOHYDRATE AS FUEL DURING EXERCISE

Exercise requires the ability to generate a continuous supply of energy (ATP) in order for skeletal muscle to contract and activity to continue. Because muscle can store only small amounts of ATP, other fuel sources are required, namely, glucose, fatty acids, and to a limited extent, amino acids. Glucose can be used to produce ATP for skeletal muscle contraction via partial oxidation of the glucose molecule (glycolysis) or complete oxidation of the glucose molecule (aerobic metabolism). Remember that complete glucose oxidation includes three steps that occur in the following order: glycolysis, TCA cycle, and the electron transport chain (see chapter 2). The source of glucose for exercising muscle primarily comes from stored muscle glycogen but can also come from blood glucose and gluconeogenesis. Exercise intensity plays a key role in determining how much and when glucose is used for a given activity (table 3.5). In general, glucose use is increased

> whenever exercise intensity increases beyond a steady state (e.g., includes the onset of exercise) and
> whenever steady-state exercise intensity increases (26).

ROLE OF CARBOHYDRATE IN EXERCISE FATIGUE

Muscle fatigue during exercise typically occurs as a result of three far-different circumstances: (1) muscle cannot produce enough force to meet the demands of the activity, (2) high ATP demand (high-intensity exercise) prevents the complete oxidation of glucose, causing lactate accumulation, or (3) energy reserves in muscle become depleted. The first situation does not involve carbohydrate. The second situation is known as metabolic fatigue and occurs when exercise intensity rises to the level that it prevents glucose from being aerobically oxidized, thereby causing lactate to accumulate in the cell. Lactate gets converted to lactic acid, and the hydrogen ions produced in the process create an acidic environment in the muscle cell that disrupts

Table 3.5 ATP Produced From Glucose During Exercise at Varying Intensities

Exercise intensity	% of ATP produced
Rest	35
Light to moderate	40
High and short duration	95
High and long duration	70

Data from McArdle, Katch and Katch 2013.

ATP production and muscle contraction, thus producing symptoms of fatigue. Once metabolic fatigue has occurred, the exerciser will have to slow down or stop so the body can work to clear the excess hydrogen ions from the muscle. Lactate is not only a metabolic by-product, it is also a fuel source for many cells throughout the body, so clearing excess lactate and subsequent hydrogen ions is simply a matter of time. Once these metabolic products are cleared, which is a fairly rapid process, the fatigue dissipates and the skeletal muscle can once again contract and perform. Note that endurance-trained individuals are better able than sedentary people to use lactate for energy (7, 25, 26, 31, 40).

The third situation is called **substrate fatigue**, which occurs when skeletal muscles essentially run out of substrate (i.e., glucose). When glycogen reserves in the skeletal muscles become significantly reduced, no glucose is available to produce ATP to any meaningful extent, exercise must slow down or stop entirely, and cannot recommence until more glucose is introduced into the system via consumption or gluconeogenesis (7, 25, 26, 31, 40). Substrate fatigue is a real concern for endurance athletes and is discussed in greater detail in chapter 11.

CARBOHYDRATE RECOMMENDATIONS

The Food and Nutrition Board of the Institute of Medicine issues **Dietary Reference Intakes (DRIs)** that serves as a recommendation of carbohydrate intakes for healthy people. The DRIs include recommendations for women who are pregnant and breastfeeding, infants, children, and adults. DRIs are not designed to replace medical nutrition therapy for persons with certain nutrition-related diseases and conditions. These values take into consideration age and gender but do not account for activity or disease states. Special recommendations exist for these unique populations (22).

Recommendations for the General Population

The Acceptable Macronutrient Distribution Range (AMDR) for carbohydrate is 45 to 65 percent of total energy intake; this range applies to males and females in all age brackets and life stages (pregnancy and lactation are life stages) (43). The Recommended Dietary Allowance (RDA) for carbohydrate is based on the minimum requirement needed for brain function and is currently set at 130 grams per day for toddlers, children, adolescents, and adults of all ages. This value does not reflect the amount needed for daily activities and purposeful exercise. Women who are pregnant need at least 175 grams per day, and women who are breastfeeding need at least 210 grams per day. The RDA is lower in infants, with those under 6 months of age needing at least 60 grams per day, and those between 7 and 12 months needing at least 95 grams per day. The majority of the daily carbohydrate intake should come from high-quality food sources such as whole grains, fruits, vegetables, beans, and legumes, while limiting added sugar intake to 10 percent of energy consumption or less (44).

Fiber is a type of carbohydrate with its own set of recommendations because fiber can have unique health benefits different from the other types of carbohydrate. The DRI for fiber is 38 grams per day for males aged 14 to 50, and 25 grams per day for females aged 19 to 50. Pregnant and lactating women need more—28 and 29 grams per day, respectively (22). Average intake in the United States is approximately 15 grams per day. The DRIs for fiber are currently set based on the available data examining the relation between fiber and cardiovascular disease, but research examining fiber's relation to other aspects of health is emerging. Until that research

DO YOU KNOW ?

When you first start an exercise program or engage in a tough bout of exercise, the muscle soreness you feel 1 to 3 days later is not caused by lactic acid. The soreness you experience is caused by overexerting your muscles, resulting in microtrauma and inflammation, which causes pain. Once healing takes place, soreness should subside after a few days. During this time, it is usually best to perform light activities. If the soreness or pain persists, seek the advice of a physician before resuming your normal routine.

exists, the current DRIs are the best guidelines we have for daily fiber intake (22). If an individual wishes to increase fiber intake to improve health, it is recommended to do this gradually and with a concomitant increase in fluid. Increased fiber intake without adequate fluid could result in constipation (22, 36).

Recommendations for Active Individuals and Athletes

For athletes, the absolute quantity of carbohydrate in grams and g/kg body weight consumed is more important than considering total carbohydrate intake as a percentage of total energy. As an example, due to their high calorie intake, some endurance athletes may consume up to 70 percent of their total energy intake in the form of carbohydrates while still meeting their total protein and fat requirements. In general, athletes should consume from 3 to 12 g/kg carbohydrate per day (table 3.6) (39). This is a large range intended to accommodate athletes of all sizes and states of training.

> The low end of the range, 3 to 5 g/kg, is usually best for athletes undergoing a light training regimen, playing a skill-based sport, having a large body mass, or attempting to lose body fat via an energy-restricted diet (39).

> The middle range of 5 to 7 g/kg should be used for athletes exercising at a moderate intensity for approximately an hour per day or those in high-intensity, short duration type sports (39).

> The range of 6 to 10 g/kg is recommended for those engaged in high-intensity exercise between 1 to 3 hours per day (39).

> The upper end of the range, 8 to 12 g/kg, is usually reserved for extremely committed athletes exercising at the highest intensity or for greater than 4 to 5 hours per day (39).

Again, note that these are general recommendations and not meant as prescriptions for individuals. Values will vary depending on total energy expenditure, specific training regimens, and personal experience with strategies that optimize performance. Athletes tend to know their physiological responses to diet and training, and their practice may deviate from these general recommendations. These guidelines should serve as a starting point for *healthy* athletes and be fine-tuned to meet the specific needs of each athlete. If these guidelines are not working, or if an athlete has a nutrition-related medical condition, the athlete may need to obtain sport- and training-specific carbohydrate recommendations from a Certified Specialist in Sports Dietetics (CSSD). The CSSD can tailor

Table 3.6 Daily Carbohydrate Recommendations for Trained Athletes

Carbohydrate recommendation	Exercise intensity and duration	Daily amount for 59-kg (130 lb.) athlete (g)	Daily amount for 79-kg (175 lb.) athlete (g)
3–5 g/kg	Low-intensity training	177–295	237–395
5–7 g/kg	More than 60 minutes per day of low-intensity training / 60 minutes per day of moderate-intensity training / Up to 30 minutes per day of high-intensity training	295–413	395–553
6–10 g/kg	1–3 hours per day of moderate- to high-intensity training	354–590	474–790
8–12 g/kg	4–5 hours per day of moderate- to high-intensity training	472–708	632–948

Assumes adequate energy intake and that carbohydrate is spread throughout the day, depending on training schedule.
Data from Thomas, Erdman, and Burke 2016.

meal planning to the individual and take into account any issues that warrant a balance in carbohydrate need and medical nutrition therapy (e.g., celiac disease, lactose intolerance, and irritable bowel syndrome).

Table 3.7 provides the estimated number of grams of daily carbohydrate needed to maintain glycogen stores for athletes of varying body weights. Athletes should time the intake of carbohydrate at appropriate intervals throughout the day, taking into account when practice and competition occur during the day.

Percentages of total energy do not always align with absolute quantity of carbohydrate. For example, large individuals with more muscle mass often have a higher energy requirement and might

be able to meet carbohydrate needs with a lower total percentage of energy. An athlete consuming 4,000 kilocalories per day, 50 percent of that from carbohydrate, would be eating 500 grams of carbohydrate. This would be equivalent to 7.4 g/kg for a 150-pound (68 kg) man—well within the recommendation. On the contrary, a 120-pound (54.5 kg) woman consuming 1,400 kilocalories per day, 65 percent from carbohydrate, would actually be eating 4.2 g/kg, which may or may not be adequate for her training (figure 3.10). From these examples you can see that a lower percentage of carbohydrate, 50 percent, could be adequate, while a higher percentage, 65 percent, might not be ideal for a person who is endurance training at moderate to high intensity.

Table 3.7 Daily Carbohydrate Needs by Target Intake Level and Body Weight

Weight (lb.)	Weight (kg)	3 g/kg	4 g/kg	5 g/kg	6 g/kg	7 g/kg	8 g/kg	9 g/kg	10 g/kg	11 g/kg	12 g/kg
100	45	136	182	227	273	318	364	409	455	500	545
105	48	143	191	239	286	334	382	430	477	525	573
110	50	150	200	250	300	350	400	450	500	550	600
115	52	157	209	261	314	366	418	470	523	575	627
120	55	164	218	273	327	382	436	491	545	600	655
125	57	170	227	284	341	398	455	511	568	625	682
130	59	177	236	295	355	414	473	532	591	650	709
135	61	184	245	307	368	430	491	552	614	675	736
140	64	191	255	318	382	445	509	573	636	700	764
145	66	198	264	330	395	461	527	593	659	725	791
150	68	205	273	341	409	477	545	614	682	750	818
155	70	211	282	352	423	493	564	634	705	775	845
160	73	218	291	364	436	509	582	655	727	800	873
165	75	225	300	375	450	525	600	675	750	825	900
170	77	232	309	386	464	541	618	695	773	850	927
175	80	239	318	398	477	557	636	716	795	875	955
180	82	245	327	409	491	573	655	736	818	900	982
185	84	252	336	420	505	589	673	757	841	925	1,009
190	86	259	345	432	518	605	691	777	864	950	1,036
195	89	266	355	443	532	620	709	798	886	975	1,064
200	91	273	364	455	545	636	727	818	909	1,000	1,091

Data from Thomas, Erdman, and Burke 2016.

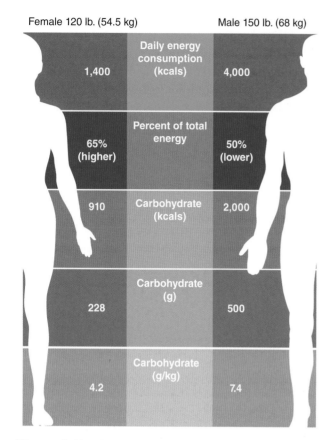

Female 120 lb. (54.5 kg)   Male 150 lb. (68 kg)

	Daily energy consumption (kcals)	
1,400		4,000
65% (higher)	Percent of total energy	50% (lower)
910	Carbohydrate (kcals)	2,000
228	Carbohydrate (g)	500
4.2	Carbohydrate (g/kg)	7.4

Figure 3.10 Example of percentage of energy from carbohydrate versus amount of carbohydrate.

CARBOHYDRATE CONTENT OF FOODS

Figure 3.11 lists some popular foods and their associated carbohydrate content. When reading Nutrition Facts panels, keep in mind there might be more than one serving per package (46).

CARBOHYDRATE AND HEALTH

Much of this chapter has focused on carbohydrate as an energy source for athletes, but carbohydrate can also have an important role in overall health and well-being. While athletes might have an immediate need of performance optimization for a specific event or competitive season, long-term health is also of concern. Some types of carbohydrate, such as whole grains that contain fiber, might promote health and prevent disease. Other types, such as simple sugars and processed flours, might contribute negatively to health. Some of these topics have been investigated for years, while others have more limited data. In either case, more research is needed in these areas to best understand the relation of carbohydrate consumption to health.

The Nutrition Facts Panel is an easy way to check the fiber content of foods. The label discloses the amount of dietary fiber in each serving, as well as the percent daily value (%DV).

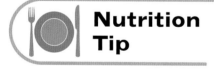

Nutrition Tip

High-fiber diets might reduce the risk of developing type 2 diabetes mellitus or may help manage marked fluctuations in blood glucose. Fiber absorbs fluid and expands in the intestine, slowing digestion. Fiber also stimulates the release of hormones that increase satiety (8). All of these factors have been cited as explanations for the association between diets higher in fiber and whole grains and both lower body weight and prevention of weight gain (12, 52). However, a systematic review of the research examining thirty-eight types of fiber found the majority of short-term fiber treatments did not enhance satiety or reduce food intake (52).

Despite the conflicting evidence regarding the role of dietary fiber in weight control, research suggests that the type of fiber matters, and that the form of food might matter as well (i.e., liquid vs. solid food). Beta-glucan (from oats and barley), lupin kernel fiber, whole-grain rye, rye bran, and a mixed diet of specific fiber-containing foods (5–8 grains, legumes, vegetables, and fruits) have all been shown to enhance satiety. However, increases in satiety do not necessarily correspond to a decrease in food intake, total calories, and weight loss. Oat and barley beta-glucan might be superior to other types of fiber for reducing total calorie intake (12).

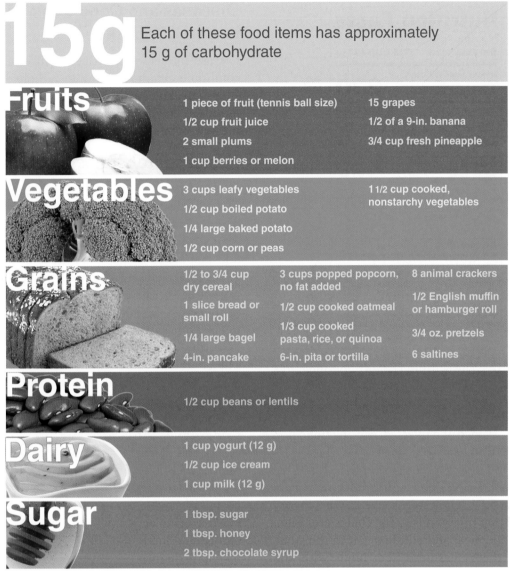

Figure 3.11 Carbohydrate content of selected foods.

Data from American Diabetes Association 2014.

In general, a low-fiber food is one that has 5 percent or less of the DV, and a high-fiber food is one with 20 percent or more of the DV (figure 3.12) (46).

Health Benefits of Fiber

Although **dietary fiber** is not digested, it might be beneficial in the fight against diseases of the digestive tract, cardiovascular disease, and diabetes mellitus. Through its action of binding toxins in the **colon** and facilitating their elimination from the body, fiber might reduce the risk of developing colon and rectal cancer. Other cancers with a possible healthy relation to fiber include cancer of the mouth, pharynx, larynx, esophagus, and stomach (2). Fiber also increases stool bulk, and with adequate fluid intake, keeps stool smooth and easy to eliminate. This ease of elimination may reduce the chance of developing the painful condition known as **diverticulosis**, which occurs when small pockets form in the intestinal walls caused by the high pressure required to eliminate small, hard stools from the colon. These pockets

Nutrition Facts

8 servings per container

Serving size   2/3 cup (55g)

Amount per 2/3 cup

Calories   230

	% Daily Value*
Total Fat 8g	**10%**
Saturated Fat 1g	**5%**
Trans Fat 0g	
Cholesterol 0mg	**0%**
Sodium 160mg	**7%**
Total Carbohydrate 37g	**13%**
Dietary Fiber 7g	**20%**
Total Sugars 12g	
Added Sugars 10g	**20%**
Protein 3g	
Vitamin D 2mcg	10%
Calcium 260mg	20%
Iron 8mg	45%
Potassium 235mg	6%

* The % Daily Value (DV) tells you how much a nutrient in a serving of food contributes to a daily diet. 2,000 calories a day is used for general nutrition advice.

Figure 3.12   The Nutrition Facts Panel indicates the amount of dietary fiber in a serving of food.

become inflamed and infected, causing transition to **diverticulitis** (36, 40).

Fiber might also play a role in the prevention of cardiovascular disease, by reducing serum total and LDL cholesterol levels. One theory suggests that fiber binds to the cholesterol eaten in the same meal and eliminates it in the stool. Another theory assumes fiber binds with and eliminates **bile** from the gut, which stimulates the liver to synthesize new bile to replace what is lost in stool. Bile itself contains cholesterol, so synthesizing new bile requires cholesterol to be removed from the blood and incorporated into newly produced bile, thereby reducing serum cholesterol levels over time. Without this function of fiber, bile is recycled and not eliminated from the body. Newer research is emerging that suggests fiber might also reduce inflammatory markers for heart disease and blood pressure. Given this promising body of evidence, increasing fiber intake from whole grains, fruits, vegetables, or supplements likely provides a protective health benefit for reducing the risk of developing certain diseases (36, 40).

Diseases and Conditions Related to Carbohydrate

Lactose intolerance and celiac disease are two conditions that have a link to carbohydrate consumption and usually require afflicted persons to modify their dietary intakes, and possibly their lifestyle habits, to compensate for the disease.

Lactose Intolerance

Recall that carbohydrates must be digested into their simplest form, monosaccharides, in order to be absorbed into the small intestine. **Lactose intolerance** is a condition in which the small intestine does not produce enough of the enzyme lactase, so the disaccharide lactose present in dairy foods cannot be digested (13, 40). Because the lactose cannot cross the intestinal cell wall, it progresses to the **large intestine**, where gut bacteria act on it to produce gas, watery stools, and diarrhea. The condition can be quite uncomfortable, but generally does not require medical attention (40).

Not all of those with lactose intolerance experience the same level of symptoms. Some people are mildly intolerant and can consume milk, yogurt, cheese, and related foods in small quantities. Others might not tolerate milk but can consume yogurt and cheese; because these products have already been fermented, they contain less lactose than milk. Still others are severely intolerant and cannot consume any dairy products at all. This is important to understand, as milk is often recommended for athletes as a recovery beverage because of its ideal composition of carbohydrate and protein. Milk is also a key source of calcium and vitamin D. Fortunately, over-the-counter products are available that contain the enzyme lactase that can be consumed along with dairy foods to reduce the amount of lactose ultimately delivered to

DO YOU KNOW ?

Don't confuse lactose intolerance with a milk allergy, which is an allergy to the protein in milk. Lactose intolerance involves symptoms of the gastrointestinal tract, whereas milk allergies involve an immune response.

gut bacteria. In addition, some brands of milk are lactose free. For those who prefer no dairy, there are many vegetarian-based products on the market that have varying levels of carbohydrate, protein, and calcium (35, 40).

Figure 3.13 presents a list of foods that contain lactose.

Celiac Disease and Other Gastrointestinal Disturbances

Celiac disease is an autoimmune disease that involves an interaction between genetics (one must have the gene) and environment (exposure to the protein gluten). **Gluten** contains a specific sequence of amino acids located in the prolamin fraction of wheat. Barley and rye contain proteins related to gluten (though all of these proteins are typically referred to as gluten). Prolamins are storage proteins found in many grains, but it is the amino acid sequence in those grains that are harmful to those with celiac disease. When gluten is consumed, an immune response is triggered, resulting in damage to the small intestinal mucosa, which alters the absorptive surface area and compromises the absorption of nutrients in the small intestine. Over time, this can progress to the malabsorption of both macronutrients and micronutrients. This is different from a wheat allergy, which is an immediate immune system allergy reaction to the protein molecule in wheat. Some food allergy reactions require immediate medical attention.

People with celiac disease require medical nutrition therapy and should seek the advice of a RDN. They must consume a gluten-free diet, avoiding wheat, barley, and rye in any form, as well as other grains, such as triticale. Some other grains and flours can be tolerated, such as corn, potato, rice, amaranth, quinoa, and buckwheat (buckwheat is a vegetable). Fortunately, gluten-free products are becoming easy to find, though many of them are higher in kilocalories and sugar than their counterparts with gluten.

Many individuals now prefer a gluten-free diet even in the absence of a wheat allergy or celiac disease. Some people suffer from gluten sensitivity, which is not the same autoimmune disease as celiac disease and is not a protein allergy. These individuals report feeling better when they avoid gluten. While there is not enough evidence to support the gluten-free approach for athletes or other individuals without celiac disease, gluten sensitivity, or wheat allergy, it is certainly possible to eat a balanced diet without gluten (35, 40).

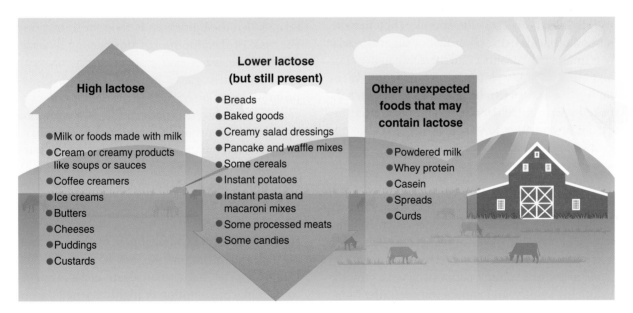

Figure 3.13 Foods containing lactose.

Data from Cleveland Clinic 2016.

More recent research has confirmed that foods containing gluten often also contain compounds called fermentable oligo-, di-, and monosaccharides and polyols (FODMAPs). These compounds also cause gastrointestinal distress even without being in the presence of gluten. These molecules are most commonly found in fructose (e.g., apples, pears, honey), lactose (e.g., milk, cottage cheese), fructans (e.g., wheat, garlic, onions), galactans (e.g., beans, lentils, soy), and polyols (e.g., sweeteners). These all have an osmotic effect, pulling water into the small intestine, which results in bloating, abdominal pain, and diarrhea. If they go undigested and travel to the large intestine, gas is usually another side effect. People have different tolerances to different foods high in FODMAPs. If one has chronic gastrointestinal issues, it is important to seek medical attention before trying to self-diagnose or treat the problem. Low FODMAPs diets are therapeutic for many different diseases and conditions that may require both medical and dietary treatment. Individuals without a specific disease may also follow this diet if undesirable side effects are a consequence of eating a diet rich in high FODMAPs (29).

Health Effects of Nutritive Sweeteners

Nutritive sweeteners contain carbohydrate, usually sugar, and provide energy. They may be monosaccharides, disaccharides, or sugar alcohols (e.g., mannitol, sorbitol). Nutritive sweeteners can be found naturally in foods such as fruits, vegetables, and dairy; can be added to foods such as baked goods, salad dressings, and peanut butter; or can be consumed by themselves (15).

Sugar

The most common nutritive sweeteners, or "sugars," are glucose, fructose, galactose, sucrose, maltose, and corn-based sweeteners such as high-fructose corn syrup. While providing sweetness is a key function of these products, sugars also play a role in texture, volume, supporting yeast growth, balancing acidity, and enhancing crystallization. The Food and Nutrition Board of the Institute of Medicine recommends that no more than 10 percent of total energy intake should come from added sugars (22). Foods high in sugar tend to be processed, and though energy-dense, they usually are not nutrient-dense. It would be difficult to consume a large percentage of energy from sugar and still meet other macronutrient and micronutrient needs. The most common source of sugar in the U.S. diet is from sweetened beverages (20). On average, one 12-ounce can of soda contains almost 10 teaspoons of sugar. When you consider that many "servings" of soda available at fast-food restaurants, theaters, amusement parks, and other venues are 16 or 24 ounces, or even larger, you can see how the amounts of sugar really add up. Even moderate sugar consumption may contribute to a significant number of adverse health conditions, including cardiovascular disease, inflammation, diabetes, and obesity (15, 35, 40). Note that most research studies support a relationship between sugar consumption and health issues, and more data are needed to distinguish between added sugars, excess energy, and other dietary factors.

Dyslipidemia Some evidence indicates that overconsumption of sugar and other processed carbohydrates are associated with increased levels of low-density lipoprotein (LDL) cholesterol and triglycerides (blood fats), both risk factors for cardiovascular disease, and a reduced level of high-density lipoprotein (HDL) cholesterol—the kind that removes LDL from the arteries. This pattern, called **dyslipidemia**, is thought to increase the risk of developing cardiovascular disease. While there is not enough evidence to say with certainty that sugar or processed carbohydrates promote heart disease, it is prudent to be concerned if one has this pattern (35, 40). Note that dyslipidemia is primarily a concern for individuals who are overconsuming sugar and carbohydrates compared to their energy expenditure. The concern might not apply (at least not to the same degree) to athletes consuming large quantities to fuel a sport or activity.

Inflammation Though much of the research on diet and **inflammation** has focused on fats, it does appear that carbohydrate plays a role as well. High consumption of highly **refined carbohydrates**—that is, those made from white flour and sugar—are associated with increased blood glucose levels and accompanying inflammatory

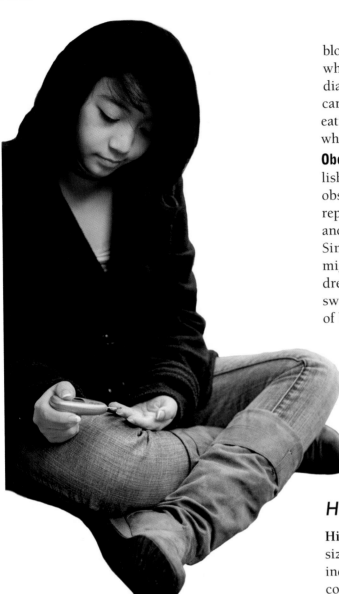

Careful monitoring of blood sugar along with regular exercise and a healthy diet can help people with diabetes.

messengers called cytokines. On the other hand, it also appears that replacing refined carbohydrates in the diet by consuming larger quantities of plants in the form of fruits and vegetables may help limit these inflammatory markers (18, 35).

Diabetes No indisputable scientific evidence implicates sugar consumption as a direct cause of diabetes mellitus; however, people who already have diabetes must learn to modify their carbohydrate intake and balance it with insulin or oral medications and exercise in order to keep their blood glucose levels under control. Some athletes who participate in rigorous sports also have diabetes, yet they still require large amounts of carbohydrates and have the unique challenge of eating enough carbohydrates to fuel their activity while maintaining blood glucose balance (40).

Obesity While more data are needed to establish a cause-and-effect relationship (30), some observational and controlled research studies report weight loss with reduced intake of sugars, and weight gain with increased intake (20, 38). Similarly it appears that sugar consumption might play a role in obesity development in children, with those consuming one or more sugar-sweetened beverages a day having a higher risk of becoming overweight (20). Many of the studies agree that it is the excess energy from the sugar contributing to the weight gain rather than the chemistry of the sugar molecules themselves (38). Excess energy in any form can contribute to weight gain, so if a person is consistently consuming more sugar than they are using as fuel or storing as glycogen, fat gain will result over time.

High-Fructose Corn Syrup

High-fructose corn syrup (HFCS) is a synthesized product derived from cornstarch. HFCS is inexpensive to produce and results in a stable, concentrated, sweet product with a long shelf life. Currently, the FDA does not have a formal definition for the term "natural," but when it comes to food labeling, the FDA considers "natural" to mean that nothing artificial or synthetic has been included in, or has been added to, the food item in question (51). HFCS does not contain artificial ingredients or color additives, and thus meets the FDA's requirements for use of the

DO YOU KNOW ?

Data from the United States Department of Agriculture suggest that consumption of high-fructose corn syrup (HFCS) has been declining over the years but that obesity and diabetes rates continue to rise. In other parts of the world, HFCS is limited in the food supply, yet obesity rates are still rising in those areas (15).

term *natural*. HFCS also makes food more palatable and is currently found in a seemingly endless number of food and beverage products, although this trend is reversing because of the negative publicity associated with HFCS (15, 35, 40).

Much attention has been given to HFCS and

DO YOU KNOW ?

Contrary to its name, high-fructose corn syrup is not extremely high in fructose, at least not relative to other ingredients. HFCS is between 42 and 55 percent fructose, depending on the processing, and the remainder is glucose. This composition is nearly identical to sucrose and honey and is apparently metabolized the same way in the body (15, 35, 40).

the development of diabetes and obesity; however, evidence is insufficient to support the notion that HFCS is less healthy than any of the other nutritive sweeteners. Some evidence strongly suggests that consumption of excess sugar, in *any* form, can contribute to excess energy intake and fat gain, which, in turn, increases the risk of developing type 2 diabetes, metabolic syndrome, and cardiovascular disease. But obesity is a multifactorial disease affected by overall lifestyle, and sugar intake is only one contributor (15, 35, 40).

Sugar Alcohols

Sugar alcohols are carbohydrates present naturally in some fruits and vegetables, and also made in laboratories. These alcohols are less sweet than sugar, contain 2 kilocalories per gram (kcal/g) instead of the 4 kcal/g found in sugar, and they do not promote tooth decay. They are not readily available on supermarket shelves, but they are abundant in manufactured products such as candy, frozen desserts, gum, toothpaste, mouthwash, and baked goods. They are often combined with nonnutritive sweeteners to enhance the sweet taste in a food product. Sugar alcohols are called by many names on food labels, but the most common are xylitol, maltitol, mannitol, sorbitol, or simply "sugar alcohol." Moderate doses of 10 to 15 grams per day are probably tolerated, but higher doses of 30 grams per day or more might result in undesirable gastrointestinal effects such as flatulence

or diarrhea. However, each individual's tolerance is different, so a trial-and-error approach might be best. When comparing sweet products made with sugar alcohols to those made with glucose or sucrose, the sugar-alcohol products produce a lower glycemic response and so are often promoted for people with diabetes (15, 16, 40).

Health Effects of Nonnutritive Sweeteners

Because they are generally not digested, **nonnutritive sweeteners** (NNS) such as saccharin and sucralose contain very little or no energy. They are considered high-intensity sweeteners because their sweetness-to-energy ratio is much greater than sugar. In addition, they generally do not cause a significant rise in blood glucose. They can be used alone as a tabletop sweetener or added to foods and beverages that traditionally contain sugar. Though sweet in taste, they often do not offer the same desirable food science properties as sugar. Some nonnutritive sweeteners do not contribute the bulk that sugar contributes to a recipe and do not aid in browning or crystallization, so they might not be ideal for baking (15, 45, 48).

Most nonnutritive sweeteners are regulated as food additives by the FDA. An exception is made for substances **generally recognized as safe (GRAS)** because these substances are recognized by qualified scientists as safe for consumption for their intended use. This makes them exempt from the food-additive approval process. Companies wishing to manufacture and market a new nonnutritive sweetener must conduct significant research on the product and present all of the required safety data to the FDA in consideration of approval. Research includes the extent of the absorption of the substance, any distribution in tissues, mechanisms and rates of metabolism, and rates of elimination of the substance or any metabolites. The FDA examines probable intake of the population, cumulative effects from using the product, and toxicology data. The FDA sets an acceptable daily intake (ADI) for a human, which is defined as the amount considered safe for daily consumption

PUTTING IT INTO PERSPECTIVE

DOES ASPARTAME AFFECT ENERGY BALANCE OR APPETITE?

Significant evidence suggests that using food items and products sweetened with aspartame as part of a comprehensive weight-management program might assist individuals with weight loss and weight maintenance over time by helping them lower total calorie intake. There is also good evidence suggesting aspartame does not increase appetite or total food intake in adults; however, there is limited evidence in children. Use of any nonnutritive sweetener may only be useful in improving energy balance if it is replacing a more energy-dense choice, and the consumer is not compensating for the lower-energy product consumption with overindulgence of other items in the same meal or another time in the day (15).

over the course of a lifetime without adverse health effects. This value takes into account even the estimated intake of a "high-consumer." The FDA may request additional consumption or safety data during the post-approval period. Note that FDA approval holds only in the United States. It is possible to purchase other, sometimes unapproved, products from other countries. Currently, six high-intensity sweeteners are FDA approved as food additives: saccharin, aspartame, acesulfame potassium (Ace-K), sucralose, neotame, and advantame. Two other types of high-intensity sweeteners have been submitted to the FDA as GRAS: Stevia rebaudiana Bertoni and Luo Han Guo (monk fruit). See table 3.8 for a summary of the most common nonnutritive sweeteners approved for use in the United States (45, 48, 49).

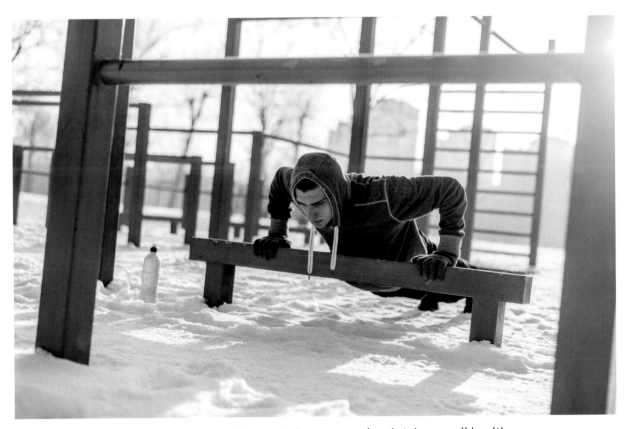

Keep added sugar in your diet to a minimum to improve and maintain overall health.

Table 3.8 Common Nonnutritive Sweeteners in the United States

Name of NNS	Description	Sweetness (number of times sweeter than sucrose)	ADI (mg/kg body weight) per day	Number of packets equivalent to ADI	FDA approval status and common uses
Saccharin*	Oldest NNS on the market Not metabolized and heat stable May not be desirable for cooking and baking Some experience a bitter aftertaste	200–700	15	250	Approved for limited use: <12 mg/fl. oz., 20 mg/packet, 30 mg/serving in foods
Aspartame	Dipeptide of phenylalanine and aspartate Provides 4 kcal/g but need such small quantity for sweet taste Metabolized to aspartic acid, phenylalanine, and methanol Persons with PKU should not consume** Degrades and loses sweetness during heating	160–220	50	165	Approved as a sweetener and general flavor enhancer
Acesulfame potassium	Approximately 95% is excreted unchanged in the urine and therefore does not provide significant energy Stable for cooking and baking Usually combined with another NNS	200	15	165	Approved as a sweetener and general flavor enhancer except meat and poultry
Sucralose	Often marketed as "made from sugar" 3 chloride molecules replace OH groups on sucrose Approximately 85% is not absorbed and excreted in the feces unchanged. The 15% absorbed is excreted unchanged in the urine. Heat stable for cooking and baking	600	5	165	Approved as a sweetener and general flavor enhancer
Neotame	Heat stable for cooking and baking	7,000–13,000	0.3	200	Approved as a sweetener and general flavor enhancer except for meat and poultry
Stevia (steviol glycosides)	Extract from the leaves of the Stevia rebaudiana Bertoni plant Different from whole stevia leaves May be bitter in large quantities Stable in dry form; may be more stable than others in liquid form	200–400	4	29	GRAS*** Rebaudiana extract approved as food additive; other is considered a dietary supplement
Luo Han Guo	Marketed as powdered "monk fruit extract" Heat stable for cooking and baking	100–250	Not specified	Not determined	GRAS***
Advantame	Does not yet have a brand name Chemically related to aspartame but much sweeter Does not carry the PKU warning	20,000	32.8	4000	Approved as a sweetener and general flavor enhancer except for meat and poultry

*In 2000, the National Toxicology Program of the National Institutes of Health concluded that saccharin should be removed from the list of potential carcinogens. Saccharin containing products no longer need to carry a warning label regarding cancer risk.

**Phenylketonuria (PKU) is an inborn error of metabolism where the person cannot metabolize the amino acid phenylalanine. The phenylalanine would build up and become toxic. People with PKU cannot consume phenylalanine and require special diets.

***GRAS = generally recognized as safe. There must be "a reasonable certainty of no harm" to earn this category.

Adapted from U.S. Food and Drug Administration 2015.

SUMMARY

Carbohydrate is an essential fuel source for the human body and abundant in many foods. Virtually all ingested carbohydrates absorbed in the small intestine are ultimately converted to glucose, which is the usable form of carbohydrate by the cells of the body. Blood glucose level is normally tightly regulated by hormones that work via modulating glycogenolysis and gluconeogenesis as needed. Glucose reserves in the body are stored in the form of glycogen primarily in skeletal muscle, and to a lesser extent in the liver.

While everyone needs a minimal amount of carbohydrate for normal physiological function, it is a particularly important fuel source for the exercising skeletal muscle. Many athletes need more dietary carbohydrate than a sedentary person in order to meet the physical demands of training. The AMDR for carbohydrate is 45 to 65 percent of total energy intake from high-quality sources and with minimal added sugar. Carbohydrate recommendations for athletes are better expressed in absolute terms ranging from 3 g/kg to 12 g/kg body weight depending on the day-to-day training volume.

The quantity of sugar, refined starch, and fiber consumed in the diet may impact overall health and well-being. Certain diseases and conditions are related to carbohydrate consumption, and managing these conditions may require the help of a RDN or CSSD. Nutritive and nonnutritive sweeteners are widely used in manufactured food and beverage products and may have effects on overall health.

Remember that sports nutrition is a young science, with new research emerging on a regular basis. Principles and guidelines presented in the chapter are based on current available evidence and may change or expand as new information becomes available. These guidelines are designed for healthy individuals. Those with a disease or nutrition-related condition may need to seek specific medical nutrition therapy from an RDN or CSSD.

FOR REVIEW

1. Describe the classification of carbohydrate.
2. How is carbohydrate absorbed?
3. Once carbohydrate gets to the liver as glucose, what are its possible metabolic fates?
4. Describe how blood glucose is regulated. Include the organs and hormones involved.
5. Describe the fuel used at rest and at high-intensity exercise.
6. What is the cause of metabolic fatigue?
7. What are the dietary carbohydrate recommendations for the general population?
8. What are the dietary carbohydrate recommendations for athletes? How do these differ from the general population?
9. List the sources of dietary carbohydrate (food groups that contain carbohydrate). How much carbohydrate is in a serving size of these groups?
10. Describe the differences in carbohydrate quality.
11. How does carbohydrate quality affect health?
12. Does sugar intake cause obesity and chronic diseases?
13. What is the difference between nutritive and nonnutritive sweeteners?
14. How are nonnutritive sweeteners regulated?

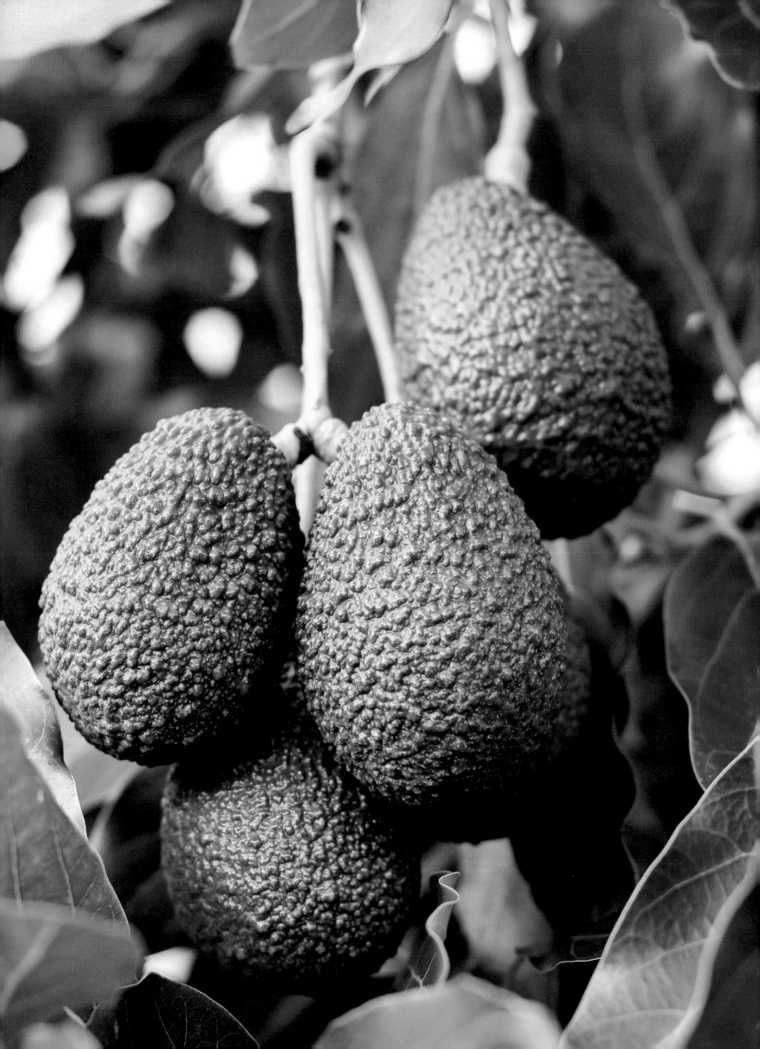

CHAPTER 4

Fat

> **CHAPTER OBJECTIVES**

After completing this chapter, you will be able to do the following:

> Discuss the main types of dietary fats and their health implications.

> Distinguish between dietary fats and dietary fatty acids within each category.

> Discuss the importance of dietary cholesterol in the body.

> Summarize the health implications of excess blood cholesterol and how various dietary fats and dietary cholesterol affect blood cholesterol levels.

> List dietary fat recommendations for the prevention of cardiovascular disease.

Dietary fats are composed of a mixture of saturated, monounsaturated, and polyunsaturated fat. Each type of fat contains an array of fatty acids, some of which have positive or negative effects on various aspects of health, including risk factors for cardiovascular disease. Only two dietary fatty acids are essential to be consumed in the diet. The human body can make all other fats from carbohydrate and protein. In the body, fat serves as a source of energy, helps with the absorption of fat-soluble vitamins and certain plant-based compounds, and plays an important structural and functional role in cell membranes, the brain, and myelin, the protective layer covering nerve cells. Though some athletes prefer a high-fat diet or believe it improves performance, no clear performance advantage is evident from following this approach. Ultraendurance athletes, who train and compete at a relatively slow pace, rely on more fat as percentage of energy (calories) used during activity and might be able to get away with a diet higher in fat; however, research has yet to show that this approach is advantageous for performance. A high-fat, low-carbohydrate diet will likely have deleterious effects on training and performance for athletes participating in high-intensity training programs or competing in high-intensity sports such as football, tennis, basketball, or rugby.

LIPIDS AND DIETARY FAT

Lipids are a category of macronutrients that are insoluble in water. Collectively, lipids have various biological functions in the body. There are three main categories of lipids, including triglycerides, sterols, and phospholipids; each has different functions in the body (figure 4.1). **Dietary fat** is composed primarily of triglycerides, with smaller amounts of phospholipids and sterols. Cooking oils, butter, animal fat, nuts, seeds, avocados, and olives are all significant sources of triglycerides in the diet (123). Dietary fats and oils provide energy and aid in the absorption of fat-soluble vitamins

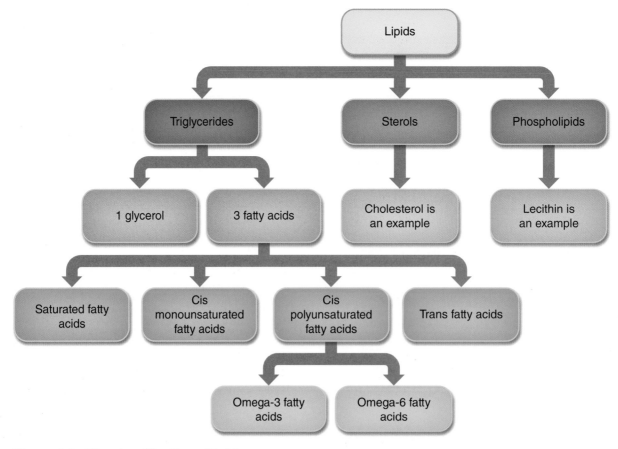

Figure 4.1 The classification of lipids.

A, D, E, and K, as well as certain food components such as carotenoids (90). Dietary fats and oils also have a textural role in foods, increasing palatability (130).

Triglycerides

Triglycerides are composed of one glycerol molecule and three fatty acid molecules. Fatty acids are either saturated, containing no double bonds, or unsaturated, containing one or more double bonds. Saturated fatty acids are the building blocks of saturated fat. **Saturated fatty acids** can stack together, making them solid at room temperature. **Unsaturated fatty acids** are the building blocks of unsaturated fat. Because of kinks at the double bonds (figure 4.2), unsaturated fatty acids do not stack neatly on top of one another and are therefore liquid at room temperature. **Monounsaturated fatty acids (MUFA)** contain one double bond, and **polyunsaturated fatty acids (PUFA)** contain more than one double bond and are identified based on the location of their first double bond. So, for instance, omega-3 fatty acids have their first double bond at the third carbon from the methyl end of the FA structure, whereas omega-6 fatty acids have their first double bond at the sixth carbon (figure 4.3). The majority of animal fats are high in saturated fat and therefore solid at room temperature, whereas plant-based fats (such as nut and fruit-based oils, including walnut oil and olive oil) tend to be liquid at room temperature because of their higher unsaturated fatty acid content. However, coconut oil and palm kernel oil are plant-based fats that are more solid, yet soft (due to their shorter carbon chains) at room temperature and have a high content of saturated fat (130). Regardless of the source, 1 gram of fat contains approximately 9 kilocalories.

Fatty acids vary in the number of double bonds they contain, the structure or configuration of the double bonds, and carbon chain length (130, 131). Although fatty acids are often referenced by their saturation status—saturated, monounsaturated (containing one double bond), or polyunsaturated (containing more than one double bond), individual fatty acids that are members of the same category can have very different effects on health. The carbon chain length and structure of a fatty acid determines how it functions in

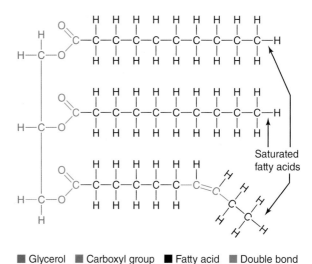

■ Glycerol ■ Carboxyl group ■ Fatty acid ■ Double bond

Figure 4.2 Triglycerides contain one glycerol molecule and three fatty acids.

food and cooking, its role in the body, and how it impacts health and disease (131).

In addition to differences in location and number of double bonds, there are two chemical configurations of unsaturated fatty acids. Those in the **cis configuration** have hydrogen ions on the same side of the double bond, whereas unsaturated fatty acids in the trans configuration have hydrogen ions on the opposite side of the double bond (130) (figure 4.4). The carbon chain can range from 2 to 40 carbons in length, though the majority of dietary fatty acids contain 12 to 20 carbons (47). Short-chain fatty acids contain up to 6 carbons, medium-chain from 8 to 12 carbons, and long-chain fatty acids contain more than 12 carbons (131).

Fatty acids are necessary for cell signaling and the expression of genes involved in carbohydrate and fat metabolism. Fatty acids also influence inflammation, insulin action, cell signaling, and neurological functioning. The body can produce all necessary fatty acids in the liver from dietary fat, carbohydrate, and protein with the exception of **linoleic acid (LA)** and **alpha-linolenic acid (ALA)**, which are "essential" fatty acids, meaning they must be consumed in the diet (90).

Glycerol is the backbone of triglycerides. In the human body, glycerol is released in the bloodstream from the breakdown of stored body fat. Like fatty acids, glycerol can be used to build

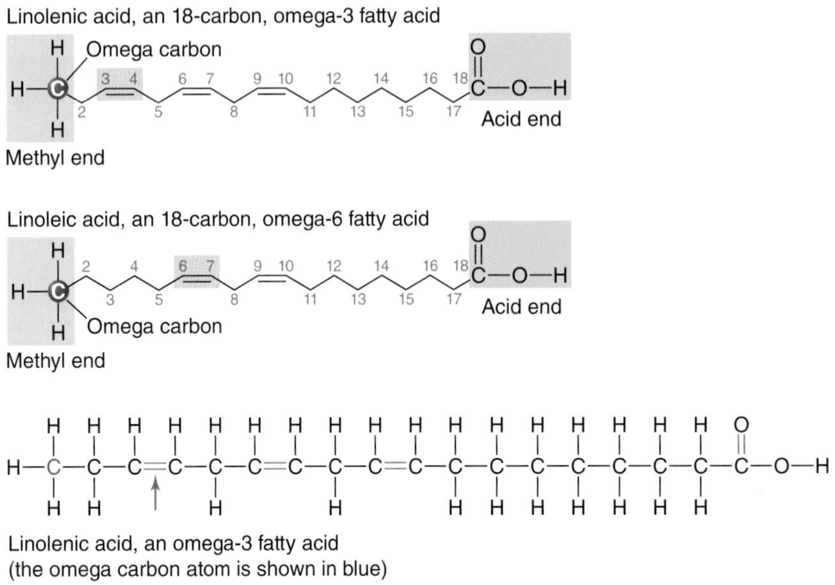

Linolenic acid, an 18-carbon, omega-3 fatty acid
Omega carbon
Methyl end
Acid end
Linoleic acid, an 18-carbon, omega-6 fatty acid
Omega carbon
Methyl end
Acid end
Linolenic acid, an omega-3 fatty acid
(the omega carbon atom is shown in blue)

Figure 4.3 Chemical structure of omega-3 and omega-6 fatty acids. Polyunsaturated fatty acids are identified by the location of their first double bond from the CH_3 (methyl group).

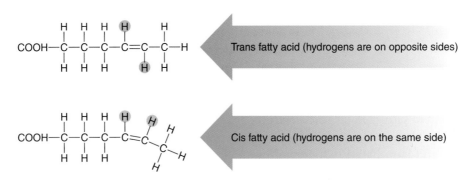

Trans fatty acid (hydrogens are on opposite sides)
Cis fatty acid (hydrogens are on the same side)

Figure 4.4 Cis and trans configuration of unsaturated fatty acids.

molecules necessary for membranes or stored in body fat for later use. Glycerol can also be converted to carbohydrate through glycolysis or gluconeogenesis (13). Glycerol (glycerin) is produced synthetically or derived from plants and is used as an ingredient in food and pharmaceuticals (128). Glycerol is a colorless, thick liquid with a mild odor and sweet, warm taste. It is a sugar alcohol (sugar alcohols are not completely absorbed in the body and so provide fewer calories than sugar) (121).

Sterols

Sterols are compounds with a multiple-ring structure found in both plants and animals. **Cholesterol**, the most well-recognized sterol in food (figure 4.5), is a component of all animal tissues and found only in animal-based foods such as eggs, meat, poultry, cheese, and milk (123). Humans absorb 20 to 80 percent of cholesterol from food. Genetic variations in cholesterol absorption can influence blood cholesterol levels (104). In the body, cholesterol is essential for all cells; it is a structural component of cell membranes, helps repair and form

DO YOU KNOW ?

Humans do not need to consume cholesterol in food because the body makes enough to meet physiological requirements.

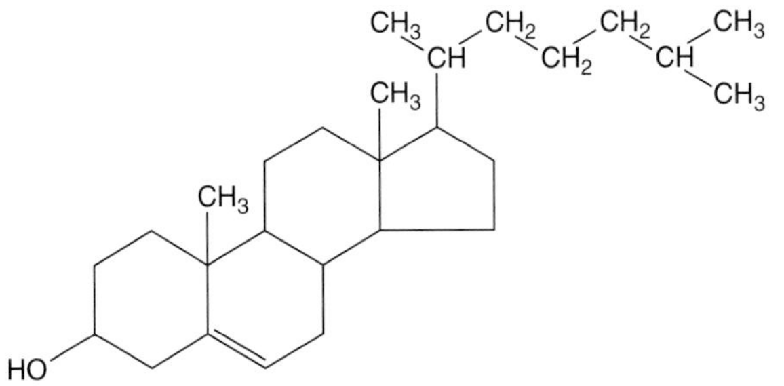

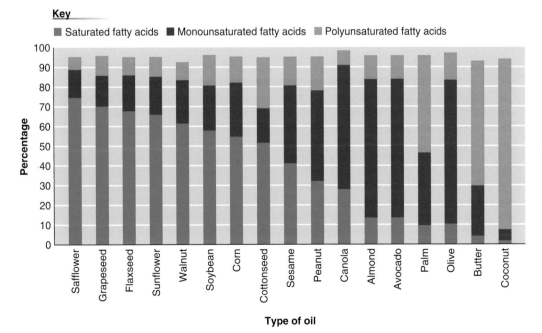

Figure 4.5 Chemical structure of cholesterol.

new cells, and is necessary for synthesizing steroid hormones (such as testosterone, androgen, and estrogen) and bile acids (which facilitate lipid digestion and absorption and are important for regulating cholesterol in the body). High levels of total and LDL cholesterol in the blood are considered risk factors for cardiovascular disease because they contribute to the formation of plaque in arteries.

Plant sterols, compounds naturally found in plants, are similar in structure to cholesterol and interfere with the body's absorption of cholesterol (46). Though not consumed in high enough doses through food to have an appreciable effect on blood cholesterol levels, supplemental doses of plant sterols can help lower blood cholesterol levels yet also decrease the bioavailability of beta-carotene and alpha tocopherol (96, 104).

Phospholipids

Phospholipids are comprised of glycerol, fatty acids, phosphate, and inositol, choline, serine, or ethanolamine (84). Phospholipids are naturally found in some foods and added to others as emulsifiers (helping liquids stay mixed, such as oil and vinegar as a salad dressing). Lecithin (phosphatidylcholine) is a naturally occurring phospholipid found in several foods, including eggs, liver, soybeans, wheat germ, and peanuts. In the body, phospholipids are structural components of cell membranes and lipoproteins *lipo* meaning lipid; lipoproteins contain both proteins and lipids and are transporters of cholesterol and fats in blood) (84). Phospholipids are necessary for the absorption, transport, and storage of lipids and aid in the digestion and absorption of dietary fat (139).

TRIGLYCERIDES AND HEALTH

The majority of fats found in food, including oils, contain a mixture of fatty acids (figure 4.6). Though many studies have focused on the health effects of fatty acids based on their saturation status (saturated, monounsaturated, or polyunsaturated), fatty acids within a particular group can have different actions in the body. In addition, determining the health effects stemming from

Figure 4.6 Fatty acid content of oils.

intake of a specific fatty acid can be difficult. A fatty acid's impact on health may be influenced by the food matrix (the combination of nutrient and nonnutrient compounds found in food and their chemical bonds to each other), how the fat is processed and cooked, and a person's health status and overall dietary intake (21, 124, 131). More recent research is teasing out the effects of individual fatty acids from the category of fats they belong to while also emphasizing the impact of certain foods, versus just the fat within the food, on health.

Saturated Fatty Acids

Saturated fatty acids are a source of energy and a structural component of cell membranes; some saturated fatty acids are necessary for normal protein functioning. Saturated fatty acids can be made in the body, there is no dietary requirement for them (124, 130). Most saturated fatty acids contain 14 or more carbon atoms.

The main sources of saturated fat in the U.S. diet are mixed dishes containing cheese or meat, such as burgers, sandwiches, tacos, and pizza; rice, pasta, and grain dishes; and meat, poultry, and seafood dishes (124). Saturated fats are typically more resistant to oxidation and therefore less likely to spoil.

There is no indication at this time that saturated fats prevent chronic disease. For decades consumers were told to decrease their intake of foods high in saturated fats because these fats increase total and LDL cholesterol as well as the risk of coronary heart disease (CHD) (130). Yet population-based studies, in which dietary intake was accessed through 24-hour recalls and food frequency questionnaires, found no relation between saturated fat intake and fatal heart attacks and stroke (108). However, relying on population-based studies for data is problematic. In many of these studies, a single 24-hour dietary recall, taken at one point in time, was used, which does not reflect long-term dietary intake (118). Also, 24-hour dietary recalls and food frequency

DO YOU KNOW ❓

A crossover study is a type of longitudinal study (people are studied over a period of time rather than at one point in time) in which all study subjects go through each type of treatment. If treatment options are a high-fat diet, moderate-fat diet, or low-fat diet, for instance, each subject will rotate through each diet for a set period, followed by a "washout period," during which they are not on any of the treatment diets, before progressing to the next diet.

PUTTING IT INTO PERSPECTIVE

THE FOOD MATRIX AND HOW FOODS HIGH IN SATURATED FAT AFFECT BLOOD CHOLESTEROL

In addition to varying effects from different saturated fatty acids, the food matrix influences how saturated fat affects blood cholesterol levels. Dairy foods are a good example. Though all full-fat dairy products have a high percentage of saturated fat, they have differing effects on blood cholesterol. Several studies show aged cheeses have a relatively minor impact on LDL-cholesterol or no impact at all (15, 40, 117). By way of explanation, some scientists point to the calcium content of the cheese, or the fermentation of aged cheeses (111). Full-fat yogurt also appears to affect cholesterol levels less than would be expected. However, the research on yogurt is inconsistent, possibly because of differences in types of yogurt used in studies (54, 67). Some scientists believe yogurt with live and active cultures may be responsible for the positive research results.

Whole milk raises LDL to the same extent as butter, but milk contributes substantially less fat per amount consumed compared to butter. Butter raises LDL cholesterol and should be replaced with oils rich in polyunsaturated fat, such as olive oil.

questionnaires (a series of questions asking how often standard serving sizes of common foods and beverages are consumed) depend on a subject's memory of their dietary intake, including how their food is typically prepared and portion sizes (118). In addition, all saturated fatty acids are grouped together regardless of the food they are in; therefore, the food matrix isn't taken into account. Also, each saturated fatty acid affects blood cholesterol differently (some have little to no effect on blood cholesterol while others raise total and LDL cholesterol). Finally, population studies cannot be used to determine cause and effect because they aren't designed to answer the question "do higher levels of intake of saturated fatty acids increase risk of coronary heart disease?" (107). Taken together, these factors are sufficient to make some researchers dubious about the efficacy of population-based studies, particularly when the results of such studies are not supported by clinical trials.

When substituting other energy-yielding macronutrients for saturated fat in the diet, clinical trials show that replacement strategy matters. When saturated fat is taken out of the diet, the specific macronutrient used to replace saturated fat determines changes in cholesterol levels, triglycerides, and risk of coronary heart disease (108). Replacing saturated fats with unsaturated fats, particularly PUFAs, is associated with a reduction in total and LDL cholesterol (124). Replacing saturated fat with PUFAs is also associated with a reduction in heart attacks and death from heart attacks (124) (figure 4.7). In addition, randomized controlled trials show replacing saturated fat with PUFAs decreases coronary heart disease events (81). Additional benefits might also be associated with this strategy. A crossover study in adults with type 2 diabetes as well as healthy obese and nonobese adults found that PUFAs improved insulin sensitivity and LDL levels compared to diets high in saturated fats (112). Also,

The replacement strategy

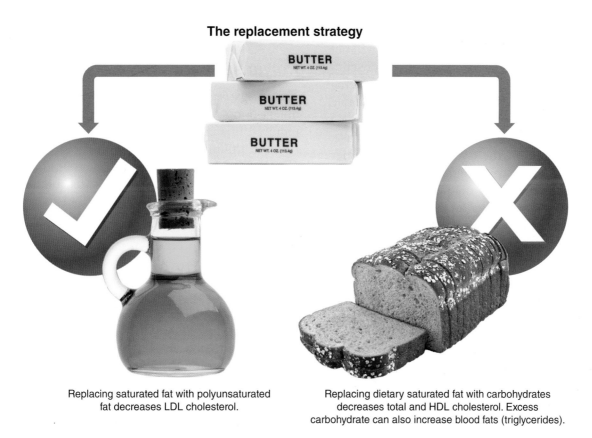

Replacing saturated fat with polyunsaturated fat decreases LDL cholesterol.

Replacing dietary saturated fat with carbohydrates decreases total and HDL cholesterol. Excess carbohydrate can also increase blood fats (triglycerides).

Figure 4.7 The replacement strategy matters. The strategy presented here is a generalization and may result from choosing low-fiber, refined carbohydrates, such as candy and cookies, not fiber- and nutrient-right carbohydrates, such as squash.

a study in healthy nonoverweight and nonobese adults found overeating saturated fat, as opposed to overeating polyunsaturated fat, increased liver and visceral fat storage. (Visceral fat wraps around organs like a blanket and is associated with insulin resistance and increased risk of type 2 diabetes and cardiovascular disease.) Overeating polyunsaturated fat, and not saturated fat, led to greater gains in muscle, as opposed to fat (101). Note that considerable differences exist among individuals in their response to saturated fat intake (14, 53). In addition to the potential for intrinsic genetic differences in lipid metabolism among individuals (89), higher weight and insulin resistance may reduce the beneficial effects of a reduction in saturated fat intake on LDL cholesterol.

Though not as strong as the evidence for replacing saturated fat with polyunsaturated fat, the evidence for replacing saturated fat with monounsaturated fat (olive oil, nuts) suggests this strategy may also be associated with a reduction in cardiovascular disease (124). Replacing saturated fats with carbohydrates can reduce total and LDL cholesterol, yet also decrease HDL cholesterol and increase triglycerides—this strategy will not decrease risk of cardiovascular disease. More clinical trials are needed to determine how replacing saturated fat with different types of carbohydrate (whole grains as opposed to sugar, for instance) affects risk factors for cardiovascular disease. Studies examining the association (these studies cannot determine cause and effect) between different types of carbohydrate and cardiovascular disease risk show higher intakes of whole grains are associated with lower risk of coronary heart disease, whereas refined starches and added sugars are positively associated with coronary heart disease risk. Given the state of the current evidence, whenever possible, foods high in saturated fats should be replaced with foods higher in polyunsaturated fats or whole grains (63, 124).

Though saturated fat should be replaced with polyunsaturated fats and monounsaturated fats, there are distinct differences in types of fatty acids. The atherogenic (artery clogging) potential of specific saturated fatty acids varies depending on carbon chain length (table 4.1), fats eaten concurrently, overall diet, carbohydrate intake,

and overall health (44). Saturated fat is listed on the food label.

Monounsaturated Fatty Acids

There is no known requirement or health benefit associated with the consumption of monounsaturated fatty acids. Monounsaturated fats can be synthesized by the body (90). As noted in the previous section, some research shows replacing saturated fat with monounsaturated fats lowers total and LDL cholesterol (57, 70). Monounsaturated fat can also increase HDL and lower triglycerides compared to carbohydrates (106). The average American diet contains more monounsaturated fats than saturated or polyunsaturated fats. The monounsaturated fatty acid oleic acid is the most abundant fatty acid in the American diet (122).

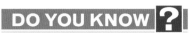

DO YOU KNOW ?

Monounsaturated fat supplements are available alone and in mixtures with omega-3 and omega-6 fatty acids. There is no reason to take these supplements (131).

Polyunsaturated Fatty Acids

The omega-6 polyunsaturated fatty acid LA and omega-3 polyunsaturated fatty acid ALA are required in small amounts for structural integrity and fluidity of membrane lipids, synthesis of **eicosanoids** (hormone-like agents), and as substrates for biological pathways that produce metabolic products necessary for structural and functional roles within the human body (figure 4.8) (4, 25).

Omega-6 Fatty Acids

Omega-6 fatty acids are important to epithelial cell function and regulation of gene expression (130). Epithelial cells are "barrier cells" that make up epithelial tissue, which lines most of the body's surfaces, including the skin, blood vessels, and organs. Linoleic acid is the only essential omega-6 fatty acid; the body cannot make this fatty acid, so it must be consumed in the diet. Insufficient LA can lead to scaly rash and reduced growth. In developed countries, linoleic acid deficiency is not

Table 4.1 Types of Fatty Acids Found in Common Foods

Fatty acid	Common food sources (not all inclusive)
CIS POLYUNSATURATED FATTY ACIDS (PUFA)	
Omega-3 PUFAs	
Alpha-linolenic acid (ALA)	Flaxseeds, chia seeds, walnuts, canola oil, soybean oil, flaxseed oil
Stearidonic acid (SDA)	Sardines, herring, algae, GMO soybean oil
Eicosapentaenoic acid (EPA)	Seafood, especially fatty fish such as salmon, mackerel, herring, and halibut
Docosapentaenoic acid (DPA)	Seafood, especially fatty fish such as salmon, mackerel, herring, and halibut
Docosahexaenoic acid (DHA)	Seafood, especially fatty fish such as salmon, mackerel, herring, and halibut
Omega-6 PUFAs	
Linoleic acid (LA)	Soybean oil, corn oil, meat, sunflower oil, safflower oil
Gamma linolenic acid (GLA)	Black currant seed oil, evening primrose oil
Arachidonic acid (ARA)	Meat, poultry, eggs
CIS MONOUNSATURATED FATTY ACIDS (MUFA)	
Palmitoleic acid	Macadamia nuts, sea buckthorn oil, some blue-green algae
Oleic acid*	Olive oil, canola oil, beef tallow, lard, avocado
Erucic acid	Available in low quantities in food, including rapeseed, kale, and broccoli
TRANS FATTY ACIDS (UNSATURATED)	
Elaidic acid**	Partially hydrogenated vegetable oils
Vaccenic acid**	Butterfat, meat
Conjugated linoleic acid (CLA)**	Ruminant meat, dairy, CLA supplements; food typically contains more cis 9, trans 11 18:2, whereas supplements often contain an equal mix of both isomers
SATURATED FATTY ACIDS (SFA)	
Caprylic acid (MCT)	Coconut oil, palm kernel oil
Capric acid (MCT)	Coconut oil, palm kernel oil
Lauric acid (MCT)	Coconut oil, palm kernel oil
Myristic acid	Several types of cheese, coconut meat, coconut oil, beef fat
Palmitic acid	Beef, pork, and bacon fat; butter; several types of cheese; whipped cream; whole milk; egg yolks; palm oil; palm kernel oil; most fats and oils contain some palmitic acid
Stearic acid	Beef and pork fat; Brazil nuts; lamb; cashew nuts; fully hydrogenated vegetable oil

GMO = genetically modified organism; MCTs = medium-chain triglycerides.

*Oleic acid is the most common monounsaturated fatty acid, accounting for approximately 92 percent of MUFAs found in the diet.

**In high doses (3.7% of calorie intake), trans fatty acids from industrial sources and naturally occurring trans fatty acids both increase LDL cholesterol and decrease HDL cholesterol (76).

Based on Vannice 2014; U.S. Department of Agriculture 2013; U.S. Institute of Medicine 2002.

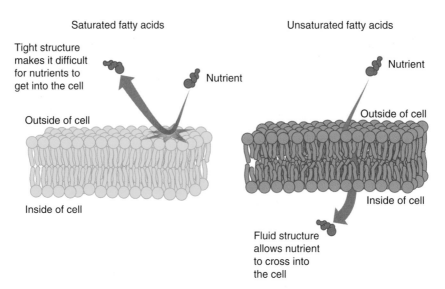

Figure 4.8 Cell membrane.

only rare, but also most adults consume several times more linoleic acid than they need (130). LA is a precursor for arachidonic acid, a fatty acid that is a part of membrane structural lipids, serves as a substrate for eicosanoid production, and is necessary for cell signaling pathways (90, 130). However, arachidonic acid can also lead to an inflammatory cascade in the body (59).

Omega-3 Fatty Acids

Three primary omega-3 fatty acids are consumed in the diet: alpha-linolenic acid (ALA), **eicosapentaenoic acid (EPA)**, and **docosahexaenoic acid (DHA)** (figure 4.9). Each omega-3 fatty acid has a different role in the body and impact on health. **Stearidonic acid (SDA)** is an omega-3 fatty acid found in some seed oils; some fish, including sardines and herring; algae; and GMO (genet-

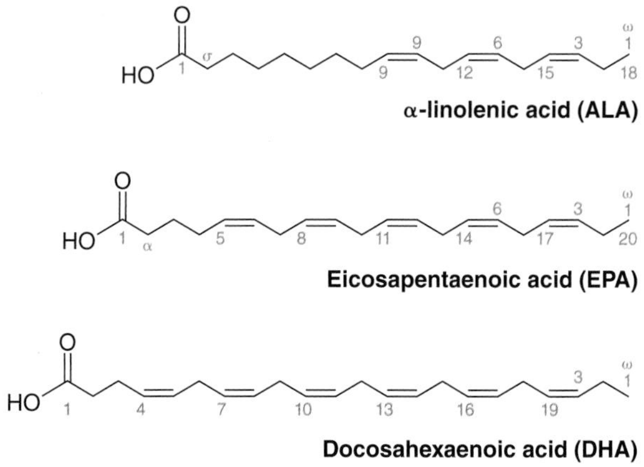

Figure 4.9 Structure of ALA, EPA, and DHA, all polyunsaturated fatty acids. ALA has 18 carbons and 3 double bonds, EPA has 20 carbons and 5 double bonds, and DHA has 22 carbons and 6 double bonds.

PUTTING IT INTO PERSPECTIVE

HOW FAT AFFECTS CELL MEMBRANES AND CELL FUNCTIONING

Fats are incorporated into cell membranes, and both saturated fat and unsaturated fat are necessary for optimal cell membrane functioning. Saturated fatty acids stack neatly on top of each other in cell membranes. If a membrane were composed of all, or mostly, saturated fatty acids, the tight structure would make it difficult for nutrients to get into cells, compromising cell health and increasing the likelihood of cell injury. Unsaturated fats do not pack neatly on top of each other in cell membranes. They provide a more fluid structure, allowing nutrients to easily cross the cell membrane into the cell and allowing receptors in nerve cells to recognize neurotransmitters (chemical messengers).

ically modified organisms) soybeans used to create SDA-enriched soybean oil (126, 135). SDA-enriched soybean oil increases red blood cell EPA to a greater extent than ALA, though much less than taking EPA directly (60, 135). Compared to taking EPA directly, conversion of SDA to EPA from SDA-enriched soybean oil is about 17 percent efficient, according to a study in healthy, overweight adults (35). At this rate of conversion, SDA does not improve blood lipids, including triglycerides and HDL cholesterol (60). Consuming SDA does not increase tissue levels of DHA (35, 49). At this time it is not clear if consuming SDA has any independent effect on cardiovascular disease risk factors or other aspects of health.

Alpha-Linolenic Acid Alpha-linolenic acid is found in soybeans, soybean oil, canola oil, flaxseed oil, black walnuts, flaxseeds, and chia seeds (123). ALA has no known function in the body other than serving as a precursor to EPA and DHA (5, 90). However, ALA deficiency can

result in scaly dermatitis (130). ALA-rich foods are beneficial for cardiovascular disease risk as a result of the ALA, other compounds found in these foods, or a synergistic effect between the ALA and these compounds (28, 77). Compared to EPA and DHA, there is much less research-based evidence suggesting ALA is beneficial for cardiovascular disease risk (28). ALA is converted into EPA and DHA in the body. However, studies show only 5 to 21 percent of ALA is converted to EPA, and less than 0.5 to 9 percent of ALA is converted to DHA (18, 93). Diet, health status, genetics, gender, and fatty acid competition for elongase and desaturase enzymes (figure 4.10) influence the conversion rate (131).

Eicosapentaenoic Acid and Docosahexaenoic acid Sources of EPA and DHA in the diet include fatty fish such as salmon, mackerel, herring, and halibut. Supplemental sources of EPA and DHA are typically sourced from sardines, anchovies, and some types of algae and krill.

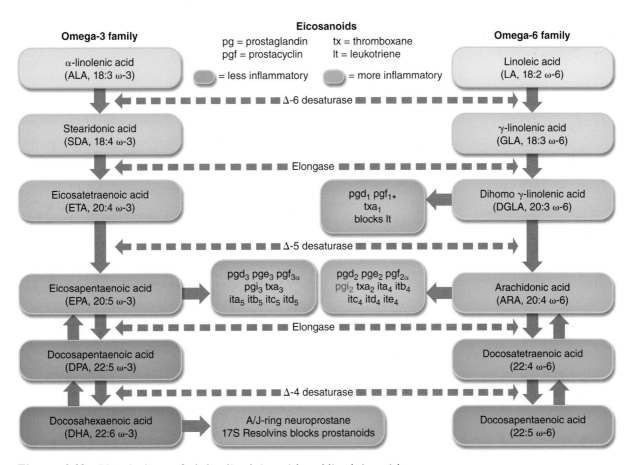

Figure 4.10 Metabolism of alpha-linoleic acid and linoleic acid.

At the top of the food chain there is increased risk of mercury contamination among certain fish. Shark, king mackerel, swordfish and tilefish tend to live longer and feed on smaller fish, accumulating more methylmercury over their lifetime (figure 4.11). These fish should be avoided, especially by pregnant women, children, the elderly, and those with a compromised immune system (129).

EPA and DHA have distinct roles in the body. EPA is a precursor to eicosanoids, including a group of eicosanoids (series-3 prostaglandins) that may be protective against heart attacks and strokes. EPA helps decrease inflammation by inhibiting the production of pro-inflammatory compounds. DHA is the major fat found in the brain and important for brain development and function. DHA is necessary for the production of compounds that help reduce inflammation in the brain from reduced blood flow (strokes for instance). In addition to their distinct roles, together, EPA and DHA decrease triglycerides in a dose-dependent manner (triglycerides decrease in greater amounts with more fish oil consumed) (24), increase HDL cholesterol (24), improve blood vessel functioning (85), reduce inflammation (62), and lead to a small decrease in blood pressure (72).

Population-based studies and randomized controlled trials examining cardiovascular health and fatty fish or EPA and DHA indicate the following:

> Consuming small amounts of fish is associated with a 27 percent decrease in risk of nonfatal heart attack (56).

> Consuming at least one serving of fish per week is associated with a reduced risk of sudden death from coronary heart disease (CHD) (137) and a 17 percent decrease in risk of CHD mortality, while each additional serving per week decreases risk an additional 3.9 percent (56).

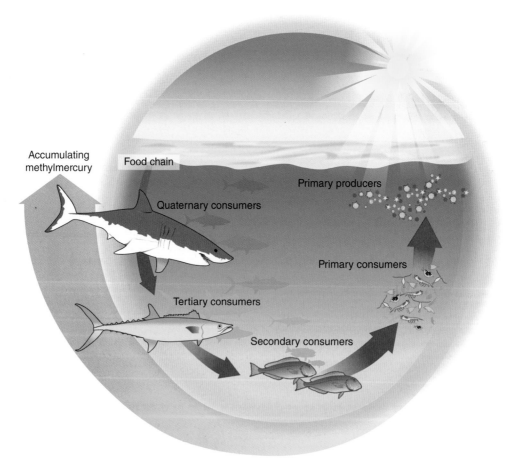

Figure 4.11 Fish that live longer and eat smaller fish contain more methylmercury.

> Consuming fish at least once per week is also associated with a decrease in CHD death rate when compared to never eating fish, while consuming fish five or more times per week is associated with a 38 percent decrease in CHD mortality (38).

> A pooled analysis of randomized controlled trials found one to two servings of fatty fish per week or approximately 250 mg of EPA plus DHA per day resulted in a 36 percent decrease in CHD death (78).

> Modest consumption of fish (one or two servings per week or approximately 250 mg of EPA plus DHA per day) reduces risk of CHD by 36 percent and all-cause mortality by 17 percent (82).

> Two weekly servings of fatty fish reduced risk of death by ischemic heart disease and reduced all-cause mortality by 29 percent in men with a previous history of heart attack (20).

> One capsule containing 850 EPA and DHA reduced the risk of all-cause mortality, sudden death, and coronary death in adults with a recent history of heart attack compared to no intervention (31).

> 850 to 882 mg EPA and DHA reduced incidence of death and CHD hospitalizations in those with heart failure (116).

Though some studies found EPA and DHA do not affect cardiovascular disease risk or events, a number of factors might have influenced the results of these studies, including low levels of supplementation; a short duration of study; higher baseline dietary omega-3 intake of the population studied (a higher intake before the start of the study will decrease the potential impact of supplementation); and improvements in cardiovascular disease care and therapies, including use of statin drugs (which lower blood cholesterol), which may mask the effects of EPA and DHA (16, 34, 48, 58, 66, 95, 133, 144).

Omega-3 Fatty Acids and Joint Health, Sport, and Exercise EPA and DHA improve joint functioning, particularly in those with rheumatoid arthritis; decrease the damaging effects caused by concussions (in rat studies); and appear to help reduce excess soreness after muscle-damaging exercise in untrained individuals. In addition, studies show EPA and DHA can improve muscle mass and muscle functioning in older adults.

According to a meta-analysis of 17 randomized, controlled trials, EPA and DHA supplementation, in doses ranging from 1.7 to 9.6 grams per day for 3 to 4 months, reduced patient-reported joint pain intensity, minutes of morning stiffness, and number of painful and/or tender joints in those with inflammatory joint pain from rheumatoid arthritis, inflammatory bowel disease, or painful menstruation (32). Additional research shows EPA and DHA supplementation decreased global assessments of pain and disease activity, while also decreasing the need for nonsteroidal anti-inflammatory drugs in those with rheumatoid arthritis (71).

DO YOU KNOW ❓

It is currently unclear if there is an ideal ratio of omega-6 to omega-3 fatty acids for health or human performance. In any case, most Americans consume plenty of omega-6 fatty acids, while many need to consume more omega-3 fatty acids.

There are several mechanisms through which EPA and DHA may benefit recovery after a concussion (a type of traumatic brain injury). DHA makes up 97 percent of the omega-3 fatty acids in the brain and is essential for normal brain functioning (103). EPA and DHA increase fluidity of cell membranes, reduce inflammation, and increase blood flow to the brain. Concussion causes a reduction in blood flow to the brain for up to a month or longer (68). Cell membrane fluidity is important because membranes that are more fluid allow substances to more easily enter cells. Several animal studies show EPA and DHA supplementation before or after a traumatic brain injury helps limit structural damage and a decline in brain functioning (73, 74, 138, 140-143).

A randomized double-blind placebo-controlled trial in healthy older adults found 6 months of supplementation with omega-3 fatty acids (1.86 g of EPA plus 1.50 g of DHA—equivalent to 200 to 400 g of fatty fish) increased muscle mass (thigh muscle volume) and function (handgrip strength, 1 RM strength composite score for leg press, chest press, knee extension, and knee flexion). Compared to the control group, the group supplemented with omega-3 fatty acids had a 3.5 percent improvement in muscle volume and a 6 percent improvement in muscle strength. It isn't clear how the fish oil supplements improve muscle mass (110). An older study by the same authors found omega-3 fatty acids augment increases in muscle protein synthesis in older adults (109). In addition, the authors suggest omega-3 fatty acids may improve mitochondrial functioning in muscle (110). It is not clear if younger adults will experience the same muscle-related benefits as older adults.

Untrained individuals may also benefit from omega-3s. When taken for 30 days before and 48 hours after eccentric exercise, omega-3s helped decrease inflammatory markers of muscle damage in untrained individuals, suggesting a decrease in inflammation. However, the study did not measure actual inflammation-related muscle damage (115). Two other studies found EPA plus DHA decreased muscle soreness after exercise. In one study, 24 men were given 600 mg of EPA and 260 mg DHA per day for 8 weeks prior to exercise and 5 days after. Compared to the placebo, the supplement group had greater muscle functioning and range of motion for several days after the exercise. Three days after the exercise, muscle soreness was also greater in the placebo group compared to the supplemented group. These results suggest, when consumed regularly, omega-3s might help decrease muscle damage and soreness, thereby allowing for greater range of motion, improved muscle functioning, and, thus, better workouts in the days after a damaging bout of exercise. However, these results may be applicable only to those who are engaging in a very damaging bout

of eccentric exercise that they are not used to performing (and therefore not adapted to through regular training). In this study, the subjects were healthy men who were not engaging in strenuous exercise, while the exercise itself was not an activity commonly performed in everyday life: five sets of six repetitions of bicep exercises at maximal weight (119). In another study, healthy male athletes who competed in summer Olympic sports for 2 years or more, trained over 12 hours a week, and did not regularly consume fish were given omega-3 plus vitamin D supplements (375 mg EPA, 230 DPA, 510 DHA, 1000 IU vitamin D_3) or 5 ml of olive oil as a placebo for 21 days. During this time, they continued their regular training program and were asked to refrain from eating more than three servings of fish per week and not to take any additional omega-3 supplements. After the 21 days, plasma EPA was higher in the supplemented group, though EPA and DHA were not significantly different. The only positive effect noted in the omega-3 supplement group was a suggested improvement in neuromuscular functioning (61).

Trans Fatty Acids

Trans fatty acids are unsaturated fatty acids, though they behave differently from other unsaturated fatty acids (90). Two trans fatty acids—vaccenic aid and elaidic acid—are made by bacteria in the rumen (one of the four chambers of the ruminant stomach) of ruminant animals (animals that have a stomach with four complete chambers or cavities; cows, goats, and sheep are ruminant animals) from polyunsaturated fatty acids. These trans fatty acids are found in beef and dairy

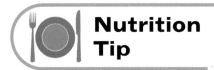

Nutrition Tip

Omega-3 supplements, in doses up to 3 grams per day, are generally recognized as safe (125). Supplemental fish oil does not increase risk for clinically significant bleeding (134). However, doses over 3 grams per day should only be taken under the care and guidance of a medical doctor. Though there is some absorption of EPA and DHA on an empty stomach, for greater absorption, EPA and DHA should be taken with a meal. Adverse side effects related to fish oil or ALA supplements are typically minor (such as diarrhea) and resolved by lowering the dose or discontinuing the supplement (136).

products. Trans fatty acids make up less than 9 percent of ruminant fat (7, 88). The majority of trans fatty acids found in the diet are produced from partial hydrogenation of oils. Hydrogenation involves bubbling hydrogen gas through edible oils in the presence of high heat and a catalyst (22). Partial hydrogenation converts some of the unsaturated fatty acids to saturated fatty acids, and some of the unsaturated fatty acids from a cis (hydrogen atoms on the same side of the double bond) to a trans configuration (hydrogen atoms are on opposite sides of the double bond) (figure 4.12). Hydrogenated oils are more resistant to spoilage and rancidity (124). Modifying the conditions of hydrogenation alters the amount of trans fatty acids formed, which affects the properties of the end product (solid or semi-solid, melting point, mouth feel, etc.) (22). The chemical configuration of trans fatty acids lets them pack neatly on top of each other, forming a semi-solid to solid compound.

DO YOU KNOW ?

Man-made trans fatty acids are the worst type of dietary fat; even small amounts increase cardiovascular disease risk. No amount of trans fat is considered safe for consumption.

Industrial Trans Fatty Acids

Clinical trials show industrial-produced (i.e., man-made) trans fatty acids negatively affect several risk factors for coronary heart disease, while observational studies show an association between industrial trans fatty acid consumption and increased risk for coronary heart disease (79). Trans fatty acids from partially hydrogenated oils increase LDL cholesterol, reduce HDL cholesterol, and reduce LDL particle size, all risk factors for coronary heart disease (8, 10, 52, 64, 80). Some, though not all, studies suggest trans fatty acids increase triglycerides (9, 80). Trans fatty acids from partially hydrogenated oils also increase inflammation (11) and were found in a randomized trial in overweight postmenopausal women to increase body fat more than other dietary fats (10).

Given the abundance of data indicating that man-made trans fatty acids are harmful for health, in 2015 the FDA removed generally recognized as safe (GRAS) status for partially hydrogenated oils (127). Manufacturers and restaurants have reduced use of industrially produced trans fatty acids in foods over the past several years. However, as of 2016, trans fatty acids were still found in some processed foods, including desserts,

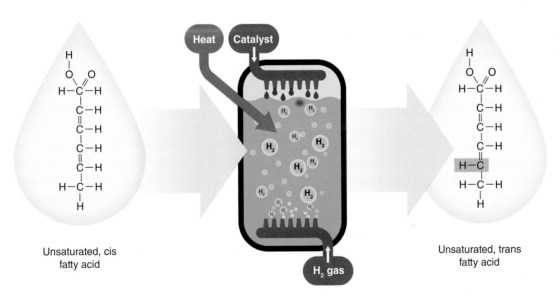

Figure 4.12 Unsaturated fats, which are liquid at room temperature, are made solid by bubbling hydrogen gas through them with a catalyst at a high temperature.

microwave popcorn, frozen pizzas, margarines, and coffee creamers (124).

Trans Fatty Acids in Dairy and Meat

Trans fatty acids make up 2 to 5 percent of total fatty acids in dairy products and 3 to 9 percent of total fatty acids in beef and lamb (table 4.2) (7, 88). The amount varies based on feeding practices and geographical and seasonal changes (88, 94).

Total daily intake of vaccenic acid and c9, t11-CLA ranges from 0.4 to 0.8 grams per day and 0.14 to 0.33 grams per day, respectively (120). In the human body, vaccenic acid can be converted to c9, t11-CLA. The conversion rate ranges from 0 to greater than 30 percent, with an average of 19 percent (1, 26, 75, 120). Therefore, estimation of dietary intake of c9, t11-CLA alone may not reflect the synthesis of CLA from the vaccenic acid in the body (120).

DO YOU KNOW ?

According to the World Health Organization, observational studies suggest ruminant trans fatty acids (those found in dairy and meat) do not increase coronary heart disease risk in typical amounts consumed (22, 86).

It isn't clear what effect, if any, ruminant trans fatty acids, vaccenic acid, and elaidic acid have on cardiovascular disease risk factors. The data are mixed, possibly because of differences in study design. However, some studies suggest that lower doses of ruminant trans fatty acids do not affect lipids in lipoprotein, but at higher doses, which are not attainable through diet but instead through supplemental intake, these fatty acids may have effects similar to man-made trans fatty acids, increasing LDL and decreasing HDL (30).

In a very well-designed, double-blind crossover study in healthy men, four different experimental diets (all contained 2,500 calories; all food was provided) were given to participants for 4 weeks: (1) high in ruminant trans fats (10.2 g; butter and milk specifically designed for this study to contain high amounts of trans fatty acids), (2) moderate in ruminate trans fats (4.2 g), (3) high in industrial (man-made) trans fats (10.2 g), and (4) low in trans fats from any source (2.2 g). High intake of trans fats, whether from ruminants or industrially produced, increased LDL. Also, HDL cholesterol concentrations were significantly lower after the diet high in ruminant trans fats compared to the diet containing a moderate amount of ruminant trans fats. There was no significant difference in changes in cholesterol between the diet containing a moderate amount of ruminant trans fat and the diet containing low trans fats from any source. This study suggests moderate amounts of trans fats from dairy will not have a substantial effect on blood cholesterol. But trans fats, whether from dairy or industrial production of partially hydrogenated oils, are not heart healthy when consumed in high amounts. Note that the high amount of ruminant trans fats used in this study were beyond the amount of typical human consumption (76).

Supplemental CLA is discussed in more detail in chapter 9.

Interesterified Fats

Interesterified fats have been used for decades in margarines, cooking oils, and infant formulas (145). Interesterification typically involves blending fats high in saturated fatty acids, which are solid at room temperature, with liquid edible oils (114). Interesterification leads to chemical

Table 4.2 Trans Fatty Acid and Conjugated Linoleic Acid Content of Dairy and Meat

Food	TFA content per serving	CLA content per serving
Cheddar cheese, 1 oz.	240 mg	36.7 mg
Milk, whole, 1 cup	210 mg	41.6 mg
Yogurt, plain, low-fat, 1 cup	60 mg	37.8 mg
Meat, beef, ground, 20.8% fat, raw, 4 oz.	910 mg	103.8 mg

Data from Gebauer 2011.

or enzymatic rearrangement of fatty acids along the glycerol backbone. By altering the chemical structure of a fat and inserting a saturated fatty acid (typically stearic acid), interesterification produces customized fats ranging in melting points and solidity to fit the needs of various food preparations (22).

No trans fatty acids are formed during the production of **interesterified fats**. Though older studies suggested interesterified fats do not affect blood lipids, any untoward health effects might depend on the type of fatty acid inserted and where it is inserted (12, 43, 69, 87). Altering the position of fatty acids along the glycerol backbone may affect lipoprotein metabolism and atherogenesis (37). Additionally, the type of interesterification—chemical or enzymatic—and weight status of the person consuming the fat—obese or nonobese—may determine how interesterified fats affect blood lipids. In a randomized crossover study, obese and nonobese adults consumed 50 grams of carbohydrate from white bread in addition to 1 gram of fat per kilogram body mass of (1) noninteresterified stearic acid-rich fat spread, (2) chemically interesterified stearic acid-rich fat spread, (3) enzymatically interesterified stearic acid-rich fat spread or (4) no fat. Interesterification had no effect on post-meal blood glucose, insulin, free fatty acids, or cholesterol in either group. However, obese subjects had an 85 percent increase in triglycerides after consuming the fat that was modified through chemical interesterification compared to noninteresterification. Nonobese subjects' triglycerides were not affected by either fat treatment. Given the extremely large consumption of fat in one sitting, 91 grams for a 200-pound adult, it is unclear if the results would be different when given lower quantities of the chemically interesterified fat in a meal (98).

A 4-week, crossover study examined the effects of different fats on blood lipids and blood glucose when incorporated into a whole-food diet, including a man-made trans-fat rich partially hydrogenated soybean oil (containing 3.2% trans fat), palm olein (an unmodified fat naturally rich in saturated fat), and an interesterified fat. Both the partially hydrogenated soybean oil and interesterified fat decreased HDL compared to the palm olien and

increased fasting blood glucose (almost 20% in the interesterified group). The interesterified fat meal led to a significant rise in post-meal blood glucose (113). Though the results of this study may lead one to believe all interesterified fats are harmful for blood glucose and insulin, the effect a modified fat has on glucose and insulin might depend on the position of the fatty acids and the health status of the study subjects. In a crossover trial, healthy men and women aged 20 to 50 years were fed a controlled diet (providing the same percentage of macronutrients and foods) containing (1) palm olein, (2) interesterified palm oil, or (3) high oleic acid sunflower oil, for 6 weeks each. The interesterified palm oil did not adversely impair insulin secretion or glucose (27). It remains unclear at this time if any long-term health effects are associated with consuming interesterified fats (55).

DIETARY RECOMMENDATIONS

The AI for dietary fat for infants up to 6 months of age and from 6 to 12 months of age is 31 and 30 grams per day, respectively. Inadequate fat intake can lead to poor growth (130). There is no AI, RDA, or UL for dietary fat for anyone above 12 months of age because of a lack of data regarding risk of inadequacy, prevention of chronic disease, or a known dietary fat intake level at which a person will experience adverse health effects (90). If a diet contains adequate calories, carbohydrate can serve as an energy source in place of dietary fat (130). As mentioned in chapter 1, the acceptable macronutrient distribution range (AMDR) for dietary fat is 20 to 35 percent of energy. The lower end of this range was set based on concern of decreased HDL cholesterol and increased triglycerides following a low-fat, high-carbohydrate diet, while the upper end of the range allows for adequate intake of other nutrients (130). Some populations following low-fat diets have a low rate of chronic disease (90).

As of the latest DRI report for fat (2002), no DRI is available for MUFAs, saturated fat, cholesterol, or trans fatty acids (130). The Dietary Guidelines for Americans 2015–2020 recommend consuming less than 10 percent of calories from saturated fat based on evidence showing that replacement of saturated fats with unsaturated fats reduces risk of cardiovascular disease (124). Monounsaturated fat should comprise up to 20 percent of total calorie intake (83). The guidelines do not include a recommendation for cholesterol, though the report refers to the Institute of Medicine recommendations to eat as little dietary cholesterol as possible (124).

An AI is available for the essential fatty acids (both polyunsaturated fats) linoleic acid and alpha-linolenic acid. The AI for linoleic acid (an omega-6 polyunsaturated fatty acid) ranges from 4.4 grams per day in infants 0 to 6 months of age to 13 grams per day in pregnant and lactating women. The lower end of the range was set based on an amount at which deficiency does not exist in healthy individuals. The upper end of the range was set based on a lack of evidence of long-term safety and cell studies showing increased lipid peroxidation (breakdown of lipids) and free radicals formed with higher intakes. Lipid peroxidation is considered a potential component in the development of plaque in arteries (130). The AI for alpha-linolenic acid (an omega-3 polyunsaturated fatty acid) ranges from 0.5 grams per day in infants 0 to 12 months of age to 1.6 grams per day in males over the age of 14. The AMDR ranges from 0.6 to 1.2 grams per day for people of all ages. The AMDR is based on maintaining a balance of omega-6 fatty acids, lack of long-term safety data, and cell studies performed in a lab that showed increased free radical production and lipid peroxidation with higher intakes of omega-6 fatty acids (130). The DRIs do not include a recommendation for EPA or DHA. Some organizations list recommendations for EPA plus DHA or fatty fish. For instance, the World Health Organization recommends 250 mg per day EPA and DHA for adults (51). The American Heart Association recommends eating at least two 3.5-ounce servings of fatty fish per week (3).

> **DO YOU KNOW ?**
>
> Any incremental intake of industrially produced trans fatty acids increases the risk of coronary heart disease (130), thus there is no safe level of intake of trans fatty acids (124).

DIGESTION AND METABOLISM

Dietary fat digestion starts in the mouth with the enzyme lingual lipase, but this part of the digestion process is minor. When dietary fat enters the small intestine, the gallbladder releases bile, and the pancreas releases lipases. Bile mixes partially digested fat so enzymes can further hydrolyze (break down) the fat into free fatty acids, glycerol, cholesterol, and phospholipids, all of which are almost completely absorbed into the intestinal lining.

After absorption, free fatty acids, glycerol, cholesterol, and phospholipids are packaged into chylomicrons. Chylomicrons are a type of lipoprotein composed of 85 to 92 percent triglycerides, 6 to 12 percent phospholipids, 1 to 3 percent cholesterol, and 1 to 2 percent protein. Chylomicrons are triglyceride-transport vehicles (45). Chylomicrons leave the small intestine and eventually enter the blood, where the enzyme lipoprotein lipase takes them apart. The fatty acids are delivered to fat cells for storage or muscle cells for energy. Some fat and cholesterol are held by fiber and exit the body through feces.

Because of their shorter carbon chain length, short-chain fatty acids and medium-chain saturated fatty acids (referred to as **medium-chain triglycerides**, or **MCTs**) are not converted to chylomicrons. Medium-chain triglycerides are absorbed in the blood and transported to the liver, where they are quickly broken down into fatty acids and glycerol. Supplemental medium-chain triglycerides can cause gastrointestinal side effects, including abdominal cramps, diarrhea, and nausea (65, 132).

Storing Fat in Adipose Tissue

All energy-yielding macronutrients—carbohydrate, protein, and fat—can be stored as body fat. When more calories are consumed than are burned, excess is stored in adipose tissue (body fat) for later use. The enzyme lipoprotein lipase breaks down triglycerides from lipoproteins in the bloodstream. Fatty acids, diglycerides, and monoglycerides are delivered to adipose cells,

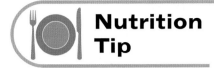

where enzymes reassemble these parts into triglycerides for storage (25). While the majority of excess fat is stored in adipose tissue (fat tissue), small amounts are stored in skeletal muscle (105).

Using Body Fat

Skeletal muscle and adipose tissue, as well as the heart, lungs, kidney, and liver, break down stored body fat. Stored triglycerides are degraded into free fatty acids and glycerol by the enzyme lipoprotein lipase. The fatty acids are transported in the blood and taken up by cells. Most of the cells in the human body can oxidize fatty acids to produce energy, but the brain and nervous tissue cannot use fatty acids for fuel. The fatty acids can also be repackaged into triglyceride molecules and stored until needed. The glycerol released from the breakdown of body fat is transported to the liver, where a phosphate is added. The resulting compound can be used as triglyceride by the liver or be converted into a compound that enters glycolysis or gluconeogenesis (25).

DIETARY FATS AND EXERCISE

Although the human body has a limited capacity to store carbohydrate, fat stores are vast, even in lean athletes, providing enough energy to fuel several back-to-back marathons (36). For instance, a 160-pound athlete with 4 percent body fat has approximately 22,400 calories stored in fat tissue (33). Despite significant fat reserves in the human body, fat is a slow source of fuel; it takes time and requires oxygen to break down fat—a process called lipolysis—for use as energy during exercise. At rest and during low-intensity exercise (walking for instance), fat is the primary source of energy used (100). Low-intensity exercise is not calorically demanding; the body does not need as many calories to walk as it does to run. Thus the rate of fat breakdown can easily meet energy needs during low-intensity exercise. As exercise intensity increases from low to moderate, the amount of fat released from adipose tissue into the bloodstream decreases, while intramuscular triglyceride use increases (91). Increasing intensity from moderate to high decreases the percentage of fat used as energy, while carbohydrate (from glycogen and glucose) use increases.

DO YOU KNOW ?

Consuming more calories than needed drives the storage of fat in adipose cells. However, the acute (i.e., short term, such as after a large meal) storage of fat is not as important as calorie balance over time. Even if more calories are consumed than needed over the course of a few hours or a day, the body will pull fat from adipose tissue for energy during periods when fewer calories are consumed than needed.

Though higher-intensity exercise shifts fuel use from fat to carbohydrate as the preferred source of energy, training and diet also influence the type of energy used. Consistent aerobic training increases the muscle's capacity to use fat as a source of energy (50). In addition to training, the body will adapt to greater reliance on fat for energy when a higher-fat, lower-carbohydrate diet is consumed consistently over a period of time (39, 50). Adapting to a

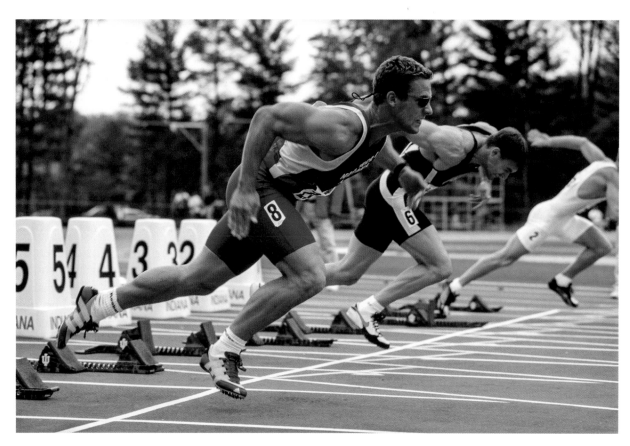

There is no known performance advantage to a high-fat, low-carbohydrate diet; in fact, this strategy is detrimental to athletes engaging in high-intensity activity.

higher-fat, lower-carbohydrate diet does not necessarily translate to improved performance (42, 92, 97, 102). In addition, training with low glycogen stores can suppress immune and central nervous system functioning (19, 39).

SUMMARY

Dietary fats and oils are sources of energy and aid in the absorption of fat-soluble vitamins A, D, E, and K, as well as certain food components such as carotenoids. However, only two types of fatty acids—linoleic acid (LA) and alpha-linolenic acid (ALA)—are considered essential, while the human body can make other fatty acids as needed. Small amounts of LA and ALA are necessary for the structural integrity of cell membranes, synthesis of eicosanoids, and cellular communication. Although not considered essential, because the body can make them from ALA (though this process is inefficient), EPA and DHA are beneficial for cardiovascular health. EPA and DHA also help decrease inflammation, and DHA is necessary for optimal brain development and function. Emerging evidence supports a role for EPA and DHA in joint health, particularly for those with rheumatoid arthritis, decreasing inflammation and restoring muscle function after damaging bouts of resistance exercise in untrained individuals, and improving strength and muscle mass in the elderly.

Industrially produced trans fats, found in partially hydrogenated oils, are harmful. Man-made trans fats also have a negative impact on cholesterol, yet they are not consumed in large amounts in the diet and are thus considered safe in the amounts typically consumed. Certain saturated fatty acids increase LDL and total cholesterol risk factors for cardiovascular disease. Substituting polyunsaturated fatty acids for saturated fat can help lower total cholesterol and LDL cholesterol, a strategy associated with a reduction in heart attacks and death from heart attacks and improved insulin sensitivity.

Excess calories from protein, carbohydrate, or fat can be stored in fat tissue. However, excess calories coming from dietary fat are more likely to be stored as body fat. Although fat can be used as a source of energy during exercise, it is a slow source and can thus meet energy demands only during low-intensity exercise. There is no known performance advantage to a high-fat, low-carbohydrate diet; in fact, this strategy is detrimental to athletes engaging in high-intensity activity.

■ FOR REVIEW ▶

1. How does saturated fat affect risk factors for cardiovascular disease?
2. Should saturated fat be replaced in the diet? If so, with what nutrients and why?
3. How does high blood cholesterol affect risk for cardiovascular disease?
4. What factors influence how much fat is used during exercise?
5. Why are the essential fatty acids important for health?
6. Describe the cardiovascular benefits associated with fatty fish and fish oil supplements.
7. How does overeating dietary fat compare to overeating carbohydrate?
8. Describe how EPA and DHA can influence muscle.
9. Where is stearidonic acid (SDA) found? Is SDA beneficial for health?

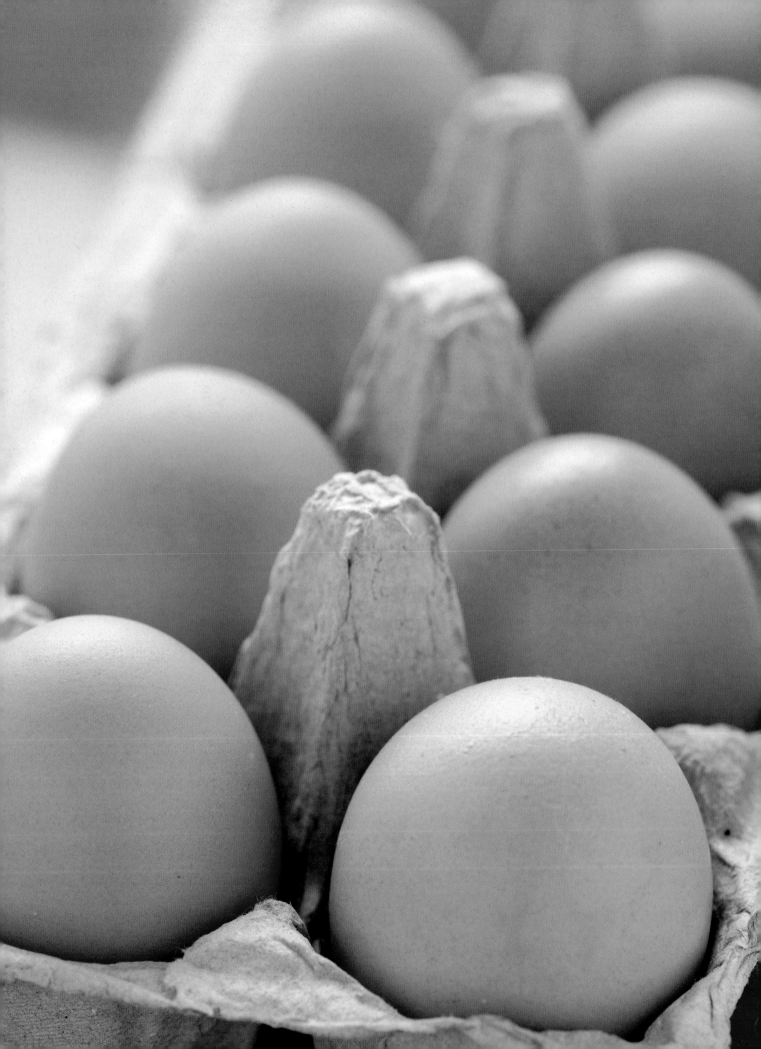

CHAPTER 5

Protein

After completing this chapter, you will be able to do the following:

> Explain the types and basic functions of amino acids.

> Outline the classification of proteins.

> Explain the digestion, absorption, and metabolism of proteins.

> Describe the metabolic fates of proteins.

> Summarize the concepts and factors affecting protein synthesis.

> Describe the differences between general protein guidelines and those for athletes.

> Define vegetarianism and veganism, and explain how these dietary practices affect athletes.

Foods from both animals and plants contain dietary protein. Protein helps build structures in the body and is involved in multiple chemical reactions. The body is efficient at recycling amino acids from proteins broken down through the body. However, this process cannot meet all of the human body's amino acid needs, so dietary protein is necessary to prevent excess breakdown of protein in skeletal muscle to meet the need for amino acids. In this chapter we describe several aspects of protein from amino acid and protein classification to digestion, absorption, and metabolism. We also delve into the unique protein needs of those who are physically active and how dietary protein can be manipulated to support health, training adaptations, and competition goals of athletes. Finally, we look at vegetarianism, veganism, and other dietary practices and their implications for athletes.

AMINO ACIDS

Amino acids are the building blocks of protein and make up the sequences of peptide bonds to form protein structures (figure 5.1). In biochemistry, there are multiple ways to classify hundreds of amino acids and simple compounds made of amino acids found in nature. In human nutrition, the primary way to classify amino acids is based on the amino acid's ability to create proteins or serve as precursors to proteins. These amino acids are referred to as **proteinogenic**, and 23 amino acids fit this classification, of which 20 are used by the human body to make a variety of proteins that work to properly support all structure and function in human physiology. With the exception of the amino acid proline, all amino acids contain carbon and are considered organic compounds. These amino acids are comprised of a nitrogen ($-NH_2$) and a carboxylic acid ($-COOH$) functional group as part of their main structure. Also present is a side chain (R) specific to each individual amino acid. These R chains can vary from a simple hydrogen atom found in glycine to a complex ring of carbon and hydrogen atoms, as in phenylalanine. The R chain gives the amino acid its identity, distinguishing its unique features. Because of these side chains, each amino acid differs in shape, size, composition, electrical charge, and pH.

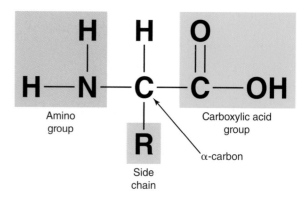

Figure 5.1 All amino acids consist of this basic frame and a unique side chain.

Within any of the many complex classes of amino acids, considerable differences occur in shape and physical properties, so amino acids are often grouped into their functional subgroups (figure 5.2), of which there are several types. Amino acids with an aromatic group (phenylalanine, tyrosine, tryptophan, and histidine) are often grouped together. The **branched chain amino acids (BCAAs)** consist of leucine, isoleucine, and valine. These amino acids are found in food sources of protein but are most abundant in complete sources of protein that contain all the essential amino acids needed by the body (e.g., animal sources of protein such as beef, poultry, dairy, eggs, fish, and the plant-based protein soy) (7). BCAAs are an important subgroup of amino acids that are unique in muscle physiology as the only amino acids that can be directly taken up by muscle tissue and oxidized for energy. BCAAs also play an important role in supporting muscle adaptation to exercise by triggering the activation of anabolic machinery in the muscle to promote muscle protein synthesis (MPS) and a net positive balance in muscle protein accretion. When studying amino acids in biochemistry, classification can occur in many categories related to their charge, size, and optical activity.

Amino Acid Roles in Metabolism

Amino acids are diverse in their activities in different metabolic pathways and can have fates based on the metabolic needs of the body. As discussed in chapter 2, an amino acid can be oxidized for energy by disposing of its nitrogen

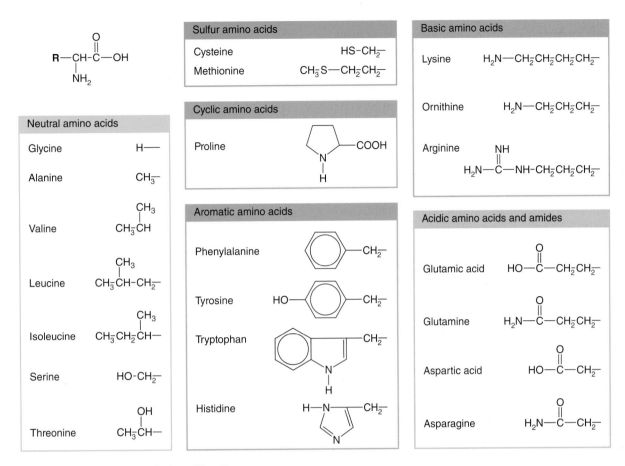

Figure 5.2 Amino acid classification.

group and donating its carbon skeleton to the TCA cycle or can be processed into glucose in the liver. While retaining their nitrogen group, amino acids can be incorporated into proteins in the body or used in the formation of other nitrogen-containing compounds, which includes the synthesis of **nonessential amino acids**. Of the 20 amino acids incorporated into human protein, an important distinction is whether or not the amino acid is essential in the diet or can be made by the body. Nonessential amino acids are also known as "dispensable" because they can be removed from the diet and still be made from other amino acids or from simpler precursors. For several other amino acids, no synthetic pathway exists in the body; these amino acids are termed "essential," or "indispensable." Nine essential amino acids are found in our diet, eight of which are clearly indispensable for adults. These eight **essential amino acids** are phenylalanine, valine, threonine,

tryptophan, isoleucine, methionine, leucine, and lysine. The ninth, histidine, is essential for infants and believed to be essential for adults in small amounts but has not been documented in healthy adults (16). All other amino acids are considered either nonessential—alanine, asparagine, aspartic acid, glutamic acid, and serine; conditionally essential—arginine, cysteine, glutamine, glycine, proline, and tyrosine; or are categorized as simple ammonium (carnitine), nitrogenous (creatine), or gamma (glutathione) compounds. "Conditionally essential" means that particular amino acids are normally synthesized in adequate amounts but become limited when adequate amounts of precursors are unavailable to meet the needs of the body. These amino acids can become essential during times of stress, injury, or illness (8). For example, many conditionally essential amino acids are abundant in seafood and meat and can also be synthesized from other amino acids, but the body has trouble meeting synthetic demands, without help from the diet, as a result of trauma, infection, and kidney failure. Glutamine, a normally nonessential amino acid, provides fuel for rapidly dividing cells and is a preferred fuel for intestinal cells. However, after trauma or periods of critical illness, the body has an increased need for glutamine, which must be met by the diet. In addition to the essential and nonessential amino acids described that are incorporated into protein, other amino acids appear in the body and have important physiological functions. Hydroxyproline and hydroxylysine are two examples of modifications of amino acids that are produced when proline and lysine are hydroxylated in collagen. **Collagen**, which is discussed later in the chapter, is the most abundant protein in the human body and provides the scaffolding to provide strength and structure to hold the body together. Other examples of nonproteinogenic amino acids involve amino acid incorporation into the neurotransmitters GABA and L-Dopa.

Note that other sources discussing amino acids will list 9 essential amino acids but might classify the remaining 11 amino acids under different categories, and perhaps also include other amino acids–like nitrogenous compounds as amino acids. This explains why some sources cite more than 20 amino acids as important to human physiology. In summary, under normal conditions the adult body has the ability to manufacture the 11 nonessential (includes those classified as conditionally essential) amino acids. Amino acids can be arranged in many different combinations; if cells have all 20 amino acids at their disposal, it's possible for the body to make a bewildering number of combinations to create tens of thousands of different protein chains.

Nine Essential Amino Acids

- Histidine (essential at least for infants and perhaps for adults)
- Isoleucine
- Leucine
- Lysine
- Methionine
- Phenylalanine
- Threonine
- Tryptophan
- Valine

Eleven Nonessential Amino Acids

- Alanine
- Arginine*
- Asparagine
- Aspartic acid
- Cysteine*
- Glutamic Acid
- Glutamine*
- Glycine*
- Proline*
- Serine
- Tyrosine*

*Conditionally essential amino acids during stress, illness, or injury

Amino Acids as a Fuel Source

Although the human body prefers to burn carbohydrate and fat to create ATP, protein can also be broken down by the body (catabolized) to be used as an energy source or to make new glucose in the liver (a process known as gluconeogenesis, discussed in chapter 2). While it is important to understand that metabolism is complex and that no metabolic pathway, including protein oxidation, is ever shut down, the use of carbohydrate and fat as energy sources allows protein to be used for protein synthesis and the other essential bodily functions. If we do not consume enough energy to sustain vital functions, such as maintaining our blood glucose levels, the body will readily sacrifice its own protein, preferentially from skeletal muscle tissue, to make glucose for use by our nervous system and other vital organs. In order for protein to be used for energy production, amino acids must be released from their protein structures from a body source or through the process of digestion from the protein foods we eat. Free amino acids from the bloodstream derived from digestion and absorption or from endogenous protein catabolism must then go through a process called deamination to remove their nitrogenous functional unit and free up the carbon skeleton backbone that can enter energy transfer pathways, such as the

TCA cycle, within many cells in our body. The roles of amino acids in energy metabolism are further discussed in chapter 2. Figure 5.3 shows several entry points for amino acids into the TCA cycle to help meet the ATP demands of working cells. In the absence of severe metabolic stress and trauma, fortunately, the oxidation of protein as an energy source is minimal and takes a backseat to the oxidation of fat and carbohydrate in production of ATP. This allows for protein to be conserved for structural, metabolic, and homeostatic roles within the body.

DO YOU KNOW ?

Diets high in protein have a low risk profile for harming the body and can be quite healthy, especially if you are pursuing an active lifestyle. The healthy body is very efficient at handling waste products associated with protein metabolism. The key to maintaining a healthy high-protein diet is to focus on consuming a variety of foods from all food groups.

CLASSIFICATION AND FUNCTION OF PROTEIN

Amino acids come together to make protein, and protein is second only to water as a component of all plant and animal tissues. Protein plays an integral role in every human cell, vital to the structure, function, and health of the human body. In many ways, proteins are intricate molecules that can constantly change in response to various stimuli the body encounters daily. Body proteins are constantly broken down, and amino acids from the amino acid pool are used to supply our body with the majority of the new amino acids required to support constant body protein turnover—thus, more of the amino acids are recycled than are supplied in the diet. The largest portion of protein demands come from body proteins that are broken down via catabolism as a part of normal protein turnover to provide building blocks to synthesize body proteins. This is the primary reason we need relatively little protein in our diet when

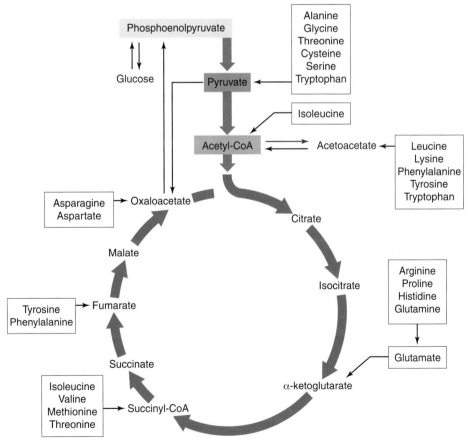

Figure 5.3 Entry points of amino acids.

we are not physically active and have minimal physiological stress. That said, dietary protein remains extremely important; when inadequate, increased catabolism of body protein occurs to replenish the amino acid pool, which can lead to the breakdown of essential body tissue. This importance is obviously magnified in times of metabolic stress, such as infection, inflammatory

PUTTING IT INTO PERSPECTIVE

AMINO ACID POOL

The free amino acids distributed throughout the body in the extracellular fluids and blood make up the amino acid pool (figure 5.4), which is available for protein synthesis at any given time. Amino acids that constantly enter the pool are those that have been catabolized from other tissues, those made in the liver, and those from protein digestion. In addition to protein synthesis, amino acids from the pool can also be broken down to participate in other metabolic pathways. By being broken down, they produce energy and unstable molecules known as amino groups ($-NH_2$). The $-NH_2$ is quickly converted into ammonia (NH_3) and expelled by the cells as a toxic by-product taken up for processing by the liver. The liver can detoxify this molecule by combining it with another amino group in the presence of carbon dioxide to generate urea and water. This process is a component of the metabolic pathway known as the **urea cycle**. The nitrogen-rich urea compound is released by the liver and travels to the kidneys, where it is filtered from the blood to form urine, which is then sent to the bladder for excretion. Other nitrogen-containing compounds are also excreted in the urine in small amounts, such as ammonia, uric acid, and creatine. The primary source of nitrogen lost by the body is present in the form of urea, but some nitrogen is also lost through skin and nails, sloughed-off gastrointestinal cells, mucus, and other body fluids. The cycling of amino acids in the amino acid pool is determined based on the metabolic demands of the body. For example, the liver regulates the blood level of amino acids based on tissue needs and breaks down and converts excess amino acids to carbohydrates for energy production.

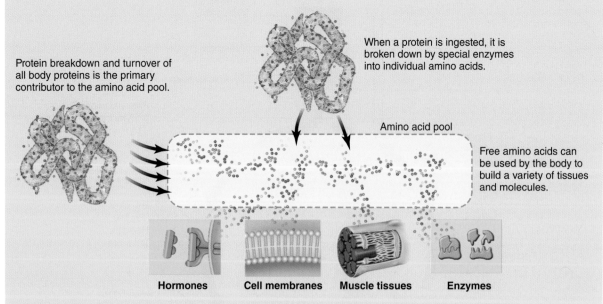

Protein breakdown and turnover of all body proteins is the primary contributor to the amino acid pool.

When a protein is ingested, it is broken down by special enzymes into individual amino acids.

Amino acid pool

Free amino acids can be used by the body to build a variety of tissues and molecules.

Hormones   Cell membranes   Muscle tissues   Enzymes

Figure 5.4 The makeup of the amino acid pool is derived primarily from endogenous protein breakdown and supplemented by protein ingestion.

disease and trauma but is also of key importance for athletes who desire to maintain sufficient levels of different proteins in the body that are crucial to health and performance.

Although the primary sources of protein in the average American diet are beef and poultry (21), all meat, cheese, milk, fish, and eggs are high-quality sources of animal protein. High-quality protein sources contain all the essential amino acids that the body cannot synthesize on its own and are largely found in animal foods. Some plant foods are also a good source (10–19% of daily needs) or high source (>20% of daily needs) of protein (34). Beans, peas, grains, nuts, seeds, and vegetables all contribute protein to the diet, while also providing vitamins, minerals, and phytonutrients; they typically have the bonus of being low in fat and high in fiber. However, not all grains and vegetables are good sources of protein, containing a complete profile of essential amino acids. Table 5.1 presents some common high-protein food sources.

Protein Formation

All protein consumed in our diet, regardless of the source, is digested, absorbed as amino acids, and reassembled in our bodies. Digested animal and plant sources of protein contribute a wide array of amino acids to the "protein pool" in the body to make new proteins. In order to support human growth and repair, as well as protein turnover, the proper amount and proportion of amino acids is required. To form protein in our body, amino acids are joined together in long strings by covalent chemical bonds known as **peptide bonds** (figure 5.5). These bonds form when a **carboxyl group** of one amino acid reacts with the amino group of another to form peptide chains that are arranged in a biologically functional way to form proteins. Their structure and function serve as the centerpiece for the biochemical reactions of life.

When amino acids start linking together via peptide bonds, and eventually form a protein,

Table 5.1 High-Protein Foods

Food	Protein (g)	Kilocalories from protein (%)
3 oz. lean beef steak	26	53
3 oz. skinless chicken breast (grilled)	16.3	74
3 oz. tilapia filet	15	88
3 oz. salmon	17	68
3 oz. pork loin	24	54
1 cup lentils	9	32
1 cup black beans	15	26
1 cup peas (cooked)	9	27
3 oz. tofu	9	40
1 large egg	6.3	32
1 cup milk (1%)	8	31
1 cup soy milk	7	28
1 cup chopped broccoli (raw)	2.6	34
1 cup cooked white rice	4.4	14
1/2 cup quinoa	4	14
2 tbsp. peanut butter	7	15
1/4 cup almonds	7	16

Data from U.S. Department of Agriculture and U.S. Department of Health & Human Services 2015.

Figure 5.5 A protein peptide bond.

all the polypeptide chains making up the protein. An example of a quaternary protein structure important in sports nutrition is hemoglobin, an iron containing protein that is a component of red blood cells. Hemoglobin binds oxygen from the lungs to be delivered throughout the body, including exercising muscles, while picking up carbon dioxide to shuttle back to the lungs for drop-off and exhalation.

Dietary proteins, as well as protein that make up the body, are long polypeptides, with peptide bonds linking hundreds of amino acids. Proteins,

the complex characteristics work together to determine the specific function of that protein. The number of bonds formed determines the name of the bond. Dipeptides and tripeptides are two and three amino acids joined together by peptide bonds, respectively. A **polypeptide** contains more than 10 amino acids. Strands of proteins (made from polypeptide chains) can be linked together by peptide bonds in up to hundreds of amino acids long. The vast number of biological functions that proteins perform depends on their structural arrangement. Proteins can fold into one or more specific spatial conformations through many biochemical interactions. Protein structures can contain tens to several thousand amino acids and can vary greatly in size (4). Additionally, when performing their biological function, these complex protein structures can go through many structural changes, called conformational changes, to effectively modify their function.

Amino acid residues come in several levels of protein structures, referred to as primary, secondary, tertiary, and quaternary structures (figure 5.6). When referring to a protein's primary structure, its sequence of amino acids forms one or more polypeptide chains. The secondary structure of a protein is the coiling or folding of its polypeptide chains and is primarily a result of hydrogen bonding between amino acid chains. The tertiary structure of a protein refers to its three-dimensional shape caused by weak interactions among side groups and interactions between side groups and the fluid environment. Finally, the quaternary structure of a protein is the final three-dimensional structure formed by

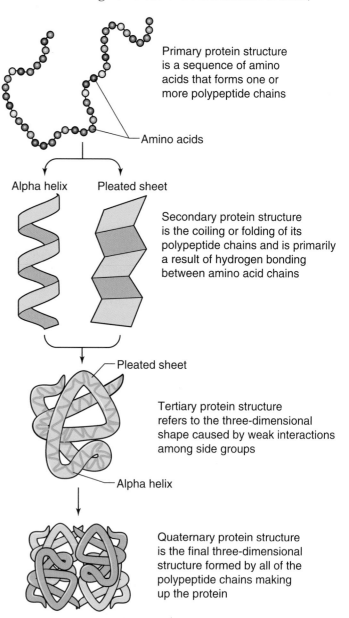

Primary protein structure is a sequence of amino acids that forms one or more polypeptide chains

Amino acids

Alpha helix Pleated sheet

Secondary protein structure is the coiling or folding of its polypeptide chains and is primarily a result of hydrogen bonding between amino acid chains

Pleated sheet

Tertiary protein structure refers to the three-dimensional shape caused by weak interactions among side groups

Alpha helix

Quaternary protein structure is the final three-dimensional structure formed by all of the polypeptide chains making up the protein

Figure 5.6 Protein structure hierarchy.

both small and large, reside in every part of the body participating in key physiological functions. The largest source of protein in the human body is found in muscle, where a large and diverse family of proteins form contractile fibers and a structural framework that make up muscle tissue. Contractile protein fibers slide alongside each other, shortening and lengthening to contract and relax the muscle tissue.

Protein Functions

Intact body proteins are very diverse in human physiology, serving a structural role for muscles, skin, bones, and connective tissue. In fact, the human body contains thousands of different proteins, each with a specific function determined by its shape. For example, **enzymes** work to speed up chemical reactions, whereas **hormones** serve as chemical messengers. **Antibodies** are proteins that make up our immune system and protect us from foreign pathogens. Proteins also serve as regulators by helping to pump molecules across cell membranes. They can serve as fluid regulators by attracting water to keep body water in the right place and can influence acid-base balance by releasing or gaining hydrogen ions as needed. Finally, proteins can play a key structural role in serving as transporters of oxygen, vitamins, and minerals for delivery to target cells throughout the body. Key characteristics of the structural and mechanical functions of proteins, enzymes, and hormones, and the role of protein in immune function, fluid, and acid-base balance, as well as their role in blood transport, are shown in figure 5.7 and described in detail later in the chapter.

Structure

The most abundant single protein in the body of all mammals is collagen. This protein serves as the major constituent of bones and teeth and helps to maintain the structure of every connective tissue within the human body. Collagen relies on its densely packed structure to contribute elastic strength to bones and skin. Keratin is another structural protein that primarily serves to provide the anatomical structure for hair and nails. Motor proteins, such as the contractile fibers described earlier, also provide structure and make up a significant portion of skeletal and smooth muscles. These proteins initiate mechanical movement by harnessing the body's chemical form of energy (ATP) into mechanical work to make muscles contract.

Enzymes

Enzymes are proteins that function to speed up or catalyze chemical reactions in the body to make or change substances that are often referred to as products. There are thousands of enzymes within each cell of our body, each with its own purpose to drive a reaction forward. Enzymes can be thought of as shepherds that steer and regulate a reaction. Enzymes interact with the substrates of a chemical reaction to form new biological products affected by the chemical reaction (figure 5.8). Substrates can bind to the enzyme's active site, causing the active site to change shape, resulting in a better fit for multiple substrates to interact. The enzyme can then maneuver the substrates so they bind and form the product. The product is then released and the enzyme can return to its normal shape to interact with other substrates and keep the metabolic processes moving. For example, our skeletal muscles contain hundreds of enzymes to catalyze a series of reactions that allow them to break down fuel sources (carbohydrate, protein, and fat) to eventually generate the ATP that facilitates muscle contraction. As discussed in chapter 2, multiple enzymatic reactions work to help decide the fate of pyruvate. Proteins working as enzymes are also very prominent every time we digest our food. Multiple enzymes work to target food proteins, carbohydrates, and fats and break them down into smaller particles to prepare them for absorption in the small intestine. Lactase is an excellent

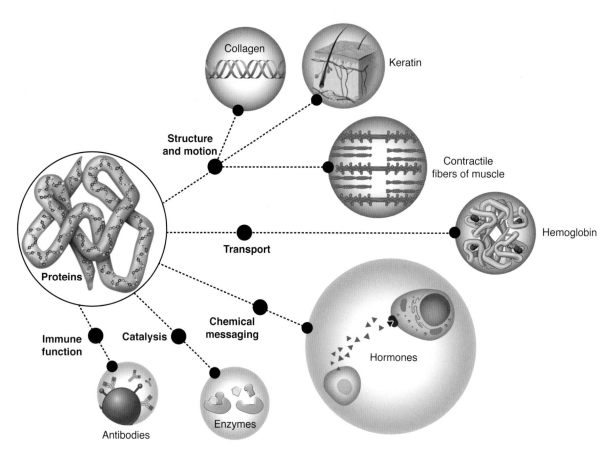

Figure 5.7 Proteins have multiple functions throughout the body.

example of a digestive enzyme that breaks down the carbohydrate lactose into smaller sugars.

Just as amino acids build proteins that create complex polypeptide bonds that in turn form complicated protein structures, these proteins structures are also constantly turning over (i.e., broken down and replaced). A process called protein denaturation is the initial catabolic event responsible for destabilizing a protein's shape. Several forms of stimuli can initiate this cascade of events in the body. Outside of the body, many examples of denaturation can be observed by how we prepare the protein foods in our diet for eating. Treating a food with acid, alkalinity, heat, alcohol, oxidation, and agitation can all disrupt a protein's three-dimensional shape, causing it to unfold (**denature**) and lose its shape and function. A good visual example is an egg cooking in a skillet. The heat causes the protein bonds in the egg to break and unfold. The broken proteins then crowd each other and crowd tightly to form an opaque egg solid. When lemon juice is added to milk, the milk proteins denature and curdle because of the acid in the juice. In human nutrition, the best example of an acid denaturing dietary protein occurs in the stomach during digestion as hydrochloric acid (HCL) is released by parietal cells found in the stomach lining. This acid denatures dietary proteins, uncoiling them into simpler chains with greater surface area for digestive enzymes to attack their peptide bonds. The process of protein digestion is covered in more detail later in the chapter.

Chemical Messengers

Proteins also play an instrumental role as chemical messengers, called peptide hormones, which interact with cells to signal intracellular events. Insulin (figure 5.9) and growth hormone are two examples of many peptide hormones made in specific parts of the body that act on cells in other parts of the body. Many of these proteins have important regulatory functions, are relatively

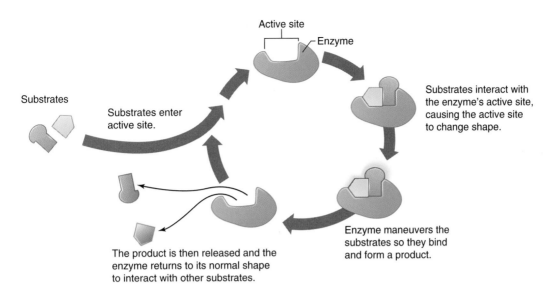

Figure 5.8   Enzyme binding. Enzymes with the addition of a substrate forms a product.

fragile, and have a fairly short half-life so that their breakdown can limit the degree of chemical signaling that occurs.

Immunity

Proteins play a key role in bolstering our immune defense against pathogenic invaders such as bacteria and viruses. Antibodies are blood proteins that attack and deactivate these invaders to prevent infection. Antibodies are produced in response to a previous infection so the body can quickly respond the next time that germ invades. Immune cells can keep a memory of each previous viral invasion to mount a faster response during future invasions.

Fluid Maintenance

In addition to serving an important role in immune function, proteins also function in promoting fluid and acid-base balance. In the human body, fluids are found in two basic areas: inside of cells (intracellular) or outside of cells (extracellular). For the body to function properly, a healthy balance of fluid in each space is partially maintained by specific proteins (figure 5.10). Proteins called globulin and **albumin** are large in size, attract water, and remain inside the blood. They function to attract water within this space to help balance fluid that is lost through the force

of the heart pumping blood and pushing the fluid fraction of the blood outside of the blood vessels. Hospitalized patients who experience severe metabolic and catabolic stress resulting from trauma many times become deficient in the blood protein albumin. Albumin deficiency disrupts normal fluid balance and control and results in a form

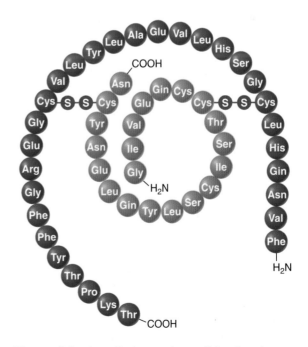

Figure 5.9   Insulin is a polypeptide structure.

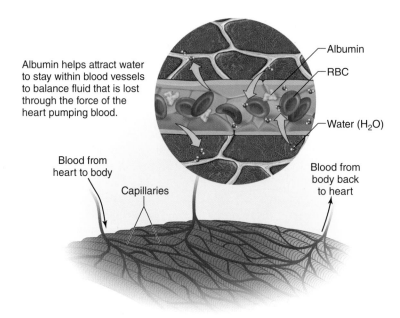

Albumin helps attract water to stay within blood vessels to balance fluid that is lost through the force of the heart pumping blood.

Albumin

RBC

Water (H_2O)

Blood from heart to body

Capillaries

Blood from body back to heart

Figure 5.10 Proteins such as albumin assist in the balance of fluid through attraction of water and serve to regulate vascular pressure.

of tissue swelling known as edema. Proteins can also function to stabilize the body's pH by serving as a buffer to pick up extra hydrogen ions when acidity increases (pH decreases). On the other hand, when blood composition becomes slightly basic (rise in pH), proteins can donate hydrogen ions in an effort to neutralize blood pH. The body works hard to keep the pH in tight check, at a neutral measure close to 7.4 on a scale of 0 (acidic) to 14 (basic). Having a blood pH too far outside the range of 7.35 to 7.45 can cause disastrous consequences and has been observed clinically as a result of severe hyperglycemia or trauma. If left unchecked, the unbalance can lead to acidosis and cause death within a matter of hours, primarily by altering the function and activity of many proteins throughout the body.

DO YOU KNOW ?

Influenza (flu) vaccines are an example of a public health initiative that provides individuals with a small amount of a dead or deactivated virus that does not cause an infection but does cue the body to make antibodies to prepare for the potential of a future invasion of the virus. Immune cells retain memory of the protein material provided in the vaccine to mount a fast response if the flu virus invades.

Cell Transporters

All body cells allow substances to pass into their intracellular space, while also working to excrete various substances. These functions are maintained by protein transporters that act as channels and pumps to regulate intra- and extracellular movement. Protein channels typically work by a process known as diffusion, during which substances freely pass in and out without requiring energy. On the other hand, protein pumps utilize **active transport** that requires energy in the form of ATP to move substances across cellular membranes. Sodium-potassium pumps, often introduced in undergraduate physiology classes, use a significant amount of ATP as a chemical energy source to move sugars and amino acids and to control cell volume and nerve impulses. Proteins also act as carriers to transport important substances to tissues throughout the body. An example of an important protein carrier is a **chylomicron**. This protein carrier is a type of **lipoprotein** that packages lipids from the fats that we consume so that these fats can be carried in the blood to peripheral tissues. Have you ever heard the phrase oil and water do not mix? This would be the case with the fat in our water-filled blood without lipoproteins. The chylomicron lipoprotein functions to engulf lipids in the center of its sphere-like core while embedded hydrophilic (water loving) protein tails toward the outside of this protein molecule to be water-soluble and not "separate" from the blood. Figure 5.11 shows an example of a protein transporter used in amino acid intestinal absorption and a chylomicron.

It is clear that protein serves many diverse roles and is of significant importance to human health, function, and athletic performance (table 5.2).

In order to meet these responsibilities, the diet must provide adequate amounts of amino acids. In addition, the body must have an adequate source of energy (calories) to allow dietary protein to optimally serve in these important roles instead of being used (oxidized) as an energy source. Although a very small portion of the protein in the body contributes to ATP synthesis, the proportion of protein used as a fuel source can increase through various stimuli, such as pro-

longed endurance exercise or starvation. During prolonged endurance exercise (typically greater than 90 minutes), small increases in protein oxidation occur, particularly if limited carbohydrate is consumed (13). The use of protein as an energy source can be problematic in cases of starvation or anorexia nervosa and in chronic situations of inadequate energy intake. In these scenarios, the chronic effect of elevated protein breakdown and oxidation for fuel has deleterious effects on health.

DIGESTION AND ABSORPTION

To fully appreciate how energy-yielding macronutrients are integrated during metabolism, we must first understand how they are digested and absorbed by the body. The body must first address these important tasks before it can use protein from food to make body protein (figure 5.12). Protein digestion begins in the mouth, where protein in foods is mechanically altered by chewing.

Digestion in the Stomach

In the stomach, proteins are unfolded into long polypeptide chains by the action of hydrochloric acid (HCL). This stomach acid also has a secondary, but equally important, responsibility. HCL interacts with a **proenzyme** called **pepsinogen** that is released by the cells of the stomach lining. In the stomach cavity, HCL works to unfold and cut off some of the amino acids that make up pepsinogen to change its form and function.

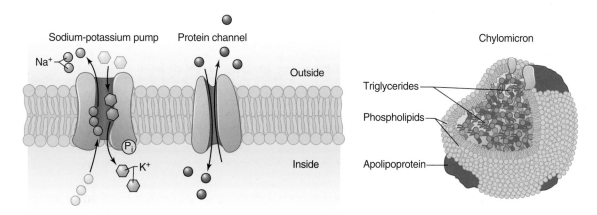

Figure 5.11 The chylomicron is a lipid-containing protein transporter used in the intestinal absorption of fat.

Table 5.2 Protein Functions in the Body

Component	Role
Hormones	Serve as chemical messengers.
Regulators	Help pump molecules across cell membranes to preserve cellular function.
Transporters	Move oxygen, vitamins, and minerals for delivery to target cells throughout the body.
Immune function	Proteins compose antibodies that protect the body from bacteria and viruses.
Fluid and acid-base balance	Attract water and release hydrogen ions; can influence acid-base balance by releasing or gaining hydrogen ions.
Enzymes	Initiate or speed up chemical reactions.
Structure	Cellular integrity; muscle contraction.

This process activates pepsinogen to its active protein digesting form, called **pepsin**. This enzymatic activation step within the gastric cavity and small intestine is common and strategic in the protein-digestion process. The activation of these enzymes at the proper time ensures that dietary protein is digested at the right stage of digestion. This process also protects the cells that create the proenzymes, because if each cell created only active forms of these enzymes, the cell would end up digesting itself! In addition to the pathways that activate pepsin, the pepsin generated from this reaction is very efficient at clipping peptide bonds of the proteins we consume and will activate more pepsin from additional pepsinogen released into the stomach cavity. When digesting dietary protein, pepsin begins breaking down polypeptides into shorter amino acid chains called peptides. As a result of HCL and pepsin action in the stomach, dietary proteins are digested into smaller polypeptides and approximately 15 percent free amino acids.

Digestion in the Small Intestine

As polypeptides and smaller peptide chains leave the stomach, they enter the small intestine to complete the next phase of digestion and prepare for protein absorption. As partially digested protein enters the small intestine, the **duodenum** detects protein in the partially digested food and signals duodenal cells to release the hormones **secretin** and **cholecystokinin** (CCK) into the bloodstream. These hormones trigger the pancreas to release

REFLECTION TIME

PROTEIN IS FOR MUSCLES BUT WHAT ELSE?

We know the importance of skeletal muscle proteins to athletic performance. Now consider several other proteins made in the body that are key to an athlete's success, such as collagen's role in connective tissue and all the protein containing immune regulators needed to maintain healthy immune function. Without proper formation and function of these proteins, it won't matter if your muscles are bigger and stronger—performance will ultimately suffer. New protein intake guidelines for athletic performance (30) take this into account. While athletes do need more protein than their nonathlete counterparts, it is important not to overdo protein consumption. Consuming healthy foods from all food groups is important in order to maintain diet quality.

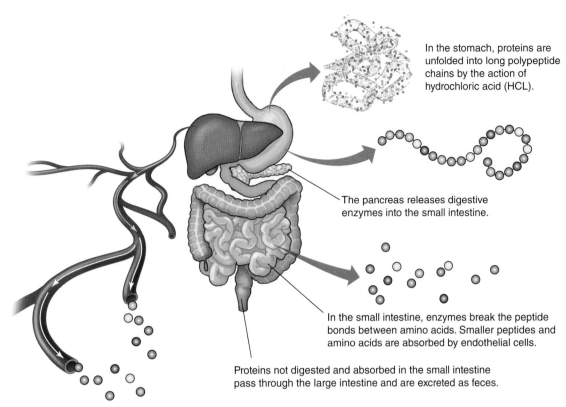

In the stomach, proteins are unfolded into long polypeptide chains by the action of hydrochloric acid (HCL).

The pancreas releases digestive enzymes into the small intestine.

In the small intestine, enzymes break the peptide bonds between amino acids. Smaller peptides and amino acids are absorbed by endothelial cells.

Proteins not digested and absorbed in the small intestine pass through the large intestine and are excreted as feces.

Following intestinal absorption, amino acids are transported via the portal vein to the liver and then released into general circulation.

Figure 5.12   Protein digestion.

other digestive substances into the small intestine. At the same time, duodenal cells facing the inside of the gastrointestinal (GI) tract release **enterokinases** in the **luminal brush border** to activate additional enzymes to break other peptide bonds. Collectively, these events signal what is called the **protease activation cascade** in the duodenum. Secretin signals the pancreas to release water and bicarbonate in the intestine to neutralize the acidic **chyme**, whereas CCK signals the pancreas to release a family of enzymes that have high specificity for breaking specific amino acid-amino acid peptide bonds. As a result of enzymatic digestion of protein in the stomach (pepsin) combined with the action of pancreatic enzymes (**trypsin**, chymotrypsin, elastase, and carboxypeptidase A and B) and the enterokinases found at the brush border of the small intestine, the protein that was originally consumed now consists of more than 90 percent free amino acids combined with less than 10 percent small peptide chains.

Absorption

All along the small intestine, short peptide chains and single amino acids can be absorbed by intestinal endothelial cells. These cells are aligned back to back on the surface of the intestinal villi. On the brush border membrane of these endothelial cells are at least six different amino acid carriers, also known as channels or transporters, which have overlapping specificity for different amino acids based on their physical and chemical characteristics. Transporters requiring sodium also require ATP to move the amino acid to within the cell. This form of absorption is known as active transport. Other amino acids diffuse across transporters through a process called facilitated diffusion. Most amino acids are transported by more than one transport system (figure 5.13). Normally, proteins in foods supply a healthy mix of several amino acids, so amino acids that share the same transport system are absorbed equally. As amino acids are absorbed in

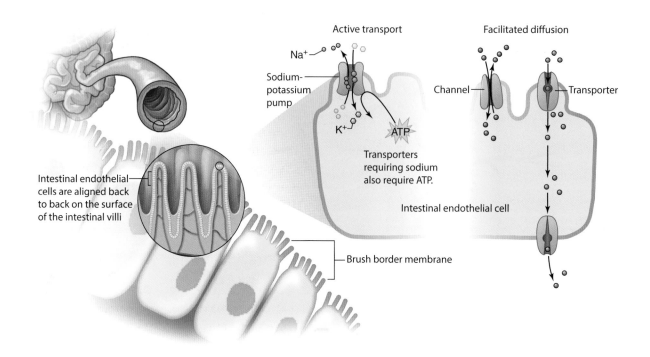

Figure 5.13 The transport of protein can occur through active transport and facilitated diffusion.

absorptive endothelial cells, other peptidases within the absorptive cells are present to completely break down di- and tripeptides into single amino acids. The individual amino acids are then absorbed into the bloodstream by leaving the endothelial cell and absorbed into the capillaries of the larger villi structure and transported to the liver via the **portal vein**. Proteins not digested and absorbed in the small intestine pass through the large intestine and are excreted as feces. In the absence of GI diseases such as celiac disease and cystic fibrosis, generally more than 90 percent of protein is absorbed from the diet in the enterocytes that line the duodenum and jejunum, of which 99 percent enters the blood as individual amino acids. Following absorption, most amino acids and a few absorbed peptides are transported via the portal vein to the liver and then released into general circulation (figure 5.14).

METABOLIC FATE OF PROTEIN IN THE BODY

Various metabolic processes use amino acids derived from the liver and the bloodstream fol-

lowing intestinal absorption. As described earlier, these amino acids contribute to what is generically called the liver and blood amino acid pool of the body (see figure 5.4). In the bloodstream, amino acids from this pool are transported throughout the body and are available for synthesizing new proteins. In this section we will discuss how the body uses this amino acid pool for various synthetic and catabolic processes.

Protein Synthesis

As previously described, cells use peptide bonds to link amino acids and build proteins. The nucleus of every cell provides the blueprint for the synthesis of thousands of proteins our bodies need to stay healthy and function properly. Our cells store this important genetic information in the form of **deoxyribonucleic acid (DNA)** in each cell's nucleus. To make new protein, cells signal a specific section with a very specific pattern of the DNA, called a gene, to make a special type of **ribonucleic acid (RNA)** called **messenger RNA (mRNA)** (figure 5.15). This mRNA carries the blueprint sequence of amino acids needed in the

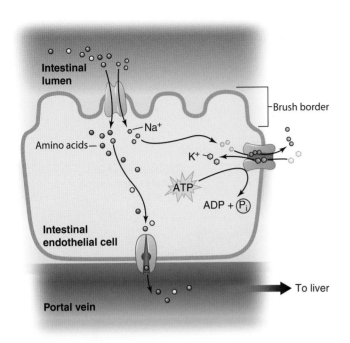

Figure 5.14 Amino acid entry into a portal vein.

protein to be synthesized. The mRNA leaves the nucleus and attaches itself to one of the protein-making factories of the cell, called ribosomes, in the cell's cytoplasm. During synthesis, the 20 amino acids that are incorporated into human protein are carefully selected from the body's amino acid pool for protein synthesis when coupled to another type of RNA called **transfer RNA (tRNA)**. Transfer RNA gathers the necessary amino acids in the cytoplasm of the cell and carries them to the mRNA. To synthesize protein, strands of DNA are transcribed into mRNA, and then tRNA binds to mRNA in three-base groups, where enzymes attach each amino acid to the growing protein chain in the cell's ribosomes. Different combinations of three consecutive RNA molecules in the mRNA provide a code for the synthesis of different tRNA molecules. However, the three-base combinations of mRNA are recognized by only 20 different tRNA molecules, and 20 different amino acids are incorporated into protein during protein synthesis. During protein synthesis, thousands of tRNAs each carry their own specific amino acid to the site of protein synthesis, but only one mRNA controls the sequencing of the amino acids for a specific protein. A third type of RNA resides in the ribosome (rRNA) and serves as a ribonucleic acid that is prevalent in the ribosomes that provide a structural framework for protein synthesis and coordinate the many steps involved in protein synthesis.

Protein synthesis requires all the amino acids required to build a specific protein; an insufficient amount of any one might impede or slow formation of a polypeptide chain. If one nonessential amino acid is missing during protein synthesis, the cell can either make that amino acid or obtain from the pool of amino acids in the liver via the bloodstream. If an essential amino acid is missing, the body may break down some of its own protein to supply the missing amino acid. Without the particular essential amino acid, synthesis of that specific protein will halt, and the incomplete protein that is made will be tagged for breakdown

PUTTING IT INTO PERSPECTIVE

AMINO ACID COMPETITION FOR ABSORPTION

Consuming a large amount of one particular amino acid can compromise the absorption of other amino acids that share the same transporter. For instance, taking a dietary supplement consisting of a large dose of one amino acid, such as lysine, might be interfering with the absorption of other amino acids from the diet. Lysine is classified as a basic amino acid (i.e., nonacidic) and has a specific transporter shared with other basic amino acids, such as arginine. If arginine is consumed in low quantities combined with lysine supplementation, the minimal arginine available will have limited access to absorption transporters saturated with lysine. While it is possible that taking single-amino-acid supplements can cause imbalances that might interfere with normal absorption of food-derived amino acids, particularly essential amino acids, there is not enough research in humans to know exactly at what dosage this can be a problem.

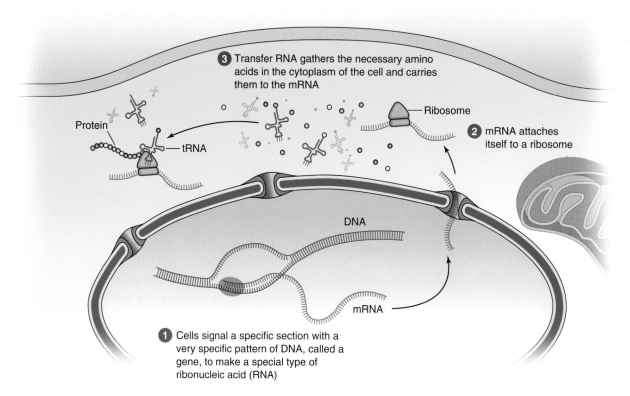

Figure 5.15 Gene expression occurs from DNA transcribed into mRNA, which is translated into a protein.

to recycle the amino acids to the amino acid pool. The body then must decide which proteins are most important to make, while sacrificing the structure and synthesis of others. A greater portion of skeletal muscle protein would be expected to be catabolized to contribute to the amino acid pool, while some muscle-specific protein-synthetic pathways may be compromised.

Protein Catabolism

On the other side of the protein metabolism equation is protein catabolism, or breakdown. When proteins of a cell are catabolized, the protein's amino acids return back to circulation to contribute to the amino acid pool. The resulting amino acids can also be classified according to the products they produce when metabolized to generate ATP. Amino acids can participate in gluconeogenic (to make glucose) or ketogenic (to make ketones) pathways. There are three metabolic entry points for amino acids following deamination. They include conversion of the

amino acid to pyruvate in the cytosol of the cell, conversion to acetyl-CoA in the mitochondria, or conversion to a TCA cycle intermediate. Some of these amino acids may be used again for protein synthesis, while others may have their amino groups removed in the liver to produce energy or make molecules such as glucose, DNA, RNA, neurotransmitters, hormones such as thyroxine, histamine, and many other important compounds.

Nitrogen Balance

Traditional attempts to evaluate whether the body is getting enough protein have involved a rudimentary method known as nitrogen balance. Because nitrogen is excreted as proteins are recycled or used, we can estimate the balance of nitrogen in the body. The nitrogen balance equation takes the grams of nitrogen consumed (dietary protein is 16% nitrogen) subtracted by the grams of nitrogen lost (primarily as urea) over the timeframe of 24 hours to determine if someone is in a positive or negative nitrogen balance.

Classical nitrogen balance work has been useful for determining protein requirements to prevent deficiency in sedentary humans in energy balance (37). However, this technique has also long been recognized as a flawed method due to several methodological limitations (23) that minimize its utility in present-day nutrition science. It should be recognized that the nitrogen balance technique is only a snapshot of what is occurring with nitrogen at the whole-body level and disregards the fact that protein metabolism and turnover is a very complex and dynamic process that is always changing in all the different areas of the body. The nitrogen balance technique assumes that all proteins in all body systems and tissues are behaving the exact same way and relies on very rough estimates of nitrogen excretion that is usually only in the form of a 24-hour urine collection.

Note that determining "need" to prevent deficiency is very different from assessing dietary protein amounts that are necessary for proper adaptation to exercise and athletic performance. In the world of physical fitness and sport, athletes do not meet this profile, and achieving nitrogen balance is secondary to an athlete whose primary goal is adaptation to training and performance improvement (23). The nitrogen balance technique cannot provide insight into the kinetics of body proteins or account for rapidly turning over body tissues. Finally, this technique certainly cannot provide accurate insight on dietary protein intake recommendations for athletes and has created some confusion.

Despite these limitations, the nitrogen balance technique has been used for years to help determine a need or requirement for dietary protein to replaces losses and thus prevent deficiency and thus still has some purpose. A positive nitrogen balance suggests nitrogen intake exceeds the sum of all sources of nitrogen excretion and has been historically interpreted as achieving adequate protein status to prevent protein malnutrition. This positive balance suggests the body is adding protein effectively, such as in the case of pregnancy or in supporting child and adolescent growth. Conversely, a negative nitrogen balance implies nitrogen intake is less than the sum of all sources of nitrogen excretion. Those in a negative balance are thought to be losing protein and may be experiencing starvation, severe illness with fever and infection, extreme weight loss, or recent trauma (23, 26).

General Equation

N intake – (24-hr UUN* + 4**) = nitrogen balance

Adding Protein Effectively

$$14 - 12 = + 2.0$$

Losing Protein

$$14 - 16 = - 2.0$$

*UUN = urine urea nitrogen; **+ 4 refers to grams of nitrogen from feces, hair, skin, and other body fluids.

PROTEIN IN THE DIET

Many organizations worldwide have recommendations regarding the amount of protein required to contribute to a healthful diet. When we think about the major food groupings that make up our diet, only fruits and fats contain minimal amounts of protein and are not considered protein sources. In the United States and Canada, the Recommended Dietary Allowance (RDA) is the accepted dietary standard for setting protein needs. The RDA for protein was calculated to meet the nutrition needs of most healthy people; however, it is important to note that the RDA assumes people are consuming adequate energy and other nutrients to allow their bodies to use the protein they consume for synthesis, rather than for energy. As mentioned earlier, when discussing protein recommendations for athletes, some

DO YOU KNOW ?

Nitrogen assessment measures are commonly used to measure protein content in protein powder supplements for food-labeling purposes. To take advantage of this, many manufacturers have been accused of adding other nitrogen-containing ingredients, such as individual amino acids like glycine and taurine, and portraying them as grams of protein on the label, despite the fact that these are incomplete proteins. How can you avoid amino acid spiking of protein powders? Read the ingredients to look for added amino acids and cheaper, incomplete protein sources.

PUTTING IT INTO PERSPECTIVE

CALCULATING PROTEIN NEEDS BASED ON THE RDA

For a college freshman male who weighs 175 pounds, follow these steps to determine the gram amount of protein intake based on the RDA.

1. Convert pounds to kilograms: 175 lb. / 2.2 kg = 79.5 kg
2. Multiply kg body weight × 0.8 g/kg body weight: 79.5 kg × 0.8 g/kg = 63.6 g

This means a male who weighs 175 pounds needs a minimum of 63.6 grams of protein to prevent protein deficiency, assuming he is both healthy and sedentary. Based on new protein intake guidelines for athletic performance, if this college freshman participates in regular exercise or sport, his protein needs rise 1.2 to 2.0 grams per kilogram (30).

confusion has surrounded the phrase "protein needs." The RDA, for instance, is meant to prevent protein deficiency and does not take into account additional dietary protein that might be needed to prevent age-related sarcopenia or enhance physiological adaptations to exercise (14, 24).

Based on studies suggesting increased heart disease risk when diets are low in fat and high in refined carbohydrate (sugar), and increased risk of overweight, obesity, and heart disease when diets are high in fat, the Food and Nutrition Board set the acceptable macronutrient distribution range (AMDR) for protein in adults as 10 to 35 percent of total protein calories consumed (10). So if an individual requires 2,000 kilocalories per day in their diet to maintain their weight, their protein intake recommendations would range from 50 to 175 grams per day:

$$2{,}000 \text{ kcals} \times (0.10 \text{ or } 0.35) / 4 \text{ calories per gram of protein}$$

This range of protein intake is typically higher than the RDA.

Protein historically provides about 15 to 16 percent of energy for adults in North America (5). Although the AMDR recommendations for protein are quite wide, and in many cases not very specific, for the first time, the AMDR allows for flexibility when considering protein needs for active individuals. This range is broad enough to cover the needs of most active individuals (15) and is elevated beyond the RDA to match the physical stress that increases the body's need for additional

protein. Exactly how much? This is a question that generates conversation and debate among many interested in the scientific community and continues to spark scientific inquiry, primarily in exercise science, but also for aging and specific clinical conditions. Many factors affect the protein needs of physically active individuals, and these elevated needs are linked to supporting various outcomes that may be very important to the athlete. Although training is now widely recognized to increase protein needs, the amount is often much less than most people think. However, it should not be assumed that adequate protein consumption in athletes is always the case, particularly in female athletes (23).

How much protein does an individual normally consume, and how does this amount compare to the RDA? For a comprehensive assessment of how much protein an individual needs, it is important not only to understand variables, such as physiological stressors or the need of growth and recovery, but also how much protein is normally consumed. The most accurate method is to rely on food labels that list the quantity of protein (in grams) in a serving of food. By using food labels, the grams of protein consumed in one day can simply be added together. Clearly, not all foods have food labels, so using other methods to assess the protein quantity of these foods is essential. One method, used for decades, is to rely on food exchange lists. These lists provide serving sizes for most foods and combine this information with a corresponding number of exchanges for carbohydrate, protein, and fat. For example, one protein exchange equals one ounce, which corresponds to 7 grams of protein. So a 3-ounce chicken breast equals three exchanges and is estimated to contain 21 grams of protein. Other protein-containing food groups also have exchanges that can be used to estimate protein intake. A vegetable exchange provides 2 grams of protein, whereas a milk exchange provides 8 grams. A starch exchange contributes 3 grams of protein, whereas fat and fruit exchanges contribute zero protein. For those who prefer not to use food exchange lists, other strategies are commonly used. Food composition tables and "protein calculators" are prevalent online, and computer software programs are available for purchase. The most prudent strategy to ensure accuracy per the RDA is to visit the United States Department of Agriculture's website at www.choosemyplate.gov.

PROTEIN QUALITY

Protein quality measurement is an assessment of the ability of a dietary protein source to fulfill our body's requirement for indispensable (or essential) amino acids. The better the score, the better the food protein meets our body's needs. Generally, protein quality refers to how well or poorly the body uses a given protein. Protein quality can also be defined by how well the essential amino acid (EAA) profile of a protein matches the requirements of the body, the digestibility of the protein, and the bioavailability of the amino acids. Although both animal and plant foods contain protein, the quality of protein in these foods differ. Meat, poultry, fish, eggs, milk, and milk products are all high-quality complete proteins that have at least 20 percent of their calories from protein. Protein isolated from soybeans also provides a

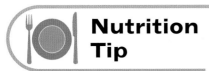 **Nutrition Tip**

When whole-food protein sources are not convenient, third-party tested supplemental protein powder is an alternative way to meet protein-intake needs. Look for these protein sources:

- Whey—milk protein that is the richest source of BCAAs and has the quickest digestion rate (20), leading to a quick rise in blood amino acids to help muscles adapt to exercise.
- Casein—a milk protein similar to whey but with slower absorption. Casein protein consumption helps stimulate muscle protein synthesis like whey protein but occurs at a slower rate (caused by slow digestion) that might take several hours (22).
- Egg—a high-quality protein with high biological value; a good option for those who prefer to avoid milk products.
- Vegetable (soy, pea, etc.)—a viable option for vegetarians, vegans, or others. Many soy and hemp products are beneficial because they supply antioxidants, vitamins, minerals, and many essential amino acids. However, few plant sources of protein are considered complete because of low levels of certain essential amino acids and lower digestive bioavailability affecting protein quality.

complete protein that is equal to animal protein, with a slightly lower proportion of the amino acids cysteine and leucine. Soy protein may also offer unique health benefits, making it a good choice as a replacement for some of the protein we consume from animal sources. Soy protein does not contain saturated fat and has been linked to the reduced risk of several chronic diseases (38). Table 5.3 describes several methods available to measure the protein quality of food.

Besides ensuring energy intake is adequate with a wide variety of foods, a strategy to circumvent protein-quality concerns for those who choose to consume a more plant-based diet is to consume complementary proteins. A complementary protein is defined as two or more incomplete food proteins whose assortment of amino acids complement each other's lack of specific EAAs so that the combination provides sufficient amounts of all the EAAs. Grain products tend to be low in the EAA lysine but high in the EAAs methionine and cysteine, while legumes such as beans are low in methionine and cysteine but high in lysine. Good examples of complementary proteins found in the diet are beans with rice, peanut butter sandwiches, pasta with beans, and chickpeas with sesame paste. Each one of these food pairs contain all the EAAs required to make new protein but by themselves (e.g., the peanut butter without the bread) are limited in at least one EAA. Specific pairings of these foods do not need to be consumed together at the same time to make new body protein. Protein complementation is generally only important for people who consume little to no animal proteins. Provided that a variety of low-quality proteins are consumed as part of a healthy diet, the body will have access to all the EAA needed for optimal protein synthesis. Note that even small amounts of animal proteins

can also complement the protein in plant foods and further minimize the need for protein complementation.

In addition to assessing the general amino acid composition of foods, one can measure the quality of a protein in many other ways. We know that a high-quality protein provides all the EAAs in the amounts the body needs, provides enough other amino acids to serve as nitrogen sources for synthesis of nonessential amino acids, and is easy to digest. A protein food that provides all the EAAs but cannot be digested is useless to the body. Each technique to assess protein quality requires information about the amino acid composition and has been traditionally used to help formulate a special diet or to develop new feeding formulas for infants.

Calculating Chemical Score

Calculating the chemical score (also known as the amino acid score) of a protein is an easy way to determine a food's protein quality and refers simply to its amino acid profile rated to a standard or reference protein; each amino acid is rated on a scale indicating how much of that amino acid is present compared to the reference protein (table 5.4). The amino acid composition of the reference protein closely reflects the amounts and proportions of amino acids humans need. Currently, the pattern of amino acids required by preschool children is used as the reference (29). The idea is that if a protein meets the needs of young, growing children, it should meet the needs of all other segments of the population. In order to calculate the chemical score, the quantity of each of the EAAs in the test food (in milligrams) are divided by the quantity of each of the amino acids found in the reference protein. The resulting numbers for

Table 5.3 Protein Quality Methods and Limitations

Protein quality method	Equation	Primary outcome	Limitation of method
Biological value (BV)	$BV = N$ retained $/ N$ absorbed or $$BV = \frac{I - (F - F_0) - (U - U_0)}{I - (F - F_0)}$$	Represents nitrogen retention as a percentage of nitrogen absorption.	Tedious process that must measure urine and fecal nitrogen loss both on the test diet and the N-free diet.
Net protein utilization (NPU)	Protein ingested ÷ amount protein stored in body	Compares the amount of protein eaten to the amount stored in the body, or how much the body actually used.	Relies on animal nitrogen excretion to determine the nitrogen content retained.
Protein efficiency ratio (PER)	Gain in body mass (g) ÷ protein intake (g)	A score of 1 provides all amino acids needed and is fully digested.	May not correlate well with humans due to reliability on animals for score.
Digestible indispensable amino acid score (DIAAS)	DIAAS % = (amino acid in the protein ÷ amino acid requirement) × amino acid digestibility	Measures protein absorption at the end of the small intestine. Method measures the digestion of individual amino acids to paint a better picture of how protein meets the body's amino acid needs.	Complexity.
Chemical score	AA score = mg AA in 1 g test protein/mg AA in 1 g reference protein × 100	The lowest score for any of the essential AA's designates the limiting AA → chemical score for that protein.	Digestibility and AA availability not taken into account.
Protein digestibility corrected amino acid score (PDCAAS)	Chemical score × % digestibility of a protein	Involves calculating the ratio of amino acids of a food source against the requirements of a 2- to 5-year-old child based on the first limiting dietary EAA within the protein.	Based on young children, so may not serve as best method for determining protein quality for adults.

I = N intake; F = fecal N; U = urinary N; F_0 and U_0 = fecal and urinary N on an N-free diet; AA = amino acid.

Table 5.4 Protein Chemical Score

| | PROTEIN SOURCE | | | | | |
| | Peanut butter | | White bread | | Brie (cheese) | |
Essential amino acid	mg/g	% optimal	mg/g	% optimal	mg/g	% optimal
Lysine	36	**62**	27	**46**	89	154
Threonine	35	102	29	87	36	**106**
Amino acid (chemical) score	62		46		106	

Cheese may be lower in protein in this example but contains higher quality protein, as indicated by the chemical score.

When comparing amino acids in foods, the amino acid with the lowest percent optimal score (the chemical score) is the limiting amino acid (bolded in the table).

each of the amino acids are then multiplied by 100 to create a percentage score for each amino acid.

The amino acid with the lowest score is the limiting amino acid. This amino acid, by definition, presents in the smallest amount relative to our biological need. The chemical score of the food protein is the same score as its limiting amino acid. The weakness of the chemical score is that it is not used much anymore and is based off of an "ideal" reference protein that some suggest

Amino acids in protein help build new proteins in muscle.

serves as an antiquated concept. Further, the chemical score says nothing about digestion or how a given protein is used by the body.

Calculating Biological Value

Biological value (BV) is one of the more common methods of measuring protein quality and is simply a measure of how much of the protein absorbed by the digestive tract is retained in the body for growth and maintenance. This concept of nitrogen retention is primarily a function of nitrogen absorption, since technically nitrogen cannot be "retained." BV compares protein in versus protein out to determine nitrogen absorption as a key element. Based on the calculation used to derive a BV, the highest possible value is 100, meaning that the protein has an amino acid composition most similar to our needs. The protein that entered the bloodstream will be most efficiently retained by the body. The BV is measured through a tedious process that involves feeding subjects a protein-free diet, followed by a measured amount of protein. The amount that is excreted via urine, feces, and skin are estimated, and BV is calculated. The final value represents nitrogen retention as a percentage of nitrogen absorption. For example, the BV of corn protein is 60, meaning that only 60 percent of the absorbed corn protein is retained for use by the body. BV is typically tested at very low protein intakes and can be a source of significant misinterpretation since most adults, and especially athletes, consume adequate protein amounts. Further, the number of calories consumed has a significant effect on BV values. Despite these limitations, BV is very accurate under conditions of low protein intake, but energy intake (kilocalories) should be meticulously controlled.

Measuring Net Protein Utilization

Net protein utilization (NPU) is similar to BV but simply compares the amount of protein eaten to the amount stored in the body, or how much the body actually uses. BV takes digestion and actual absorption of protein into account, whereas NPU does not. The nitrogen content of the test food is carefully measured and given to laboratory animals as their sole protein source. Animal nitrogen excretion is then measured to determine how much of the food's nitrogen content was retained. How efficiently the animal uses the food protein to make body proteins determines the NPU score.

Measuring the Protein Efficiency Ratio

The protein efficiency ratio (PER) is a measure of the amino acid composition that accounts for digestibility. The amount of weight gain (in grams) of growing animals fed a test protein is compared to the weight gain of growing animals fed a high-quality reference protein. This method provides information on how well the body can use a test protein by understanding amino acid composition, digestibility, and availability. This PER has been most commonly used to determine the protein quality of infant formulas.

Measuring the Protein Digestibility Corrected Amino Acid Score

The protein digestibility corrected amino acid score (PDCAAS) has been used since the 1990s for scoring protein quality and until recently has been the most common method used. The PDCAAS involves calculating the ratio of amino acids of a food source against the requirements of a 2- to 5-year-old child based on the first limiting dietary EAA within the protein. This method is similar to the chemical score, as it compares the amino acid profile to a reference protein while also considering digestion efficiency by multiplying the chemical score by the percent digestibility of the food protein. Foods with the highest possible PDCAAS of 1.0 are casein, whey, egg whites, and soy proteins. Any score calculated above 1.0 is truncated because any excess protein consumed was originally thought to be of no biological value. If a protein has a chemical score of 0.70, and 80 percent of that protein is digestible, then the PDCAAS would be 80 percent of 0.70 or 0.56. The FDA has recognized the PDCAAS as the official method for determining the protein quality of most food (29), and if the %DV of protein is listed on a food label, it must be based on the food's PDCAAS. With this requirement, the total grams of protein might be the same per serving for two different foods, but their %DV could be very different because the foods do not contribute equally to the amino acid needs of the body.

Using the Digestible Indispensable Amino Acid Score

Most recently the Food and Agriculture Organization of the United Nations (FAO) has recommended a new method of assessing the quality of dietary protein. The digestible indispensable amino acid score (DIAAS) method builds on previous approaches by accurately measuring the digestion of individual amino acids rather than crude protein digestion. The DIAAS can accurately distinguish between proteins that were previously truncated to a maximum score of 1.0, using the PDCAAS method. Significant improvements in accuracy over the PDCAAS are a result of several advancements. First, measuring protein absorption at the end of the small intestine provides a more accurate assessment of the actual food protein remaining in the GI tract before endogenous proteins are added in the large intestine. This method also measures the digestion of individual amino acids to paint a better picture of how well a protein meets the body's amino acid needs. The DIAAS also does not allow for truncation of scores to 1.0 and recognizes that an excess can make up for any amino acid deficits from consuming incomplete protein foods. Finally, the DIAAS expanded the amino acid reference pattern from the ages of 2 to 5 to account for variation based on age. The DIAAS differentiates between the needs of infants and children with three reference patterns: 0 to 6 months, 6 months to 3 years, and greater than 3 years. With the development of the DIAAS, we are now able to distinguish between protein sources PDCAAS previously classified as the same. The DIAAS can be a useful tool in cases where proteins are consumed in smaller amounts, such as in aging or in clinical applications. When developing new protein formulations by blending protein ingredients, it is important to understand the true value of protein sources in order to formulate the best protein ratio to meet the body's needs.

In summary, many measurements of protein quality are available, including chemical analysis of amino acid content and biological measures of protein digestibility. Ultimately, the most important factors that determine protein quality are the protein's retention in the body to support all amino acid needs and its ability to promote growth.

PROTEIN IN EXERCISE AND SPORT

Many people think that since muscle fibers are made up of protein, building and maintaining muscle must require large amounts of protein consumed from the diet. In reality, dietary protein is just one part of the equation to promote an optimal environment for muscles to adapt to physical training. The additional amount of protein required that is beyond what is already consumed to support optimal muscle adaptation is relatively small, and many athletes are already meeting their daily protein intake goals. Athletes should note that regular, well-structured training regimens combined with a proper mix of nutrients that meet their energy demands is the cornerstone for achieving their goals. Further, many other factors such as stress, frequent alcohol consumption, and inadequate rest can sabotage even the best diet and exercise plan. This is not to say that protein is not important. Research over the last decade has provided much more detail for how dietary protein works to foster muscle hypertrophy (growth) and metabolic adaptations when combined with a proper training program. The following are the four primary roles of dietary protein in an athlete's diet related to sport performance:

1. Maximizing gains in muscle mass and strength
2. Promoting adaptations in metabolic function (an up-regulation of oxidative enzymes)
3. Preserving lean mass during rapid weight loss
4. Structural benefits to other protein-containing nonmuscle tissues, such as tendons, ligaments, and bones

New guidelines now exist for daily protein needs as well as the daily distribution of protein consumed. In this section, we delve into these details and also look at the ways protein metabolism changes during and in response to exercise and how this information melds with other sections of this chapter.

Protein Metabolism and Exercise

Although carbohydrate and fat are the primary macronutrients metabolized for energy in the muscle, protein can also be used during exercise and can be oxidized directly in the muscle. Fortunately, most protein is spared for important synthetic processes, but it is important to remember from chapter 1 that the oxidation of all energy-yielding macronutrient fuel sources is always occurring in the body during exercise. The only thing that changes is the relative proportion of the macronutrients burned. At any one time during exercise, carbohydrate and fat make up more than 85 percent of the energy-yielding macronutrient fuels oxidized, but some protein is always used.

Exercise has a strong effect on protein metabolism. During exercise, the range of protein contribution to meet energy demands (ATP) is generally less than 5 to 10 percent, and in some extreme cases up to 15 percent of total energy expenditure. Many factors affect the percentage of protein oxidized during exercise, including exercise intensity, training level (new vs. experienced), and availability of other fuels (e.g., carbohydrate). The type of exercise, or mode of exercise, also has a strong influence. During strenuous resistance training, less than 5 percent of protein is oxidized as an energy source. Conversely, prolonged endurance exercise (>90 min) might result in up to 15 percent to serve as an energy source. A significant increase in protein oxidation, within the 5 to 15 percent range, occurs when muscle glycogen is depleted. As the body's most limited fuel source (carbohydrate) becomes depleted, the body must attempt to keep blood sugar stable to fuel the nervous system. For most individuals, the process of gluconeogenesis (see chapters 2 and 3) kicks in to help stabilize blood sugar levels by making new glucose from gluconeogenic precursors, including protein. For those following a low-carbohydrate diet, the production of ketones provides more fuel to the nervous system when glucose is limited. Regardless of the amount of carbohydrate in the diet, when muscle glycogen becomes depleted, BCAA oxidation within the muscle increases and contributes to the rise in protein use as a fuel source. In such a scenario, exercise intensity decreases. Gluconeogenesis and ketone production cannot keep up with the high ATP demands of high-intensity exercise.

Gluconeogenesis

The most prominent gluconeogenic pathway is the glucose-alanine cycle (figure 5.16). In this metabolic pathway, the gluconeogenic amino acid alanine leaves the muscle to create new glucose in the liver, which contributes to new blood glucose. This process occurs simultaneously with muscle tissue oxidation of BCAAs. As BCAAs are liberated from muscle tissue, their catabolism results in donating their NH_2 group to pyruvate in a process called transamination. The carbon skeletons from the BCAAs can then enter the TCA cycle in the mitochondria of muscle cells as TCA intermediates to contribute to ATP generation. Meanwhile, pyruvate originating from glycolysis can bind with NH_2 that originated from the BCAAs deamination to form the gluconeogenic amino acid alanine. Alanine can freely leave the muscle tissue and travel through the blood to the liver. The liver can then deaminate alanine to reform pyruvate. This liver-generated pyruvate can be further metabolized to form glucose that contributes to blood glucose or liver glycogen. Gluconeogenesis is never really turned off in human metabolism; instead it may occur only at a very low capacity and increase during long bouts of exercise, particularly when carbohydrate stores become limited. A significant limitation of this pathway is that the speed at which it can create new glucose depends on the availability of enzymes needed to drive the reaction. These enzymes must go through the protein synthesis process and are thus not capable of being made fast enough to keep up with the demands of one long endurance exercise bout. As a result, hypoglycemia can eventually occur and is the primary reason exercise halts during long events. While the glucose-alanine cycle is an integral pathway in human metabolism and contributes to exercise metabolism, it is best suited for nonexercise situations during starvation, when key enzymes have time to be up-regulated to produce glucose at the expense of muscle protein.

Protein Oxidation

Besides BCAAs, other amino acids from muscle tissue provide substrates for the TCA cycle (glutamine) in working muscle. BCAAs are the only amino acids liberated by the muscle that can be oxidized directly in the muscle. There is an increased percentage of BCAA oxidation with prolonged aerobic training, with only a marginal carbohydrate-sparing effect that is most appreciable in endurance events lasting longer than 90 minutes. However, in these situations there is limited evidence to support BCAA supplementation as a strategy to enhance performance. BCAAs are oxidized at such a low capacity that supplementation has no effect on performance.

Protein needs in athletes are elevated in part to account for increased protein oxidation. This is most pronounced for endurance athletes to

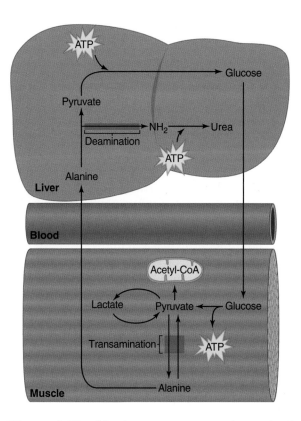

Figure 5.16 Alanine serves as an important gluconeogenic precursor.

support these metabolic activities and to allow the muscle to adapt for endurance success by synthesizing more mitochondrial enzymes, producing more and larger mitochondria, and making new capillaries and hemoglobin to transport oxygen to working muscle. For other athletes, those who focus more on strength and power, much less protein is oxidized during exercise. However, because of the nature of their sport and sport-specific training, breakdown of contractile proteins is greater than what is observed with endurance training.

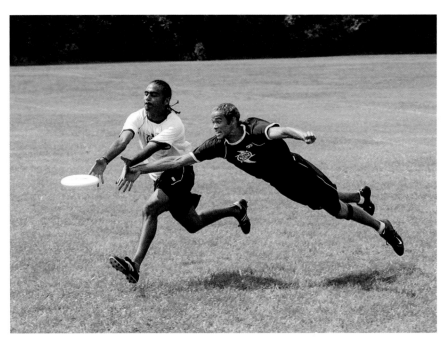

Protein provides the building blocks (amino acids) needed to build and repair muscle.

Since these protein structures (i.e., the protein fibers that make muscles move) are larger than oxidative enzymes, and at times the breakdown can be significant, protein needs tend to be higher in athletes who participate in strength and power sports. While these distinctions are clear from a scientific standpoint, from a practical sense, exercising athletes are much more complicated. For instance, many athletes rely on strength, power, and endurance to be successful in their sport and often rely on one aspect more than the others during specific phases of their training. The most prudent strategy to minimize protein oxidation is to have a well-chosen diet that meets both carbohydrate and energy demands of both the endurance athlete (e.g., runners and cyclists) and any athlete involved in a sustained competition where endurance is a key component (e.g., soccer).

Daily Protein Needs for Athletes

Current data suggest that dietary protein intake necessary to support an athlete's needs generally ranges from 1.2 to 2.0 g/kg per day (30). This daily amount is thought to support metabolic adaptation, repair of muscle and connective tissue, remodeling, and protein turnover in athletes. It

is this range that appears to support the optimal amount of protein for the athlete to repair and replace damaged proteins; remodel proteins within muscle, bone, tendon, and ligaments; maintain optimal function of all metabolic pathways that use amino acids; support accretion of lean mass; support immune function; and support the optimal rate of production of plasma proteins. It is also recognized that at any given time, based on training demands, goals, or other physiological stressors, an athlete's protein needs might fluctuate within this range from day to day, week to week, or month to month. In some scenarios, short-term intake of protein exceeding 2.0 g/kg might be indicated for athletes during intensified training or when reducing energy intake (17, 25). Protein needs of athletes are higher when on a lower calorie diet to minimize the breakdown of skeletal muscle (8).

Periodization

The aforementioned daily protein intake guidelines provide a general range of daily targets that should be based around adapting to specific sessions of training or competition within a periodized training program. The aim of periodization is to reach the best possible performance in the most important competition of the year and involves progressive cycling of various aspects of a training program during a specific period. These various aspects also include nutrient periodization and certainly involve protein as a nutrient, with changing needs underpinned by an appreciation of the larger context of athletic goals, nutrient needs, energy considerations, and food choices. Generally, within the 1.2 to 2.0 g/kg protein range, requirements can fluctuate based on "trained" status (experienced athletes requiring less), training (sessions involving higher frequency and intensity, or a new training stimulus at the higher end of protein range), carbohydrate availability, and most importantly, energy availability (2, 28). Maintenance of normal bone metabolism and menstrual function are just two of the many body functions that can be negatively affected by low energy and carbohydrate availability in athletes. For athletes in heavy training and competition, the consumption of adequate energy, particularly from carbohydrates, to match energy expenditure is important so that amino acids are spared for protein synthesis and not oxidized (27). In cases of energy restriction or sudden inactivity as a result of injury, elevated protein intakes as high as 2.0 g/kg per day or higher (17, 30, 35) spread over the day at different mealtimes might be advantageous in minimizing fat-free mass (FFM) loss from skeletal muscle (25).

Recommendations for Protein Intake

As shown in table 5.5, the modern view for establishing recommendations for protein intake in athletes clearly extends beyond the DRIs and the AMDR. Focus has shifted to evaluating the benefits of providing enough protein at optimal periodized times to support tissues with rapid turnover and augment metabolic adaptations initiated by a training stimulus. Given the wide range the AMDR provides for protein intake, the use of the AMDR to determine protein needs in athletes should generally be used only as a way to double-check to ensure maximal diet quality (from other energy-yielding macronutrients). The AMDR can also be used after protein needs by body weight (grams per kilogram) are determined to evaluate if an athlete is consuming a minimal protein amount to meet health needs while not consuming an excessive amount that may displace the intake of carbohydrate and fat. Gram per kilogram recommendations are superior to the AMDR and help to fine-tune protein recommendations for athletes depending on their individualized needs during the various training cycles. These recommendations are more specific to the athlete's training demand and goals and are more practical to prescribe. Take, for instance, an athlete who may require 6,000 kilocalories during heavy training and 3,000 kilocalories while trying to make competition weight. The daily protein amounts needed based solely on the AMDR would vary greatly for these two calorie requirements combined, with added variability of having to choose a value to use between 10 and 35 percent, and these calculations may either fall significantly short or exceed g/kg recommendations that are currently recommended. As another example, a competitive athlete might consume as many as 5,000 kilocalories per day. If that athlete weighed 80 kilograms, and if his diet contained only 10 percent of calories as protein, he would be getting about 125 grams of protein daily—about 1.6 g/kg body weight. This level of protein is

Table 5.5 Protein Intake Recommendations for Athletes and Individuals With a High Volume of Vigorous Activity

RECOMMENDATIONS BASED ON 1.2 G/KG TO 2.0 G/KG OF BODY WEIGHT	
Lower end of range	**Higher end of range**
Light- to moderate-intensity physical activity with low to moderate weekly volume	High-intensity training periods During reduced energy intake Recovering from injury or during rehabilitation
Recovery protein	**15 to 25 g (0.25–0.30 g/kg) of high biological value protein**

likely adequate to meet the needs of this athlete and would need to be only slightly modified to reach goal intake amounts specific to the current needs described in the literature.

Factors Affecting Protein Synthesis

Body proteins are constantly turned over through both synthesis and degradation pathways. While it is important to implement strategies that can augment muscle protein synthesis (MPS), it is also important to minimize muscle protein breakdown (MPB) in order to promote a net increase in muscle protein accretion. Several factors other than protein consumption can affect protein synthesis, including the type, volume, and intensity of exercise. For example, resistance training is the most potent stimulus for muscle building. Progressive resistance training allows athletes to consistently train to complete lifts at higher loads (i.e., weights) and repetitions. It is largely the damage to contractile proteins that result from this training that triggers the body to adapt to synthesize more muscle protein to accommodate the increasing loads placed on the dumbbells or barbells. This muscle adaptation associated with exercise occurs with most exercise, albeit to a lesser extent than with progressive resistance training. Exercise is an important variable that can stimulate MPS but is also a moving target, given the wide range of exercises, training volume, intensity, and duration commonly found in any one training program. In addition, the familiarity of the exercise, training program, or sport also is a strong influencer of maximal MPS response. Athletes who complete the same training program and are very efficient with the physical movements associated with their sport have a lower MPS response compared to athletes who are new to an intense resistance-training program. The hormonal environment is another factor that works alongside dietary protein and a well-structured exercise program to maximize MPS. Several endogenous hormones, such as insulin-like growth factor-1 (IGF-1), growth hormone, testosterone, and insulin facilitate the anabolic response. The role of these anabolic hormones is essential to facilitate hypertrophy, but the effect is significant only when maintaining normal hormone levels as a result of youth and exercise. Targeted exercise and nutrition strategies to target these hormones to enhance their ability to promote MPS have been underwhelming, and their effect seems to be maximized but not enhanced by proper exercise and nutrition. The negative effect of an unfavorable hormonal environment on MPS is most pronounced as a result of aging, illness, and injury. The major players that initiate significant MPB are malnutrition, inactivity, illness, and injury. These factors promote acute muscle loss from MPB, and one could argue that minimizing

DO YOU KNOW ?

Many athletes and those who are recreationally active tend to "backload" their energy intake. This means they tend to consume most of their calories in the evening or night. Optimal use of protein occurs when smaller, but adequate, amounts of dietary protein are consumed throughout the day. This simple strategy will optimize skeletal muscle protein synthesis in adults as opposed to eating a little here and there throughout the day and one large protein meal at night.

PUTTING IT INTO PERSPECTIVE

MUSCLE PROTEIN SYNTHESIS

Muscle protein synthesis (MPS) helps individuals adapt to exercise by promoting muscle growth, which can further help to increase overall muscle mass and support optimal muscle function. This is accomplished through exercise programs, timing, and ingestion of protein after exercise. BCAAs, particularly leucine, are key players in stimulating MPS, and consuming a full complement of essential amino acids is important to maximize muscle growth over time (6).

these variables is as important as optimizing variables associated with MPS.

While the extremes of these MPB variables are most commonly observed in clinical environments where people are extremely ill from infection or trauma, lesser forms of these variables can significantly contribute to muscle loss in athletes. For example, athletes who train and compete with low energy availability or practice fasting after exercise will experience sustained MPB. Inactivity also serves as the opposite of exercise by removing the exercise stimulus that drives the intracellular MPS machinery to be activated and use proteins from the amino acid pool to make new muscle tissue. Athletic injury (e.g., ACL tear, bone break) and illness promote MPB via two mechanisms. The first is by promoting inactivity or a significant reduction of activity less than required to maximize MPS. Second, illness and injury can negatively affect the hormonal environment and promote inflammation that elicits an elevated immune response requiring additional MPB to provide amino acids to support the body's defense of illness or recovery from injury.

Several factors besides total daily protein can affect the body's ability to gain skeletal muscle mass. Other negative factors, including unhealthy lifestyle habits such as smoking and alcohol consumption, can limit MPS, along with high levels of the hormone cortisol, associated with stress and lack of sleep, and inadequate recovery time between workout sessions (3). Diminished blood flow to muscle tissues, such as that observed with peripheral vascular disease also limits MPS (1). Other positive factors for increasing and maintaining muscle mass include maintaining a positive energy balance (consuming more calories than expended), a consistent meal pattern, pre- and postexercise sports nutrition strategies to spare muscle protein, and adequate rest to promote recovery between training sessions. The complex nature of MPB can make overly simple recommendations such as "eat more protein" shortsighted.

Dietary Protein as a Trigger for Muscle Metabolic Adaptation

Dietary protein has been well chronicled to interact with exercise, providing both a trigger and a substrate for the synthesis of contractile and metabolic proteins (23, 25). Adaptations are thought to occur by (a) turning on MPS in response to the amount of leucine consumed in a meal and (b) providing an additional outside source of amino acids for incorporation into new proteins and to keep this process running (6). A sample of foods high in leucine is listed in table 5.6.

Optimal Protein Source for Athletes

High-quality dietary proteins are effective for the maintenance, repair, and synthesis of skeletal muscle proteins (31). Chronic training studies have shown that the consumption of milk-based protein after resistance exercise is effective in increasing

Table 5.6 Leucine Content of Foods

Food	Leucine (g)
36 g of whey protein isolate	3.2
36 g soy protein isolate	2.4
4 oz. sirloin steak	2.0
4 oz. chicken breast	2.0
1 cup low-fat yogurt	1.1
1 cup fat-free milk	0.8
1 egg	0.5
2 tbsp. peanut butter	0.5
1 slice wheat bread	0.1

Data from U.S. Department of Agriculture and U.S. Department of Health & Human Services 2015.

muscle strength while also promoting favorable changes in body composition (9, 11, 12). Other studies suggest increased MPS and muscle building with whole milk, lean meat, and dietary supplements, some of which provide the isolated proteins whey, casein, soy, and egg. To date, dairy proteins appear to be superior to other tested proteins, largely because of their leucine content and the digestion and absorptive kinetics of branched-chain amino acids in fluid-based dairy foods (22). Amino acids from whey protein, for example, can appear in the plasma in less than 30 minutes, whereas amino acids from intact animal proteins (beef, fish, etc.) can take 90 minutes or more. This might suggest that easily digested, quickly absorbed proteins such as whey are ideal for promoting a favorable anabolic response immediately after exercise.

In summary, an athlete's protein needs should be expressed using body weight guidelines (per kg body mass) to allow recommendations to be scaled to the large range in body sizes of athletes. Sports nutrition guidelines for protein intake should also consider the importance of the timing and distribution of daily protein intake rather than focusing only on general daily targets. Note that excess protein may contribute to excess calories, and excess protein can add more weight as fat, not muscle, which can slow down an athlete's performance. Most weekend athletes and recreational athletes can easily meet slightly elevated protein needs by simple changes in their diet, and there is no reason that protein supplements will help their performance. Competitive athletes should choose adequate calories from a wide variety of foods to help ensure adequate protein intake.

VEGETARIANISM AND VEGANISM

Vegetarians all share the common practice of limiting or completely avoiding meat and meat products; they can, however, differ significantly in their particular dietary choices.

Others may choose a semi-vegetarian diet by minimizing red meat consumption, very similar to the Mediterranean diet. Those who follow this diet focus on consuming grains, pasta, vegetables, cheeses, olive oil, and small amounts of chicken and fish. Table 5.7 lists good sources of protein for lacto-ovo-pesco vegetarians. Figure 5.17 lists meatless food options that are high in protein.

Although there are certainly many health benefits of a vegetarian diet, certain types of vegetarian choices might pose unique nutrition risks. Vegan diets are the most susceptible to these individual nutrient concerns because the best sources of these nutrients are from animal foods, and vegan diets contain higher amounts of oxalates and phytates. These compounds are plant-based food constituents that can bind some minerals in the GI tract, making them less available for absorption. Lacto-ovo-pesco vegetarians can easily have a nutritionally complete diet providing all protein requirements, but such a diet might also be high

Table 5.7 Example Protein Sources for Lacto-Ovo-Pesco Vegetarians

Protein source	Biological value (BV)	Protein (g)	Serving size
Whey isolate	159	16	1 scoop (28.7 g)
Whey concentrate	104	25	1 scoop (28.7 g)
Egg	100	6	1 egg
Milk	90	8	1 cup
Fish	83	22	1 filet (3 oz.)
Soybeans	73	9	1 cup
Brown rice	57	5	1 cup
Lentils	50	18	1 cup

Data from U.S. Department of Agriculture and U.S. Department of Health & Human Services 2015.

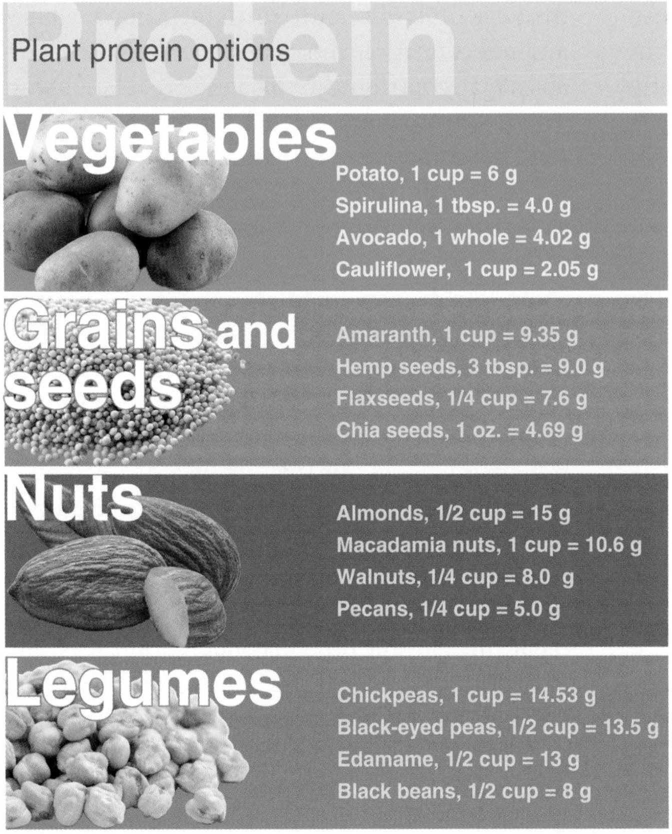

Plant protein options

Vegetables

Potato, 1 cup = 6 g
Spirulina, 1 tbsp. = 4.0 g
Avocado, 1 whole = 4.02 g
Cauliflower, 1 cup = 2.05 g

Grains and seeds

Amaranth, 1 cup = 9.35 g
Hemp seeds, 3 tbsp. = 9.0 g
Flaxseeds, 1/4 cup = 7.6 g
Chia seeds, 1 oz. = 4.69 g

Nuts

Almonds, 1/2 cup = 15 g
Macadamia nuts, 1 cup = 10.6 g
Walnuts, 1/4 cup = 8.0 g
Pecans, 1/4 cup = 5.0 g

Legumes

Chickpeas, 1 cup = 14.53 g
Black-eyed peas, 1/2 cup = 13.5 g
Edamame, 1/2 cup = 13 g
Black beans, 1/2 cup = 8 g

Figure 5.17 Numerous nonmeat food options are sources of protein.

in fat and low in iron, particularly if a large part of the diet is made up of dairy products. While vegetarian diets can be adequate for most people, followers should be thoughtful of their food choices, taking care to pursue a varied diet and be cautioned against vegan diets that exclude multiple food groups.

Vegetarian athletes committed to frequent training, competition, and success should also be cognizant of the benefits and challenges associated with a vegetarian diet. Vegetarian athletes might have an increased risk of lower bone mineral density and stress fractures (36). Additional practical challenges include gaining access to suitable foods during travel, at restaurants, and at training camps and competition venues. Without proper planning, it is not uncommon for these athletes to limit their energy and protein intake, which can significantly affect their performance. Vegetarian athletes might benefit from compre-

hensive dietary assessments and education. This helps to ensure their diets are nutritionally sound to support training and competition demands, while also functioning to identify nutrient gaps that can be addressed to support both health and performance.

In order to meet protein needs, vegetarian athletes and nonathletes alike should focus on protein quality, while striving to consume protein at every meal. Several vegetarian foods have a high PDCAAS score, including eggs, low-fat yogurt and milk, and soy, as well as tofu, edamame, and soy milk and yogurt. Consuming multiple small meals and snacks per day also provides the opportunity to add more variety to the diet to include protein-containing foods such as vegetables, legumes, whole grains, and nuts and seeds. Finally, it is generally accepted that vegans who avoid all animal products should supplement their diets with a reliable source of vitamin B_{12}, such as fortified soy milk, other fortified foods, or a dietary supplement. A more detailed discussion of vegetarian diets is provided in chapter 14.

PROTEIN DEFICIENCY AND EXCESS PROTEIN

Given the important role of protein to virtually all body systems and processes, it is no surprise that protein deficiency can create several problems affecting normal human physiology. As a reminder, a lack of essential amino acids will stop the synthesis of body proteins, leading to increased rates of body protein catabolism to meet the body's amino acid demands. Protein deficiency occurs when energy or protein intake is inadequate to meet and sustain the nitrogen demands of the body. While protein provides essential nitrogen for synthetic processes, adequate energy intake protects protein from being removed from its important synthetic role. Specifically, adequate energy intake spares both dietary and body proteins so they can be used for the synthesis of new protein. Inadequate energy intake leads the body to oxidize protein for energy and for glucose generation. Protein deficiency can also occur in those who appear to be eating adequate daily amounts of protein if the protein they consume is not digested well or is of poor quality. Further, a risk of protein deficiency exists in situations when protein needs are elevated without being met by the diet. During growth and development, childhood and adolescent dietary protein deficiency can lead to inadequate growth (stunting). Risk of protein deficiency can also become elevated as a result of physiological stress presenting in the form of an injury, trauma, pregnancy, or other medical conditions. Protein consumption that was adequate prior to the onset of these physiologic stressors might not be adequate once they are present and can result in suboptimal physiological adaptation, as the need for elevated protein synthesis might be compromised.

While protein deficiency is widespread in poverty-stricken communities in underdeveloped countries, in North America it is most common in clinical settings where patients experience severe metabolic stress and do not have the ability to meet their elevated protein needs through their diet. In industrialized countries, most people face the opposite problem of protein excess, which in many cases is a product of consuming more calories than needed. However, dietary protein excess is more difficult to define in terms of specific daily intake of protein and cut-points above the RDA and the Food and Nutrition Board has not provided an upper intake level for protein because of insufficient evidence to support the link to chronic health problems (19). Despite the lack of a clear definition of "excess protein intake," we know that the average American consumes well above the RDA for protein. As described earlier, in many cases this is justified, but note that if the diet contains more protein than is needed for synthesis, much of the protein excess is converted and stored as fat. As a result, individuals who consume protein supplements or eat a very high-protein diet in hopes to gain muscle mass might be contributing more to their fat mass, especially if the extra protein consumed is above and beyond the calorie intake needed to maintain body weight. Although chronic high-protein intakes have been linked to chronic

disease, it is difficult to determine a cause-and-effect relationship. Several confounding variables may contribute to this negative relationship. Those who consume higher protein intakes also tend to consume higher amounts of saturated fat and fewer fruits and vegetables, and in some cases they might adopt other lifestyle factors that influence a negative relationship. When examining specific protein intakes in relation to body weight, anecdotal reports of dehydration and kidney stress have been associated with protein intakes greater than 2.0 g/kg per day, but there is no consensus in the scientific literature that protein intakes at this level are harmful. Although the kidney must excrete the products of protein breakdown, high protein intake is only thought to strain kidney function in people with diabetes or kidney disease. The most significant concern regarding chronic protein consumption at greater than 2.0 g/kg is that the protein foods, and in some cases the protein supplements consumed to reach this level of protein intake, might be displacing the opportunity to consume a variety of nutrient-dense foods from multiple food groups that have a strong connection to chronic disease prevention and longevity of life. Many of these displaced foods also tend to be higher in fiber, contain fewer calories and fat, and are more protective against obesity and cancer.

SUMMARY

Amino acids are the building blocks of both body and dietary protein. Protein is the key structural component that makes up not only muscle but also all other connective and organ tissues. Protein also has an essential role in making up hormones, enzymes, and antibodies and can also be used as an energy source to make ATP. High-quality dietary proteins are essential and effective for repair, synthesis, and maintenance of all body proteins. Protein consumed at appropriate amounts and at the right times is particularly important to help skeletal muscle recover and adapt to exercise. Dietary proteins can be obtained through animal and vegetable sources, as well as in supplement form, and must be digested and absorbed before being utilized. Vegetarians can meet their protein needs by planning a well-chosen diet. Most individuals can easily meet their protein needs by consuming a source of dietary protein with every meal and snack. For athletes, special attention should be given to the total amount of protein consumed per day, the type of protein, and the timing of intake. Careful planning of protein feedings for the athlete allows for optimal skeletal muscle utilization of these food-derived amino acids.

▇▇ FOR REVIEW ⟫

1. Describe the different functions and roles of protein.

2. What is an enzyme? How does it function?

3. Can essential amino acids be made by the body? What amino acid group is important for promoting MPS?

4. Describe the primary, secondary, tertiary, and quaternary structure of proteins (if necessary, review figure 5.6).

5. Describe protein digestion.

6. How would you begin to recommend protein intake for a sedentary, active, and extremely active individual? Explain the steps you would take.

7. What are the benefits of consuming vegetable protein sources? What are potential concerns for athletes trying to meet their protein needs with a vegetarian diet?

8. What is gluconeogenesis? List the gluconeogenic precursors.

PART III

ROLE OF MICRONUTRIENTS, WATER, AND NUTRITIONAL SUPPLEMENTS

This section of the book covers vitamins (chapter 6), minerals (chapter 7), water and electrolytes (chapter 8), and nutrition supplements (chapter 9). Vitamins and minerals do not provide energy, but they facilitate chemical reactions in the body that help generate energy. In addition, vitamins are important for growth and development, organ functioning, and building and maintaining structures in the body, including protecting the body from damage. Minerals help build structural components of the body and are necessary for a wide variety of functions that support health and athletic performance. Deficiencies in certain vitamins and minerals can impair health and athletic performance.

Because minerals are electrolytes, they conduct electricity in the body and affect fluid balance and muscle pH and function. Electrolytes and water go hand in hand as overconsumption or underconsumption of fluid can alter electrolyte balance. Water is also a medium for transportation in the body. Dietary supplements may include macronutrients, micronutrients, or a wide variety of compounds intended to support good health, athletic performances, or dietary gaps.

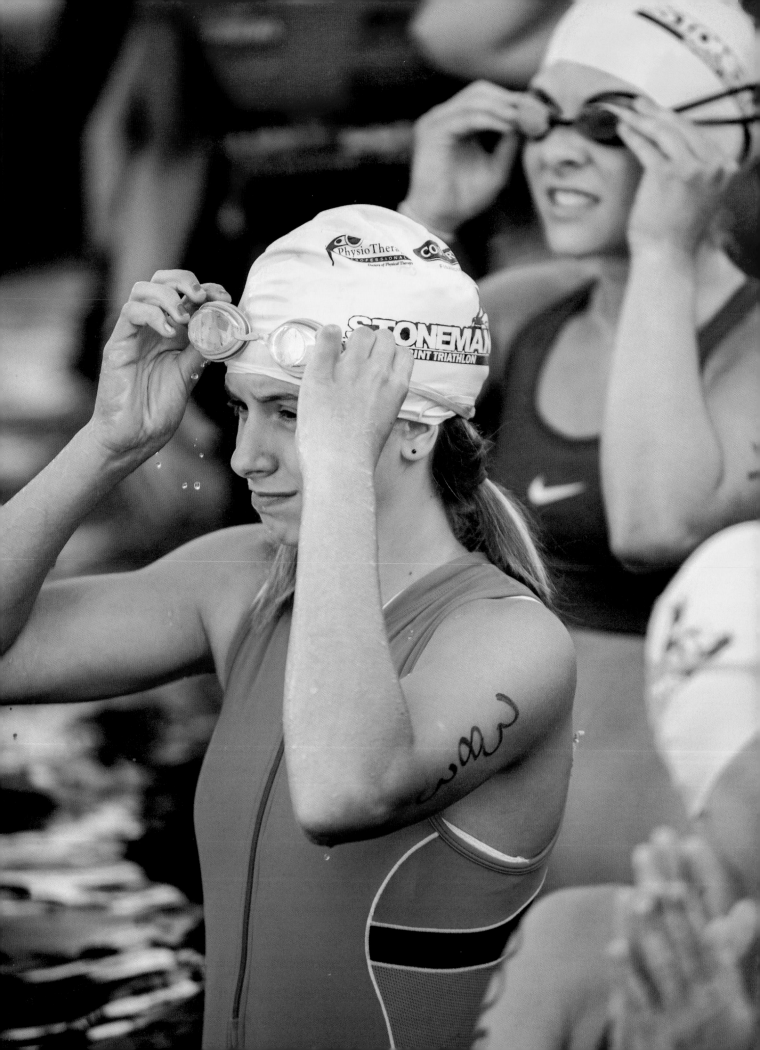

CHAPTER 6

Vitamins

After completing this chapter, you will be able to do the following:

> Discuss why vitamins are important for overall health and training.

> Describe how training and exercise affect vitamin needs.

> List the vitamins that most people are not getting enough of through their diet.

> List the vitamins that are toxic when consumed in excess.

> List a few good food sources for each major vitamin.

> Explain factors that may increase a person's need for a specific vitamin.

Vitamins are necessary for metabolism, proper growth and development, vision, and organ and immune functioning. They also aid human performance by facilitating energy production; supporting muscle contraction and relaxation, as well as oxygen transport; building and maintaining bone and cartilage; building and repairing muscle tissue; and protecting the body's cells from damage. The human body can make vitamins D and K; all other vitamins must be consumed in the diet to meet dietary requirements. Although deficiencies or insufficiencies in certain nutrients can impair training adaptations and performance, no current data indicate that excess nutrient intake, beyond the requirements for general health, will improve athletic performance (94). In some cases, excess consumption of specific vitamins may interfere with performance, training adaptations, and recovery. Figure 6.1 illustrates the importance of many vitamins discussed in this chapter.

FAT-SOLUBLE VITAMINS

Vitamins A, D, E, and K are **fat-soluble** vitamins. They are stored in the body's fat tissues and more easily absorbed when consumed with dietary fat.

Vitamin A

Vitamin A helps form healthy teeth, bones, soft tissue, skeletal tissue, mucous membranes, and skin. Vitamin A also promotes good vision, particularly night vision, and is necessary for growth, development, cellular communication, and immune system functioning, as well as the formation and maintenance of several organs, including the heart, lungs, and kidneys (158). The active form of vitamin A in the body is retinol. Two types of vitamin A are found in food:

> **Preformed vitamin A** is found in some animal foods. Retinol is a type of preformed vitamin A found in animal liver, whole milk, and some fortified foods.

> **Provitamin A carotenoids**, including beta-carotene, alpha-carotene, and beta-cryptoxanthin, are the dark-colored pigments found in red palm oil and in several fruits and vegetables, notably carrots, mango, cantaloupe, squash, sweet red bell peppers, seaweed, and

spinach. These carotenoids are converted to the active form of vitamin A in the body, a process that depends on several factors, including the food matrix, food processing, and dietary fat intake, as well as genetic differences (90, 146). Approximately 45 percent of the Western population are considered "low converters" of beta-carotene to the active form of vitamin A in the body, a factor that can affect vitamin A levels over time if a large portion of vitamin A intake comes from carotenoids (90). See figure 6.2 for sources of provitamin A carotenoids.

There are over 600 types of carotenoids found in nature; many, though not all, have provitamin A activity. Nutrition data exists for alpha-carotene, beta-carotene, and beta-cryptoxanthin, all of which are pro-vitamin A carotenoids and act as **antioxidants**. Certain antioxidants protect plants from pests and disease (170, 175) and protect cells in the human body from **free radical** damage (57). Figure 6.3 shows the interaction between free radicals and antioxidants.

Free radicals are reactive oxygen and nitrogen species generated in the body through metabolism and exposure to various physiological conditions or disease states. Free radicals are essential for health, but they can be harmful when they go into overdrive. For normal physiological functioning, the body must maintain a balance between free radicals and antioxidants (not getting too much or too little of either; supplemental antioxidant intake may actually increase oxidative damage to cells or impair adaptations to resistance training). Overproduction of free radicals, when combined with an inability to regulate them, leads to oxidative stress and subsequent damage to cellular lipids, proteins, and DNA in addition to initiating a number of diseases (91).

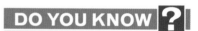

DO YOU KNOW ?

One glass of milk contains less than 10% DV of vitamin A, from a combination of preformed and provitamin A (158).

Sources of Vitamin A and the RDA

The RDA for vitamin A is given in mcg of retinal activity equivalents (RAE) to account for sources of vitamin A. While 1 mcg of retinol is equal to

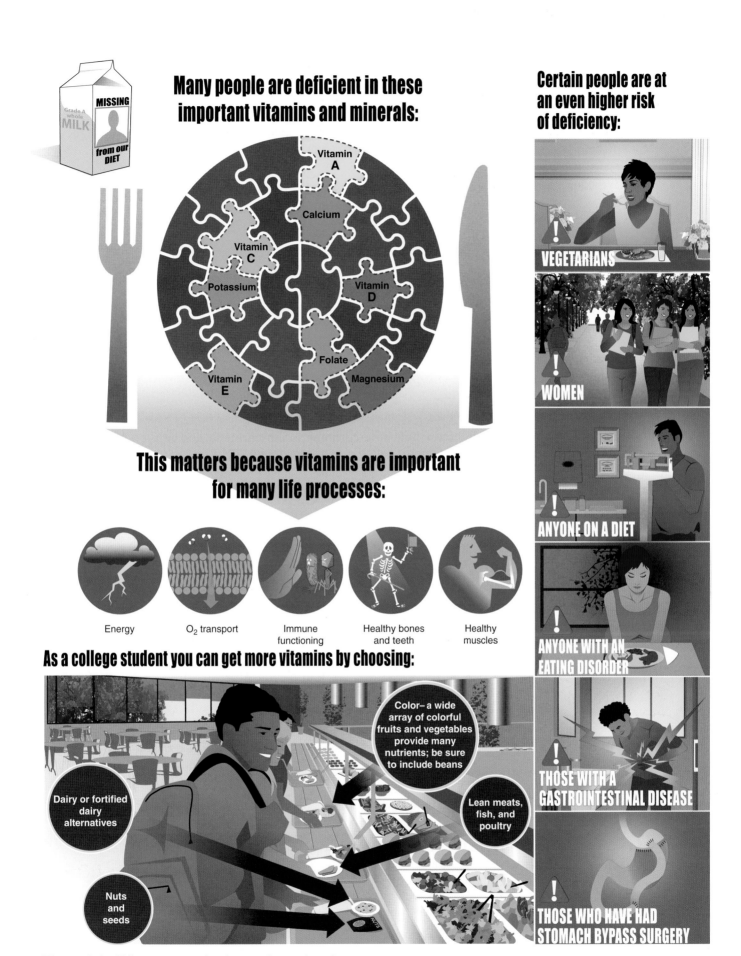

Figure 6.1 What you need to know about vitamins.

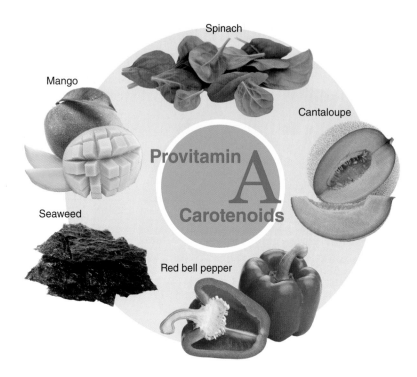

Figure 6.2 Provitamin A carotenoids include beta-carotene, alpha-carotene, and beta-cryptoxanthin. Beta-carotene is considered the most important source of provitamin A (151).

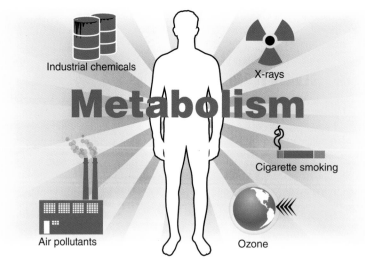

Maintaining a healthy balance of free radicals and antioxidants is essential for good health.

Figure 6.3 Free radicals are naturally produced in the body and made upon exposure to various environmental insults and diseases. Some antioxidants can help attenuate oxidative damage resulting from free radicals running amok.

1 mcg RAE, it takes 12-mcg beta-carotene or 24-mcg alpha-carotene or beta-cryptoxanthin to equal 1 mcg RAE. Making matters more confusing, vitamin A is listed on dietary foods and supplements in international units (IUs). The conversion between IU and RAE depends on the source of vitamin A (table 6.1).

Vitamin A Deficiency and Toxicity

Vitamin A deficiency is rare in North America, yet common in developing countries (44, 133), where it is a leading cause of preventable blindness in children (1, 78, 179). Xerophthalmia—dry eyes caused by inadequate tear production—which can lead to night blindness, is an early sign of vitamin A deficiency. Vitamin A deficiency can also suppress immune system functioning and increase risk of infection (141). In the United States and other developed countries, groups at risk of deficiency include premature infants and individuals with cystic fibrosis (26, 112).

Preformed vitamin A is stored in the body, particularly the liver, and can be toxic when taken in one single massive dose or in large doses over time. Acute overdose can lead to very dry skin, inflammation and cracking of the lips at the corners of the mouth (**cheilosis**), gingivitis, muscle and joint pain, fatigue, depression, and abnormal liver tests. Signs and symptoms of chronic consumption of very high intakes of vitamin A might include increased cerebrospinal fluid pressure, dizziness, blurred vision, vomiting, nausea, bone and muscle pain, headaches, and poor muscular coordination (113). Vitamin A toxicity can also lead to liver damage (that is not always reversible), coma, and death (158, 187). Excess dietary intake (from food) could potentially lead to toxicity, but most cases of vitamin A toxicity are from therapeutic retinoids (medicines prescribed in high doses for the treatment of acne, psoriasis, and other conditions). It takes a considerable amount of time for tissue stores of vitamin A to decline after discontinuing intake (158).

Provitamin A carotenoids are considered nontoxic, though over a long period of time excess beta-carotene can lead to yellow-orange skin. Skin will return to its natural shade once beta-carotene intake is discontinued (158). Though beta-carotene

Table 6.1 Excellent or Good Sources of Vitamin A

Food	Serving size	RAE per serving (mcg)	IU per serving	%DV
Beef, variety of meats and by-products, raw liver	4 oz. (113 g)	32,000	106,670	2,133
Sweet potato, baked or boiled (no skin)	1 cup mashed (145 g)	2,581	51,627	1,033
Pumpkin, canned	1 cup (245 g)	1,906	38,129	762
Goose liver (raw)	1 liver (94 g)	8,750	29,138	582
Carrots (frozen, cooked, boiled, drained)	1 cup sliced (146 g)	1,235	24,715	494
Carrots (raw)	1 cup chopped (128 g)	1,069	21,384	428
Turkey liver (raw)	1 liver (78 g)	6,285	21,131	422
Collards (frozen, chopped, cooked, boiled, drained)	1 cup chopped (170 g)	978	19,538	391
Kale (frozen, cooked, boiled, drained)	1 cup chopped (130 g)	956	19,115	382
Spinach (cooked, boiled, drained)	1 cup (180 g)	943	18,866	377
Swiss chard (cooked, boiled, drained)	1 cup chopped (175 g)	536	10,717	214

Data from U.S. Department of Agriculture 2013.

does not build up in the body, studies show very high doses (33,000–50,000 IU supplemental beta-carotene) taken over the course of 5 to 8 years increased risk of lung cancer and cardiovascular disease in current and former smokers (23, 60, 166). In a controlled supplementation trial in male smokers spanning 6 years, high-dose beta-carotene (66,600 IU beta-carotene/day) increased risk of hemorrhagic stroke (caused by rupture of a weak blood vessel), while alpha-carotene (50,000 mcg/day) increased risk of hemorrhagic stroke and death from hemorrhagic stroke, yet lowered risk of ischemic stroke (caused by a blockage in the blood vessel) (87).

Vitamin A and Exercise

Because of the body's ability to store vitamin A and a lack of data on vitamin A status in athletes, there is no evidence or plausible reason to suggest athletes or recreational gym-goers are more likely to be deficient in this vitamin (94). Further, data on vitamin A supplementation in athletes is insufficient to suggest supplementation is beneficial for

performance or recovery, especially beyond the RDA and in the absence of deficiency.

Vitamin D

Vitamin D comes from food and dietary supplements and is made in the body when skin is exposed to UVB rays from the sun (figure 6.4). All of these forms are inert and must be converted to the active form, calcitriol (1,25-dihydroxy-vitamin D). **Calcitriol** is a steroid hormone that promotes calcium absorption, helps to maintain blood calcium and phosphorus levels for normal bone mineralization, reduces inflammation, and has important physiological effects on cell growth, muscle, and immune system functioning (29, 41, 42, 105, 163). It remains unclear whether vitamin D deficiency causes inflammation or is a consequence of inflammation (95).

Vitamin D controls hundreds of genes and might have a beneficial role in outcomes related to cancer, autoimmune disease, cardiovascular disease, and diabetes, though the research on vitamin D in relation to these diseases isn't entirely clear at

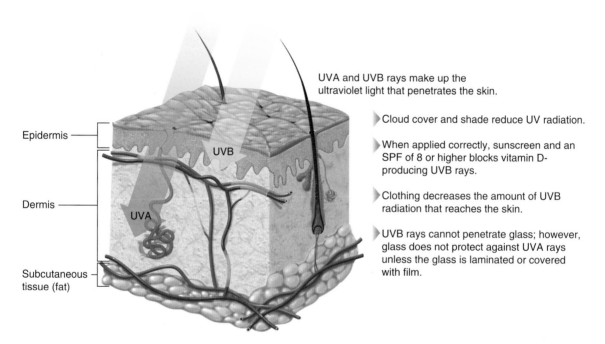

UVA and UVB rays make up the ultraviolet light that penetrates the skin.

Cloud cover and shade reduce UV radiation.

When applied correctly, sunscreen and an SPF of 8 or higher blocks vitamin D-producing UVB rays.

Clothing decreases the amount of UVB radiation that reaches the skin.

UVB rays cannot penetrate glass; however, glass does not protect against UVA rays unless the glass is laminated or covered with film.

Epidermis

Dermis

UVB

UVA

Subcutaneous tissue (fat)

Figure 6.4 UVA rays penetrate the middle layer of skin (dermis). UVB rays are shorter in wavelength and extend only to the outer layer of skin (epidermis). UVB rays, as well as combined UVB and UVA rays, increase the body's production of vitamin D. UVA rays alone lead to a decrease in vitamin D levels in the blood.

PUTTING IT INTO PERSPECTIVE

TANNING BEDS AND VITAMIN D

Tanning beds damage skin and might be worse for your vitamin D levels than no light at all. Tanning beds emit either UVA radiation only or a combination of UVA and UVB radiation (154). UVB radiation helps the body produce vitamin D. UVA plus UVB radiation (sunlight contains both) also increases vitamin D production in the body. However, UVA radiation alone leads to a significant reduction in blood vitamin D (calcidiol) (48, 131). Both UVA and UVB rays damage skin. A tan is an injury to the skin resulting from UV radiation. Tanning bed use (both newer and older models) is associated with a significant increase and risk of melanoma (a form of skin cancer that can be deadly). Therefore, tanning beds are not a safe way to get vitamin D and are not FDA approved as a way to increase vitamin D levels (25, 33, 38).

this time (18). In addition, vitamin D levels below 15 ng/ml are associated with progression of knee osteoarthritis in those with osteoarthritis (185). Though supplementation has been suggested for cartilage health, a two-year study in patients with osteoarthritis found vitamin D supplementation in a dose sufficient to increase serum vitamin D to 36 ng/ml (a level considered sufficient) did not reduce knee pain or cartilage volume loss. Thus the association between vitamin D and osteoarthritis is not clear at this time (101).

produced in the body when skin is exposed to UVB rays (see figure 6.4). See figure 6.5 for more information on sources of vitamin D.

Several studies suggest vitamin D_3 is superior to vitamin D_2 for maintaining serum 25(OH)D concentrations (5, 148). However, this has been challenged by at least one study, which found vitamin D_2 was as effective as vitamin D_3 for maintaining serum vitamin D levels (73).

Sources of Vitamin D

There are two types of vitamin D: vitamin D_2 (ergocalciferol) and vitamin D_3 (cholecalciferol). Vitamin D_2 is made from irradiating fungus, such as mushrooms, or yeast (121). This form of vitamin D is found in vegan supplements and vegan-fortified foods, including soy milk, almond milk, and other nondairy beverages. Vitamin D_2 is the form given in prescription doses (50,000 IU per week, every 2 or 4 weeks). Vitamin D_3 is naturally found in cod liver oil and oily fish, including halibut, mackerel, salmon, and trout, and in much smaller amounts in egg yolks, cheese, and beef liver. Vitamin D_3 is in fortified foods, notably milk, and made from lanolin in sheep's wool for dietary supplements (72). In addition to natural and fortified food sources of vitamin D_3, this vitamin is

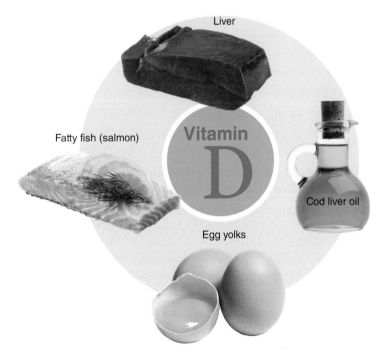

Figure 6.5 Sources of Vitamin D. In addition to food sources of vitamin D_3, mushrooms exposed to UV radiation are a source of vitamin D_2.

PUTTING IT INTO PERSPECTIVE

FOOD FORTIFICATION AND ENRICHMENT

Although many people use the terms "fortification" and "enrichment" interchangeably, they have distinct meanings. Food **fortification** refers to the addition of nutrients to food to improve the nutrition content. Fortification started with the mineral iodine in 1924 as a systematic approach to correcting nutrient deficiencies and nutrient deficiency diseases. Food manufacturers follow a "standard of identity"—an established type and level of fortification for a staple food. Enrichment refers to the addition of vitamins and minerals that are lost during food processing. For instance, white flour is enriched with iron, thiamin, riboflavin, niacin, and folic acid in levels that occur naturally in flour prior to nutrient losses during processing (155, 159).

Serum 25(OH)D [25-hydroxyvitamin D or 25(OH)D] is used to assess vitamin D status in the body.

Aside from differences in cost, there are two main reasons for choosing vitamin D_2 supplements instead of vitamin D_3:

1. Vitamin D_2 can be used as a diagnostic tool to determine if a vitamin D deficiency is caused by malabsorption (89).
2. Vitamin D_2 is vegan.

For optimal absorption, vitamin D supplements should be taken with a meal that contains fat, rather than with a fat-free meal or on an empty stomach. Absorption of a single 50,000 IU vitamin D_3 supplement was 32 percent greater when taken with a meal containing fat compared to a fat-free meal (39).

Vitamin D Deficiency and Insufficiency

Serum-circulating calcidiol—also referred to as 25-hydroxyvitamin D or 25(OH)D—is used to assess vitamin D levels. However, it isn't always easy to compare rates of deficiency or health effects based on deficiency because different values for vitamin D deficiency, insufficiency, and sufficiency have been used in scientific papers and corresponding data briefs, media reports, and other consumer-related communications (95).

In 2011, the Endocrine Society issued vitamin D guidelines based on vitamin D's role in bone and muscle health. These definitions, along with the Institute of Medicine's guidelines, are provided in table 6.2 and will be used for this chapter (74).

The National Health and Nutrition Examination Survey (NHANES) data, including a representative sample of 4,495 people in the United States from 2005 to 2006, found 41.6 percent of those tested were deficient in vitamin D. Among African Americans tested, deficiency rates were much higher (82.1%), whereas Hispanics had a deficiency rate of 69.2 percent (51). Vitamin D deficiency is also common in athletes, especially black athletes and indoor athletes with little exposure to sunshine. Two separate studies found that 38 percent and 11 percent of healthy endurance athletes were deficient, and 91 percent of Middle Eastern sportsmen were deficient. Two studies in NFL players found that 26.3 percent and 30.3 percent of players, respectively, were deficient in vitamin D (65, 67, 98, 138, 176). Several studies show higher rates of vitamin D deficiency in black athletes as compared to white athletes (98). In addition to high deficiency rates, a high percentage of athletes also have insufficient levels of vitamin D for optimal muscle and bone health (67, 98, 138). The body's production of vitamin D through exposure to sunlight (UVB rays) is a significant source of vitamin D, so athletes who test normal in the summer might be deficient in the winter months (63).

Groups with a higher risk of vitamin D deficiency or insufficiency include the following (51, 99, 160, 182):

> The elderly, as aging alters vitamin D synthesis in the body after sunlight exposure.
> Obese individuals.
> Individuals who have had gastric bypass surgery.

Table 6.2 Vitamin D Definitions

	Endocrine Society	Food and Nutrition Board, Institute of Medicine
Deficiency (ng/ml)	<20 ng/ml (50 nmol/L)	0–11 (<30)
Insufficiency (ng/ml)	21–29 ng/ml (52.5–72.5 nmol/L)	12–20 (30–50)
Sufficient levels (ng/ml)	> 30 ng/ml (75 nmol/L)	≥20 (≥50)
Toxicity (ng/ml)	It is not clear what the safe upper limit is for serum-circulating calcidiol to avoid hypercalcemia. According to the Endocrine Society, studies in both adults and children show blood levels may need to be above 150 ng/ml (375 nmol/L) before risk of harm.	>50 (>125)

Based on serum-circulating calcidiol.

Data from Holick 2011; Institute of Medicine 1998.

> Those who avoid the sun (homebound individuals), those who wear attire that covers their body and head, and those who regularly use sunscreen with an SPF of 8 or higher. Sunscreen with an SPF of 8 will not fully protect skin from the damaging effects of UV rays, but it will decrease (by 95 percent or more) the body's ability to synthesize vitamin D.

> Infants exclusively or partially breastfed.

> People who have medical conditions leading to fat malabsorption, including cystic fibrosis, celiac disease, and Crohn's disease.

> Individuals with dark skin—the pigment melanin provides natural protection from the sun, yet decreases the body's ability to produce vitamin D upon exposure to sunlight.

Additionally, athletes who live in northern latitudes and those who train primarily indoors throughout the year are at risk for poor vitamin D status. Poor dietary intake also contributes to low levels of vitamin D in athletes. In several studies, the majority of athletes surveyed do not meet the RDA for vitamin D through food alone; one study found under 5 percent of athletes surveyed obtained the RDA for vitamin D through dietary intake (14, 17, 36, 63, 186). This is in line with research in the population at large, which shows that more than 90 percent of Americans do not consume an adequate amount of vitamin D from food alone (52).

Vitamin D deficiency decreases calcium and phosphorus absorption 10 to 15 percent and 50 to 60 percent, respectively (104). In children, vitamin D deficiency can lead to rickets, a disease characterized by soft bones and skeletal deformities resulting from impaired bone mineralization (173). In adults, deficiency can lead to osteomalacia, resulting in weak bones, bone pain, and muscle weakness (124, 160). Vitamin D deficiency is also associated with chronic low-back pain, which improves after vitamin D supplementation (93, 126, 136). Maintaining vitamin D levels at or above 20 ng/ml is associated with a decreased risk of fractures, cardiovascular disease, colorectal cancer, diabetes, depressed mood, cognitive decline, and death, though the association with fractures and cardiovascular disease has not been seen in black individuals (85).

Note that, in consistency with the Endocrine Society's guidelines, prior to vitamin D treatment, current vitamin D status should be measured through a blood test.

Identifying and Treating Vitamin D Deficiency

When determining if individuals should get their vitamin D levels tested, the following factors should be considered:

> Risk factors for and symptoms of vitamin D deficiency

> Health history, including injuries, particularly stress fractures and bone and joint injuries

> Muscle pain or weakness

> Frequency of illness

PUTTING IT INTO PERSPECTIVE

WILL THE RDA HELP US MEET OUR VITAMIN D NEEDS?

The RDA for vitamin D was established primarily based on bone health (160) and obtaining adequate serum blood levels of 25-hydroxyvitamin D for skeletal health (>20 ng/ml). However, several questions have been raised about both the RDA and the range set for sufficient vitamin D status in blood. Bone researchers suggest the lowest acceptable cutoff level for optimal skeletal health should be 30 ng/ml (68), based on evidence from a large randomized controlled study showing 33 percent lower rates of osteoporotic fractures when serum vitamin D was increased from 21 to 29 ng/ml (149) as well as research in older adults suggesting risk of fractures is lower in those with vitamin D levels above 30 ng/ml, and above 40 ng/ml for certain fractures (20, 22). In addition, if dietary intake is the sole source of vitamin D (e.g., when an individual avoids the sun), the RDA is not enough to keep serum vitamin D level at 10 ng/ml—an amount far below adequacy (68).

Some scientists question if the RDA for vitamin D is adequate for the general population. High rates of vitamin D deficiency and insufficiency in a wide range of climates—from sunny California to colder areas—support the case for increasing the RDA. In most cases, the RDA is set to meet the needs of 97.5 percent of healthy individuals, which means if the RDA were adequate, 2.5 percent, or less, of the healthy population would be vitamin D deficient—yet rates are much higher than this. Two separate groups of scientists reviewed the studies and estimates used to determine the RDA. They found that an estimated daily intake of 7,000 to 8,895 IU of vitamin D from all sources, including 3,875 IU vitamin D per day from food, might be necessary to achieve adequate blood levels of vitamin D in 97.5 percent of the population (164).

> Use of medications or herbal supplements that interfere with vitamin D metabolism, such as kava kava and St. John's wort (61, 71)

High-dose loading regimens, under the guidance of a physician, might be beneficial for people who are deficient in vitamin D. Anyone with excess body fat or darker skin and those taking medications affecting vitamin D metabolism might need higher levels of vitamin D (74). Given seasonal changes in vitamin D status, anyone with vitamin D deficiency should be tested at least twice a year—in the winter and summer. According to the Agency for Healthcare Quality and Research, part of the Department of Health and Human Services, both vitamin D_2 and vitamin D_3 can be used for treatment and prevention of deficiency (74). Treatment guidelines are listed in table 6.3.

Excess Intake and Vitamin D Toxicity

As a fat-soluble vitamin, vitamin D can accumulate in tissues and become toxic when levels are very high. Toxicity can occur over time with supplemental or prescription doses. It is not possible for the human body to produce toxic levels of vitamin D from exposure to UV light (either through sunlight or tanning beds), and consumption of toxic levels through food is highly unlikely (70, 165). Patients with chronic granuloma-forming disorders, including sarcoidosis and tuberculosis; chronic fungal infections; or lymphoma might overproduce vitamin D, which can lead to high blood calcium or high levels of calcium in the urine. These patients should have their vitamin D and calcium levels monitored regularly (74). Data from animal studies suggests vitamin D_2 may be less toxic in high doses as compared to vitamin D_3 (160).

Vitamin D toxicity has a wide range of effects, including anorexia, weight loss, large volume of dilute urine, heart arrhythmias, and high blood calcium levels that can result in calcification of tissues leading to damage to the heart, blood vessels, and kidneys (160). The upper intake level (UL) for vitamin D is 4,000 IU per day for adults (160). Both low and high serum levels of vitamin D

Table 6.3 Prevention and Treatment of Vitamin D Deficiency

Age group (yr) or health condition	Treatment for deficiency (<20 ng/ml)	Maintenance plan after achieving 30 ng/ml
1–18	2,000 IU vitamin D_2 or D_3 for at least 6 weeks or 50,000 IU vitamin D_2 once per week for at least 6 weeks	600–1,000 IU/day
>18	50,000 IU vitamin D_2 or vitamin D_3 once a week for 8 weeks or 6,000 IU of vitamin D_2 or vitamin D_3 daily	1,500–2,000 IU/day
Obese, malabsorption syndromes, those on medications that affect vitamin D metabolism	At least 6000–10,000 IU/day of vitamin D	3,000–6,000 IU/day
Hyperparathyroidism	Treatment as needed; monitor blood calcium levels	Treatment as needed; monitor blood calcium levels

Data from Heaney 2011.

(in the form of calcidiol) are related to higher risk of certain diseases (11, 42, 128). Table 6.4 lists signs of vitamin D toxicity and includes information on many vitamins throughout the chapter.

Vitamin D and Exercise

Vitamin D influences muscle functioning by regulating calcium transport and uptake of inorganic phosphate, which is used to produce ATP (19, 120). In particular, vitamin D affects type II fast-twitch fibers—the kind used for short, rapid-fire bursts of activity such as jumping and sprinting (58). Vitamin D deficiency leads to weak type II fibers, impaired muscle contraction and relaxation, decreased strength, and a potential decline in athletic performance (21, 58, 64, 134, 171). Vitamin D deficiency and insufficiency are also associated with an increased risk of bone injuries, including fractures; impaired immune system functioning; and increased incidence of upper-respiratory infections (98, 104).

Higher serum vitamin D status is associated with greater muscle strength, power, and force; jumping performance; $\dot{V}O_2$max; and speed (82, 171). Higher vitamin D levels are correlated to greater $\dot{V}O_2$max, with the strongest correlation in those with low levels of physical activity (4). Improving vitamin D levels may have the greatest effect on muscle strength in those with severe deficiency (<12 ng/ml) and the elderly (10).

Professional male athletes deficient in vitamin D (<12 ng/ml or 30 nmol/L) or with insufficient vitamin D levels (12–20 ng/ml or 30–50 nmol/L) improved 10-meter sprint time and vertical jump (both recruit mainly type II fibers) after taking 5,000 IU vitamin D_3 per day for 8 weeks (raising mean levels from 11.6 ng/ml to 41 ± 10 ng/ml) compared to no change in athletes with deficient or insufficient levels who were given a placebo (37, 56, 129).

Though vitamin D deficiency can lead to musculoskeletal pain, lower levels of vitamin D are not associated with greater muscle pain or weakness after eccentric exercise (125).

Vitamin D and Illness

Vitamin D deficiency is associated with increased risk of illness, whereas maintaining sufficient levels of vitamin D can reduce risk of infectious illness (63). In one study, 27 percent of athletes with vitamin D levels above 48 ng/ml experienced one or more upper-respiratory tract infections over a 4-month period, compared to 67 percent of those with levels below 12 ng/ml. Athletes with vitamin D below 12 ng/ml also experienced more total symptomatic days compared to athletes with vitamin D levels above 12 ng/ml (67). These results are in line with studies in nonathletes; adults with vitamin D levels below 10 ng/ml had a significantly higher

Table 6.4 Vitamin Sources and Symptoms of Excess and Deficiency

Vitamin	Excellent sources (≥20% DV) based on standard serving size	Good sources (≥10% DV) based on standard serving size	Best form in food and dietary supplements	Deficiency signs and symptoms	Excess intake and toxicity signs and symptoms
Vitamin A (as preformed vitamin A, beta-carotene, alpha-carotene, beta-cryptoxanthin, or a combination of these compounds)	Beef liver, goose liver, turkey liver, sweet potato, pumpkin, canta-loupe, sweet red bell peppers, mangoes, broccoli, apricots	Herring, tomato juice, ricotta cheese	Beta-carotene	Deficiency is rare	Increased intra-cranial pressure, dizziness, nausea, headaches, skin irritation, joint and bone pain, coma, and death. Above 33,000–50,000 IU beta-carotene may increase risk of lung cancer in smokers.
Biotin	Data on the amount of biotin in food is not available, though it is found in a wide range of foods, including turkey breast, beef, whey protein, soybeans, chickpeas		Biotin	Rare unless a person is eating raw egg whites frequently	Excess is excreted.
Folic acid or folate	Beef liver, spin-ach, black-eyed peas, cooked rice, asparagus, enriched spaghetti	Cooked broccoli, raw spinach, avo-cado, white bread, kidney beans, green peas, boiled mustard greens	Found in supple-ments as folic acid; in food, it is found as folate	Though deficiency is rare, women of childbearing age have an increased need for folate or folic acid	Excess folic acid can mask a vitamin B_{12} deficiency and might interfere with certain medi-cations.
Niacin	Turkey (all parts or breast alone), pea-nuts, tuna fish, pork loin, brown or white rice, anchovies, beef, chicken, mackerel, salmon, potatoes	Greek yogurt, gluten-free pasta made with corn and rice flour, flax-seeds, chestnuts, blue cheese	Niacin	Rare; niacin is found in protein-rich foods	Flushed skin, rashes, and liver damage.
Pantothenic acid	Turkey breast, sunflower seeds, shiitake mushrooms, beef liver, lamb liver, avocado, sockeye salmon, brown or white rice, canned mushroom gravy	Sweet potato, orange juice, pro-claim, egg, black-berries, peanuts, burrito with beans, cream of potato soup, wild Atlantic salmon	Pantothenic acid	Rare	Excess is excreted though diarrhea, and water reten-tion may result.
Vitamin B_1 (thiamin)	Enriched breakfast cereals, long-grain white rice, egg noodles, pork chops, trout, black beans, muscles	Whole-wheat macaroni, acorn squash, bluefin tuna	Thiamin	Rare	Excess is excreted.
Vitamin B_2 (riboflavin)	Fortified breakfast cereals, instant oats, yogurt, milk, beef, clams	Almonds, Swiss cheese, egg, chicken, salmon, plain bagels, por-tabella mushrooms	Riboflavin	Rare except in those who are severely malnour-ished	Excess is excreted.

Vitamin	Excellent sources (≥20% DV) based on standard serving size	Good sources (≥10% DV) based on standard serving size	Best form in food and dietary supplements	Deficiency signs and symptoms	Excess intake and toxicity signs and symptoms
Vitamin B$_6$ (pyridoxine)	Chickpeas, beef liver, tuna, sockeye salmon, potatoes, banana, marinara sauce	Winter squash, cottage cheese, bulger, ready-to-heat waffles, ground beef	Pyridoxine	Rare	Large doses over time can cause nerve damage.
Vitamin B$_{12}$	Clams, trout, sockeye salmon, beef liver, haddock, some fortified breakfast cereals, sirloin	Milk, Swiss cheese, beef taco, ham, egg	Cobalamin	Strict vegetarians and the elderly are at risk	Low toxicity, no UL established.
Vitamin C	Sweet red or green pepper, orange juice, orange, grapefruit juice, kiwifruit, broccoli, Brussels sprouts, grapefruit, tomato juice, cantaloupe, cabbage, cauliflower, potato, tomato	Spinach, frozen green peas, pumpkin, prune juice, teriyaki rice bowl with chicken, peaches, hash brown potatoes, summer squash, yellow corn, edamame, okra, butternut squash	Ascorbic acid	Rare	Excess is excreted, though very large amounts (over 1,000 mg/day) may cause diarrhea and upset stomach.
Vitamin D (D$_3$ or cholecalciferol)	Cod liver oil, swordfish, sockeye salmon, tuna fish, orange juice fortified with vitamin D (check label), yogurt fortified with 20% DV vitamin D, milk	Egg (in the yolk), sardines	D$_3$ or cholecalciferol	Low intake levels are more common in individuals who are not exposed to sunlight, as well as the elderly	Excess is stored in the body and can be toxic. Quantities above 5,000–10,000 IU/day can cause hypercalcemia, hypercalciuria, kidney stones, and soft tissue calcifications.
Vitamin E	Wheat-germ oil, sunflower seeds, almonds, sunflower oil, safflower oil, hazelnuts	Peanuts, corn oil, spinach, peanut butter	Natural vitamin E (d-alpha tocopherol) is more active than the synthetic form of vitamin E (dl-alpha tocopherol); approximately 50% more of the synthetic form is needed to compare to the natural form	Very rare unless fat absorption is an issue	Few side effects have been noted, even in doses as high as 3,200 mg.
Vitamin K	Natto, collards, turnip greens, spinach, kale, broccoli, soybeans, soybean oil, edamame, pumpkin, pomegranate juice	Pine nuts, blueberries, iceberg lettuce, grapes, chicken breast, canola oil, cashews, carrots, olive oil, vegetable juice cocktail	Phylloquinone, phytonadione, menadione	Rare	Few side effects noted, though excess intake isn't recommended.

Based on Allen et al. 2006; U.S. Institute of Medicine 1998; U.S. Institute of Medicine 2001; U.S. Institute of Medicine 2011.

risk of respiratory infections when compared to adults with vitamin D levels greater than 30 ng/ml (56). A study in British adults found respiratory infections peak in the winter and decrease as the weather gets warmer, while also finding a 7 percent decrease in risk of respiratory infections with each 4 ng/ml increase in blood vitamin D up to the average study participant high of 28.8 ng/ml in September (16). Another study found blood serum concentrations of vitamin D equal to or greater than 38 ng/ml were associated with a significant reduction in risk of acute respiratory tract infections and percentage of days ill (129).

Vitamin D and Injuries

An association is evident between vitamin D insufficiency and deficiency and injuries, including stress fractures, as well as chronic musculoskeletal pain. A study examining NFL players found those with at least one muscle injury (muscle strain, tear, or pull) resulting in at least one missed practice or game during the season had significantly lower vitamin D levels compared to players with no reported muscle injuries during the same time period (19.9 ng/ml and 24.7ng/ml, respectively) (138). In another study, conducted with players from the Pittsburgh Steelers, significantly lower vitamin D levels were found in players with at least one bone fracture compared to those with no bone fractures (after correcting for total number of NFL seasons played because years played influ-

ences injuries). Also, significantly lower vitamin D levels were observed in players released during the preseason (because of injury or poor performance) when compared to levels in those who played the entire regular season. Athletes with serum vitamin D above 41 ng/ml played more seasons than those with serum vitamin D levels below 21 ng/ml (98). In addition to the association between vitamin D and risk of injury, vitamin D might also influence recovery following some kinds of surgeries. Patients with levels below 30 ng/ml (75 nmol/L) had delayed strength recovery after anterior cruciate ligament surgery (8).

Vitamin E

Vitamin E is incorporated in the body's cellular and subcellular membranes, where it helps to prevent oxidative damage to the fats in cell membranes. This oxidative damage can disrupt cell membrane structure and function as well as function of the cell overall (84, 157, 161). Vitamin E is also involved in immune functioning, cell signaling, metabolic processes, blood vessel dilation, and inhibiting platelets from clumping together (157).

Sources of Vitamin E

The eight naturally occurring forms of vitamin E are alpha-, beta-, gamma-, and delta-tocopherol and alpha-, beta-, gamma-, and delta-tocotrienol.

Though gamma-tocopherol is the most prevalent form found in the diet, only alpha-tocopherol

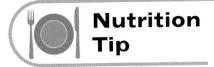

Some companies list total antioxidant capacity (TAC) scores of a food, beverage, or supplement on the label based on antioxidant testing methods such as ORAC (oxygen radical absorbance capacity). TAC scores provide a measure of the food's capacity to scavenge free radicals. Though these scores are useful for research purposes, they do not tell us anything about human health because TAC scores do not take into account how the body absorbs and uses antioxidants. So these scores should not be used as a way to compare foods, beverages, or supplements or to suggest one food is healthier than another food (118).

is maintained in human blood in significant amounts, and thus is the form considered most biologically important and the one used to estimate vitamin E requirements. See figure 6.6 for excellent sources of vitamin E.

Vitamin E Deficiency and Toxicity

Vitamin E deficiency is rare, seen only in individuals with fat malabsorption disorders and those with rare inherited disorders preventing maintenance of normal blood concentrations of vitamin E. Symptoms of deficiency may include peripheral neuropathy, loss of control of body movements (ataxia), skeletal muscle weakness, and retina damage. Vitamin E deficiency can also lead to hemolytic anemia, the type of anemia characterized by ruptured red blood cells.

No health effects have been observed from vitamin E intake through dietary sources. However, lab studies suggest large doses of vitamin E can inhibit platelet clumping and thereby increase risk of bleeding. This may be particularly dangerous when large doses of vitamin E are taken with anticoagulants, especially in conjunction with low vitamin K intake. Additionally, the Selenium and Vitamin E Cancer Prevention Trial found men who supplemented with 400 IU

DO YOU KNOW ?

National survey data suggest Americans do not consume adequate amounts of vitamin E through food; however, total vitamin E intake might have been underestimated if oil used during cooking was not accounted for in surveys assessing dietary intake (107).

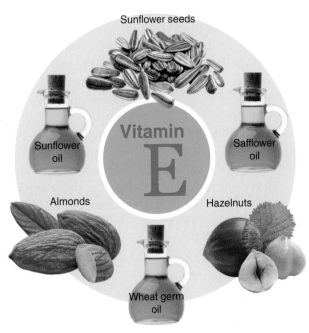

Figure 6.6 Excellent sources of Vitamin E, containing more than 20% DV per serving (151).

vitamin E each day for an average of 5.5 years had a 17 percent increased risk of prostate cancer (81). The tolerable upper limit for vitamin E in adults 19 years of age and older is 1,000 mg (1,500 IU).

Vitamin E and Exercise

Free radicals, produced in muscle, have important roles in cell signaling, production of muscle force, muscle growth, and recovery. A healthy balance is important, as excess free radicals can damage plasma membranes, impairing muscle contraction and contributing to muscle fatigue and delayed-onset muscle soreness (79, 122).

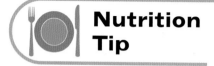

The stress of exercise, particularly exercise with high oxygen demand (high oxygen demand means more free radicals are produced) or muscle-damaging exercise, damages cell membranes—the barrier that protects cells. Vitamin E protects cells from the damaging effects of free radicals and is essential for cell membrane repair, so it might support training adaptations and recovery (122). Vitamin E–deprived muscle cell membranes do not heal properly.

Though vitamin E is critical for muscle cell health, studies examining vitamin E's role in athletics have yet to find supplemental vitamin E, above the amount provided in the average diet, improves athletic performance or decreases muscle damage (35, 53, 137, 145). In fact, in high doses, vitamin E may interfere with training adaptations as noted later in this chapter.

Vitamin K

Vitamin K is a fat-soluble vitamin composed of vitamin K_1 and several forms of vitamin K_2. In the body, vitamin K is a coenzyme involved in the synthesis of proteins necessary for blood clotting and bone metabolism. Additionally, scientists are working to determine how vitamin K_2, as part of a vitamin K–dependent protein, might reduce calcification in arteries (arterial calcification contributes to arterial plaque and blockage within arteries, which increases risk of chronic kidney disease and cardiovascular disease) (66, 135). Vitamin K is also found in the brain, liver, heart, and pancreas (158).

Vitamin E interferes with clotting activity of vitamin K, though there seems to be inter-individual differences in response to vitamin E intake that influences its effect on clotting as well as bleeding (147).

Sources of Vitamin K

There are two types of vitamin K:

> Vitamin K_1 (phylloquinone, phytomenadione, or phytonadione) is made in plants and can be converted to vitamin K_2 by bacteria in the human body. Vitamin K_1 is found in high concentrations in green leafy vegetables, soybeans, soybean oil, and canola oil. Vitamin K_1 is less bioavailable from greens than from oil or supplements. Consuming dietary fat at the same

PUTTING IT INTO PERSPECTIVE

IMPROVING JOINT PAIN

If you exercise regularly or participate in sports, you might experience joint pain. In particular, some athletes feel pain or stiffness in their knees, especially if sitting for a long time with knees bent (in a lengthy class lecture, movie theater, or on an airplane, for instance) because of worn-down cartilage. Some athletes may have osteoarthritis, a degenerative joint disease characterized by pain, stiffness, and swelling in joints. Osteoarthritis is a disease that primarily affects cartilage, the tissues that provide cushioning between joints, allowing them to move over one another smoothly. Studies suggest higher dietary intake of vitamin C, beta carotene, and vitamin E can support joint health by attenuating the development of osteoarthritis (40, 102, 169, 181).

time as vegetables improves vitamin K_1 absorption from vegetables.

> Vitamin K_2 comes in several forms (menaquinones) and is found in animal livers, some Chinese dishes, and some fermented foods, such as natto. In addition, most menaquinones are produced by bacteria in the human gut (151, 158). See figure 6.7 for good and excellent sources of vitamins K_1 and K_2.

Vitamin K Deficiency and Toxicity

Vitamin K status, as measured by the time it takes for blood to clot (prothrombin time), is not typically tested unless a person is taking anticoagulants (medicines that help prevent blood clots, which antagonize the action of vitamin K—warfarin is an example) or has a bleeding disorder. Vitamin K deficiency can cause bleeding and hemorrhage and might also decrease bone

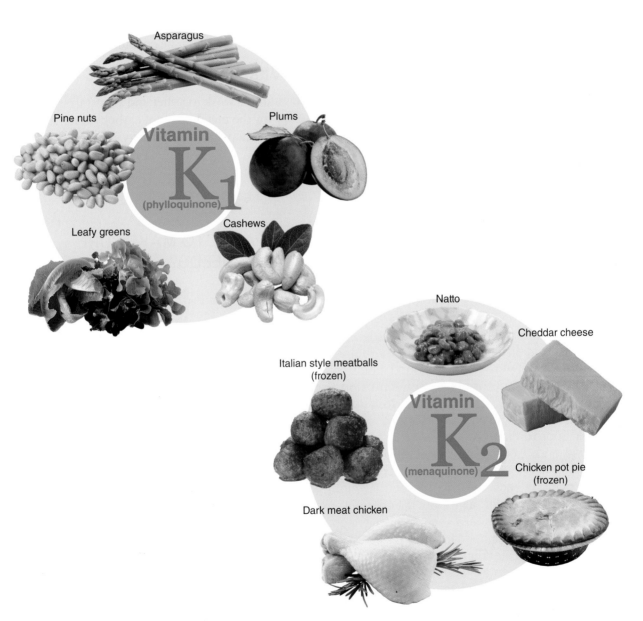

Figure 6.7 Excellent and good sources of vitamin K_1 and vitamin K_2. Note that chicken and meat products contain vitamin K_2 only if their feed contained a synthetic form of vitamin K. (The animals produce vitamin K_2 from the vitamin K in their feed.)

mineralization, thus possibly contributing to osteoporosis. Infants not treated with vitamin K at birth and those with malabsorption syndromes and GI diseases (including celiac disease, cystic fibrosis, and ulcerative colitis) are at risk for vitamin K deficiency. (Vitamin K interacts with certain medications, notably anticoagulants, a type of blood thinner.) Such individuals require close monitoring and consistent intake of vitamin K-containing foods and supplements (as directed by a physician). Note, too, that changes in vitamin K intake can increase or decrease the effectiveness of some anticoagulants (158). No evidence suggests that vitamin K interferes with a different category of blood thinners that prevent platelets from sticking together to form clots—aspirin and clopidogrel are examples. To be on the safe side, patients on blood thinners, regardless which type, should always check with a medical professional about vitamin K from dietary supplements and food.

DO YOU KNOW ?

No known association exists between vitamin K and athletic performance or recovery.

WATER-SOLUBLE VITAMINS

Unlike fat-soluble vitamins, the majority of water-soluble vitamins are not stored in the body, and any excess is excreted in the urine. Therefore, these vitamins must be consumed regularly.

B Vitamins

B vitamins work together and are catalysts necessary for the metabolism of carbohydrate, fat, and protein, as well as for energy production (156).

PUTTING IT INTO PERSPECTIVE

CAN I USE THE NUTRITION FACTS PANEL TO MAKE SURE I AM MEETING MY VITAMIN NEEDS?

The Nutrition Facts Panel (figure 6.8) can be used to compare foods that include nutrients many Americans are not getting in adequate amounts, including vitamin D, calcium, potassium, and iron. Getting enough of these nutrients helps to reduce the risk of some diseases or disease risk factors, while improving health. The FDA requires that food labels list the total content of these micronutrients on the Nutrition Facts Panel. The Daily Value (DV) was developed to help consumers see the nutrient levels in a standard serving size of food compared to their approximate requirement for that nutrient. The %DV is based on a 2,000-calorie diet and thus provides a reference you can use to compare foods, even if you consume more or less calories each day (153). A food is "high," "rich in," or an "excellent source of" a nutrient if it contains 20 percent or more of the DV for a standard serving size. It is considered a "good source," "contains," or "provides" if it contains 10 to 19 percent of the DV for a standard serving size (152). In addition to these four micronutrients—vitamin D, calcium, potassium, and iron—some companies voluntarily list the amount of other vitamins and minerals.

Nutrition Facts	
8 servings per container	
Serving size	**2/3 cup (55g)**
Amount per 2/3 cup	
Calories	**230**
	% Daily Value*
Total Fat 8g	**10%**
Saturated Fat 1g	**5%**
Trans Fat 0g	
Cholesterol 0mg	**0%**
Sodium 160mg	**7%**
Total Carbohydrate 37g	**13%**
Dietary Fiber 4g	**14%**
Total Sugars 12g	
Added Sugars 10g	**20%**
Protein 3g	
Vitamin D 2mcg	10%
Calcium 260mg	20%
Iron 8mg	45%
Potassium 235mg	6%

*The % Daily Value (DV) tells you how much a nutrient in a serving of food contributes to a daily diet. 2,000 calories a day is used for general nutrition advice.

Figure 6.8 Companies must list the DV for vitamin D, calcium, potassium, and iron on the Nutrition Facts Panel.

As such, B vitamins are critical for health and human performance. Each B vitamin also has other functions in the body. There is little data examining consistently low intake of B vitamins and the effect on athletic performance, though one study found dietary restriction of thiamin, riboflavin, and vitamin B_6 resulted in decreased peak aerobic capacity and peak power in trained male cyclists (162). No evidence suggests a greater intake of B vitamins, beyond what the body needs, improves athletic performance.

According to national survey data, few people consume below the Estimated Average Requirements (EAR) for thiamin, riboflavin, niacin, or vitamin B_6. There are no nationally representative estimates of pantothenic acid intake, but this vitamin is widely distributed in food. Low calorie intake may increase an athlete's risk for low thiamin, riboflavin, and vitamin B_6 (43, 69). Despite low intake, B vitamin deficiencies are uncommon, though certain groups have a higher risk of developing a vitamin B_{12} deficiency.

Biotin

Biotin is found in a wide range of foods, including turkey breast, beef, whey protein, soybeans, and chickpeas (151). Biotin deficiency can occur during pregnancy or with long-term tube feeding, rapid weight loss, or consumption of raw egg whites over a long period of time. Raw egg whites contain a protein called avidin, which binds biotin so it cannot be absorbed in the body (184).

DO YOU KNOW ?

Many skin, hair, and nail supplements contain biotin because a biotin deficiency can cause skin rashes and hair loss (156).

Biotin deficiency can lead to dermatitis (red, scaly, skin rash), conjunctivitis, hair loss, central nervous system abnormalities, and seizures. In infants, biotin deficiency can lead to lethargy, developmental delay, withdrawn behavior, and hypotonia (floppy baby syndrome). Biotin toxicity has not been observed in humans (156). There is insufficient research to assess the effect of biotin supplementation on athletic performance.

Choline

Americans get most of their choline in the diet from milk, meat, poultry, fish, eggs and egg-based dishes, bread, and grain-based dishes such as pasta (34). Eggs, turkey, beef, soybeans, chickpeas, and lima beans are excellent sources of choline (151).

Choline is a methyl donor necessary for lipid metabolism and transport, cell functioning, brain development and functioning, and creatine formation. Choline is the precursor for the neurotransmitter acetylcholine, phospholipids, and betaine (132, 156). National survey data suggest that many people are falling short of their choline needs; mean choline intakes for children and for all age ranges of men and women are below the AI (34).

Choline deficiency leads to fat infiltration in the liver and to liver and muscle damage (49). High supplemental doses of choline (10 g/day) might slightly reduce blood pressure. High dietary intake of choline, especially choline magnesium trisalicylate, is associated with potential side effects that include ringing in the ears and mild liver toxicity.

Though humans placed on a choline-deficient diet for three weeks experienced a decline in muscle functioning, (183) there is no evidence of choline deficiency caused by exercise, and choline supplementation does not benefit either brief, high-intensity anaerobic exercise or prolonged aerobic exercise (142).

Dietary Folate and Folic Acid

Dietary folate is found naturally in food. Excellent dietary sources of folate include beef liver, dark green leafy vegetables, beans and peas, rice, fortified cereals, and wheat germ (151). Folic acid is the term used for the synthetic form of folate found in dietary supplements and fortified foods. For our purposes, we will call both folate and folic acid "folate" unless otherwise specified. Folate is necessary for metabolism and healthy red blood cells (156).

Folate status can be assessed by measuring red blood cell (erythrocyte) folate levels. Deficiency can lead to megaloblastic or macrocytic anemia, a type of **anemia** characterized by large, immature (not completely developed) red blood cells (figure 6.9). Anemia is when blood fails to carry enough oxygen throughout the body. Signs and symptoms of megaloblastic anemia include fatigue, shortness of breath, weakness, pale skin, and sore mouth and tongue. Babies born to pregnant women deficient in folate have an increased risk of neural tube or spinal defects. In addition to consistently low intake of dietary folate or folic acid, malabsorptive diseases, chronic heavy alcohol intake, smoking, and genetic variations in folate metabolism can contribute to the risk of folate deficiency. Many women and adolescent females capable of becoming pregnant do not meet their folate needs (7). Several medicines may interfere with folate metabolism, including long-term therapeutic doses of nonsteroidal anti-inflammatory drugs (NSAIDs), such as ibuprofen (156). The Institute of Medicine encourages every women who could become pregnant to get 400 mcg of folic acid every day from fortified foods, supplements, or a combination of both to decrease the risk of birth defects (http://pediatrics.aappublications.org/content/104/2/325).

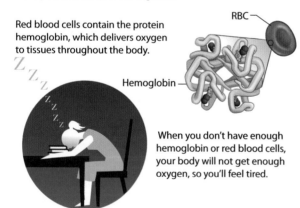

Anemia

A blood disorder characterized by an inadequate supply of red blood cells (RBCs) or hemoglobin.

Red blood cells contain the protein hemoglobin, which delivers oxygen to tissues throughout the body.

RBC

Hemoglobin

When you don't have enough hemoglobin or red blood cells, your body will not get enough oxygen, so you'll feel tired.

Deficiencies in several vitamins and minerals can lead to anemia including:
- Vitamin B_6 (pyridoxine)
- Vitamin B_{12}
- Folate
- Iron
- Vitamin E

Figure 6.9 Deficiencies in several nutrients can result in anemia.

No adverse effects are associated with folate consumption through food. Excess folic acid intake can mask a vitamin B_{12} deficiency, thereby correcting megaloblastic anemia without addressing the side effects caused by a B_{12} deficiency.

Though folate status in athletes appears to mirror the general population, with women more likely to be deficient than men (9, 47, 100, 156, 178), folic acid supplementation in athletes deficient in folate, yet not anemic, does not improve athletic performance (100).

Niacin

Niacin is important for metabolism, digestive system function, and skin and nerve function. Niacin is found in a wide variety of foods, including beef, milk, eggs, legumes (including peanuts), poultry, fish, and rice (151). Niacin deficiency leads to the disease pellagra. Symptoms of pellagra include inflamed skin,

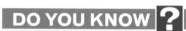

DO YOU KNOW ❓

Consuming high amounts of niacin can lead to flushing or a warm, itchy, or tingly feeling of the face, neck, arms, and upper body, as well as to GI effects and vision changes.

mental impairment, and digestive issues. Niacin toxicity is associated with nausea, vomiting, and liver toxicity (156).

No evidence suggests that niacin supplementation is necessary for athletic performance. In fact, niacin supplementation might block the release of fatty acids from fat tissue, increasing the body's reliance on carbohydrate, which could potentially lead to faster depletion of muscle glycogen and impaired endurance performance (15, 114, 144).

Pantothenic Acid (Vitamin B_5)

Pantothenic acid is an important part of a coenzyme involved in fatty acid metabolism. Deficiency is very uncommon under normal circumstances and has been observed only in experimental conditions in those fed a diet void of pantothenic acid. There is no evidence of toxicity from pantothenic acid. Major sources of pantothenic acid include chicken, beef, potatoes, tomato products, whole grains, and egg yolks (156).

We have no reason to believe that pantothenic acid, beyond that obtained from dietary intake, is necessary for athletic performance (172).

Riboflavin (Vitamin B₂)

Riboflavin (figure 6.10) is a component of two coenzymes necessary for metabolism, energy production, cellular function, growth, and development.

Most Americans consume enough riboflavin through their diet, so riboflavin deficiency is rare in the United States (52), though endocrine abnormalities can lead to deficiency. Signs and symptoms of deficiency include skin issues, edema in the mouth and throat, cracks at the corners of the mouth (called angular stomatitis or angular cheilosis), hair loss, sore throat, itchy red eyes, liver and nervous system abnormalities, and reproductive problems (103, 156).

Exercise might increase riboflavin needs, which can be met through increased calorie intake of nutrient-dense foods. Athletes who are dieting may fall short of their riboflavin intake (12, 50, 96, 178). Little research has looked at the effect of riboflavin supplementation on performance, though one study found correcting low riboflavin status improved endurance performance in adolescents aged 12 to 14 (143).

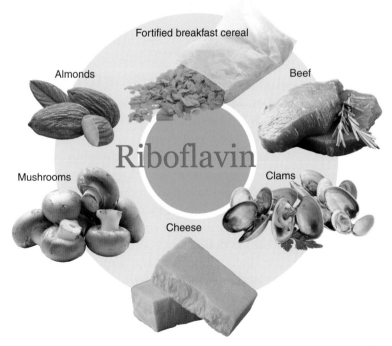

Figure 6.10 Good or excellent sources of riboflavin (151, 156).

Thiamin (Vitamin B₁)

Thiamin (figure 6.11) is essential for the activity of enzymes involved in carbohydrate, lipid, and amino acid metabolism. In the United States and many other countries, grain products, including breads and cereals, are fortified with thiamin. Cooking food decreases thiamin content to about 50 to 60 percent of precooked levels. The greatest thiamin losses are from boiling, followed by baking, poaching, and frying. High temperature, high pH, and high chlorine content in water all accelerate thiamin losses (80).

Thiamin Deficiency and Toxicity The majority of people in the United States consume enough thiamin. Thiamin deficiency, often caused by chronic alcoholism, leads to the neurological disorder Wernicke-Korsakoff syndrome (75). Thiamin deficiency can also lead to beriberi, a disease that is now very rare in the United States because of thiamin fortification in grains. Older adults have a higher risk of thiamin deficiency, which may be caused by low dietary intake, chronic diseases, nutrient-drug interactions, or a decrease in thiamin absorption (167, 174). Individuals with HIV or AIDS, diabetes, or those with a history of bariatric surgery have a greater risk of developing thiamin deficiency (24, 76, 130, 180). Signs of thiamin deficiency include weight changes, mental changes, apathy, impaired short-term memory, confusion, irritability, muscle weakness, and enlarged heart (156).

Thiamin and Exercise Studies in athletes on calorie-restricted diets indicate they might be consuming less than the RDA for thiamin (46, 92, 139). Therefore, anyone on a reduced calorie diet should include foods that are a good or excellent source of thiamin. Several studies show no benefit for muscle strength or endurance performance from thiamin supplementation (45, 50, 172, 177).

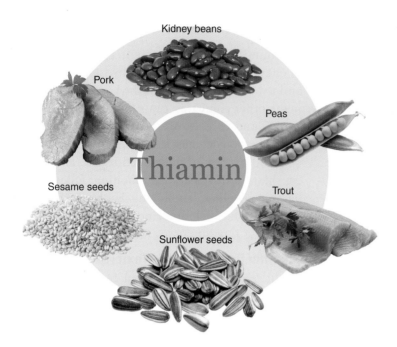

Figure 6.11 Excellent sources of thiamin (151).

Pyridoxine (Vitamin B₆)

Pyridoxine is necessary for metabolism and immune functioning (156). Excellent sources of pyridoxine include chickpeas, tuna, salmon, chicken breasts, and fortified cereals (151). Most people in the United States consume adequate amounts of pyridoxine. Pyridoxine deficiency is rare by itself but instead typically occurs alongside other B vitamin deficiencies. Deficiency leads to microcytic anemia, characterized by small, pale red blood cells; abnormalities in the electrical activity of the brain; dermatitis; cheilosis; swollen tongue (glossitis); depression; confusion; and suppressed immune functioning. Kidney diseases, malabsorption diseases, autoimmune diseases, alcoholism, and some genetic diseases can cause a pyridoxine deficiency. No toxic effects of vitamin B₆ from food sources are known, but chronic high-dose supplemental intake can lead to neuropathy, loss of control of body movements, painful dermatological lesions, sensitivity to sunlight, and GI symptoms (13, 54, 140, 156).

Exercise increases pyridoxine losses, so athletes on reduced calorie diets might fail to meet the RDA for pyridoxine (50, 86, 96, 97, 127).

It remains unclear if supplemental pyridoxine intake will enhance performance, as few studies have assessed this.

Vitamin B₁₂ (Cobalamin)

Vitamin B₁₂ is necessary for the formation of red blood cells, neurological functioning, and DNA synthesis (156). Vitamin B₁₂ is naturally found in many animal foods. Excellent sources include clams, beef, beef liver, salmon, haddock, trout, and tuna fish, as well as fortified breakfast cereals and some types of nutritional yeast (151, 156).

Vegetarians, particularly vegans (those who eat no animal foods) who do not take a multivitamin containing vitamin B₁₂ or a separate vitamin B₁₂ supplement, and who do not regularly consume foods fortified with vitamin B₁₂, have an increased risk of developing marginal vitamin B₁₂ status or deficiency (117), which can lead to megaloblastic anemia. Individuals with pernicious anemia—caused by an autoimmune disease that affects the stomach lining, infections, surgery, medicine, or diet—cannot absorb vitamin B₁₂ (62, 156) and require vitamin B₁₂ shots. Without shots, they will develop megaloblastic anemia and neurological disorders (3, 156). Individuals with reduced stomach acid or intestinal disorders might have problems absorbing vitamin B₁₂ from food, putting them at risk for deficiency (30). Elderly women are more likely than men and younger women to have malabsorption, putting them at greater risk of developing a B₁₂ deficiency or marginal B₁₂ status (6, 88).

Signs and symptoms of pernicious and megaloblastic anemia include pica (the desire to eat

> **DO YOU KNOW** ❓
>
> Vitamin B₁₂ is the only water-soluble vitamin stored in the body. Rather than being excreted in the urine, it can be stored in the liver for several years.

nonfood items such as ice or clay), diarrhea or constipation, nausea, poor appetite, loss of appetite, pale skin, pale nail beds and gums, difficulty concentrating, lightheadedness, dizziness, shortness of breath during exercise, swollen red tongue, and bleeding gums. Chronic vitamin B$_{12}$ deficiency can lead to nerve damage and related symptoms, including tingling and numbness in the hands and feet, difficulty walking, irritability, memory loss, dementia, depression, and mental illness (108). No evidence suggests vitamin B$_{12}$ supplementation, beyond correction for deficiency, improves athletic performance (123). However, there is a scarcity of data on vitamin B$_{12}$ and athletic performance.

Vitamin C (Ascorbic Acid)

Vitamin C is an antioxidant that

> protects cells in the body from free radical damage,

> helps regenerate other antioxidants, including vitamin E (31),

> affects immune system functioning,

> produces collagen,

> helps repair and maintain cartilage and bone (157),

> keeps capillary and blood vessel walls firm, which helps prevent bruising,

> keeps skin and gum tissue healthy, and

> helps the body absorb plant sources of iron (non-heme iron; this form is not absorbed by the body as well as heme iron, the kind found in animal foods).

Excellent sources of vitamin C include oranges, grapefruit, tomatoes, bell peppers, peaches, kiwi, strawberries, and broccoli (151).

Does Vitamin C Prevent Illness?

Though vitamin C is necessary for immune system functioning (157), several studies show vitamin C supplementation may not benefit

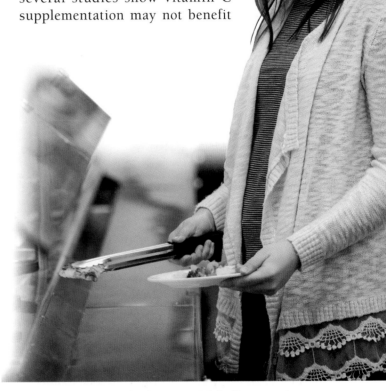

Look for nutrient-packed options including a variety of steamed vegetables, grilled chicken, and potatoes in college dining halls.

Nutrition Tip

Water, light, and heat decrease the vitamin C content in foods. Instead of boiling vegetables (and throwing out a good amount of vitamin C in the water they are boiled in), consider microwaving or steaming vegetables or eating them raw. Try cutting fruits and vegetables soon before you eat them instead of buying precut produce or leaving cut produce out of the refrigerator for long periods prior to eating. The more surface area (smaller pieces of produce) exposed to heat and light, the greater the amount of vitamin C lost. If you are in a dorm room, consider vegetables you can microwave or eat raw.

PUTTING IT INTO PERSPECTIVE

CAN ANTIOXIDANTS IMPROVE RECOVERY AND DECREASE MUSCLE SORENESS?

Muscles produce free radicals (reactive oxygen and nitrogen species), compounds that are necessary for cell signaling, production of muscle force, muscle growth, and recovery. A healthy balance of free radicals is necessary because high levels can damage cells, impair muscle contraction, and contribute to muscle weakness, fatigue, and dysfunction (27, 168). Dietary intake of antioxidants, including vitamins C and E, as well as carotenoids, might protect against excess muscle cell damage caused by free radicals (122). Though consuming a diet rich in antioxidants might help protect muscles from the damaging effects of excess free radicals, no evidence supports supplemental doses for this purpose, and taking high doses of antioxidant supplements, particularly vitamins C and E, can shortcut the essential actions of free radicals (27, 59, 106, 111, 145, 168). Daily supplements of 1,000-mg vitamin C plus 235-mg (261 IU) vitamin E (as dl-alpha tocopherol acetate) interferes with cell signaling after resistance training, impairs increases in muscle strength in response to strength training, and interferes with cellular adaptation to endurance training (115, 116). Supplemental doses of greater than 1,000 mg of vitamin C alone impaired sports performance in at least four studies (28).

such functioning (83, 109, 110). In athletes, the research is mixed and might depend on regular dietary intake of vitamin C, supplemental vitamin C dose and duration, and the level of exercise stress. A double-blind, placebo-controlled study found daily supplementation with 600 mg of vitamin C for 21 days prior to a 90-km race reduced self-reported symptoms of upper-respiratory tract infections during the 2-week period after the race, compared to placebo. Nonrunning controls also benefited. Other foods consumed at the same time as those taking vitamin C supplementation reduced the duration and severity of self-reported symptoms of upper-respiratory tract infections, compared to placebo (119). Another randomized, double-blind, placebo-controlled study showed no differences in immune markers between runners who took 1,500 mg of vitamin C daily for 7 days prior to an 80-km race, compared to those who took a placebo (110). Additionally, a randomized, double-blind study found 500 mg of vitamin C consumed 3 times a day for several days prior to a 120-minute bout of indoor cycling at a moderate pace in a hot and humid environment did not affect incidence of upper-respiratory tract infections or immune system functioning, as measured by salivary immunoglobulin A (32).

Vitamin C and Exercise

Regular exercise can increase vitamin C needs, and low vitamin C status negatively affects performance (55). Correcting a vitamin C deficiency or suboptimal intake can increase work capacity and aerobic power (77, 162).

SUMMARY

Exercise stresses many vitamin-dependent pathways. Vitamins are important for health and have several important roles related to exercise and athletic performance, including energy production, oxygen transport, immune functioning, building and maintaining bone density, and synthesizing and repairing muscle tissue. The body can make vitamins D and K, although vitamin D production depends on exposure to UVB rays and the ability to convert vitamin D to its active form in the body. Many Americans are not making adequate amounts of vitamin D in their body or getting enough from food. Other vitamins commonly underconsumed include vitamins A, C, E, and folate. Athletes who are dieting or cutting out food groups or who generally consume a nutritionally poor diet have an increased risk of deficiency in one or more vitamins. Water-soluble vitamins, with the exception of vitamin B_{12}, need to be replenished daily, as excess is excreted in urine. Several vitamins, including folate and vitamins B_6 and B_{12}, are important for oxygen transport throughout the body, including to muscle tissues. In addition to monitoring overall dietary intake, the effect of cooking methods on water-soluble vitamin content should be considered. Supplemental intake must also be considered to get a good overall picture of a person's vitamin intake. Though vitamin deficiencies can negatively affect performance, excess intake has not been shown to enhance performance and in some cases might be detrimental.

◼◼ FOR REVIEW ⟫

1. Discuss the vitamins affected by cooking methods and cooking methods that contribute to vitamin losses.
2. List some of the signs and symptoms associated with vitamin C deficiency.
3. Discuss methods to help the body absorb antioxidants from food.
4. How does vitamin D deficiency or insufficiency affect athletes?
5. Discuss how excess intake of antioxidants might affect muscle.
6. List a day's worth of vitamin-rich meals.

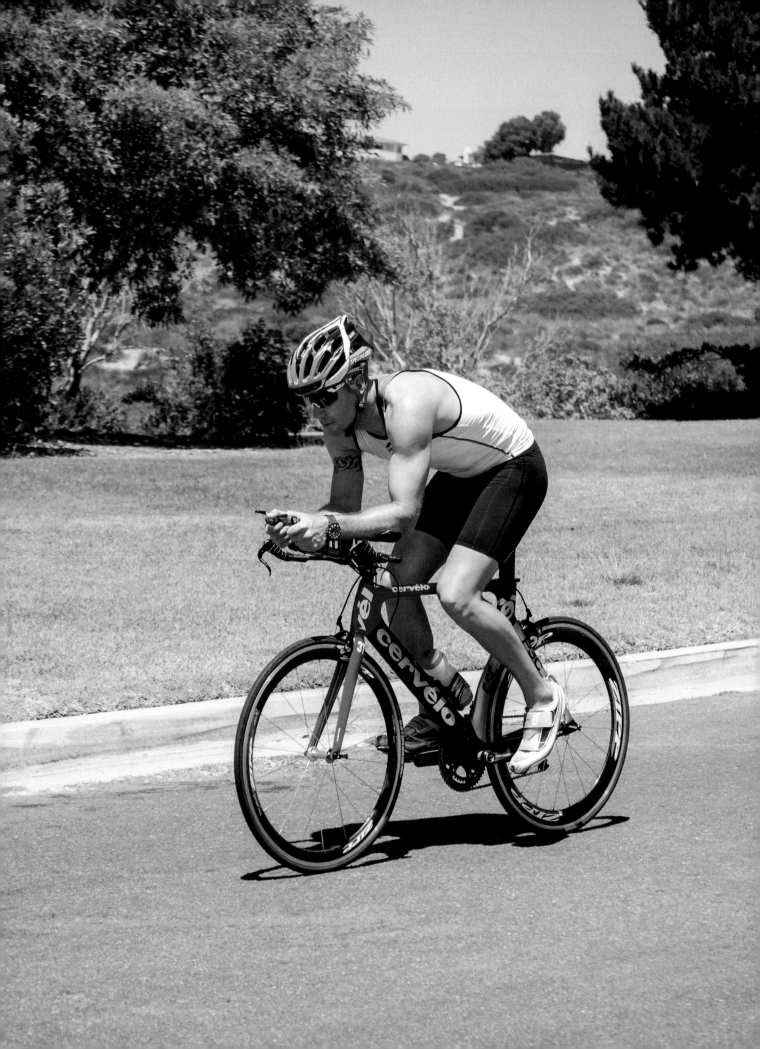

CHAPTER 7

Minerals

> ▶ **CHAPTER OBJECTIVES**
>
> After completing this chapter, you will be able to do the following:
>
> > Discuss why minerals are important for overall health and training.
> > Explain how training and exercise affect mineral needs.
> > List the minerals that athletes are most likely not getting enough of through their diet.
> > Discuss potential hazards of excess mineral intake.
> > List a few good food sources for each major mineral.

Minerals help regulate fluid balance, muscle contraction (including heartbeat), nerve impulses, oxygen transport, immune functioning, muscle building and repair. Minerals are structural components of many body tissues, including bones, nails, and teeth. Additionally, they are part of enzymes that facilitate several metabolic functions (66). Sodium, chloride, potassium, calcium, magnesium, and phosphorus are electrolytes—they conduct electricity in the body. Electrolytes affect fluid balance, muscle pH, and muscle functioning (140).

Minerals are essential for health and athletic performance; deficiencies can lead to health consequences and performance decrements (66). Mineral needs depend on gender and life stage (pregnancy, lactation, etc.). Table 7.1 includes the Dietary Reference Intakes (DRIs) for adults aged 19 to 30. Though vital, there is no evidence to suggest that increased intake of minerals, beyond the DRIs, will improve training adaptations or measures of performance (91).

MACROMINERALS

Minerals needed by the body in larger amounts are called macrominerals. These include calcium, phosphorus, magnesium, sodium, potassium, chloride, and sulfate. Each mineral, with the exception of sulfate, has a DRI. Sulfur-containing amino acids provide the body with enough sulfate to meet dietary requirements, so there is no EAR, RDA, or AI for sulfate. In addition, there isn't enough data to establish a UL (121).

Calcium

All cells require calcium. Calcium is involved in hormone secretion and nerve transmission, constricting and dilating blood vessels, and acts as an intracellular messenger supporting muscle contraction. Calcium keeps bones and teeth strong and functioning properly. Ninety-nine percent of calcium is stored in bones and teeth in the form of **hydroxyapatite**. Less than 1 percent of total body calcium is found in blood, muscle, extracellular

Table 7.1 Dietary Reference Intakes for Minerals for Adults 19 to 30 years old

Mineral	Males	Females	Pregnancy	Lactation
Calcium	**1,000 mg	**1,000 mg	**1,000 mg	**1,000 mg
Chloride	*2.3 mg	*2.3 mg	*2.3 mg	*2.3 mg
Choline	*550 mg	*425 mg	*450 mg	*550 mg
Chromium	*35 µg	*25 µg	*30 µg	*45 µg
Copper	**700 µg	**700 µg	**800 µg	**1,000 µg
Iodine	**95 µg	**95 µg	**160 µg	**209 µg
Iron	**6 mg	**8.1 mg	**22 mg	**6.5 mg
Magnesium	**400 mg	**310 mg	**350 mg	**310 mg
Manganese	*2.3 mg	*1.8 mg	*2.0 mg	*2.6 mg
Molybdenum	**34 µg	**34 µg	**40 µg	**36 µg
Phosphorus	**580 mg	**580 mg	**580 mg	**580 mg
Potassium	*700 mg	*700 mg	*700 mg	*700 mg
Selenium	**45 µg	**45 µg	**49 µg	**59 µg
Sodium	*1.5 g	*1.5 g	*1.5 g	*1.5 g
Zinc	**9.4 mg	**6.8 mg	**9.5 mg	**10.4 mg

All values are estimated average requirements (EAR) unless otherwise indicated.
*Specifies adequate intake (AI).
**Specifies recommended dietary allowances (RDA).
Data from U.S. Institute of Medicine 1997; U.S. Institute of Medicine 2001; U.S. Institute of Medicine 2011.

fluid, and other tissues. The endocrine system keeps calcium in the blood within a tight range (typically ranging from 8.5 to 10.2 mg/dl, though some labs use a slightly different range) (84, 134). All organs, but particularly nerves and muscles, depend on an adequate supply of calcium in blood and cells (159). When blood calcium drops, the body pulls this mineral from bone to keep a constant concentration of calcium in blood, muscle, and intracellular fluids to maintain critical metabolic processes (135, 167) Therefore, high or low levels of calcium in the blood are primarily due to certain health conditions affecting calcium regulation (167).

Sources of Calcium

Excellent sources (foods containing 20% or more of the DV per standard serving) of calcium include dairy foods such as milk, cheese, and yogurt. The DV for calcium and other minerals is shown in table 7.2. Dairy foods are the top sources of calcium in the diets of Americans over the age of 2 years (70). Calcium-fortified orange juice, soy beverages, almond drinks, and tofu prepared with calcium sulfate are excellent or good sources of calcium (157). Some leafy green vegetables contain relatively small amounts of calcium. For instance, one cup of raw spinach contains 30 mg of calcium—far below the RDA for men and women aged 19 to 50 years, which is 1,000 mg calcium per day (157, 167). See figure 7.1 for the calcium content in common foods. Approximately 30 percent of calcium from food is absorbed, though the exact amount varies by the type of food consumed (167). Several factors affect calcium absorption, as noted in figure 7.2. For instance, the bioavailability of calcium from spinach is poor because of its high oxalate content, a compound that reduces the absorption of minerals from food (180). Phytic acid in plant-based foods might also decrease calcium absorption (121). The DRI takes into account potential factors that decrease mineral absorption.

In addition to compounds that affect calcium absorption, other factors can increase calcium excretion. Caffeine has a very minor effect on calcium excretion; studies show one cup of coffee resulted in a 2 to 3 mg calcium loss (8, 97). Phosphorus intake has a

DO YOU KNOW ?

If raw spinach were the only source of calcium in your diet, you would need to eat 33 cups a day to meet the DV for calcium.

Table 7.2 Daily Values for Minerals

Food component	DV
Sodium	2,400 mg
Potassium	3,500 mg
Calcium	1,000 mg
Iron	18 mg
Iodine	150 ηg
Magnesium	400 mg
Zinc	15 mg
Selenium	70 ηg
Copper	2 mg
Manganese	2 mg
Chromium	120 ηg
Molybdenum	75 ηg
Chloride	3,400 mg

Data from U.S. Food and Drug Administration 2013.

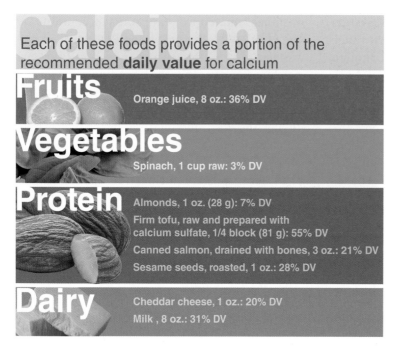

Figure 7.1 Calcium content of commonly eaten foods.

Text based on U.S. Department of Agriculture.

minor impact on excretion (64). A high-protein diet increases both calcium excretion and absorption and appears to have no detrimental impact on bone (39, 63, 79, 152). Additionally, protein is a component of bone tissue, and dietary protein intake is associated with a marker of bone formation and a decrease in bone breakdown (26, 63).

Several forms of calcium appear in fortified foods and dietary supplements. Calcium carbonate and calcium citrate are two of the more common forms found in supplements. Calcium absorption decreases as the amount of calcium consumed at one time increases. Calcium absorption also decreases with aging (121). For maximum absorption, up to 500 mg of calcium should be taken at once (167).

Calcium Deficiency and Inadequacy

Calcium deficiency is not uncommon, but consistently low calcium intake can lead to health consequences over time. If calcium intake is insufficient to meet physiological needs, the body will withdraw calcium from its backup supply in bone to keep levels within the blood constant. Consistently low calcium intake affects bone health, as too many withdrawals weakens bone (figure 7.3) (159).

The skeleton is an organ that provides support, mobility, and protection for the body and stores the essential minerals calcium and phosphorus. The brittle bone disease osteoporosis is characterized by low bone mass, which can lead to structural abnormalities, including bent posture (159).

Bone is a dynamic, metabolically active tissue responding to genetics, exercise, and diet. Lifestyle choices have a profound impact on bone, influencing 20 to 40 percent of peak bone mass (175). During childhood and adolescence, bone is sculpted by **modeling**; new bone is formed at one site within bone, and old bone is removed at another site on the outside of bone. During this process, bones shift and grow longer, denser, and stronger. During puberty, bones become thicker as formation occurs both inside and on the outer surface of bone (159). Up to 90 percent of **peak bone mass**, maximum bone strength and density, is attained during late adolescence (66), but 100 percent peak bone mass is generally not reached until the early 20s to about age 30 (111, 159). In children, consistent inadequate dietary calcium intake or poor calcium absorption can lead to rickets, a disease characterized by weak bones that do not grow properly. Remodeling, removal of old bone and replacement with new bone at the same site, occurs throughout life; the adult skeleton is replaced approximately every 10 years (159). Remodeling repairs small cracks or deformities in bone and prevents buildup of older bone, which can become brittle (159). In older adults, bone breakdown (**resorption**) exceeds bone formation, leading to a net loss in bone mass and increased

DO YOU KNOW ❓

For optimal absorption, take calcium carbonate with food. You can take calcium citrate at any time of the day, with or without food (150).

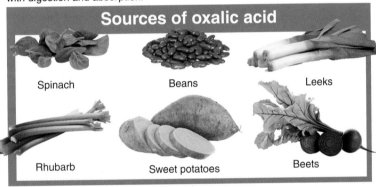

Vitamin D
It can be made when skin is exposed to UVB rays, is also naturally found in a few foods and added to others, and increases the body's absorption of calcium.

Calcium
Absorption decreases as the amount consumed at one time increases.

Absorption inhibited ⚠
Foods from plant seeds contain phytic acid, a form of phosphorus that is not well absorbed in humans. Calcium can combine with phytic acid and interfere with digestion and absorption.

Sources of oxalic acid

Spinach   Beans   Leeks

Rhubarb   Sweet potatoes   Beets

Figure 7.2 Factors that affect calcium absorption.

Based on U.S. Institute of Medicine 1997.

risk of developing brittle bones, termed **osteoporosis** (167). To prevent or delay the onset of osteoporosis, it is critical to build peak bone mass during the early years and slow bone loss after peak bone mass is reached. Figure 7.4 provides information on food that helps to build peak bone mass.

Despite the detrimental effects associated with low calcium intake, national survey data show over 40 percent of Americans do not meet the EAR for calcium (figure 7.5) (46, 70). Though females have higher calcium density than males—more calcium per the amount of calories they consume—they consume fewer overall calories) and therefore less total calcium (70). Females, particularly preteens and teenagers, are most likely to consume inade-quate amounts of calcium (135). Average calcium intake is lower for African Americans than for whites or Hispanics. Those from lower-income households also consume less than individuals from higher-income households (70).

Excess Calcium Intake

High calcium intake can cause constipation and interfere with iron and zinc absorption. Also, some studies suggest supplemental calcium intake is related to risk of kidney stones (167).

Although typically associated with primary hyperparathyroidism, very high intakes of calcium can cause high blood calcium, **hypercalcemia** (100, 167), which can lead to vascular and

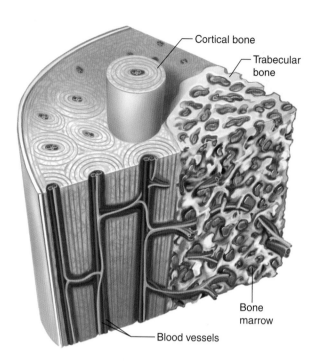

Figure 7.3 The two types of bone are cortical and trabecular. Trabecular bone, sometimes called spongy bone, has a honeycomb-like structure that makes up the inside of bone. Cortical bone is hard and forms the outer layer of bone.

soft tissue calcification, high calcium in the urine, kidney stones, and renal insufficiency (167).

Calcium and Exercise

Because of its role in bone health, calcium is extremely important for fitness enthusiasts and athletes. Among other variables, including training, biomechanics, and overall nutrition intake, chronically low calcium intake can lead to low bone mineral density, resulting in an increased risk of stress fracture (10). In addition to calcium's role in bone health, low bone mineral density and subsequent fracture risk are both increased by chronically low energy availability (not con-

suming enough total calories to meet one's needs) combined with delayed menarche (first menstrual cycle), a history of oligomenorrhea (light or infrequent menstrual cycles or cycles more than 35 days apart), or amenorrhea (absence of three or more menstrual cycles in a row) (29).

Phosphorus

Phosphorus is essential for the formation of bones and teeth, helps the body use carbohydrates and fats, and is important for growth, maintenance, and repair of cells and tissues, as well as for maintaining normal pH. Phosphorus plays an essential role in nerve signaling, blood vessel functioning, regular heartbeat, and muscle contractions (as part of ATP and PCr). All cells throughout the body contain phosphorus and rely on this mineral for functioning (159). Bones and teeth contain the majority of the body's phosphorus stores (163). When phosphorus is in short supply, the body takes it from bone to meet physiological demands (159).

Think of bone like a bank account—calcium and phosphorus are deposited in bone and removed by hormones when levels are insufficient to meet vital functions in the body. Removal decreases the amount of calcium and phosphorus stored for later use, unless you deposit (consume) more. Over time, constant withdrawals with no, or minimal, deposits leads to weaker bones (figure 7.6) (159).

Sources of Phosphorus

Phosphorus is found in a wide variety of foods, including poultry, seeds, nuts, beans, dairy, meat, poultry, and fish. The standard American diet, the typical dietary pattern of most Americans, contains roughly two to four times more phosphorus than calcium, and national survey data

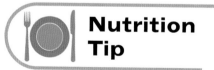

Nutrition Tip

Use it or lose it. Whether you are in a cast, on prolonged bed rest, in a wheelchair, on a space flight, or on your couch watching TV, too much immobilization leads to rapid bone loss (159). The best way to ensure your bones will allow you to be active in your 70s, 80s, and 90s is to use them when you are younger.

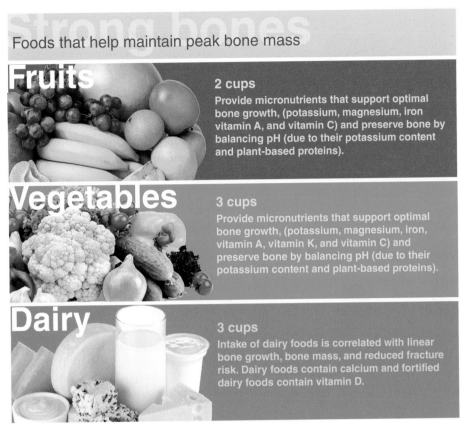

Figure 7.4 Recommended servings of dairy, fruits, and vegetables for peak bone mass for adults aged 19 to 30.

Based on Weaver et al. 2016.

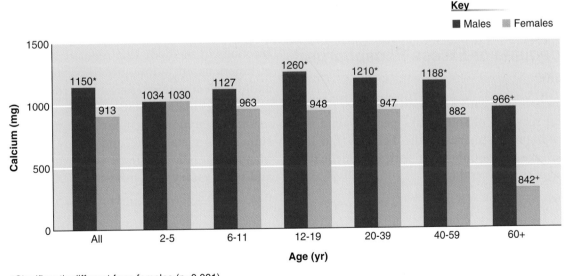

*Significantly different from females (p<0.001)
+Within gender, significantly different than other age groups combined (p<0.001)

Figure 7.5 Calcium intake of the U.S. population.

Reprinted from U.S. Department of Agriculture 2014. Available: http://www.ars.usda.gov/SP2UserFiles/Place/80400530/pdf/DBrief/13_calcium_intake_0910.pdf

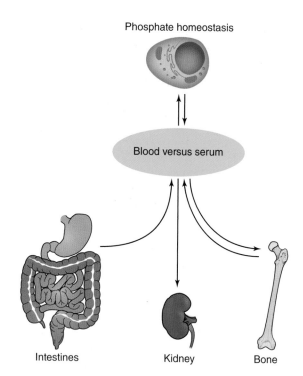

Figure 7.6 Phosphorus homeostasis.

indicate many Americans get more than enough phosphorus in their diet, suggesting sources of phosphorus are both popular among and readily available to U.S. consumers. That said, not all groups have an adequate intake of phosphorus.

Inadequate or Excess Phosphorus Intake

Individuals who eat a lot of dairy foods or drink several servings of soft drinks per day tend to have a high phosphorus intake. Females 9 to 18 years of age are the only group with an inadequate intake of this mineral (106).

Hypophosphatemia, low blood phosphate, is not common, though it is possible from starvation or in those recovering from an alcoholic bout or diabetic ketoacidosis. Hypophosphatemia can lead to anemia, muscle weakness, bone pain, rickets, osteomalacia, general physical weakness, increased risk of infection, paresthesia (a tingling or pricking feeling), ataxia (loss of body movements), confusion, anorexia, and possible death (163).

Excess phosphorus intake can lead to **hyperphosphatemia**, abnormally high phosphorus levels in blood. Risk of hyperphosphatemia is greatest in those with end-state renal disease or vitamin D intoxication. Hyperphosphatemia can lead to decreased calcium absorption and calcification of nonskeletal tissues, such as the kidneys (163).

Phosphorus and Exercise

Given the many roles phosphorus performs in the body, including in muscle, a deficiency of this mineral could, theoretically, impair athletic performance. However, because phosphorus deficiency is rare, implications of low phosphorus intake or deficiency and potential impact on athletic performance have not been studied.

Magnesium

Magnesium is a cofactor in over 300 biochemical reactions in the body that regulate a wide array of functions, including protein synthesis, nerve and muscle function, glucose control, and blood pressure regulation. Magnesium is essential for maintenance of intracellular calcium and potassium levels, metabolism, and energy production. Magnesium is a structural component of bone, and is necessary to synthesize RNA, DNA, and

PUTTING IT INTO PERSPECTIVE

HOW DO I KNOW IF I'M MEETING MY MINERAL NEEDS?

To determine if you are meeting your needs for each mineral, regularly monitor the foods you are eating. Keep a food diary for at least 3 days without changing your normal eating habits. Are you eating foods that are good or excellent sources of each mineral?

glutathione, an antioxidant that suppresses muscle fatigue resulting from prolonged exercise (5, 163). Approximately half of the body's magnesium stores is in bone. The remaining amount is in soft tissues, with less than 1 percent of the body's magnesium stores found in blood. The amount of magnesium in blood is tightly regulated and has little correlation to the amount of magnesium found within specific tissues (163). When more magnesium is consumed, the body absorbs less. Likewise, lower magnesium intake leads to an increase in absorption (121).

Several disease states have been linked to low magnesium intake, among them hypertension (high blood pressure). A meta-analysis examining the effect of magnesium supplementation on blood pressure found 22 trials with 3 to 24 weeks of follow-up and a supplemented elemental magnesium range of 120 to 973 mg (mean dose 410 mg). Combined, the trials found a small yet clinically significant mean decrease in systolic blood pressure, 3 to 4 mmHg, and diastolic pressure, 2 to 3 mmHg. Results were greater in crossover trials with a supplemental intake of >370 mg per day (77). Another meta-analysis of 34 trials found a median magnesium dose of 368 mg per day for a median duration of 3 months significantly reduced systolic blood pressure by 2 mmHg and diastolic blood pressure by 1.78 mmHg (183).

Higher magnesium intake is associated with lower fasting insulin concentrations (lower concentrations of the hormone insulin are measured during fasting) in both adults and obese children. Fasting insulin at lower levels may correspond with greater insulin sensitivity (greater insulin sensitivity means muscle, fat, and liver cells respond better to insulin; insulin absorbs glucose from the bloodstream) (47, 71,

89, 148). Additionally, approximately 25 to 38 percent of people with type 2 diabetes have low magnesium levels (27). Despite the associations between dietary magnesium intake, fasting insulin concentrations, and type 2 diabetes, clinical trials examining how magnesium supplements affect fasting blood glucose and insulin sensitivity in type 2 diabetics have led to mixed results (30, 54, 122, 123, 132, 181).

Sources of Magnesium

Magnesium is found in nuts, seeds, legumes, leafy green vegetables, and whole grains (figure 7.7). Excellent dietary sources of magnesium (those containing 20 percent or more of the DV) include pumpkin seeds, almonds, boiled spinach, soybeans, cowpeas, Brazil nuts, and cashews. Good sources of magnesium include kidney beans, peanuts, brown rice, wild rice, and walnuts (99, 157).

When examining a magnesium supplement, the total amount of actual magnesium (referred to as "elemental magnesium"), as well as the body's ability to absorb the specific source of magnesium, should be considered. Dietary supplements contain varying amounts

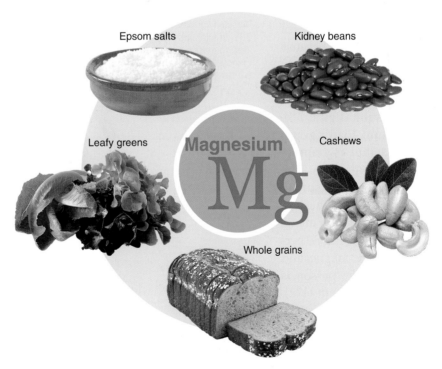

Figure 7.7 Sources of magnesium, including Epsom salts, which is absorbed through the skin during a bath and should not be eaten.

of magnesium. Manufacturers are required to list the amount of elemental magnesium on the supplement label, which is a fraction of the magnesium-containing compound. The absorption of supplemental forms of magnesium also varies. Magnesium aspartate, citrate, lactate, and chloride are better absorbed and more bioavailable then magnesium oxide and magnesium sulfate (41, 87, 107, 128, 173). Magnesium is a large mineral, so single-pill multivitamin mineral supplements do not contain anywhere near 100 percent of the DV for magnesium.

Inadequate Magnesium Intake

Poor magnesium intake is prevalent among several groups in the United States (42, 48, 170). A large percentage of American teenagers, along with men and women 71 years of age or older, are consuming below EAR for magnesium (106). National survey data show that African American women in all age groups had the lowest intake. Those who consume dietary supplements are more likely to meet their magnesium needs, yet many women who use supplements still fall short of the RDA (6, 42).

There are no nationally representative estimates of magnesium status because this electrolyte is rarely tested, and there are no universally accepted methods of testing (figure 7.8). Magnesium loading is a good test but is impractical and expensive. The test involves measuring the percent of magnesium retained by the body after a loading protocol. If 80 percent or more magnesium is retained, the person is considered deficient (172). Symptomatic magnesium deficiency in otherwise healthy individuals is rare. Gastrointestinal diseases, type 2 diabetes, alcoholism, and regular use of

specific medications can lead to magnesium deficiency (21, 131, 154). Those with cardiovascular disease, neuromuscular disease, malabsorption syndromes, renal disease, and osteoporosis may have an increased risk for depleted magnesium levels (121). In addition, older adults have an increased risk of deficiency caused by decreased magnesium absorption and increased excretion. Older adults are also more likely to have chronic diseases or take medications that affect magnesium status (7, 109). Symptoms of magnesium deficiency include decreased appetite, nausea, vomiting, fatigue, weakness, numbness, tingling, muscle contractions and cramps, twitches or spasms, seizures, personality changes, abnormal heart rhythms, hypocalcemia (low serum calcium), hypokalemia (low serum potassium), and coronary spasms (22, 50). Magnesium deficiency can disrupt muscle cell functioning, impair carbohydrate uptake by muscle cells, lead to impaired cardiovascular functioning, muscular fatigue, muscle cramping, and impair athletic

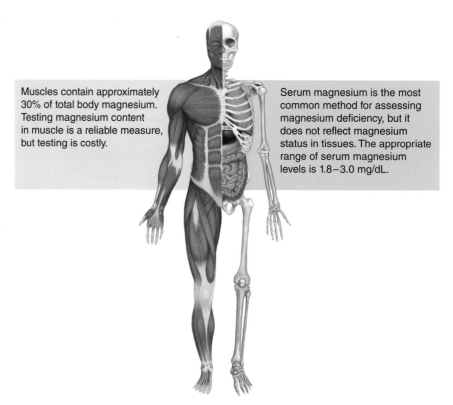

Muscles contain approximately 30% of total body magnesium. Testing magnesium content in muscle is a reliable measure, but testing is costly.

Serum magnesium is the most common method for assessing magnesium deficiency, but it does not reflect magnesium status in tissues. The appropriate range of serum magnesium levels is 1.8–3.0 mg/dL.

Figure 7.8 Red blood cell magnesium might be the best method for testing magnesium status, but it does not correlate well with total body magnesium status.

Based on Elin et al. 1994.

performance (20, 93, 113, 139). Low magnesium levels are also associated with chronic inflammation (81, 176). Based on animal research, magnesium deficiency may lead to structural and functional damage to proteins and DNA, as well as decreased antioxidant capacity (32, 43).

Excess Magnesium Intake

In healthy individuals, excess magnesium is typically excreted. No adverse effects have been noted from magnesium intake through food (121). Excess magnesium intake from supplements, magnesium-containing antacids, or medications can lead to nausea, stomach cramping, and diarrhea (121). Magnesium toxicity is associated with nausea, vomiting, facial flushing, fatigue, muscle weakness, breathing difficulty, extreme hypotension (low blood pressure), irregular heartbeat, and cardiac arrest (109). Poor kidney functioning increases risk of magnesium toxicity caused by a decline in the body's ability to remove excess magnesium (109).

Magnesium and Exercise

Given magnesium's many roles in the body that affect athletic performance, including ATP synthesis, carbohydrate and fat metabolism, bone strength, and muscle functioning, this mineral is clearly important for athletic performance (32, 43, 163). That said, relatively few studies have examined the effects of magnesium supplementation on sports performance (172).

Observational data accessing dietary recalls from adolescent athletes, ultraendurance athletes, rhythmic gymnasts, young adult male athletes (aged 19 to 25 years old), male collegiate soccer (football) players, male collegiate rugby players, and elite female athletes from a wide variety of sports suggest that many athletes are not meeting their magnesium requirements (28, 65, 72, 75, 117, 145, 178, 182).

Research indicates that even marginal magnesium deficiency can impair exercise (114). A study in postmenopausal women found low magnesium intake led to lowered magnesium stores in muscle and red blood cells; the women required more oxygen during exercise and were more likely to fatigue quickly during submaximal work (93). In another study of elite male basketball, handball, and volleyball players, magnesium intake, as assessed via a 7-day diet record, was directly associated with maximal isometric trunk flexion, rotation, handgrip, jumping performance tests, and all isokinetic strength variables, independent of calorie intake (139). Despite the associations between magnesium and factors that affect performance, only a few studies suggest magnesium supplementation, particularly in the absence of low magnesium status as identified through testing, can improve athletic performance (172).

In a double-blind, 7-week strength-training study, untrained males aged 18 to 30 were given a magnesium oxide supplement, a poorly absorbed form of magnesium (to bring total intake to 8 mg/kg body weight per day based on dietary intake as

---

REFLECTION TIME

IF YOU USE DETOX DIETS OR CLEANSES, READ THIS FIRST!

Many detox diets and cleanses rely on a combination of ingredients, foods, or beverages that often include laxatives and diuretics. Magnesium is a common ingredient in some laxative products (53). If your detox diet or cleanse contains magnesium carbonate, chloride, gluconate, or oxide, you are more likely to experience diarrhea (128). Also, very large doses of magnesium can lead to magnesium toxicity, particularly in those with impaired kidney functioning (163).

assessed via a 3-day diet record) or placebo. (In a double-blind study, both the researchers and participants are unaware of the intervention. In this study, the researchers and participants didn't know if they were using the supplement or placebo.) At the end of the 7-week period, quadriceps torque was measured. Both groups gained strength, but the supplemented group had a greater gain in absolute torque, relative torque as adjusted for body weight, and relative torque as adjusted for lean body mass, compared to the placebo group (14). Twenty-five professional male volleyball players were given either 350 mg magnesium or 500 mg of maltodextrin each day for 4 weeks. The group supplemented with magnesium experienced a significant decrease in lactate production and up to 3-centimeter increases in countermovement jump and countermovement jump with arm swing (the athlete stands upright, flexes knees, moves arms back while squatting, and then swiftly extends knees and hips to jump vertically), while there was no change in the placebo group, suggesting improvement in immediate energy anaerobic metabolism (144). A randomized, controlled trial in elderly women attending a fitness program found supplementing with 300 mg magnesium oxide daily led to improvements in performance, particularly in women consuming lower than the RDA for magnesium (171).

Potassium

Potassium helps maintain fluid volume inside and outside of cells, making this mineral important for proper cell functioning, smooth and skeletal muscle (including muscle contraction) functioning, acid-base balance, and nerve transmission. A diet rich in potassium can help decrease the adverse effects sodium can have on blood pressure, reduce the risk of recurrent kidney stones, and potentially decrease bone loss. Potassium levels must be maintained within normal limits, as either high or low levels of potassium can lead to serious health effects (166).

Sources of Potassium

The average American consumes 2,640 mg of potassium per day, far below the recommended AI of 4,700 mg each day (69). Like many other nutrients, potassium intake is related to calorie intake. Those who consume more calories each day generally consume more potassium as well. Average total daily potassium intake is greater in men than women due to higher total daily calorie intake (69). National dietary survey data suggest less than 1 percent of women consume at least 4,700 mg of potassium per day. Non-Hispanic black females consumed the least amount of potassium, followed by Hispanic women and non-Hispanic white females (69).

PUTTING IT INTO PERSPECTIVE

A POTASSIUM-RICH DIET MIGHT HELP LOWER BLOOD PRESSURE

Population-based research shows higher potassium intake is associated with lower blood pressure (58). Additional evidence supporting the role of potassium in healthy blood pressure comes from randomized clinical trials that show increasing dietary potassium intake leads to a small, though statistically significant, decrease in blood pressure in those with normal blood pressure or hypertension (177), particularly when dietary sodium intake is high (105).

Potassium decreases blood pressure by relaxing smooth muscle, which opens up blood vessels to allow for greater blood flow and a subsequent drop in blood pressure (56). In addition, supplemental potassium intake increases the excretion of sodium chloride in urine (56). The next time you drink a cup of potassium-packed, 100 percent orange juice or add slices of tomatoes to your sandwich, you will be supporting healthy blood pressure levels.

Vegetables, beans, and fruits are among the highest dietary sources of potassium. All beans (soybeans, lima beans, mung beans, white, black, kidney, pinto, etc.) are excellent sources of potassium, containing more than 25 percent of the AI per half-cup serving. Potatoes, apricots, tomatoes, orange juice, prunes, and beet greens are also some of the highest dietary sources of this nutrient (157). In the average American diet, the highest contributors of potassium include fruits and vegetables (20%), milk and milk drinks (11%), meat and poultry (10%), and grain-based mixed dishes (10%) (69).

Inadequate Potassium Intake

Moderate potassium deficiency can lead to increased blood pressure, salt sensitivity, increased risk of kidney stones, and a potential increase in cardiovascular disease, especially stroke. Severe potassium deficiency, called hypokalemia, can lead to muscle weakness, glucose intolerance, and abnormal heart rhythm. Excess intake of diuretics or laxatives, prolonged vomiting or diarrhea, as well as kidney and adrenal disorders, contribute to potassium deficiency (143, 166). Sodium intake, as tested up to 3.2 grams per day, does not increase potassium excretion (90). However, at levels above 6.9 grams per day, there is a net loss of potassium (at least over the short term—it isn't clear if the body adjusts to consistently higher sodium intake) (137).

Excess Potassium Intake

There is no UL for potassium consumption because the kidneys excrete excess intake through urine, helping prevent high blood potassium (166). However, potassium can build up in the blood, a condition called hyperkalemia, in those with poor kidney functioning and impaired ability to excrete excess potassium. Potassium-sparing diuretics, hemolytic anemia (premature destruction and removal of red blood cells), severe bleeding in the stomach or intestines, tumors, excess potassium intake from salt substitutes or dietary supplements, and certain heart medicines (ACE inhibitors, angiotensin receptor blockers) can also lead to hyperkalemia. Nonsteroidal

anti-inflammatory drugs (NSAIDs) such as ibuprofen, aspirin, and naproxen may also increase risk of hyperkalemia, particularly in those with poor kidney functioning. Hyperkalemia can lead to nausea, slow or irregular heartbeat, sudden collapse, and cardiac arrest (95). Those who have an impaired ability to excrete excess potassium should keep their total daily intake below 4.7 grams (166).

Potassium and Exercise

Relatively small changes in extracellular potassium levels can affect nervous system function, muscle contraction, and blood vessel function (166). Potassium's role in athletic performance is discussed in chapter 8.

Sodium

Sodium regulates the amount of fluid in blood and extracellular fluid balance (blood volume), is necessary for nerve and muscle functioning, helps transport molecules across cell membranes, and is involved in the electrical potential across cell membranes. Combined with sodium, chloride helps maintain fluid and electrolyte balance and makes up sodium chloride, otherwise known as table salt (121). The AI for sodium is 1.5 grams per day (3.8 g/day sodium chloride, or table salt) for young adults, 1.3 grams per day for those 50 to 70 years of age, and 1.2 grams per day for anyone 71 years of age or older. This level ensures the diet provides enough sodium to cover normal sweat losses in those not acclimated to the heat yet exposed to high temperatures, while also ensuring adequate intake of other nutrients. The AI is not applicable for those who are competitive athletes, workers exposed to extreme heat stress, or anyone else who loses large volumes of sodium through sweat (121).

The body regulates fluid balance by monitoring blood volume and sodium level. When blood volume or sodium is too high, the kidneys increase sodium excretion. Additionally, the pituitary gland releases antidiuretic hormone in response to low blood volume. Antidiuretic hormone triggers the kidneys to conserve fluid. If blood volume drops too low, the kidneys secrete the hormone aldosterone to retain sodium and excrete potassium. Increased sodium retention leads to a decrease in urine production and subsequent rise in blood volume.

As people age, fluid balance isn't as well regulated. Older adults are more likely than younger adults to have an altered thirst mechanism, and thus are less inclined to drink enough fluids. Kidney function changes with age, excreting more fluid in urine. Older adults have less total body water, so a slight drop in body water can lead to more serious health consequences than would occur in younger adults. Also, older adults are more likely to take multiple medications, which can increase fluid excretion, and to have diseases or conditions (impaired walking, swallowing difficulty, dementia) that alter their ability or desire to drink a sufficient amount of fluid.

Sources of Sodium

The majority of sodium consumed in the United States comes from salt, and the greatest source by far is processed foods, contributing to approximately 77 percent of salt intake. Only 6 percent of the average person's salt intake comes from the salt shaker, and only 12 percent is from the sodium chloride naturally found in food (121).

Inadequate Sodium Intake

The human body has a remarkable ability to adapt to low intake of sodium by conserving sodium in the body (121). Low blood sodium chloride levels are rare in healthy individuals. Severe vomiting may lead to excess sodium chloride losses, low chloride levels, and metabolic alkalosis from hydrochloric metabolic alkalosis. Prolonged or intense exercise, particularly in the heat, can lead to dangerously low blood sodium levels, a condition called hyponatremia (121), which will be discussed in chapter 8.

Excess Sodium Intake

Healthy individuals excrete excess sodium intake. However, continuous high sodium chloride (table salt) intake over a period of time is associated with an increase in blood pressure, a risk factor for stroke, heart disease, and kidney disease (121). This increase in blood pressure appears to be greatest in older adults, African

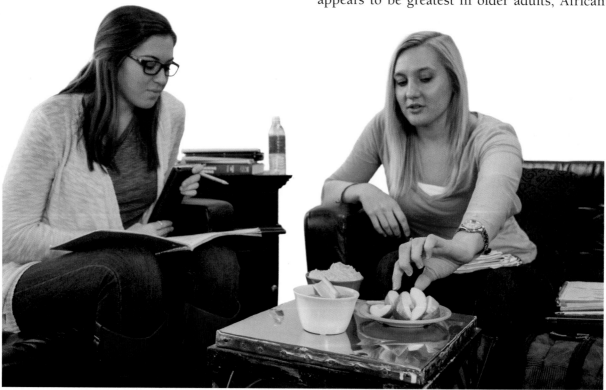

Reach for healthy snacks like fruits, vegetables, and hummus to keep up your energy for long study sessions.

Americans, and those with chronic kidney disease (121). Higher dietary potassium intake increases sodium excretion, reducing the rise in blood pressure associated with sodium intake (121). Higher potassium intake has the greatest impact on blood pressure when sodium intake is high (121).

Changes in blood pressure in response to changes in sodium intake can vary tremendously among individuals (24). Salt sensitivity refers to the change in blood pressure after a reduction or increase in salt intake (166). Older adults, African Americans, and those who are obese or have metabolic syndrome are more likely to be salt sensitive; their blood pressure increases in response to an increase in sodium intake and decreases in response to a lower sodium diet (23, 61, 141). Both genetic and environmental factors appear to influence salt sensitivity (52). Twenty-five to 50 percent of those with normal blood pressure are salt sensitive; in this group, salt sensitivity seems to predict future high blood pressure (24, 120). Forty to 75 percent of those with high blood pressure are salt sensitive (120). Those who are salt sensitive and have high blood pressure are more likely to experience changes in blood pressure in response to salt intake (24).

Based on the association between higher sodium intake and blood pressure, the *2015-2020 Dietary Guidelines for Americans* recommend that those 14 years of age and older consume less than 2,300 mg sodium per day, while those with high blood pressure consume less than 1,500 mg sodium per day (158). However, these guidelines are controversial. The Institute of Medicine reviewed the research on sodium intake and health outcomes and found a positive relation between higher sodium intake and risk of cardiovascular disease (CVD); however, no benefit is associated with a sodium intake below 2,300 mg per day in the general population. The Institute also found no evidence for benefit, but perhaps for a greater risk of harm, with sodium intakes between 1,500 and 2,300 mg per day in those with diabetes, kidney disease, or CVD (168). In addition, a study examining over 100,000 people found a sodium intake between 3 and 6 grams per day was associated with lower risk of death and CVD events compared to higher or lower sodium diets (118). Average daily sodium intake in the United States is approximately 4,400 mg per day for men 19 years of age and older and 3,090 mg per day for women 19 years of age or older (73).

Independent of its impact on blood pressure—that is, whether it raises blood pressure or has no effect—a high-sodium diet (though there is no universal definition for "high sodium") might have other adverse effects in the body. In those with normal blood pressure, 4,600 mg of sodium per day decreased nitric oxide activity—the molecule that opens blood vessels for greater blood flow (156). Nitric oxide is an important molecule for healthy blood pressure and one that is a target of active individuals—arginine and beetroot juice increase nitric oxide activity to help increase blood flow to working muscles. Adults with normal blood pressure experienced a temporary decrease in blood vessel dilation after a single high-salt meal (1,500 mg sodium) (33), while overweight or obese adults with normal blood pressure saw improvements in blood flow while on a low-sodium diet (1,150 mg sodium), compared to when on a high-sodium (3,450 mg) diet (34). High sodium intake seems to damage the inner lining of blood vessels (endothelial lining), which is involved in blood clotting, nitric oxide release, immune function, and other important processes (24), while also increasing artery stiffness (stiff arteries do not expand as well as normal arteries to accommodate increases in blood pressure) (38). Also, a link exists between high dietary salt intake, increased inflammation among immune system cells, and impaired immune regulation (120).

Sodium and Exercise

Sodium chloride has two main functions during exercise—it helps the body retain fluid consumed (98) and helps restore electrolytes for proper muscle functioning. Sodium is the top electrolyte lost through sweat, followed by chloride. Sodium chloride losses vary tremendously among athletes, so sodium chloride recommendations should be individualized as much as possible (25, 85, 140), a topic revisited in chapter 8.

IF I EAT TOO MUCH SALT NOW, WILL I GET HIGH BLOOD PRESSURE LATER IN LIFE?

Many factors contribute to high blood pressure, including genetics and obesity. There is no evidence that a high-sodium diet causes high blood pressure in healthy individuals with normal blood pressure. However, according to the Institute of Medicine, the majority of Americans consume too much salt—and not enough potassium—for health and reducing risk of some chronic diseases (166). Recall that potassium can help diminish the possible deleterious effects of a high-sodium diet on high blood pressure.

Chloride

Chloride is essential for maintaining extracellular fluid volume and plasma osmolarity. The majority of dietary chloride comes with sodium in the form of salt (sodium chloride). As a part of hydrochloric acid, chloride is also a component of gastric fluid. Approximately 98 percent of sodium chloride is absorbed. In healthy individuals with little sweat loss, the majority of sodium chloride leaves the body through urine, with the amount excreted almost equal to the amount consumed (121). Because chloride is bound to sodium, the AI for chloride is based on the AI for sodium (i.e., the AI equals the amount of chloride in the quantity of salt containing the AI for sodium). Much more sodium chloride is derived from processed foods than from salt added to food from the salt shaker. Chloride deficiency is rare, caused mainly by a loss of hydrochloric acid. Diuretics can increase sodium and chloride losses in addition to water. Those with cystic fibrosis have an unusually high sodium and chloride content in sweat and thus require more sodium and chloride. Excess intake is related to high blood pressure in those who are salt sensitive (121).

Sulfur

Many metabolic intermediates, including the antioxidant glutathione, contain sulfur. Sulfur is found in the diet through sulfur-containing amino acids and water. Sulfur is also created in the body from the amino acids methionine and cysteine. Deficiency is rare in those with adequate protein intake. There is no UL for sulfur due to an absence of sufficient data. Excess sulfur intake, from water high in inorganic sulfate, can lead to osmotic diarrhea (121).

TRACE MINERALS

Trace minerals are those the body needs in small amounts. They include iron, manganese, iodine, zinc, chromium, copper, selenium, and fluoride. Table 7.3 summarizes sources and signs of deficiency and excess intake of some minerals.

Iron

Iron is necessary for growth, development, cell functioning, immune functioning, and the synthesis and functioning of some hormones. Iron is also essential for the proteins hemoglobin and myoglobin. Hemoglobin transfers oxygen throughout the body; myoglobin transports oxygen to muscles (36, 45, 49, 57, 82).

Sources of Iron

Two types of iron are found in food: heme iron and non-heme iron (figure 7.9). Heme iron, derived from hemoglobin, is found in foods that contain hemoglobin—animal foods such as red meat, fish, and poultry. Approximately 15 to 35 percent of heme iron is absorbed (104). Dietary factors do not affect heme iron absorption (121). Vegetables, grains, iron-fortified breakfast cereal and other nonmeat-based foods contain non-heme iron; 2 to 20 percent of non-heme iron is absorbed (151). Phytic acid (the storage form of phosphorus in plants), polyphenols, phytates (legumes, whole grains), vegetable proteins, and calcium

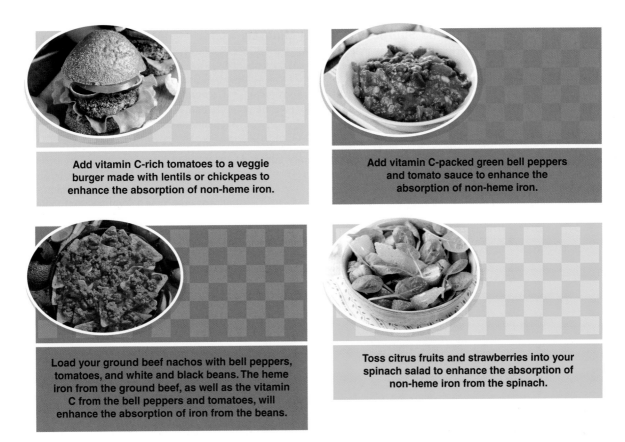

Figure 7.9 Are you getting enough iron each day? Here are some easy ways to incorporate more iron in your diet and enhance the absorption of non-heme iron.

inhibit non-heme iron absorption (59, 121, 126, 174, 179), whereas vitamin C enhances non-heme iron absorption (121). Animal protein appears to increase non-heme iron absorption (121).

Inadequate Iron Intake

Iron deficiency is the most prevalent nutrient deficiency in the world, largely because of iron-poor diets in developing countries (108). In the United States, higher rates of iron deficiency and iron-deficiency anemia are seen in infants and toddlers, women of childbearing age, teenage girls, women aged 20 to 49, pregnant women, and female endurance athletes, partially because of poor dietary iron intake (94, 130). The following individuals have a higher risk of developing iron-deficiency anemia:

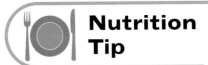

Nutrition Tip Ibuprofen, aspirin, and other nonsteroidal anti-inflammatory drugs (NSAIDs) are commonly used to prevent and treat pain, inflammation, fever, arthritis, and other conditions. Long-term use of these drugs can damage the lining of the small intestine, causing inflammation, upset stomach, and bleeding, which can lead to iron-deficiency anemia (2, 124). If you experience adverse side effects or have concerns, talk to your physician. Iron supplements can also cause upset stomach; do not take iron supplements with an NSAID unless directed to do so by your physician.

Table 7.3 Excellent and Good Sources for Select Minerals

Mineral	Excellent sources (≥20% DV) based on standard serving size	Good sources (≥10% DV) based on standard serving size	
Calcium	Yogurt, cheese, milk, calcium-fortified orange juice, calcium-fortified soy milk, some brands of tofu made with calcium sulfate (157)	Canned salmon with bones, cottage cheese, boiled turnip greens, raw kale, soybeans	
Chromium*	Chromium is in a wide array of foods typically in small amounts; meats, whole grains, some fruits, vegetables, spices, grape juice, potatoes (4)	There are no reliable methods to accurately determine the chromium content of grains, fruits, and vegetables because agricultural and manufacturing processes have a significant influence on chromium content (4)	
Copper	Lamb liver, veal liver, sesame seeds, oysters, cocoa powder, cashew nuts, pink or red lentils, sunflower seeds, Brazil nuts, chestnuts, hazelnuts, radishes kidney beans, walnuts, mashed potatoes	Blackberries, beef macaroni and cheese with tomato sauce, pecans, peas, peanuts, figs, cooked spinach	
Iron	Oysters, white beans, dark chocolate	Sardines, kidney beans, ground beef, tofu, spinach, lentils, chickpeas	
Magnesium	Pumpkin seeds, almonds, boiled spinach, soybeans, cowpeas, Brazil nuts, cashews (99, 157)	Kidney beans, peanuts, brown rice, wild rice, walnuts (99, 157)	
Phosphorus	Turkey, pumpkin seeds, sunflower seeds, cheese (Swiss, cheddar, provolone), Brazil nuts, sesame seeds, milk, beans (white, yellow, pink, navy, pinto, lima), quinoa, almonds, wild rice	Sirloin steak, beef, ricotta black bean soup, edamame	
Potassium	Radishes, beans (white, black, lima, pink, kidney, pinto, soybeans, French), turkey breast, orange juice, peaches, potatoes, bananas, yam, tomatoes	Dried apricots, canned chili, cod, halibut, Brussels sprouts, milk, artichokes, vegetable juice, brown rice, winter squash, pumpkin, spaghetti with meatballs and tomato sauce	
Zinc	Oysters, red meat	Poultry, fish, baked beans, cashews; diets high in protein provide substantial amounts of zinc	

*No DV

196

Deficiency signs and symptoms	Excess intake and toxicity signs and symptoms
Though true deficiency is not common, even mild deficiencies over time can lead to bone loss	Impaired kidney function and decreased absorption of other minerals.
Rare (4)	Chromium can interact with certain medications (4).
Rare; excess zinc intake can impair copper absorption	Copper is fairly nontoxic, but long-term excessive intake can lead to organ damage (88).
General weakness, fatigue, irritability, poor concentration, headache, decreased athletic performance, hair loss, dry mouth (11, 15, 68)	Risk of excess iron intake from dietary sources is low. High-dose iron supplements can cause constipation, nausea, vomiting, or diarrhea. Acute iron toxicity can lead to alterations in functioning of the cardiovascular system, central nervous system, kidney, and liver.
Decreased appetite, nausea, vomiting, fatigue, and weakness; as magnesium deficiency worsens, numbness, tingling, muscle contractions and cramps, seizures, personality changes, abnormal heart rhythms, and coronary spasms can occur	Doses over 350 mg per day can cause loose stools and diarrhea (163).
Anorexia Anemia Bone pain Rickets Osteomalacia General debility Increased risk of infection Paresthesia Ataxia Confusion Possible death	Decreased calcium absorption and calcification of non-skeletal tissues, especially the kidneys.
Constipation Skipped heartbeats Palpitations (heart racing or pounding) Abnormal heart rhythm (which may lead to feeling faint or lightheaded) Fatigue Muscle damage Muscle weakness or spasms Tingling or numbness If potassium levels are very low, the heart can stop	Muscle fatigue Weakness Paralysis Slow, weak, irregular pulse Arrhythmias (abnormal heart rhythms) Sudden collapse due to slow heartbeat or no heartbeat Nausea (76) Dietary supplements typically contain very tiny amounts of potassium because high potassium can be very dangerous.
Rare in the U.S.	Excess zinc may decrease magnesium balance and copper absorption, so monitor the number of zinc lozenges you take, especially when combined with a multivitamin mineral supplement with over 100% DV for zinc (138, 149).

Based on Allen et al. 2006; Otten, Hellwig, and Meyers 2006; U.S. Department of Agriculture 2013; U.S. Food and Drug Administration 2016; U.S. Institute of Medicine 1997; U.S. Institute of Medicine 1998; U.S. Institute of Medicine 2001; U.S. Institute of Medicine 2011.

> women because of blood loss during menstruation,

> endurance athletes due to depletion through exercise, and

> vegetarians because of inadequate dietary intake (94, 130).

Additionally, individuals with excessive intake of antacids, anyone who has had bariatric surgery (weight-loss surgery involving the stomach or intestines), and those with digestive diseases, such as celiac disease, have an increased risk of developing iron-deficiency anemia (153, 165).

Iron deficiency alters immune system functioning and the immune system's response to inflammation and infection. Iron deficiency is also associated with an increased risk of infection (9). Given iron's role in the formation of hemoglobin and myoglobin, low levels of iron commonly lead to fatigue (figure 7.10).

Iron deficiency occurs in three progressive stages: depletion, marginal deficiency, and anemia (80, 110). Marginal iron deficiency and iron-deficiency anemia can lead to general weakness, fatigue, feeling cold, irritability, poor concentration, headache, decreased athletic performance, hair loss, and dry mouth (11, 15, 68).

Excess Iron Intake

Risk of excess iron intake from dietary sources is low. High-dose iron supplements can cause constipation, nausea, vomiting, or diarrhea. Acute iron toxicity can lead to alterations in functioning of the cardiovascular system, central nervous system, kidney, and liver. Though there is some question about excess iron intake (through food or supplements) and coronary heart disease and cancer, the association, if any, remains unclear (121). Individuals at greater risk for developing high iron levels include those with hereditary hemochromatosis, chronic alcoholics, those with cirrhosis caused by alcoholism, and those with blood disorders (thalassemias) (121).

DO YOU KNOW ?

Footstrike hemolysis is the destruction of red blood cells in the bottom of the foot caused by activities involving running or jumping. Footstrike hemolysis might explain the association between greater exercise duration and intensity and lower hemoglobin, hematocrit, and ferritin (the storage form of iron in the body) in trained athletes (67).

Iron and Exercise

Either marginal iron deficiency or anemia can impair endurance performance and reduce exercise capacity (11, 31, 49, 68). Improving iron status through supplementation improves work capacity during exercise in athletes with marginal iron deficiency and anemia (16, 91). Iron deficiency might also affect cognitive functioning. A study of 127 females aged 18 to 35 found those with better iron status had better reaction time and faster planning time (142).

REFLECTION TIME

I'M TIRED—SHOULD I TAKE AN IRON SUPPLEMENT?

If you feel tired and grouchy, have difficulty concentrating, or notice exercise is tougher than usual, you could have marginal iron deficiency or iron-deficiency anemia. Review the best sources of iron in table 7.3. On average, are you are getting enough iron in your diet each day? If you are not meeting your iron needs, increase your intake of iron-rich foods and consider taking a multivitamin that has 100 percent (or less) of the DV for iron. Consider seeing your physician for a diagnosis. Never take high doses of iron without consulting your doctor first. In addition to the side effects associated with iron supplements, acute iron toxicity is very harmful to the body.

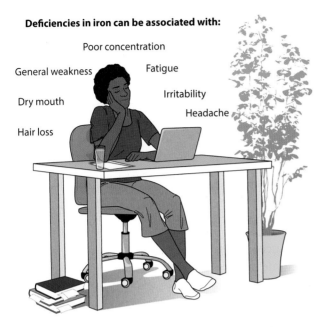

Deficiencies in iron can be associated with:

Poor concentration

General weakness   Fatigue

Dry mouth   Irritability

Headache

Hair loss

Figure 7.10   Marginal iron deficiency and iron-deficiency anemia might make studying more difficult.

Manganese

Manganese is important for bone formation and enzyme activity involved in amino acid, carbohydrate, and cholesterol metabolism. Manganese has no AI because of insufficient data to set an EAR. Grain products and vegetables make up large amounts of the manganese in the American diet (121). Beef, nuts, and beans are among the highest dietary sources of manganese (157). Clinical symptoms associated with low intakes are generally not observed, even among those with poor dietary intake of manganese (40, 121). Symptoms of manganese deficiency include dermatitis, decreased levels of clotting proteins, and low blood cholesterol. Miners exposed to manganese-laden dust have developed symptoms of toxicity, including neurological symptoms classified as manganese-induced Parkinsonism (note that Parkinsonism is different from Parkinson's disease), involving tremors, involuntary muscle contractions, impaired postural reflexes, and slow movements (40, 119).

Iodine

As a component of thyroid hormones, iodine is important for proper thyroid function. Thyroid hormones regulate a number of processes in the body, including metabolism and protein synthesis. Thyroid hormones affect several organs, including the brain, muscles, heart, pituitary gland, and kidneys. Seafood contains high amounts of iodine. Dairy products, fruits, and vegetables contain lower levels. The amount of iodine in fruits and vegetables can depend on iodine content in soil, fertilizer used, and irrigation. The addition of iodine to salt is mandatory in Canada and optional in the United States, where approximately 50 percent of salt is iodized. Iodized salt is one of the main sources of iodine in the U.S. and Canadian diet. Seafood might contain more iodine than many other foods because of the iodine content of seawater. Processed foods might also contain higher amounts of iodine because of the addition of iodized salt or other additives that contain iodine.

Excess iodine intake through food and dietary supplements is highly unlikely. Though rare, overt symptoms of iodine deficiency can lead to impaired cognitive development in children and hypothyroidism and goiter (enlarged thyroid) in adults. Iodine deficiency is particularly damaging to the developing brain, as it can lead to neurological damage. Excess intake of iodine can alter thyroid function (hypothyroidism or hyperthyroidism) and cause inflammation of the thyroid gland (121).

Zinc

Zinc is essential for immune system functioning. This mineral promotes wound healing and helps maintain skin integrity, one of the first lines of defense against pathogens. Zinc is essential for the metabolism of carbohydrates, proteins, and fats, gene expression, red blood cell functioning, normal taste and smell, and growth and development. Zinc is not stored in the body and thus must be consumed daily (129).

Sources of Zinc

Many foods are good or excellent sources of zinc. Oysters are among the highest sources, containing nearly 500 percent of the DV for zinc in just 3 ounces. Red meat is another excellent source, whereas poultry, fish, baked beans, and cashews are good sources. Diets high in protein provide substantial amounts of zinc (157).

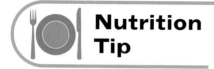

Nutrition Tip

Some, though not all, studies show that zinc gluconate lozenges taken within 24 hours of the onset of cold symptoms may be helpful for decreasing the duration and severity of the symptoms (19, 35, 127, 146, 155). Other studies have used different forms of zinc, so it remains unclear what dose, formulation, and duration of zinc is best (125, 146). When using a zinc lozenge or other zinc supplement, consume the zinc according to package directions for a few days at the early onset of symptoms. Do not take a zinc supplement long term, as this can lead to adverse side effects, including suppressed immune system functioning (55, 165).

Inadequate and Excess Zinc Intake

National survey data suggest that few people consume below the EAR for zinc (46), but several studies in athletes show low dietary intake or low zinc status. This research shows various athletes were not consuming enough zinc through their diet, including a small group of competitive male swimmers in Brazil, male and female adventure race athletes, male and female U.S. national figure skaters, trained female cyclists, and female high school gymnasts (51, 69, 78, 182, 184). Vegetarians, athletes consuming very high-carbohydrate, low-fat diets, and those who don't meet their daily calorie needs are more likely to fall short of recommended intake levels for zinc (101, 125, 184). Because of lower overall energy intake, female athletes are less likely than male athletes to meet their zinc needs (60, 136).

Although zinc deficiency is considered rare (121), inadequate zinc intake can impair energy production and measures of athletic performance (83, 92). The primary symptom of zinc deficiency is growth retardation. Additional symptoms include hair loss, diarrhea, eye and skin lesions, poor appetite, and delayed sexual maturation (121). Zinc deficiency can also delay wound healing, suppress immune system functioning, and cause weight loss (55, 136). Excess supplemental zinc intake over a long period of time can suppress immune system functioning, lower HDL, and inhibit copper absorption, potentially leading to copper deficiency (165).

Zinc and Exercise

Zinc is part of the red blood cell enzyme carbonic anhydrase, which picks up carbon dioxide for the lungs to exhale, an important step for chemical balance in muscle cells. Zinc deficiency leads to a decline in carbonic anhydrase activity, reduction in peak oxygen uptake, and peak carbon dioxide output, as well as a decrease in respiratory exchange ratio, suggesting the body had insufficient oxygen to use carbohydrates efficiently (92).

Low zinc levels lead to a decline in muscle strength and power output. Marginal zinc deficiency is associated with low levels of testosterone, thyroid hormones, and IGF-1, a hormone that promotes muscle growth and metabolism (17, 83). Correction of zinc deficiency with zinc or iron and zinc improve red blood cell functioning in those with anemia (115, 116).

Chromium

Chromium is important for the functioning of insulin, a hormone involved in the metabolism and storage of fat, protein, and carbohydrate. Chromium is found in small amounts throughout the food supply, though food processing can decrease the chromium content of whole grains and other foods (165). Chromium deficiency is rare and has been observed only in hospitalized patients fed intravenously (prior to chromium added to intravenous solutions). Deficiency can impair glucose tolerance leading to weight loss and neuropathy (74).

Although chromium deficiency can impair the action of insulin and glucose tolerance, the safety and efficacy of chromium supplementation as a treatment for insulin resistance and type 2 diabetes has not been backed by science (165). In a review of 15 trials, all but 1 showed chromium supplementation had no effect on glucose or insulin concentrations in nondiabetics or diabetics (3).

Copper

Copper is necessary for the functioning of several enzymes, helps the body make hemoglobin, and assists with energy production. The highest sources of copper are lamb, beef, shellfish, whole grains, beans, and nuts. Copper deficiency is rare, though it has been observed in premature malnourished infants; deficiency can lead to brittle bones, the blood disorder neutropenia, and anemia. High copper intake through dietary sources hasn't been observed in humans, though drinking water with high levels of copper has resulted in cramps, nausea, abdominal pain, diarrhea, and vomiting (121).

Selenium

Selenium-rich proteins are important for thyroid functioning and defend the body against

PUTTING IT INTO PERSPECTIVE

SHOULD YOU TAKE A MULTIVITAMIN SUPPLEMENT?

According to the *2015–2020 Dietary Guidelines for Americans*, "nutritional needs should be met primarily from foods. In some cases, fortified foods and dietary supplements may be useful in providing one or more nutrients that otherwise may be consumed in less-than-recommended amounts." This is an important point because foods also contain fiber and plant-based compounds necessary for good health. In some instances, a beneficial synergistic effect between the compounds is found in various foods that might not be replicated in a supplement. Multivitamins cannot take the place of consuming healthy foods (112).

If you want to ensure you're meeting your vitamin and mineral needs, eat a wide variety of nutrient-dense foods. Greater variety means you are more likely to get a wide array of compounds found in food that are necessary for good health. However, even with a very healthy diet, it can be tough to get enough of certain nutrients, especially if you don't consume at least 2,000 calories per day (more food means more opportunities to consume nutrients). Even if you eat enough total calories, research shows many athletes, active adults, and nonathletes are not meeting their nutrient needs (103). Women, individuals who avoid certain food groups, and those who are dieting are particularly likely to fall short of their micronutrient needs. Women consume far less than the dietary reference intakes set for calcium, iron, magnesium, and potassium. Plus, what you see isn't always what you get—food storage and processing (during production and at home) can destroy or decrease certain nutrients in your food. Also, some people have higher needs for specific vitamins and minerals because of medications, previous surgery (such as gastric bypass), or health conditions. Fortified foods or a multivitamin can help fill in dietary gaps (18, 133).

According to the National Institutes of Health, groups likely to benefit from taking certain nutrients found within multivitamin mineral supplements include the following:

➤ Women who may become pregnant might benefit from increased folic acid (400 mcg/day). Folic acid can reduce the risk of birth defects of the brain and spine in newborn babies.

➤ Pregnant women have higher iron needs, so their physicians might recommend a prenatal multivitamin mineral with iron or a separate iron supplement.

➤ Breast-fed or partially breast-fed infants, as well as infants who drink less than 1 quart of vitamin D-fortified milk or formula each day, need a vitamin D supplement.

➤ Postmenopausal women might need more calcium and vitamin D to increase bone strength and reduce fracture risk.

➤ Adults over the age of 50 might require supplemental vitamin B_{12} or higher amounts of vitamin B_{12} from fortified foods because of a potential decrease in absorption of vitamin B_{12} (112).

PUTTING IT INTO PERSPECTIVE

ARE PROCESSED FOODS UNHEALTHY?

Processed foods are not necessarily unhealthy. Though countless magazine articles and blogs are devoted to warning consumers about processed foods, many of the authors do not understand the true (FDA) definition of processed food. For example, frozen broccoli, frozen chicken breasts, dried beans, and dried pumpkin seeds are all examples of processed foods.

A processed food is "any food other than a raw agricultural commodity ("food that is in its raw or natural state, including all fruits that are washed, colored, or otherwise treated in their unpeeled natural form prior to marketing") and includes any raw agricultural commodity that has been subject to processing, such as canning, cooking, freezing, dehydration, or milling" (162). If you have a busy day ahead studying for exams, you might want to spend less time chopping, prepping, and cooking and more time studying. Enjoy a nutrition-packed, easy-to-prepare, healthy dinner that includes such processed foods as steamed frozen vegetables, a chicken breast that has been thawed from frozen and then grilled, and 5-minute whole-grain couscous with a glass of milk. Don't believe everything you hear about processed foods. They can provide diet versatility, good nutrition, and convenience, often at a great price.

---

oxidative stress, an imbalance between the production of free radicals and the body's antioxidant defenses (12). Selenium is in a wide variety of foods, including seafood, cereals, fruits, vegetables, grains, dairy, and meat. Selenium content of foods can vary tremendously based on the selenium content of soil. Selenium deficiency is rare, though possible in those with vegetarian diets consisting of food grown in low-selenium soil. Symptoms of deficiency include alteration in cardiac functioning and diseased cartilage. Selenium toxicity is also rare, though it can lead to GI disturbances, brittle hair, and nails (121).

DO YOU KNOW ?

Chelated means attached to another compound. Chelated minerals are often attached to an amino acid. In some, though not necessarily all, instances, chelation improves absorption.

Fluoride

Fluoride is essential for bone and teeth. This mineral helps protect against dental cavities and stimulates the formation of new bone. The primary source of fluoride in the U.S. diet is through fluoridated water. Other sources include beverages such as tea (fluoride builds up in tea leaves) and some marine fish (particularly if the bones are eaten). Inadequate fluoride intake can increase risk of developing cavities. Infants and children living in areas where water is not fluoridated will have difficulty meeting the AI for fluoride. Excess fluoride intake can lead to discolored or pitted teeth. Teeth might have opaque white spots or brown stains. Young children who swallow too much toothpaste or mouth rinse might get too much fluoride (121).

SUMMARY

Minerals have many essential functions throughout the body. For fitness and athletic performance, minerals are essential components of bone and help regulate fluid balance, metabolism, pH balance, oxygen transport, nerve impulses, and muscle contractions. Minerals are also important for muscle building and repair. Low intake of calcium can increase risk of developing a stress fracture. Low intake of other minerals and overt mineral deficiencies, particularly in the case of iron, can affect health and human performance and, in some instances, lead to performance decrements. Despite their importance, with the exception of iron, measuring mineral status can be challenging, as serum markers do not always reflect tissue stores. Although inadequate intake of minerals can affect health and performance, no evidence to date suggests that consuming more than the RDI will improve health or athletic performance. Also, excess intake of certain minerals, such as zinc, can be detrimental to health and affect the balance of other minerals in the body.

You can find several forms of minerals in dietary supplements. Many might interact with other supplements or medications, so anyone considering taking a supplement should talk to their pharmacist or RDN first.

FOR REVIEW

1. Name the minerals that many Americans do not consume in adequate quantities and discuss why.
2. How does iron deficiency affect fitness and athletic performance?
3. What are the stages of iron deficiency?
4. Which minerals are important for bone health?
5. List common sources of magnesium.
6. How does zinc deficiency affect physical performance?
7. Discuss the roles of sodium and potassium for blood pressure regulation.

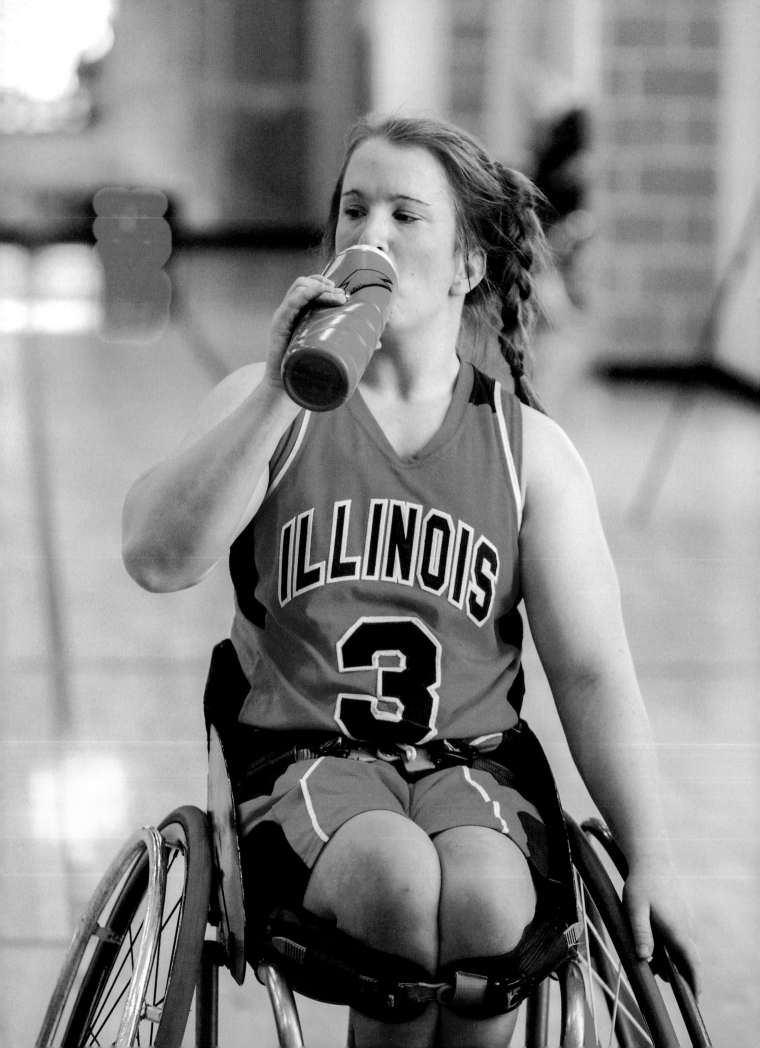

CHAPTER 8

Water and Electrolytes

> ## CHAPTER OBJECTIVES
>
> After completing this chapter, you will be able to do the following:
>
> - Discuss the role water plays in health and performance.
> - Discuss factors that affect an individual's fluid and electrolyte needs.
> - Describe the major electrolytes lost through sweat and their health and physical performance implications.
> - Calculate sweat rate.
> - Describe tools that measure hydration status, including their ease of use and efficacy.
> - Describe signs and symptoms of hyponatremia.
> - Discuss risk of developing hyponatremia.

Water and electrolytes are essential for optimal health and athletic performance. Water lost through sweat cools the body, but if it is not replaced, health and athletic performance can be compromised. When fluid losses that are not replaced reach significant levels, risk of heat illness increases. Electrolytes conduct electricity. They are essential for muscle and nerve functioning and thus critical for the heart and skeletal muscles. Several factors affect fluid and electrolyte losses, making measurements in different environments essential for developing an individualized hydration plan for each athlete.

WATER

Water is critical for **homeostasis** (a state of balance or equilibrium). Water is a solvent for biochemical reactions, helps maintain blood volume, and serves as a means to transport nutrients and remove waste products (96). Water helps regulate body temperature by absorbing heat from metabolic processes and dissipating heat through **insensible perspiration** (fluid that evaporates through pores in the skin via sweat glands before the body recognizes it as moisture on the skin) and sweating. As sweat evaporates, skin is cooled. See figure 8.1 for the functions of water in the body. Low water intake is associated with some diseases, though there isn't enough evidence to establish water intake recommendations for specific populations as a means to reduce risk of chronic disease (96).

For optimal functioning and health, total body water must be kept within a narrow range. Fluid intake, through food and beverages, increases total body water. Total body water loss stems from respiratory loss, insensible perspiration, urinary loss, gastrointestinal tract water loss (during metabolism), and fecal loss. See figure 8.2 for further information on daily fluid gains and losses. Excessive body water losses from fever, burns, diarrhea, vomiting, trauma, heat exposure, or exercise can impair health (96). **Hyperhydration** from excessive intake

of low- (or no) sodium fluids can increase body water and dilute blood sodium levels, potentially leading to **hyponatremia**—dangerously low blood sodium (96).

As the largest part of the human body, total body water comprises 45 to 75 percent of body weight in healthy individuals. Sixty-five percent of total body water is found in intracellular fluid, with the remaining 35 percent in extracellular fluid (41, 96). Differences in body water among individuals of the same body weight are typically due to variations in body composition. Muscles contain approximately 70 to 75 percent water, whereas fat tissue contains 10 to 40 percent (96). Athletes typically have high total body water compared to their sedentary counterparts because of higher levels of muscle mass and muscle glycogen (96).

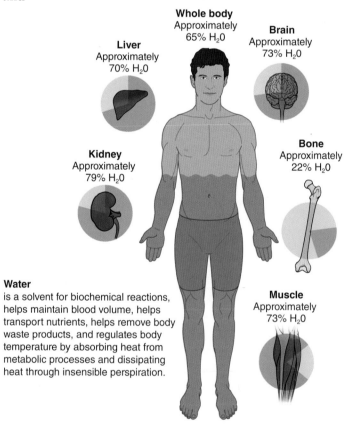

Whole body Approximately 65% H_2O

Brain Approximately 73% H_2O

Liver Approximately 70% H_2O

Bone Approximately 22% H_2O

Kidney Approximately 79% H_2O

Muscle Approximately 73% H_2O

Water is a solvent for biochemical reactions, helps maintain blood volume, helps transport nutrients, helps remove body waste products, and regulates body temperature by absorbing heat from metabolic processes and dissipating heat through insensible perspiration.

Figure 8.1 The body gains water through food and beverages, whereas typical water losses stem from respiration, insensible perspiration, metabolism, urine, and feces.

Data from U.S. Institute of Medicine 2005.

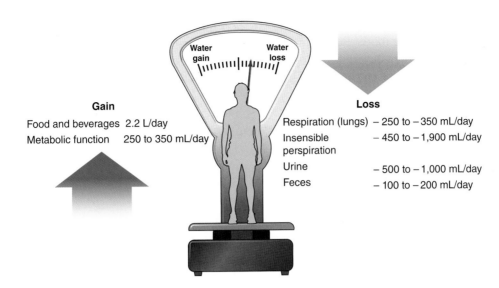

Gain

Food and beverages 2.2 L/day
Metabolic function 250 to 350 mL/day

Loss

Respiration (lungs) – 250 to – 350 mL/day
Insensible – 450 to – 1,900 mL/day
perspiration
Urine – 500 to – 1,000 mL/day
Feces – 100 to – 200 mL/day

Figure 8.2 How we gain and lose fluid.

Data from Riebl and Davy 2013; U.S. Institute of Medicine 2005.

Fluid Needs

Many factors affect fluid requirements, including age, body size, exercise, physical activity, environmental heat, altitude, health status, medications used, and use of particular dietary supplements. Individuals who exercise or live in hot climates might need more water. Additionally, fluid needs vary from day to day (68). The AI for total water intake each day from foods and beverages for healthy, sedentary adults in temperate climates is 2.7 liters (91.3 fl. oz., or 11.4 cups) for women and 3.7 liters (125.1 fl. oz., or 15.6 cups) for men. The AI for pregnant and lactating women is 3.0 liters (101.4 fl. oz., or 12.7 cups) and 3.8 liters (128.49 fl. oz., or 16.1 cups) per day, respectively. All sources of fluid contribute to meeting the AI. The majority of a person's water intake, approximately 81 percent, comes from water and beverages. The remaining amount, about 19

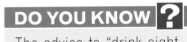

DO YOU KNOW

The advice to "drink eight 8-ounce glasses of water each day" isn't backed by science.

PUTTING IT INTO PERSPECTIVE

DO CAFFEINE-CONTAINING BEVERAGES CAUSE DEHYDRATION?

Caffeine is the most widely used legal central nervous system stimulant in the world. Caffeine temporarily increases alertness and memory, decreases fatigue, and improves mental functioning (83). Though caffeine has a small or mild diuretic effect, caffeine consumption does not lead to excessive fluid loss during exercise or at rest. Thus, caffeine is considered safe and shouldn't have a negative effect on fluid balance (104). That said, individual responses to caffeine vary tremendously because of genetics, so until you know your limits, be mindful of your caffeine intake. Caffeine can cause anxiety or jitteriness, especially in large doses (70, 103). Caffeine is completely absorbed within 45 minutes, though its effects peak anywhere between 15 and 120 minutes. The half-life of caffeine—that is, the amount of time it takes for caffeine concentration to decrease by half—is between 1.5 and 9.5 hours, a wide range that can be affected by several factors, including oral contraceptives, obesity, smoking, altitude, genetics, and intake of other stimulants (93). Although caffeine might help you study, it might do more harm than good if it interferes with sleep.

percent, comes from food (96). Table 8.1 shows the amount of water in select foods. Regardless of its source (food, water, other beverages), fluid is absorbed and treated the same in the body (96).

Body Fluid Regulation

Water and electrolytes are tightly regulated through coordination of neural pathways in the brain, kidneys, heart, sweat glands, and salivary glands. When dehydrated, sensors in the brain, kidneys, and heart detect increases in plasma osmolarity (the concentration of solutes, particularly sodium, in the blood), as well as decreases in fluid volume, and set off a cascade of actions to increase fluid volume (figure 8.3).

Dehydration, the process of losing body water, causes a drop in blood volume (61, 96). When blood

DO YOU KNOW ?

The kidneys are responsible for filtering blood and urine. On average, 1.5 liters of urine is produced each day. Urine contains water, electrolytes, and waste products (96). The kidneys function best when water is abundant (65).

volume is low, the kidneys set off a cascade of steps to maintain healthy blood pressure. Blood vessels are constricted, increasing blood pressure; sodium and water are reabsorbed from the water filtered by the kidneys so that less urine is produced; blood volume starts to rebound, leading to an increase in blood pressure; and a message is sent to the brain to stimulate thirst. However, during dehydration, thirst can lag behind fluid loss. Also during dehydration, stretch receptors in the aorta and carotid arteries detect a decrease in blood pressure and signal antidiuretic hormone (ADH) release to maintain blood volume and, in turn, sufficient blood pressure for adequate blood delivery to tissue (96).

When blood volume is higher than normal, stretch receptors in the heart send a signal inhibiting ADH release. The thirst mechanism is inhibited, and the kidneys excrete more water.

Dehydration and Hypohydration

Whereas dehydration refers to the process of losing body water, **hypohydration** is the uncompensated loss of body water (88). Depending on the amount of body fluid lost, hypohydration

Table 8.1 Water Content of Selected Foods

Food or drink	Oz. of water	% water based on weight
Water, 8 oz.	8	100
100% vegetable juice, 8 oz. (243 g)	7.7	94
Watermelon, 1 cup diced (152 g)	4.7	92
Milk, 1% fat, 8 oz. (236 g)	7.2	90
Soup, garden vegetable, 1 cup (246 g)	7.2	87
Yogurt, plain, Greek, nonfat, approximately 1 cup (200 g)	5.7	85
Grapes, American, 1/2 cup (46 g)	1.2	81
Egg, scrambled, 1 whole, large (61 g)	1.6	76
Chicken breast, sliced, 3 oz. (85 g)	2.1	74
Banana, medium (118 g)	2.6	64
Fish, salmon, Atlantic, cooked in dry heat, 3 oz. (85 g)	1.7	60
Bread, wheat, 1 slice (29 g)	0.3	34
Peanuts, raw, 1/4 cup (36.5 g)	0.1	7

Percentage water calculated based on the amount of water in the food (in gram weight) as compared to the total weight of the food.
Based on U.S. Department of Agriculture 2013.

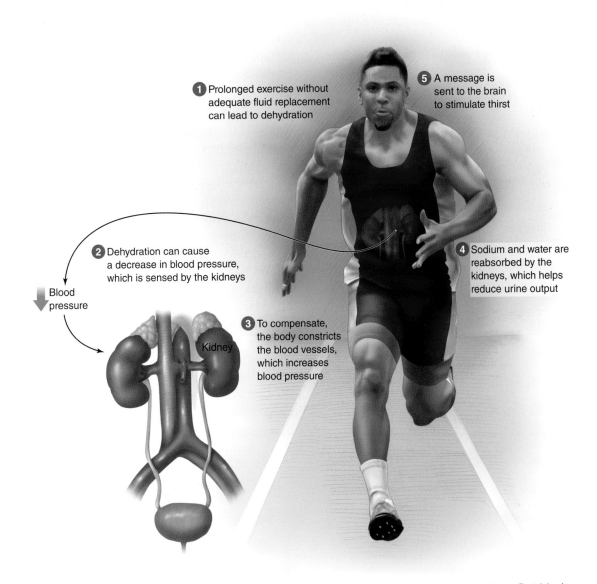

1. Prolonged exercise without adequate fluid replacement can lead to dehydration

5. A message is sent to the brain to stimulate thirst

2. Dehydration can cause a decrease in blood pressure, which is sensed by the kidneys

Blood pressure

Kidney

3. To compensate, the body constricts the blood vessels, which increases blood pressure

4. Sodium and water are reabsorbed by the kidneys, which helps reduce urine output

Figure 8.3 The human body has several feedback mechanisms in place to regulate fluid balance.
Based on Popkin 2010; U.S. Institute of Medicine 2005.

can be mild, moderate, or severe. Symptoms of mild to moderate hypohydration include thirst, dry mouth, low urine production, dry and cool skin, headache, muscle cramps, and dark urine (not to be confused with bright yellow or orange urine from B vitamins, carotene, or certain medications). Signs and symptoms of severe hypohydration include

- increased core body temperature,
- decreased blood pressure (hypotension),
- decreased sweat rate,
- rapid breathing,
- fast heartbeat,
- dizziness or lightheadedness,
- irritability,
- confusion,
- lack of urination,
- sunken eyes,
- shock,
- unconsciousness,
- delirium,

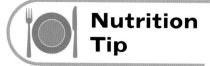

> dry, wrinkled skin that doesn't "bounce back" quickly when pitched,

> reduced stroke volume and cardiac output,

> reduced blood flow to muscles,

> exacerbated symptomatic exertional **rhabdomyolysis** (serious muscle injury), and

> increased risk of heat stroke and death (22, 36, 74, 96).

During exercise, hypohydration occurs when fluid intake doesn't match water lost through sweat (71). Risk for hypohydration is greater in hot, humid environments and at altitude (20, 50, 55). Clothing, equipment, heat acclimatization, exercise intensity, exercise duration, body size, and individual variations in sweat rates all affect risk of hypohydration (71). With repeated exposures to hot environments, the body adapts to heat stress, and cardiac output and stroke volume returns to normal, sodium loss is conserved, and the risk for heat-related illness is reduced.

DO YOU KNOW ?

Dehydration might reach a 2 to 3 percent decrease in body weight before you feel thirsty.

Sickle cell trait, cystic fibrosis, diabetes medications, diuretics, and laxatives increase risk of dehydration. Children and the elderly also have an increased risk of dehydration (10, 90).

Several studies suggest children are at greater risk than adults for dehydration and heat illness. Children have more body surface area relative to their body weight, leading to greater heat gain from the environment. They have a lower sweat rate, and thus a decreased ability to dissipate heat through sweat (though this conserves body water) and higher skin temperature. Children also take longer to acclimatize to heat (24, 27, 71, 91). Some studies suggest that children rehydrate as well as, if not better than, adults (11, 16, 69, 72), whereas other studies show children, like adults, do not drink enough to adequately replace fluid losses in warm temperatures, even when they have sufficient access to fluids (11, 37, 101). However, sweat sodium concentration is lower in children than in adults, a factor that may help children retain fluid (51). Signs and symptoms of heat illness are presented in figure 8.4.

Older adults do not have a sensitive thirst mechanism, so they generally drink less fluid than younger adults. In addition, the kidneys do not conserve water as well with age. Older individuals on certain medications might have increased fluid requirements or increased fluid losses. Some elderly people have limited access to food and fluids because of impaired motor skills, injuries, diseases, or surgeries that limit mobility. All these factors put the elderly at greater risk for heat stress, dehydration, and hypohydration.

Hyperhydration

Hyperhydration, sometimes referred to as overhydration or water intoxication, is an excess of total body water resulting from excessive intake of low- or no-sodium fluids, such as water (96). Hyperhydration is rare in healthy individuals. Those with heart, kidney, or liver disease, as well as individuals who have damage to the thirst mechanism, have an increased risk of hyperhydration because of the kidneys' reduced ability to excrete excess water. Athletes, particularly those competing in prolonged endurance events, and consuming only water or low-sodium beverages, might also be at risk for hyperhydration (100).

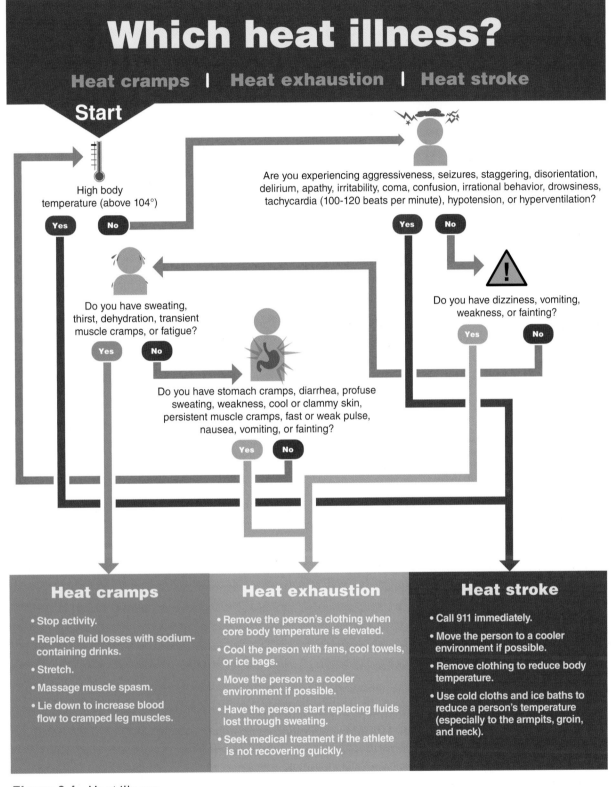

Figure 8.4 Heat illness.

Based on Binkley 2002.

WHY DOES ALCOHOL GIVE YOU A HANGOVER?

We all know that drinking too much alcohol can lead to a hangover. But why? And how can we prevent it? Hangover symptoms include fatigue, headache, poor sleep, thirst, nausea or vomiting, dizziness, and sensitivity to light, among others. Unfortunately, the mechanisms that lead to a hangover are not entirely clear. Although alcohol causes hangovers, there appears to be no way to prevent them other than the obvious—not drinking or drinking less. However, among the factors that can reduce the severity of a hangover, two are in our control: getting enough sleep and not smoking (64).

In addition to hangovers, an acute bout of heavy alcohol consumption can harm the body in other ways. Alcohol decreases the amount of ADH produced, leading to a larger volume of urine and increased dehydration (87). Alcohol shrinks and disrupts brain tissue, throwing neurotransmitters off course, so you feel sleepy and function in slow motion—both physically and verbally. A single night of heavy drinking can also compromise your immune system, decreasing the ability of white blood cells to handle harmful bacteria (57).

To prevent or reduce some of the negative side effects of overdrinking, try these strategies for drinking less. Know how much alcohol is in your drink (figure 8.5), and alter your pace accordingly. Drink a glass of water after each alcoholic drink. Eat something—eating slows down the absorption of alcohol so you have more time to metabolize what you are drinking. Also, for academic performance, don't drink, or at least limit drinking, the night before tests, exams, or days of intense studying.

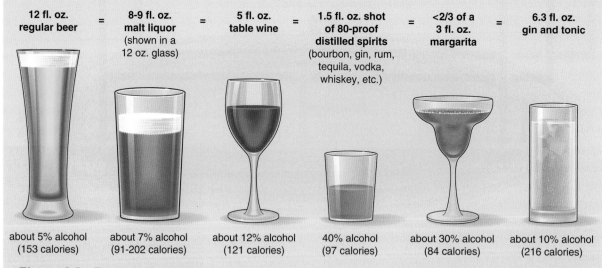

| 12 fl. oz. regular beer | = | 8-9 fl. oz. malt liquor (shown in a 12 oz. glass) | = | 5 fl. oz. table wine | = | 1.5 fl. oz. shot of 80-proof distilled spirits (bourbon, gin, rum, tequila, vodka, whiskey, etc.) | = | <2/3 of a 3 fl. oz. margarita | = | 6.3 fl. oz. gin and tonic |

| about 5% alcohol (153 calories) | about 7% alcohol (91-202 calories) | about 12% alcohol (121 calories) | 40% alcohol (97 calories) | about 30% alcohol (84 calories) | about 10% alcohol (216 calories) |

Figure 8.5 Percent alcohol by volume in alcoholic beverages. To find out the amount of alcohol in a drink, multiply the percent alcohol by the volume of the drink. Each one of the drinks pictured above contains 0.6 oz. of alcohol. Interactive calculators to help you determine both the caloric content and amount of alcohol in various drinks are available online.

Adapted from National Institute on Alcohol Abuse and Alcoholism.

WILL SUPPLEMENTS MAKE ME DEHYDRATED?

Certain ingredients commonly found in detox products, cleanses, and weight-loss supplements will increase water lost through urine. Some of these products include uva ursi, dandelion (Taraxacum officinale), burdock root, horsetail, and hawthorn. Though many people believe creatine increases dehydration, no research supports this (23, 38).

REFLECTION TIME

Signs and Symptoms of Hyperhydration (28, 59)

> Confusion

> Inattentiveness

> Blurred vision

> Muscle cramps or twitching

> Poor coordination

> Nausea or vomiting

> Rapid breathing

> Acute weight gain

> Weakness

> Paralysis

Hyperhydration can result in cellular edema and hyponatremia, which is a dangerously low blood sodium level, defined by plasma sodium below 135 mmol/L (96). When blood sodium levels fall below 125 mmol/L, an individual might experience intracellular swelling, headaches, nausea, vomiting, muscle cramps, swollen hands and feet, restlessness, and disorientation. When blood sodium drops below 120 mmol/L, risk of developing cerebral edema, seizures, coma, brainstem herniation, respiratory arrest, and death increases (3, 5, 74, 97). Hyponatremia can occur during an event or up to 24 hours after. In athletes, hyponatremia might result from high water intake during prolonged endurance or ultraendurance events, particularly for athletes with slower race times (97).

Signs and Symptoms of Hyponatremia

> Core body temperature less than 40 °C (104 °F)

> Nausea

> Vomiting

> Swelling of the hands and feet

> Low blood sodium level

> Progressive headache

> Confusion

> Lethargy

> Altered state of consciousness

> Apathy

> Pulmonary edema

> Cerebral edema

> Seizures

> Rhabdomyolysis (skeletal muscle injury)

> Coma

Based on Coris 2004; Sawka et al. 2007; U.S. Institute of Medicine 2005.

ELECTROLYTES

Electrolytes are essential for muscle contraction and nerve conduction, so an electrolyte imbalance could certainly impair athletic performance (22, 74). **Electrolytes** lost in sweat include sodium, chloride, potassium, calcium, and magnesium (figure 8.6) (74).

Because of the high amount lost through sweat, sodium losses are the greatest concern, ranging from 230 to greater than 2,277 mg/L (10 to 99 mEq/L), followed by chloride, which is lost along with sodium (22, 74, 96). Sodium influences fluid regulation by helping the body retain more of the fluid consumed (less fluid consumed is lost through urine) (49). With greater sodium losses, risk of muscle cramping increases (14, 84). Athletes who exercise intensely or for several hours and hydrate excessively with only water or a

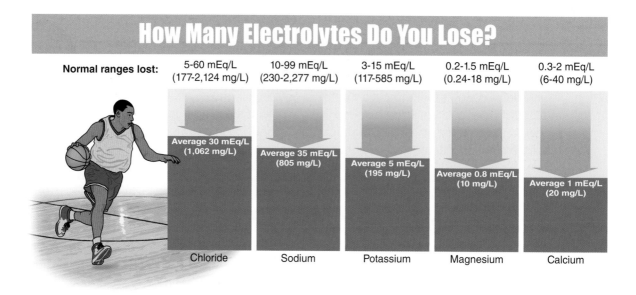

Figure 8.6 Average amounts of electrolytes lost through sweat.

Data from Coris 2004; American College of Sports 2007; Institute of Medicine 2005.

no- or low-sodium beverage can dilute their blood sodium levels, increasing risk of cramping and possibly developing hyponatremia (3, 5, 74). To avoid hyponatremia, fluid intake shouldn't exceed sweat losses, and athletes should consume sodium via food or sports drinks (62, 74).

Hypernatremia, elevated blood sodium, is defined as a blood sodium concentration greater than 145 mmol/L. Hypernatremia is typically associated with dehydration and can be extremely dangerous, even causing death (2, 21).

Some sports drinks provide very small amounts of potassium, while others provide no potassium (via pills). In a healthy individual, blood potassium is well regulated. High doses of supplemental potassium can be very dangerous, possibly fatal (96).

Calcium is lost in sweat in very small quantities. When blood calcium levels drop, the body can pull calcium from bone tissue to maintain blood calcium within a tight range. Though magnesium is lost in sweat and urine during exercise,

it is redistributed in the body to accommodate metabolic needs (58). In addition, the average amount of magnesium lost through sweat, approximately 10 mg/L, is a tiny fraction of a person's magnesium needs each day (240–420 mg/day for those 9 years old and up, depending on life stage) (74, 95).

WATER, ELECTROLYTES, AND EXERCISE PERFORMANCE

During exercise, muscular contractions produce heat, which must be dissipated through sweat to help cool skin and body temperature. When fluids are consumed to maintain normal body water (**euhydration**), sweating remains an effective compensation for increased core temperatures. However, as discussed earlier, thirst lags behind fluid needs. It might take a 2 to 3 percent loss in body mass from fluid before thirst kicks in (37). Thus thirst might not be a sufficient stimulus to prevent significant dehydration during exercise, particularly in hot, humid conditions (figure 8.7) (71). If sweat losses are not replaced with fluid, hypohydration will lead to a decrease in sweat rate and evaporative heat loss, an increase in core body temperature, a drop in blood volume, a decrease in blood pressure, and cardiovascular strain, as

Heat index
As humidity increases, air can feel hotter than it actually is.
This chart shows how hot it feels as humidity rises.

Relative humidity (%)	70	75	80	85	90	95	100	105	110	115	120
100	72	80	91	108	132						
90	71	79	88	102	122						
80	71	78	86	97	113	136					
70	70	77	85	93	106	124	144				
60	70	76	82	90	100	114	132	149			
50	69	75	81	88	96	107	120	135	150		
40	68	74	79	86	93	101	110	123	137	151	
30	67	73	78	84	90	96	104	113	123	135	148
20	66	72	77	82	87	93	99	105	112	120	130
10	65	70	75	80	85	90	95	100	105	111	116
0	64	69	73	78	83	87	91	95	99	103	107

Caution zone / Danger zone

Air temperature (°F)

Figure 8.7 The Heat Index is a measure of how hot it really feels outside when humidity is taken into account along with temperature.

Reprinted, by permission, from C.B. Corbin, G.C. Le Masurier, and K.E. McConnell, 2014, *Fitness for life*, 6th ed. (Champaign, IL: Human Kinetics), 76.

well as altered metabolic and central nervous system functioning (73, 88). Factors increasing dehydration risk include multiple layers of clothing, protective equipment (pads, helmets), heat, humidity, multiple practices per day, intentional dehydration, and other unsafe weight-loss practices, including diuretics, using the sauna, manipulating water and sodium balance to "make weight," excessive spitting, self-induced vomiting, laxative abuse, and inappropriate use of thermogenic aids (13, 31, 34-36, 86, 99).

Hypohydration of less than 1 percent of pre-training body weight is not likely to have a negative effect on performance, unless the athlete begins training with a significant fluid deficit (17). Sweat losses reaching 1 to 3 percent body weight loss can increase core body temperature and significantly affect athletic performance by increasing fatigue; decreasing motivation; impairing attention, psychomotor, and immediate memory skills; decreasing sprint performance; increasing rate of perceived exertion; and impairing neuromuscular control, accuracy, power, strength, and muscular endurance (1, 12, 20, 26, 39, 42, 43, 53, 75, 82).

In endurance-trained cyclists, dehydration of 4 percent of body weight in the heat decreased blood flow to muscles (36). Cardiac output, sweat

production, and blood flow to skin and muscle decrease when sweat fluid losses rise to 6 to 10 percent of body weight, while risk for heat illness increases (22, 25, 74, 88).

Substantial sweat sodium losses can increase an athlete's risk of muscle cramping (14), poor performance, and, when combined with over-hydration, hyponatremia (3, 5, 74, 97). A study in NCAA Division I football players found sweat sodium losses were two times higher in those with a history of heat cramps compared to age-, weight-, race-, and position-matched players who had never cramped (84).

Many athletes and recreational exercisers start training in a hypohydrated state, making it difficult to achieve euhydration during training (17, 19, 62, 85, 86, 98). In research studies, fluid losses ranged from 0.3 to over 4.6 L/h in athletes (62, 74). A study in NCAA Division I athletes found 66 percent started practice in a hypohydrated state and 13 percent in a significantly hypohydrated state as measured by urine specific gravity (USG). USG is a tool used to assess hydration status by measuring the concentration of particles in urine (81). Additional research studies found that many teenage male and female tennis players, female Canadian junior elite soccer athletes, and more than 50 percent of the athletes on Canada's junior men's hockey team began practice in a hypohydrated state (17, 34, 63). In addition, among those who started in a hypohydrated state did not drink enough during practice to avoid a fluid deficit (34, 63).

Pro indoor and outdoor athletes follow similar patterns as younger athletes—many start in a hypohydrated state. A study examining 29 NBA players during indoor summer league competition found 52 percent started the game in a hypohydrated state while 5 players lost more than 2 percent body mass (measured prior to the game) during the game (62). Figure 8.8 illustrates how performance suffers as dehydration increases.

Because of larger body size, equipment, and exercising outdoors in the heat, American football players, particularly linemen, have an increased risk of becoming dehydrated (22). A study in NFL players found that smaller players lost significantly less fluid through sweat during practice than larger players (figure 8.9).

In addition to the importance of hydrating before and during exercise, rehydrating after exercise takes time. In one small study, subjects had their food and fluid intake restricted and exercised in moderate heat to achieve hypohydration by 0 percent, 3 percent, 5 percent, and 7 percent of their body weight on 4 separate trials

PUTTING IT INTO PERSPECTIVE

CAN I USE DIURETICS, DETOXES, OR CLEANSES TO LOSE WEIGHT QUICKLY?

Diuretics increase urine production, so you lose water weight, temporarily. As soon as you rehydrate, you gain the weight back. Many detoxes and cleanses claim to remove toxins from your body, causing you to lose weight. Typical approaches include one or more of the following:

> Calorie restriction
> Consuming juice only or a liquid diet for several days
> Restricting food choices
> Laxatives, enemas, or colonics
> Various dietary supplements

No concrete evidence suggests that typical detoxes and cleanses remove toxins or improve health. If the detox or cleanse diet or program is lower in calories, compared to what you typically consume, you might lose weight. According to the FDA and the Federal Trade Commission, some detox or cleansing products or programs can be harmful. Both groups have taken action against several companies for selling illegal and potentially harmful ingredients, making false claims suggesting their products could treat serious diseases, or unapproved uses of medical devices for colon cleanses. Other issues identified include the following:

> Unpasteurized juices might contain harmful bacteria (pasteurization kills bacteria) that could make people sick, particularly those with weakened immune systems, the elderly, and children.
> Because of high levels of oxalate, high intake of juice could be harmful for those with kidney disease.
> Laxatives can lead to diarrhea, dehydration, and electrolyte imbalances.
> Anyone with diabetes could experience serious side effects resulting from an imbalance between prescribed medication and diet, causing low blood sugar.
> Fasting and very low-calorie diets could lead to headaches, fainting, weakness, dehydration, and other issues (56).

In chapter 13 we will look at safe and effective strategies for losing weight.

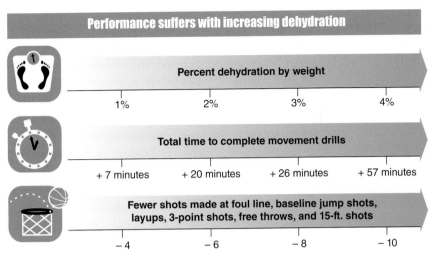

Figure 8.8 Skill decreases in basketball with progressive dehydration.

Data from Baker 2007.

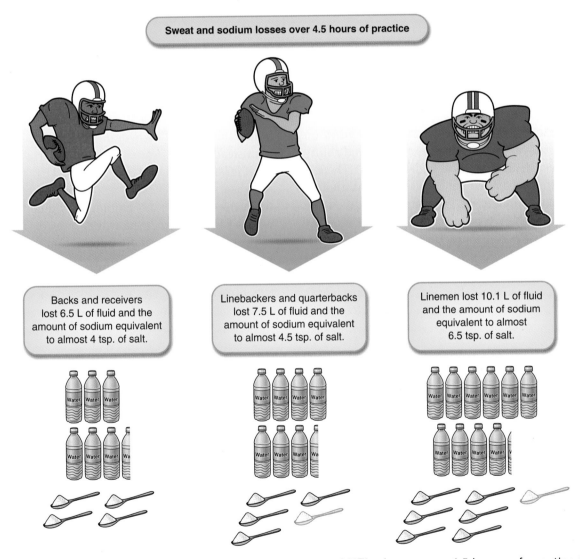

Figure 8.9 Sodium lost through sweat in three groups of NFL players over 4.5 hours of practice in the heat.

(each subject experienced each level of dehydration). For a period of 1 hour afterward, they were allowed to drink as much as they wanted. All subjects didn't consume enough fluid during this time to rehydrate back to baseline body weight, suggesting adequate rehydration after hypohydration takes time, even when subjects have access to plenty of fluid (30).

Athletes should drink enough fluid to prevent water weight losses exceeding 2 percent of body weight, while also restoring electrolytes lost through sweat to prevent adverse effects on health and athletic performance. In addition, it is important to restore fluid intake after exercise and prior to the next training session (74). Given the wide range of fluid and electrolyte losses through sweat, all athletes should have their own individualized hydration plan. The first step to developing an individualized hydration plan is an assessment of daily hydration status, as well as fluid and electrolyte losses during exercise.

HYDRATION ASSESSMENT

There are several ways to measure hydration status, all varying in cost, ease of use, and ability to detect small changes in hydration (61). There is no perfect measurement for all situations, though plasma osmolality is generally considered the most effective overall (6, 96). Plasma osmolality measures the concentration of solutes in plasma. When an athlete sweats, plasma volume and extracellular water decrease with fluid losses, while plasma osmolality increases (more fluid is lost than solutes). Plasma osmolality alters with acute changes in hydration status (96). In sports

settings, commonly used measures of hydration status include urine osmolality (UOsmol), USG, changes in body weight, sweat patches, and bioelectrical impedance analysis (6). Urine markers, including UOsmol and USG, and serum osmolality measure the concentration of particles in urine and serum, respectively. Both are sensitive (effective) indicators of hydration status (96). As discussed earlier, USG measures the concentration of particles in urine and provides an assessment of hydration status and kidney function (81). USG is easy to use, inexpensive, and practical. USG and UOsmol should be measured first thing in the morning; values may be misleading during acute periods of dehydration (as can happen when athletes sweat profusely during exercise) or if urine is assessed after rehydration (61, 74). Both devices show delayed dehydration-related changes (61). If dehydrated athletes consume a large volume of hypotonic fluid, they will produce a large volume of urine prior to becoming adequately rehydrated (euhydration). During this period of rehydration, USG and UOsmol are misleading. Both values will indicate athletes have achieved euhydration when in fact they are still dehydrated (74, 80). UOsmol is misleading and a poor indicator of hydration for at least 6 hours after exercise (46). USG values increase with increasing water deficit, though this varies considerably among individuals. USG values cannot predict the extent of water deficit (96). See table 8.2 for more information on measuring hydration with USG.

A wide range of values is normal for urine UOsmol—50 to 1,200 mOsmol/L (89). Given this range, increasing urine UOsmol can be used to determine increasing levels of dehydration,

PUTTING IT INTO PERSPECTIVE

DO RECREATIONAL ATHLETES NEED SALT?

All athletes, no matter their level of competition, should know the basics of dehydration, hyponatremia, and sodium replenishment. In fact, hyponatremia occurs more often in recreational athletes than competitive athletes. Staying well hydrated, yet not overhydrated, and replacing electrolytes will not only help you perform your best, but also help ensure that you make the most of your workout. In addition, maintaining adequate hydration could help you perform your best each day, not just while exercising or competing, but in school and during other extracurricular activities that require cognitive thinking skills.

Table 8.2 Measuring Hydration With USG

USG value	Status	% Body weight change
1.001–1.012	This may be indicative of overhydration.	Weighing more posttraining as compared to pretraining indicates overhydration.
≤1.020	Euhydration	–1 to –3%
1.020–1.030	Hypohydration	3–5% of body mass
>1.030	Severe hypohydration	>5% body mass

Some studies consider 1.010 to 1.020 as minimal dehydration and less than 1.010 as euhydration. Others consider 1.001 to 1.010 as indicative of possible overhydration.

Both USG and percent body weight change (from a state of euhydration) can be used to assess hydration status, though USG values do not correspond to or predict percent changes in body weight (for example, a USG of 1.020 does not correspond to a 3-5% change in weight).

Data from Armstrong 1994; Popowski 2001.

though it is not considered a good indicator of hydration status (8, 78, 96).

Measuring changes in weight can help identify athletes who are dehydrated. Acute changes in body weight often reflect fluid fluctuations in athletes who are in a state of caloric balance—that is, consuming enough calories each day to maintain their weight. Athletes can estimate day-to-day hydration changes by weighing in the nude or in minimal clothing each morning after using the bathroom and prior to eating or drinking. See figure 8.10 for accurately estimating sweat losses through changes in body weight. Athletes can estimate sweat-related fluid losses, and therefore sweat rate, by weighing pre- and postworkout (60, 74). Though body weight changes can be used to estimate acute changes in hydration status, over a longer period of time, food intake, bowel movements, and alterations in body composition will confound the use of weight as an indicator of changes in hydration status (60).

Athletes are sometimes advised to check their urine color to assess their hydration status; darker urine is more concentrated with solutes and a sign of dehydration or hypohydration, while pale yellow urine is less concentrated and considered a sign of euhydration. However, urine color assessment is problematic because it is subjective, imprecise, and open to interpretation (74, 96). Several food ingredients, nutrients, and medications can influence the color of urine (33, 81, 92). Also, urine color is not an accurate measure for at least 6 hours postexercise (46).

Urine will be pale in color during the immediate rehydration period after dehydration, even though the athlete is still dehydrated (74). See table 8.3 for more information on factors influencing urine color.

Sweat patches are placed on an athlete's forearm or another part of the body to collect fluid and electrolyte losses. These patches are easy to use and provide valuable information for developing an individualized hydration and electrolyte (sodium chloride) plan (29). Bioelectrical impedance analysis (BIA) is an easy, quick method of assessing hydration status. BIA uses a frequency passed through the skin. There is greater resistance to the current when water and electrolyte content in tissues is higher (48). In euhydrated and chronically hyperhydrated or hypohydrated subjects, BIA provides a good estimate of total body water and hydration status (60, 76). However, fluid shifts between intracellular and extracellular water during exercise, increased blood flow to working muscles and skin, and sweating can confound BIA measures in athletes. BIA is also independently influenced by water and

DO YOU KNOW

USG testing is often part of routine testing of urine samples. The next time you provide a urine sample at your physician's office, check the report for your USG value. USG is also measured during drug testing to determine if athletes have attempted to manipulate the test by overhydrating in an attempt to dilute their urine.

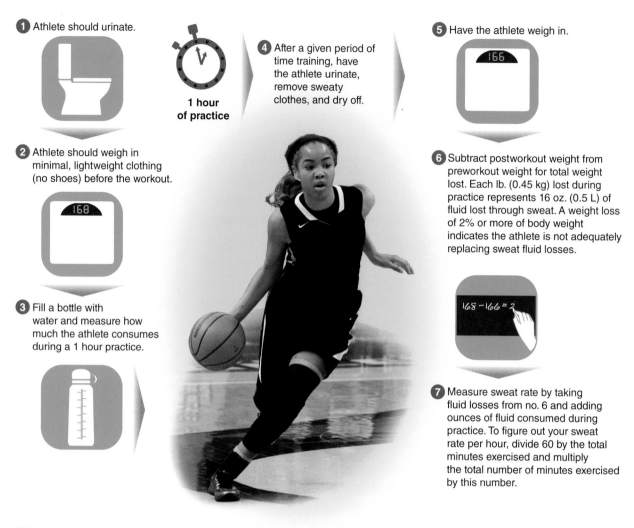

1. Athlete should urinate.

1 hour of practice

4. After a given period of time training, have the athlete urinate, remove sweaty clothes, and dry off.

5. Have the athlete weigh in.

166

2. Athlete should weigh in minimal, lightweight clothing (no shoes) before the workout.

168

6. Subtract postworkout weight from preworkout weight for total weight lost. Each lb. (0.45 kg) lost during practice represents 16 oz. (0.5 L) of fluid lost through sweat. A weight loss of 2% or more of body weight indicates the athlete is not adequately replacing sweat fluid losses.

3. Fill a bottle with water and measure how much the athlete consumes during a 1 hour practice.

168 - 166 = 2

7. Measure sweat rate by taking fluid losses from no. 6 and adding ounces of fluid consumed during practice. To figure out your sweat rate per hour, divide 60 by the total minutes exercised and multiply the total number of minutes exercised by this number.

Figure 8.10 Estimating sweat losses through weight changes.

electrolyte content, as well as changes in electrolyte content in intracellular fluid and extracellular fluid. So, for instance, when plasma (extracellular fluid) sodium concentration increases, resistance decreases, which can also confound its use for estimating hydration status (60). For these reasons, BIA is not an accurate method for assessing hydration status in athletes because they have frequent shifts in hydration status (60, 96). Table 8.4 presents methods for measuring hydration status.

HYDRATION RECOMMENDATIONS FOR EXERCISE

Given the wide variety of conditions that affect sweat fluid losses—including climate, training or athletic event, clothing, equipment, acclimation, and individual differences in sweat rates and electrolyte losses—it is impossible to develop general fluid guidelines sufficient for all individuals in all situations. However, the following research-based recommendations can be adjusted based on a thorough assessment of an individual's fluid and electrolyte losses in different environmental conditions.

Before Exercise

Many athletes and active individuals start training or exercise in a hypohydrated state, making it difficult to achieve euhydration during training (17, 19, 62, 86, 98). Thus the preexercise goal is to achieve euhydration by prehydrating, when necessary, several hours before exercise to allow

Table 8.3 Common Causes of Changes in Urine Color

Color or appearance	Medical reasons	Potential food and drug causes
Pale yellow or clear	Hyperhydration Diabetes insipidus	Diuretics Alcohol consumption Mannitol
Cloudy	UTI (urine might also smell bad) Phosphaturia (excess phosphorus in urine) Chyluria (presence of a milky white lymphatic fluid) Renal disease Hyperoxaluria (recurrent kidney and bladder stones)	Diet high in purine-rich foods such as anchovies, asparagus, liver, mushrooms, herring, gravy, sweetbreads, game meats, dried beans and peas, brains, beef kidneys, mackerel, muscles, sardines, or scallops
Milky	Bacteria (UTI) Substances in urine: • Crystals • Lipids • White or red blood cells • Mucus • Chyluria (a tropical disease more common in poverty-stricken populations)	No known food or drug causes
Brown	Bile pigments Myoglobin (a protein that carries oxygen in heart and skeletal muscles) Medications to treat Parkinson's disease or UTI Antimalarial drugs Antibiotics (flagyl)	Fava beans
Dark brown	Excess bilirubin in the urine leading to liver disorder such as acute viral hepatitis or cirrhosis Medications to treat Parkinson's disease or high blood pressure (methyldopa)	Cascara (a plant used as a laxative) Senna (a laxative) Medicine used to treat bacterial infections (metronidazole therapy) Muscle injury causing myoglobin (a protein found muscle) in urine; there are many types of muscle injury, including rhabdomyolysis (rapid breakdown of muscle tissue leading to leakage of muscle contents into blood)
Brownish black	Bile pigments Melanin Methemoglobin	Cascara, certain drugs for Parkinson's disease, certain antihypertensive medications, senna
Green or blue	Bilirubin Medications to treat depression, ulcers, allergies (Phenergan) Diuretics (triamterene) UTI	Food coloring (indigo carmine) Methylene blue (used to treat UTI) Diuretics (triamterene) Antidepressants (amitriptyline) Anti-inflammatory drugs (indomethacin)
Purple	Malabsorption and bacterial overgrowth syndromes	No known food or drug causes Purple tubing and bags in hospitals can discolor urine in long-term catheterized patients.
Orange or dark yellow	Hypohydration (especially if dark scanty urine is produced) Bile pigments Laxatives Medications such as phenazopyridine, rifampin, warfarin, pyridium, phenothiazines	Antibiotics used to treat bacterial infections (rifampicin) Carrots Cascara
Pink, red, or light brown	Hemolytic anemia Injury to the kidneys Porphyria Injury to the urinary tract or urinary tract disorders that lead to bleeding Blood in urine Medications such as phenolphthalein, rifampin (Rifadin)	Beets, blackberries, rhubarb Some food colorings Senna, anthraquinone, and phenolphthalein-containing laxatives, doxorubicin, rifampin, and phenothiazine
Bright yellow	No known medical reasons	Carrots, B vitamins

UTI = urinary tract infection

Based on Gerber and Brendler 2011; Raymond and Yarger 1988; Sharma and Hemal 2009; Simerville, Maxted, and Pahira 2005; U.S. Department of Agriculture 2013.

time for fluid absorption and urine production. If using USG, the measurement should read below 1.020 before exercise (74).

Four hours before exercise athletes should slowly drink enough fluid to urinate approximately 5 to 7 mL/kg body weight (0.076–0.108 oz./lb.) to allow for sufficient time to void excess fluid (74). The addition of sodium, through a sports drink or table salt, to a preworkout meal or snack will help the athlete retain more of the fluid consumed (54).

During Exercise

The average person loses approximately 0.3 liters per hour through insensible perspiration and sweating when sedentary (96). Sweat fluid losses during training range from 0.3 to over 4.6 liters per hour, while sodium losses range from 230 to 2,277 mg or more per liter of sweat. Given this variation, it is ideal to use an individualized hydration plan that helps limit fluid losses of greater than 2 percent, replenishes electrolyte losses, and

Table 8.4   Measuring Hydration Status

Measure	Practicality	Advantages	Measures acute or chronic hydration status or both	Normal values	Higher than normal values may suggest	Lower than normal values may suggest
Total body water (based on dilution—a lab method)	Low	Accurate, reliable	Both	<2%	Overhydration Disease state	Dehydration Disease state
Plasma osmolality	Medium	Accurate, reliable	Both	275–295 mOsm/kg	Dehydration Diabetes High blood sugar level High level of nitrogen waste products in the blood Hypernatremia Stroke or head trauma resulting in decreased ADH secretion	Hypothyroidism Hyponatremia Overhydration Adrenal gland not working properly ADH oversecretion Conditions related to lung cancer
Urine-specific gravity	High	Easy to use	Chronic	<1.020	Glycosuria Alterations in ADH Dehydration	Overhydration Diuretic use, diabetes, adrenal insufficiency, aldosteronism, impaired renal function
Urine osmolality	High	Variable—can be used to measure level of dehydration yet it isn't a good measure of hydration status	Chronic	50 to 1,200 mOsmol/L	Heart failure Dehydration Renal artery stenosis Shock Sugar in the urine Poor ADH secretion	Overhydration Damage to the kidneys Kidney failure Kidney infection
Body weight	High	Easy, quick	Both*	<1–2%	Overhydration	Hypohydration

*Chronic changes (over a few days) can be estimated in an athlete in a state of caloric balance.

Based on Kavouras 2002; Sawka et al. 2007; Tilkian, Boudreau, and Tilkian 1995.

avoids overhydration (62, 74). Most athletes can maintain adequate hydration by consuming 0.4 to 0.8 liters per hour (13–27 oz./h) of fluid. Athletes with high sweat rates (>1.2 L/h) or salty sweat or those exercising for more than 2 hours are more likely to have considerable sodium losses and should choose a beverage that contains sodium during exercise. A carbohydrate concentration of 6 to 8 percent might be ideal, as sports drinks containing more than 8 percent carbohydrate delay gastric emptying (i.e., how quickly the drink is emptied from the stomach), which could result in an upset stomach (52, 74). Cool, but not cold, beverages are recommended: 10 to 15 °C (50–59 °F) (19).

A drink containing multiple types of carbohydrate, such as glucose and fructose, or maltodextrin combined with fructose, can increase the speed of gastric emptying and thus decrease the risk of upset stomach (102). During prolonged periods of training, athletes can consume 30 to 60 grams of carbohydrate per hour to help sustain energy. Based on limited research, mainly conducted during long bouts of cycling, aerobic endurance athletes could increase total carbohydrate intake to 90 grams per hour if their sports drink contains multiple types of carbohydrates (40).

Children and Adolescents

A sports drink with flavor and sodium may increase drinking at one's pleasure. Children should be offered a choice of fluids so they can decide which one they prefer (71).

The American Academy of Pediatrics suggests enforcing periodic drinking in children to ensure adequate fluid intake during exercise. Drinks should contain a sodium chloride concentration of 15 to 20 mmol/L (1 g per 2 pints), which has been shown to increase voluntary hydration by 90 percent when compared to unflavored water (4, 15, 101). According to the Academy's guidelines:

> children weighing 40 kg (88 lb.) should drink 5 ounces (148 ml) of cold water or a flavored salted beverage every 20 minutes during practice, and

> adolescents weighing 60 kg (132 lb.) should drink 9 ounces (256 ml) every 20 minutes, even if they do not feel thirsty.

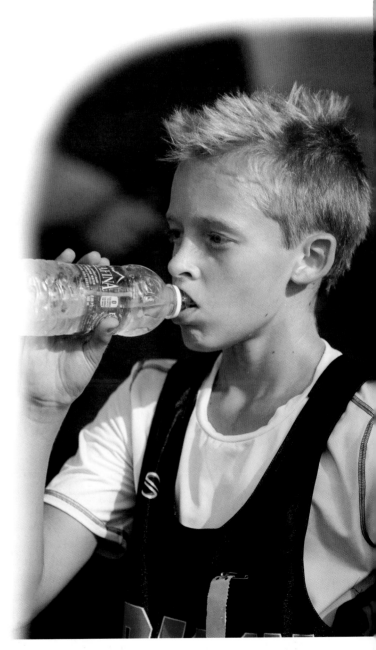

A child participating in any sport should have plenty of breaks to ensure proper hydration.

FACTORS THAT CONTRIBUTE TO GREATER FLUID CONSUMED

Given the importance of hydration and the potential adverse health effects that can result from dehydration, hypohydration, and heat illness, coaches and parents should create an environment that encourages fluid consumption. They can do this by providing access to fluids (both water and flavored sports drinks), scheduling breaks during training, and educating athletes and parents about the importance of hydration, while also providing instructions for maintaining optimal hydration (45).

Adults

Athletes should follow an individualized hydration plan. In general, a sports drinks should contain 20 to 30 mEq of sodium (460–690 mg, with chloride as the anion) per liter, 2 to 5 mEq of potassium (78–195 mg) per liter, and 5 to 10 percent of carbohydrate (94). Given the available literature on tennis players, recommendations specific to their sport suggest aiming for approximately 200 to 400 ml (approximately 7–14 oz.) fluid per changeover, with some of their fluid coming from a carbohydrate and electrolyte sports drink (47).

All guidelines for children, adolescents, and adults might need to be adjusted to fit the needs of individual athletes.

DO YOU KNOW ?

When sports drinks are ingested at high rates during intense or prolonged exercise, athletes might consume more carbohydrate than their stomach can process quickly, which could result in an upset stomach.

After Exercise

Many athletes, whether competitive or recreational, finish exercising with a fluid deficit. They might continue sweating afterward and lose additional fluid through urine. For these reasons, the athlete needs more fluid than lost through sweat to replace total fluid losses and restore fluid balance. They should aim to consume 125 to 150 percent of the fluid deficit (20–24 oz. per lb. body weight lost or approximately 1.5 L fluid for each kg body weight lost). If sodium isn't consumed with the beverage (or through food intake after exercise), much of the fluid consumed postexercise will lead to increased urine output (80). Therefore, sodium should be consumed in post-workout drinks, meals, or snacks both to replace sodium and enhance rehydration. Additional salt can be added to foods when sodium losses are substantial (74, 80, 96). This strategy helps make up for increased urine production following consumption of a large volume of fluid (74, 79).

SUMMARY

Water and electrolytes are essential to health and athletic performance, but many factors affect hydration needs, so no one recommendation fits everyone. The AI can be used as guidance and adjusted accordingly based on individual needs. Daily hydration status, as well as hydration and electrolyte losses from activity, can be measured and used to develop individual hydration strategies to ensure adequate daily hydration and prevention of an excessive loss of body fluid and sodium during exercise. In instances when hydration status is not measured (possible reasons include lack of measuring devices and sensitivity about body weight), the athlete's coach (or parent) must pay close attention to the athlete and educate them on frequency and quantity of urination, as well as symptoms of hypohydration. Despite access to fluids, many athletes and recreational exercisers start training in a hypohydrated state, lose significant quantities of sweat while training, and cannot quickly replace body fluid losses because of continued sweating and urinary losses postexercise.

■ FOR REVIEW ▶

1. Why is body water important for athletic performance, exercise, and fitness?
2. Discuss the factors that affect an individual's fluid needs.
3. Discuss the role of sodium in the body, and why it is important for athletic and exercise performance.
4. List the methods used to calculate sweat rate. Which methods are more accurate than others?
5. Discuss the symptoms associated with hyponatremia.
6. Which individuals are most at risk of developing hyponatremia? Why is their risk increased?

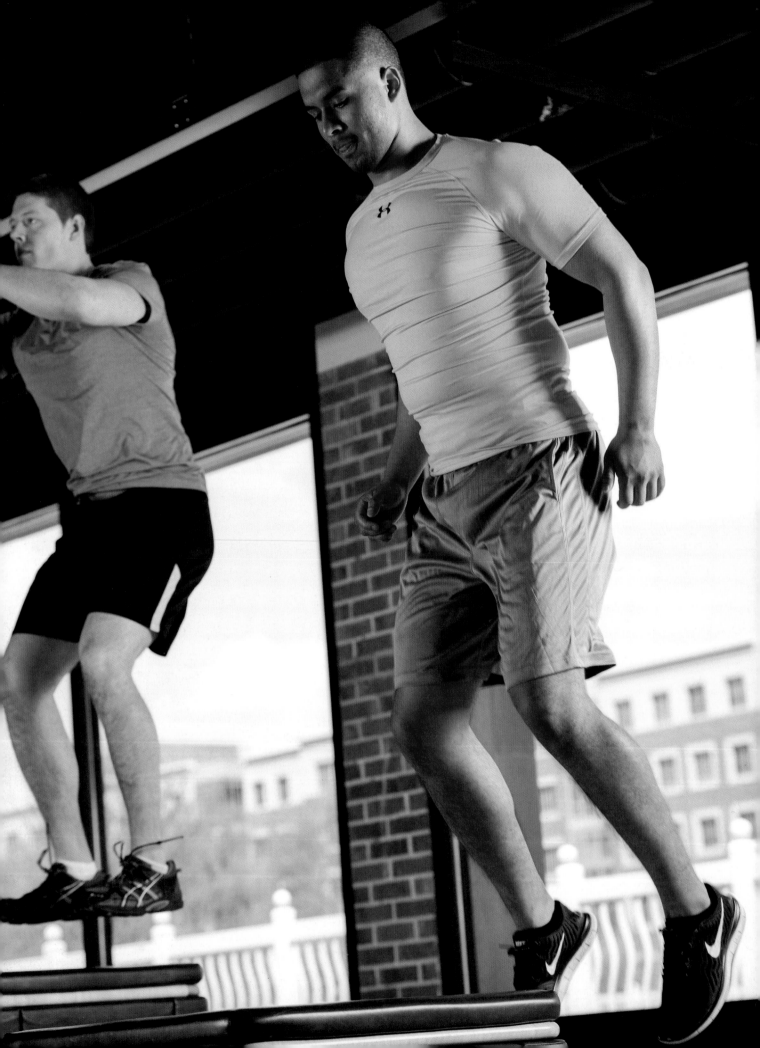

CHAPTER 9

Nutritional Supplements and Other Substances Commonly Used in Sport

▶ **CHAPTER OBJECTIVES**

After completing this chapter, you will be able to do the following:

> Explain how dietary supplements are regulated.

> Describe the categories of claims used with dietary supplements.

> Discuss the process for evaluating the safety and efficacy of dietary supplements.

> Identify the common supplements used in different sports and discuss their efficacy and safety.

> Describe the illegal drugs commonly used in sports and their consequences.

> Discuss the effects of alcohol on sports performance.

People choose to take supplements for many reasons: to improve health, boost energy levels, enhance athletic performance, change body composition, and of course to compensate for nutrients not consumed in adequate amounts through intake of food and beverages (27, 80). When used correctly, many dietary supplements can indeed support health, training, and athletic performance. However, though some dietary supplements are beneficial, others are not, and some are even harmful in certain circumstances (depending on a person's health, what else they are taking, and several other factors) (34, 53, 54, 92). For athletes, poor manufacturing practices or intentional spiking of a supplement with a prescription drug or illegal substance could result in a positive drug test. In any case, whether you are a competitive athlete or not, you must ensure the safety and other implications of any dietary supplement you choose to take.

POPULARITY OF SUPPLEMENT USE IN SPORT

The prevalence of dietary supplement use among athletes is difficult to quantify because of insufficient studies, inconsistent methodology, poor research design, and a lack of homogeneity among published studies. An estimate of supplement use internationally ranges from 37 to 89%, with the greatest use among elite and older athletes (80). A review and meta-analysis reported the prevalence of dietary supplement use among athletes using data from 159 previously published studies (44).

These data suggest that

> supplement use is higher among elite athletes compared to their nonelite counterparts,

> use is similar for men and women, with a few exceptions (men used more vitamin E, protein, and creatine, whereas women used more iron),

> prevalence of dietary supplements use has been relatively high over time (data taken from articles published up to 2014), and

> a larger percentage of athletes used supplements than the general United States adult population.

The most commonly used supplements cited from this study include vitamins and minerals, amino acids and protein, creatine, herbal supplements, omega-3 fatty acids, caffeine, and energy drinks. There are far more products on the market, with new ones being introduced on a regular basis.

REGULATION OF DIETARY SUPPLEMENTS

Dietary supplements are regulated by the FDA, whereas the **Federal Trade Commission (FTC)** protects consumers by regulating potentially unfair, deceptive, or fraudulent practices in the marketplace. The Dietary Supplement Health and Education Act (DSHEA) of 1994 legally defined a dietary supplement as "a product taken by mouth that contains a 'dietary ingredient' intended to supplement the diet. The 'dietary ingredients'

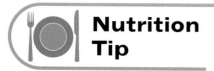

Nutrition Tip

Many supplements marketed for energy contain caffeine. However, companies are not required to list the caffeine content on the label of dietary supplements (93). According to a study conducted by the United States Department of Agriculture, the caffeine content of dietary supplements ranged from 1 mg to more than 800 mg for a daily dose—800 mg is equivalent to approximately 8 cups of coffee (96). Caffeine affects people in different ways, so consumers should use caution when taking a caffeine-containing supplement, especially if consuming other caffeinated foods or beverages (29). When taking supplements with caffeine, start slow, monitor your body's reactions, and proceed accordingly.

in these products may include vitamins, minerals, herbs or other botanicals, amino acids, and substances such as enzymes, organ tissues, glandulars, and metabolites. Dietary supplements can also be extracts or concentrates, and may be found in many forms such as tablets, capsules, softgels, gelcaps, liquids, or powders" (85). If any of these compounds are in other forms, such as a sports bar, the information provided on the product label cannot represent the product as a conventional food and cannot imply it can replace a meal or substitute for a diet comprised of foods. Under this act, dietary supplements are regulated separately and under a different set of regulations from food and drugs (85).

The FDA does not approve dietary supplements for safety or effectiveness before these products reach the store shelves for purchase by the consumer. The manufacturer is responsible for ensuring that the Supplement Facts label and ingredient list are accurate, the dietary ingredients are safe for use as intended, and the amounts of each active ingredient matches the amount declared on the label. Once a product is marketed and sold, it is the FDA's responsibility to demonstrate that a dietary supplement is harmful or unsafe before taking action to restrict the product's use or remove it from public purchase. Manufacturers and distributors of dietary supplements must record and investigate any reported adverse reactions from their product and forward any reports to the FDA. The FDA is able to review reported adverse reactions from manufacturer reports, or information reported by health care providers or consumers, to identify the potential presence of safety risks to the public. A safety alert or consumer advisory has been issued on some common products, including pure powdered caffeine, caffeinated energy drinks, red yeast rice, and botanicals added to conventional foods (86). Check the FDA website for a complete list and updates.

Marketing Supplements

Supplement manufacturers are required to notify the FDA of their intention to sell the product if it contains a "new dietary ingredient." This refers to an ingredient that meets the established DSHEA definition of a "dietary ingredient" and was not sold in the United States in a dietary supplement before October 15, 1994. If a manufacturer and distributor of the supplement intends to use a new ingredient, it is their responsibility to determine if the ingredient meets this definition and to demonstrate to the FDA their proposed ingredient has a reasonable expectation of safety for use in their product, unless it has been recognized as a food substance and is present in the food supply. Any supplements that do not contain new ingredients do not need approval from the FDA before they are marketed and sold to the consumer (85).

Manufacturers can voluntarily provide information to the FDA or consumers about safety and efficacy of their product, if they choose to do so (85). It is up to each manufacturer to establish its own policy regarding this disclosure to either the FDA or its customers.

In June 2007, the FDA published comprehensive regulations for *current* **good manufacturing practices (GMPs)** for those who manufacture, package, or distribute dietary supplement products. These regulations focus on practices that ensure the identity, purity, quality, strength, and composition of dietary supplements. The existence of GMPs may help ensure the ingredients on the label are present in listed quantities and that products are free from contaminants and impurities. These published GMPs do not govern marketing or claims made about the product, so it is the consumer's responsibility to contact the manufacturer of a product if more information is desired. The name and address of the manufacturer or distributor can be found on the dietary supplement label (85).

Supplement Facts Labels

Regulations control the information that must appear on the labels of dietary supplements. All supplement labels must include "a descriptive name of the product stating that it is a 'supplement'; the name and place of business of the manufacturer, packer, or distributor; a complete list of ingredients; and the net contents of the product" (85). The FDA further requires that most dietary supplements have a "Supplement Facts" panel on the product (figure 9.1). This panel must list each dietary ingredient contained in the product; those ingredients not included in the panel must be listed in the "other ingredients" statement printed beneath the panel. Other ingredients may include the source of dietary ingredients, other food ingredients (e.g., water and sugar), additives, colors, preservatives, flavors, or other processing aids. There are no regulations limiting a serving size or the amount of a nutrient or ingredient in the product. The recommended serving size is determined by the manufacturer and does not require FDA approval (90).

Dietary Supplement Claims

Manufacturers generally employ three types of claims with their dietary supplements (90):

1. Nutrient content claims
2. Health claims
3. Structure/function claims

Nutrient Content Claims

Nutrient content claims describe the quantity of a nutrient in a product and can be used for both foods and dietary supplements. Common examples refer to calories, fat, sugar, and sodium. Other terms, such as "light" or "healthy," are also defined. Examples include "low-fat," "sugar-free," "low-calorie," "good source," and "high potency." Some of these terms compare the level of the nutrient in a product to the Daily Value (DV) for that nutrient (e.g., "excellent source"), whereas others may compare one product to another (e.g., "reduced" or "more"). Detailed descriptions of FDA-approved nutrient content claims can be found on the FDA's website (87, 88). Check this site periodically for any changes to existing terms or the addition of new terms.

Health Claims

The second category of claims that the FDA oversees and issues regulations regarding the use of, in both foods and dietary supplements, is health claims. These claims describe a relation between a nutrient or ingredient (component of food or dietary supplement) and reduced risk of a health-related condition or disease. Both components in this relationship must be present to be a health claim. For example, the FDA-approved health claim regarding calcium and osteoporosis lists both components in its model claim: "Adequate calcium throughout life, as part of a well-balanced diet, may reduce the risk of osteoporosis" (89, 90). On the other hand, dietary guidance statements do not fulfill this requirement (e.g., regular fruit and vegetable consumption is good for health). In order for the FDA to approve a health claim for use on a food or supplement product, there must be significant scientific agreement supporting the proposed claim. A limited number of health claims have been approved for use. The complete list can be found on the FDA's website (89). Visit this site regularly to see if any new health claims have been approved. It is illegal for dietary supplement manufacturers to use any health claim not approved by the FDA. For example, manufacturers cannot promote or print on a label that the product is a treatment, prevention, or cure for a specific disease or condition.

Structure/Function Claims

The third category of claims related to foods and dietary supplements is called **structure/function claims**. Two claims are under the regulatory requirements of the DSHEA:

1. Claims of general well-being
2. Claims related to a nutrient deficiency disease

Supplement Facts

Serving Size: 1 capsule
Servings Per Container: 30

	Amount Per Serving	%DV
Ester C	50mg	83%
Vitamin E (dl-alpha tocopherol)	20IU	67%
Vitamin B6 (pyridoxine hci)	25mg	1250%
Vitamin B12 (cyanocobalamin)	25mcg	416%
Vitamin B1 (thiamine)	1.5mg	100%
Vitamin B2 (riboflavin)	1.5mg	88%
Aloe Vera Powder	50mg	-
Alpha Lipoic Acid	50mg	-
Bioperine Standardized Extract	1.5mg	-
Collagen Type II (from chicken)	250mg	-
CoQ10	10mg	-
Curcumin C3 Complex	25mg	-
Hyaluronic Acid	10mg	-

*Daily Value (DV) not established.

Other Ingredients: Vegetable Capsule (Hydroxypropyl Cellulose)

Figure 9.1 Supplement Facts label.

Structure/function claims may state how the product, nutrient, or ingredient intends to affect the normal structure or function within the body (e.g., calcium helps build strong bones) or how it acts to maintain a particular structure or function (e.g., fiber helps keep you regular; antioxidant nutrients help maintain cell integrity). Structure/function claims cannot explicitly or implicitly link or associate the claimed effect of the nutrient, component, or dietary ingredient to a specific disease or state of health leading to a disease.

These claims are not preapproved by the FDA, but the manufacturer must submit notification of the claim to the FDA no later than 30 days after marketing. It is the manufacturer's responsibility to have scientific evidence to substantiate their claim and that their claim is truthful and not misleading. If the structure/function claim is used with the product, the product must include a disclaimer stating that the claim has not been evaluated by the FDA. The disclaimer must also state that the dietary supplement product is not intended to "diagnose, treat, cure or prevent any disease" because the product is a dietary supplement, and only drugs can legally make such claims about a disease (90).

EVALUATION OF DIETARY SUPPLEMENTS

A wide array of dietary supplements are available for sale, with more arriving on the market regularly. With so many products to choose from, and so many similar products competing with each other, the risk of confusion is high. When considering a dietary supplement, use the guidelines that follow. Of course this information is not meant to replace advice given by your medical provider.

Product Labels

The first step in evaluating a dietary supplement is to view the product label. The brand, product name, claims, and name and quantity of key ingredients should be listed. This information, however, tells you nothing about the quality or efficacy of the product. The limited, and sometimes confusing, regulations associated with the DSHEA act can make the process of product evaluation very difficult for consumers. Health professionals must go above and beyond any advertising or simple label reading to determine the safety and effectiveness of a product.

Peer-Reviewed Scientific Evidence

There are many printed sources of information about dietary supplements. Laypersons might commonly turn to newspapers or magazine articles since these media tend to cover current, popular topics. Articles published in these sources may or may not be from experts in the field qualified to write about the topic, and you may not know authors' qualifications or if they have conflicts of interest (are they receiving money from a company to write a good review?). While Registered Dietitian Nutritionists and other allied health professionals possessing knowledge of dietary supplements should keep up with the lay information being presented to the public, they must stay up to date on the scientific evidence presented in peer-reviewed journals. Peer-reviewed journal articles, also called refereed or scholarly journal

REFLECTION TIME

ADVERSE SUPPLEMENT REACTIONS CAN BE REPORTED TO THE FDA

You or your health care provider can anonymously report an adverse reaction or illness suspected to be caused by a dietary supplement or problems with packaging, contamination, or other quality defects to the FDA. Visit https://www.fda.gov or call the FDA MedWatch hotline at 1-800-FDA-1088.

articles, are written by experts in the field who have conducted the research study being published or by those who are reviewing the current available literature. Not all scholarly journals go through the process of peer review.

Resources Regarding Quality and Banned Substances

Well-established resources are available for health professionals and consumers to use to minimize chances of purchasing a supplement that is adulterated or contaminated.

Independent certification programs assess various aspects of supplements, including the quality, purity, potency, and composition of the product. These programs typically have a particular seal (a stamp of approval) that supplement manufacturers include on their products, once certified. **Banned Substances Control Group (BSCG)**, Informed-Choice, ConsumerLab.com, NSF International, and the US Pharmacopeia Convention (USP) are among the organizations with assessment programs (1). An assessment should not be confused with a recommendation for use. Manufacturers who use third-party testing do so voluntarily, as testing is not required to sell products. No testing company tests for all of the substances banned by the NCAA, MLB, NFL, or WADA (World Anti-Doping Agency), and of course any list is subject to change as new substances become available.

The BSCG tests over 450 banned substances, including drugs prohibited in sports, prescription drugs, and over-the-counter drugs. They randomly test either every finished batch of supplements or one batch monthly. The BSCG database lists the supplements they have certified. Certified products carry the BSCG seal (10).

NSF International has three seals or marks that can be used with supplements. Only one of these tests for banned substances: the NSF Certified for Sport program. The NSF Certified for Sport seal indicates a supplement has been tested for over 240 banned substances. They perform ongoing testing of products that are certified, selecting certain batches to be tested (1). Under the NSF Certified for Sport program, NSF tests to ensure the supplement contains what its label says it contains. However, ingredients as listed on the label can vary by 20 percent (i.e., total sugar, calories, total fat, saturated fat, cholesterol, or sodium might be 20% higher than as listed on the label; vitamins, minerals, protein, carbohydrate, and fiber must be at least 80% of the value listed on the container) (1, 59).

Informed-Choice is a quality-assurance program specifically designed for sports nutrition products and their manufacturers and suppliers. Products that carry the Informed-Choice logo certify that the nutritional supplements and ingredients in the product have been tested for over 200 banned substances by an independent lab. The Informed-Choice website provides a

---

WHAT JOURNALS ARE PEER-REVIEWED?

REFLECTION TIME

To investigate whether or not a journal is peer-reviewed, visit the homepage of the journal on the Internet. Many state their peer-review process and also include a list of people on their editorial board. If still in doubt, a reference librarian at a university library can likely help you.

Peer-reviewed journals in the fields of nutrition and exercise sciences include the following:

> *Journal of Nutrition*

> *International Journal of Sports Nutrition and Exercise Metabolism*

> *Medicine and Science in Sports and Exercise*

search feature that allows consumers wishing to use supplements to find products that have been through this certification process (34).

The **U.S. Pharmacopeial Convention (USP)** is a scientific, worldwide, nonprofit organization that sets standards for the identity, strength, quality, and purity of medicines, food ingredients, and dietary supplements manufactured and distributed for sale. USP's drug standards are used in more than 140 countries and are enforceable by the FDA. USP offers third-party, voluntary, independent verification of dietary supplements in an attempt to limit the presence of adulterants and contaminants in supplement ingredients and final products sold to consumers (1, 95).

Products carrying the USP Verified Mark meet the criteria set by the organization, including standards of quality, purity, potency, performance, and consistency and current FDA GMPs. This mark ensures consumers of the following:

> The product contains the ingredients listed on the label, in the indicated quantities. Lower levels of ingredients may not render the intended effect or be completely useless. Higher levels can cause undesirable side effects or harm.

> The product does not contain harmful levels of tested contaminants (e.g., heavy metals or microbes).

> The product will be delivered into the body within a specified amount of time. Both digestion and metabolism factors are considered using federally recognized dissolution standards.

> The product was manufactured according to FDA GMPs, using sanitary and well-controlled procedures to ensure safety and consistent quality within and between batches (1, 95).

The FDA provides valuable resources to consumers to help them reduce the risk of encountering a product marketed as a dietary supplement containing hidden ingredient(s). The FDA's Medication Health Fraud website lists some of the potentially hazardous products with hidden ingredients marketed and sold to consumers. Products more likely to be contaminated are those

promoted for weight loss, sexual enhancement, and bodybuilding (19, 20, 92).

The FDA advises caution when considering products with these potential warning signs (19, 20, 92):

> They claim to be alternatives to FDA-approved drugs or to have effects similar to prescription drugs.

> They claim to be a legal alternative to or one step away from anabolic steroids.

> They are marketed primarily in a foreign language.

> They are marketed through mass e-mails.

> They are marketed as sexual-enhancement products promising rapid or long-lasting effects.

> They include small print about the possibility of testing positive in drug testing.

Dietary Supplement Information Specific to Athletes

Some athletes in competitive sports are tested for banned substances such as steroids. Supplements may contain prohibited substances not declared on the label, contamination of the product might have occurred because of poor manufacturing practices or sometimes through deliberate intent on the part of the athlete. Determining whether a supplement was contaminated at the outset or through a conscious choice of the athlete can be difficult to discern. It is not uncommon for athletes who test positive for a banned substance to blame the positive test on a supplement, when in reality they were taking the substance intentionally. Most sports organizations with banned substances policies have strict liability. This means even when athletes innocently ingest the substance, and then test positive, they are not allowed to compete. If the competition has already occurred, any awards, records, or other kinds of acknowledgment are nullified. Reputable organizations can be found that provide dietary supplement information specific to athletes who are concerned about testing positive.

The National Center for Drug Free Sport (**Drug Free Sport**) is a provider of drug-use prevention

> ## ARE SEALS ON SUPPLEMENT LABELS A GUARANTEE?
>
> While many of the verification and seal programs can be useful when making a supplement selection, they do not guarantee purity or safety. There are independent, third-party auditing programs that can test dietary supplements for substances that are banned or restricted by sport organizations. These testing facilities use a standard (ISO 17025 accreditation standard) that provides a better assurance that a tested supplement is free of banned substances and thus might prevent the athlete from a doping violation or loss of eligibility (80).

services for many athletic organizations and delivers strategic alternatives to traditional drug-use prevention programs. More important, Drug Free Sport is different from other third-party drug-testing companies that conduct primarily workplace and insurance testing in that they work exclusively with sports organizations and their athletes. Some of the services provided include

> blood and urine testing,
> a resource exchange center providing current and accurate information on sports supplements and prohibited substances,
> online drug education for student athletes,
> drug policy developing and consulting, and
> customized education programs and webinars (55).

The **U.S. Anti-Doping Agency (USADA)** is the national anti-doping organization for Olympic, Paralympic, Pan American, and American Games (a multi-sport event for athletes with physical disabilities held every four years after the Pan American Games). The USDA's mission is to preserve the integrity of competition, inspire true sport, and protect the rights of U.S. athletes. Their vision is "to be the guardian of the values and life lessons learned through true sport" (82). This organization manages the anti-doping program, including in-competition and out-of-competition testing, results management processes, and drug reference resources. USADA also provides education for all United States Olympic Committee (USOC)-recognized sport

national-governing bodies, their athletes, and their events. This organization contributes to the advancement of clean sport through supporting scientific research and education, as well as educational outreach initiatives focusing on awareness and prevention (82). The USADA website Supplement 411 educates athletes on how to recognize red flags indicating an increased risk, how to reduce the risk of testing positive, and how to avoid developing health problems (83).

Before competing, all athletes must know the rules regarding banned or prohibited substances in their particular sport:

> Major League Baseball Players Association (MLBPA): http://mlb.mlb.com/mlb/news/drug_policy.jsp
> National Football League Players Association (NFLPA): www.nflpa.com/active-players/drug-policies
> National Collegiate Athletic Association (NCAA): www.ncaa.org/2015-16-ncaabanned-drugs
> US Anti-Doping Agency (USADA): www.usada.org/substances/prohibited-list/
> The World Anti-Doping Agency (WADA): www.wada-ama.org/en/what-we-do/prohibited-list

Considerations for Choosing a Supplement

There are so many supplements available in the marketplace, and it is important to be able to recognize when a product's safety or efficacy is in question. First, examine the brand. Determine if the product is made by a national seller or is from a manufacturer whose products are aimed at specific populations or purposes such as weight loss, bodybuilding, or sexual enhancement. A 2014 study reported that products in these three areas had the highest level of tainted supplements (19). Many national brands have good manufacturing practices in place and want to keep a sound reputation. This does not mean smaller companies make poor products—it is only one factor to consider. Second, beware of complicated products with long lists of ingredients, unfamiliar ingredients, or **proprietary blends**. With proprietary blends, it is impossible to know the quantities of individual ingredients and compare them to the scientific literature, since the literature will specify quantity of an ingredient or ingredients.

If the proprietary blend has different amounts of ingredients than used in the research studies, a product might not have an efficacious dose of the active ingredient or ingredients. Manufacturers sometimes add useless ingredients to make a product appear more robust and appealing. Third, be concerned if a product claims to have the same effect as a prescription drug. Many such claims are false. Finally, don't be fooled by the term "natural." This is not a defined term and is not an indication of safety. Many herbal products are natural yet contain compounds that have pharmaceutical activity or that can interfere with the action of over-the-counter or prescription drugs (85). For example, kava kava should not be used with alcohol or with many of the antidepressant drugs prescribed by psychiatrists, and black cohosh might interfere with commonly prescribed statin drugs (66).

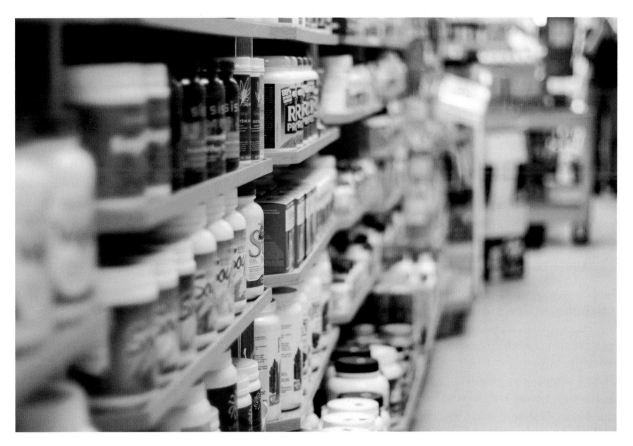

When searching for a supplement, examine the brand, beware of proprietary ingredients, and remember "natural" does not always mean the product is safe.

COMMON SPORTS FOODS AND MEDICAL SUPPLEMENTS

The most common sports foods used in endurance sports are foods and drinks containing carbohydrate and electrolytes (see chapters 3 and 8). While numerous supplements are available on the market, a few of the most popular among endurance athletes are discussed below.

Caffeine and Energy Drinks

Caffeine can be found naturally in food and beverages, can be added to food and beverage products, or can be purchased as dietary supplementals. Some of the common herbal sources of caffeine often used in weight-loss products are guarana, kola nut, and yerba mate.

Caffeine is the most widely consumed legal psychoactive agent (i.e., a substance that affects brain functioning) in the world. It occurs naturally in the leaves, nuts, and seeds of over 60 plants, yet it can also be made synthetically for use in over-the-counter medications and dietary supplements. Caffeine is consumed by billions worldwide with the major dietary sources coming from coffee, tea, and soft drinks, which contain from 30 to 200 mg of caffeine per serving. Chocolate is another common source, but the caffeine content is significantly lower (usually less than 15 mg/oz., or about 100 mg/cup) (50). Over-the-counter medications may contain 100 to 200 mg of caffeine per tablet. Quantity is listed on labels because caffeine is a drug. Caffeine can be toxic in high doses, such as 15 mg/kg body weight, and these toxic effects can be exacerbated when caffeine is combined with other stimulants (57, 84). Caffeine content is not required on food labels, so exact quantities in some products, such as coffee, are difficult to

DO YOU KNOW ?

Caffeine consumed in smaller doses (less than 180 mg/day) does not seem to significantly increase daily urine output or cause dehydration in individuals who maintain hydration status with ingestion of other fluids. Dehydration itself will result in reduced urine output but less is known about the effects of caffeine ingestion in individuals who are already dehydrated (71).

determine and can be quite variable depending on source and brewing method (50). If caffeine is added to a food or beverage, it must be included in the list of ingredients on the label, but there is no requirement to disclose the quantity of caffeine (94).

Caffeine has been studied and used for decades to improve physical performance. The original rationale for its use was related to the physiological finding of an enhanced free fatty acid (FFA) release. The assumption at that time was these FFAs would be a preferential fuel source for working skeletal muscle during exercise, and thus glycogen would be spared (28). More recent research has clarified that although FFAs are released into the bloodstream with caffeine ingestion, FFA oxidation (use) does not increase, nor is glycogen spared. In other words, the fatty acids go through circulation and then travel back to the adipose cells again to be stored and skeletal muscle (8, 74, 78).

It appears that the **ergogenic**, or performance-enhancing, benefit of caffeine is most likely related to its role as a central nervous system stimulant. Adenosine is a compound found in all cells in the body and plays an important role in energy metabolism. Adenosine prepares the body for sleep by blunting communication between nerve cells while widening blood vessels to increase oxygen flow. Caffeine and adenosine compete for the same receptors in the brain. When levels of adenosine are reduced because of higher levels of caffeine competing for binding, this results in an increased feeling of alertness. In exercise performance, the main benefit is a heightened sense of awareness and decreased perception of effort (8, 74, 78).

Caffeine is generally recognized as safe by the FDA and has been consumed for centuries as part of coffee and tea. Considerable research supports the use of caffeine as an ergogenic aid, and studies have most commonly examined doses ranging from 3 to 13 mg/kg body weight. The amount typically used to stimulate central nervous system functioning is 2 to 3 mg/kg. Some organizations ban the use of caffeine in higher doses or have limits to urinary caffeine levels. Higher doses are considered to be in the range of 10 to 13 mg/kg. For a 70-kg athlete, this is equivalent to 700 to

900 mg of caffeine, or 7 to 9 cups of coffee. This amount is greater than the average consumption. Doses in this range may come with significant side effects, including elevated heart rate and elevated levels of catecholamine, lactate, FFAs, and glycerol. Furthermore, undesirable feelings of gastrointestinal distress, jitteriness, mental confusion, problems concentrating or focusing, and sleep disturbances may accompany such doses. Symptoms might be more pronounced in individuals who usually use no or low doses of caffeine and then increase the dose for an event (8, 74, 78).

Moderate doses of caffeine (5–6 mg/kg body weight) have often been used in research studies and demonstrate an ergogenic effect on endurance performance without undesirable side effects, but other research suggests starting with even lower doses (2–3 mg/kg) can be just as ergogenic. In addition to quantity, timing is an important consideration. Caffeine is rapidly absorbed in the body, with appearance in the blood stream 5 to 15 minutes after ingestion and peak concentrations between 40 to 80 minutes (8, 74, 78).

DO YOU KNOW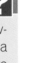

The caffeine content in beverages like coffee and tea are generally too variable to determine a specific dose. Factors such as brew time, origin and type of plant, and preparation methods can all affect caffeine content.

A final consideration is whether the ergogenic effects of caffeine use are more pronounced with acute use or chronic use. This question has not been fully resolved in the literature, and therefore must be included in trial periods. Chronic users may need a higher dose during competition to see a benefit. But caution should be taken by individuals who are not habitual caffeine users. There are genetic differences in caffeine metabolism and, if not accustomed to caffeine, a person could be sensitive to it (78). As with any change in diet, athletes who want to test their response to caffeine should experiment during the preseason or early in the training season, not during competition or precompetition.

The guidelines for the consumption of energy drinks are different from those for caffeine because energy drinks contain a variety of other ingredients, such as sugar, carbonation, herbs, amino acids, vitamins, minerals, and other stimulants (53).

Sodium Bicarbonate

Sports involving heavy use of anaerobic glycolysis as the predominant energy system result in the metabolic fatigue associated with progressive increased intracellular acidity. Athletes may consume sodium bicarbonate in an attempt to neutralize the hydrogen ions and thus extend the time of high-intensity activities before fatigue sets in. Athletes participating in sporting events of high intensity lasting 1 to 7 minutes, such as middle-distance running and swimming and high-intensity sprints, might benefit the most from bicarbonate. However, participants in other sports lasting much longer in duration (e.g., 30–60 minutes) that include surges of increased intensity, or in sports with intermittent periods of high intensity, might also benefit. While the research data do not unanimously show support for an ergogenic benefit of sodium bicarbonate, some data suggest an acute, preexercise dose of 300 mg/kg body weight might provide the blood-buffering capacity needed to see a performance benefit occur (15, 70, 80).

Sodium bicarbonate is very inexpensive and readily available in all grocery stores as baking soda, but it might not be palatable. Commercial products are available in capsules or tablets and might be more desirable. Potential side effects reported with use of sodium bicarbonate include nausea, vomiting, stomach pain, and diarrhea, which clearly result in performance impairment, not improvement (15, 70, 80).

Glycerol

Glycerol is the "backbone" that holds the three fatty acids in a triglyceride molecule. It is also a solute that, when ingested, is rapidly absorbed and evenly distributed in the body's water compartments. This causes the retention of fluid with a concomitant reduction in urine output and thus a state of hyperhydration (see chapter 8). The potential ergogenic effect stems from the extra plasma volume that in turn attenuates water loss with exercise-induced sweating. Prolonging or

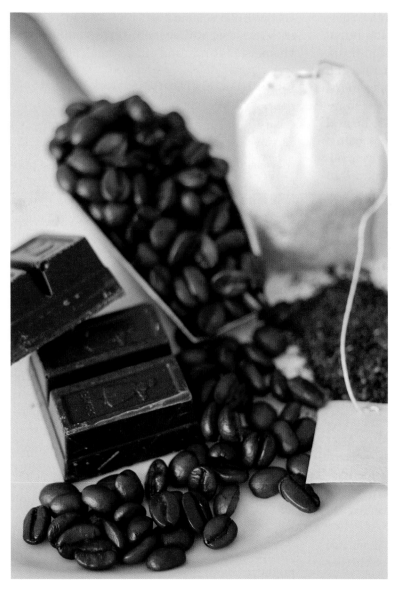

Caffeine is found in more than just coffee. Consider your intake of coffee, tea, energy drinks, and supplements claiming they will give you energy when evaluating your total caffeine consumption.

continuous exercise for a prolonged period of time, where intensities are on the higher side, and in warmer environmental conditions. It might also be beneficial in the rehydration plan. The general recommendations for glycerol use as a preparatory aid for exercise are 1.2 g/kg body weight in 26 ml/kg body weight of fluid. It is best to consume the drink over 1 hour, and then allow an additional 30 minutes before beginning exercise. If continuing glycerol consumption during exercise, the recommended dose is 0.125 g/kg in 5 ml/kg fluid. If using glycerol and a rehydration strategy, the recommendation is 1.5 liter of fluid for each kg of weight loss, with 1.0 g/kg of glycerol added to each 1.5 liter. Some users of glycerol report side effects of light-headedness and GI distress such as bloating, nausea, or diarrhea. As with other supplements, trial and error is warranted and should occur early in training rather than waiting until competition. Note that hyperhydration can result in masking illegal doping practices with other substances, and as a result, the World Anti-Doping Agency added glycerol to its list of prohibited substances in 2010 (97, 98).

Nitric Oxide

There are three main types of nitric oxide (NO) boosters. Beets and other nitrate-rich vegetables work through the nitrate-nitrite-NO pathway, one that functions when oxygen isn't as readily available (during high-intensity exercise such as sprinting up and down a soccer field). L-arginine works through a very different pathway, one that requires the presence of enzymes and oxygen and thus isn't effective during high-intensity exercise. Certain polyphenols, including those found in Concord grape juice, acai juice, cranberry juice, carrot juice, and pomegranate

preventing dehydration can have a significant positive effect on performance. Additionally, it has been proposed that glycerol can have a secondary benefit of aiding in the maintenance of blood glucose via gluconeogenesis in the liver. However, research suggests that glycerol provides an insignificant energy source during exercise (97, 98).

Some research studies suggest a performance benefit with glycerol use, while others do not. If a benefit exists, it would likely be most beneficial as a preexercise strategy in sports requiring

juice, turn on proteins that signal the endothelial cells to make more endothelial nitric oxide synthase (eNOS, one of the enzymes responsible for the majority of nitric oxide produced; eNOS helps produce nitric oxide from arginine), boosting levels of eNOS for up to a full day. The endothelial cells treated with Concord grape juice increased nitric oxide levels by 50 percent (2, 24).

Inorganic nitrate helps open blood vessels to increase blood flow, supporting cardiovascular health and athletic performance. It is naturally found in beetroot juice, green leafy vegetables, spinach, celery, commercial vegetable juices, carrot juice, and pomegranate juice (18, 80). However, the amount of dietary nitrate varies in beets and other vegetables based on growing conditions, including the nitrate content of the

fertilizer used, the level of nitrate in the water supply, soil conditions, time of year, and how the vegetables are stored (101).

Once consumed, inorganic nitrate (NO_3^-) is metabolized to bioactive nitrite (NO_2^-), which is converted to nitric oxide (NO). The initial conversion of inorganic nitrate to nitrite begins in the mouth with the help of salivary bacteria; the conversion rate is approximately 20 percent (14, 18). Antibacterial mouthwash and antibiotics kill bacteria in the mouth, which significantly reduces this initial conversion (18). Once swallowed, the conversion to nitric oxide occurs in many phases in the stomach, gut, and other organs. Though research is limited, the bioavailability (the amount that reaches the circulation) of nitrite has been reported to be 95 to 100 percent (14, 18).

Nitric oxide exerts its action by signaling the lining of blood vessels (the endothelium) to relax, subsequently enhancing blood flow. This enhanced blood flow is thought to improve exercise performance and recovery. Nitrate intake might also reduce the oxygen cost of submaximal exercise and translate to enhanced exercise tolerance and improved performance. Research has shown that both acute (2–3 hours) and chronic (3–15 days) supplementation of nitrate improve activities for men and women of all ages, including both trained and untrained (18). However, further reports suggest the positive effect is more

PUTTING IT INTO PERSPECTIVE

BAD RAP FOR NITRATE?

Nitrate is a naturally occurring chemical compound found in plants, our soil, and within the human body. Sodium nitrate is also naturally occurring and is used as a preservative in processed meats. When this compound interacts with the bacteria naturally found in meat, it gets converted to sodium nitrite. Sodium nitrite can also be added directly to meats for the purpose of preservation. Nitrites have received much attention because, when heated, they can create nitrosamines, which are reported to be carcinogenic in animals. Nitrate and nitrite are still abundant in the human diet. Vegetables are a larger source of nitrates than processed meat, and plant foods are generally considered healthy, with greater intake linked to a reduced risk of cancer and CVD. Since the initial scare, newer scientific evidence has become available that suggest these compounds might not be as detrimental as once thought. More research is needed, especially to understand the potential beneficial roles of nitrates (14, 73).

pronounced in the untrained and recreationally active, and the data are less clear for elite competitors (37, 80). Studies showing a benefit reported doses ranging from 5 to 9 mmol of nitrate (425–765 mg) ingested as a single dose or as multiple servings 3 hours prior to exercise. This quantity is equivalent to approximately 2 cups (16 oz.) of pure (nothing added) beetroot juice. For athletes choosing to stick with foods rather than traditional dietary supplements, consumption of beetroot juice and other green leafy vegetables, such as arugula and spinach, may provide some benefits. Ingestion of nitrate in typical amounts from foods does not cause adverse health consequences in healthy persons. Less is known about the safety of supplementation with high doses in the supplemental form, though there are no known safety issues with supplementation at recommended doses in healthy individuals (14, 18).

DO YOU KNOW ?

Beets and beetroot juice might turn your urine red. This is harmless. For more information on substances that change the color of your urine, see chapter 8.

L-arginine and L-ornithine are two conditionally essential amino acids known in the sports nutrition world as arginine and ornithine. The body makes them, but they become essential (and must therefore be consumed through food) during times of illness and metabolic stress. Ornithine is used to synthesize arginine, which is used to create nitric oxide (NO). Some athletes will attempt to boost their intake of these amino acids through foods or supplements in order to see a performance benefit. Both arginine and ornithine are found in fish, meat, eggs, and dairy foods. Plant sources of arginine include beans, brown rice, oats, and nuts.

Creatine

Approximately 95 percent of the body's creatine stores are in skeletal muscle, with about 60 percent of total creatine content in the form of phosphocreatine (PCr). Creatine is used in the ATP-PC energy system, where PCr is able to rapidly re-phosphorylate adenosine diphosphate (ADP) to adenosine triphosphate (ATP). ATP is then used as the energy source for the contracting muscle. This generally occurs in high-intensity activities lasting 5 to 8 seconds. Creatine can be produced by the body, primarily in the kidney and liver, though ingestion of 1 gram per day from the diet helps maintain creatine homeostasis (17, 70, 78, 80).

Primary dietary sources include meat and fish, but many athletes choose to take creatine in the supplemental form in order to maximize skeletal muscle quantities and improve performance. One common strategy begins with a 20-gram-per-day loading phase for 5 to 7 days, followed by a maintenance phase of 3 to 5 grams per day until the supplement is discontinued. Other research has found efficacy with lower doses of 5 grams per day, with maintenance doses ranging from 1 to 27 grams per day, with 3 grams per day for 28 days commonly used (41, 47). Skeletal muscle has limitations on how much creatine can be stored, and any excess gets converted to creatinine and is excreted (17, 70, 78, 80).

Creatine is a widely researched sports supplement and the subject of numerous publications in peer-reviewed journals. Much of the data support an ergogenic benefit for anaerobic performance, especially in sports with repeated short bursts of very high-intensity exercise, as seen in American football and soccer. In conjunction with resistance training, creatine supplementation might lead to greater gains in strength and lean body mass. The increased strength is likely caused by the increased ability to train at a higher intensity before fatigue. The reported increased lean body mass should not be confused with increased skeletal muscle mass. Lean body mass is comprised of muscle, water, and bone, and it is thought that much of the lean body mass increase is caused by the fluid retention required for creatine storage within the muscle. Some body composition methods are unable to detect changes to skeletal muscle, only to lean body mass as a whole, though other studies have been able to demonstrate creatine's effectiveness at the level of the muscle, using more sophisticated techniques (17, 70, 78, 80).

Creatine does not seem to have an ergogenic benefit for improving maximal aerobic capacity or improving field performance in long-

PUTTING IT INTO PERSPECTIVE

DOES CREATINE SUPPLEMENTATION LEAD TO DEHYDRATION?

It is a common belief that creatine can hinder exercise heat tolerance, muscle cramps, or hydration status. This belief stems from the fluid retention that accompanies creatine storage and dehydration reports in high school football players using creatine. However, many athletes start practice in a dehydrated state. Also, a review of the scientific literature examining randomized clinical trials show no evidence suggesting creatine impairs the body's ability to dissipate heat or contributes to dehydration when recommended doses are used (17, 70, 78, 80).

duration aerobic events such as long-distance running. While there is an abundance of scientific support for use of creatine with certain activities, the results are not unanimous. This is because of individual responses to creatine supplementation, with some people being responders and others nonresponders (17, 70, 78, 80).

Direct response to creatine cannot be determined without a muscle biopsy or sophisticated medical imaging procedure, so there is no way to feasibly screen for this. However, because of the fluid retention, weight can be accurately measured and used as an indicator of creatine retention. Furthermore, improvements in the weight room or the field can be assessed to help evaluate if a person is responding to creatine use (17, 70, 78, 80).

DO YOU KNOW ?

Though creatine supplementation is most popular among athletes, it might also have a therapeutic application. Creatine supplementation has been shown to be well tolerated and effective in improving muscle function in those with muscular dystrophy, muscle myopathies and disorders, and neuromuscular and neurometabolic disorders (43, 77, 79).

There is some controversy about the safety of creatine supplementation in those under the age of 18 years. The American Academy of Pediatrics (3) will often publish information related to creatine in adolescents and youth as well as information about other supplements. Those under the age of 18 should discuss the use of all supplements and products with parents or guardians and qualified medical professionals (70, 78, 80).

Current data indicate no short-term health risks with creatine use, but more research is needed to assess effects with long-term use (over decades). From the published literature, it appears that short-term use does not result in permanent or adverse effects in kidney, liver, cardiac, or muscle function in healthy adults (63). Caution should be used with doses greater than 3 to 5 grams per day in individuals with preexisting renal disease or those with another disease that can affect kidney function, such as diabetes and hypertension (40). Note that weight gain might be an undesirable side-effect in weight-sensitive sports and, though rare, GI stress is a reported potential side effect from some types of creatine (78, 80).

Beta-Alanine

Carnosine is a dipeptide comprised of beta-alanine and histidine and thought to serve as a buffer for skeletal muscle during high-intensity activities. Beta-alanine is a beta-amino acid, differing from the majority of alpha-amino acids found in the human diet. Synthesis of muscle carnosine is limited by the availability of beta-alanine, the rate-limiting substrate. Supplementation with beta-alanine might enhance natural carnosine production and provide an ergogenic, buffering effect during anaerobic exercise (31, 68, 70, 80).

Several research studies have reported increased skeletal muscle, carnosine content, and an ergogenic effect with beta-alanine supplementation. Supplementation of a mean dose of 4.8 ± 1.3 grams per day seems to improve perceived exertion (i.e., exercise feels like less effort) and biochemical markers of muscle fatigue (12). Common supplementation regimens vary from 1.6 to 6.4 grams per day, and beta alanine might be most beneficial during high-intensity exercise lasting 1 to 4 minutes. This is the period of time where acidity increases and therefore the best time to attempt to provide a buffering agent (31, 68, 70, 80). A meta-analysis of the literature found a total dose of 179 grams (approximately 28 days of supplementation with 6.4 g/day) resulted in a median improvement of 2.85 percent compared to placebo (31). More research is needed to examine the potential benefits for activities longer than 4 minutes. This supplement might benefit endurance athletes who have intermittent, high-intensity movements, sprinters, those engaged in repeated sprint activity (such as in soccer or American football), or those who focus on strength training. Paresthesia, tingling in the skin, is a potential side effect (31, 68, 70, 80).

Beta-Hydroxy-Beta-Methylbutyrate

Leucine is an essential, branched-chain amino acid believed to be a trigger for skeletal muscle protein synthesis. Beta-hydroxy-beta-methylbutyrate (HMB) is a metabolite of leucine and has been reported to have therapeutic effects in individuals with atrophic conditions and cachexia (wasting) (51, 102, 105). Athletes and bodybuilders have expressed an interest in using the compound in attempts to increase skeletal muscle protein strength and hypertrophy.

Early research studies reported HMB reduces skeletal muscle damage with resistance training. Unfortunately, this area of study has not significantly increased over time, so published research studies are somewhat scarce. Based on available data, it appears that 3 grams per day is the dose for maximal response, with no additional benefits from doses of 6 grams per day. The most common reported ergogenic effects include reduced muscle damage and increased strength, primarily in novice weightlifters, but minimal data support this claim. No safety concerns or significant side effects have been reported in the literature at this dosage. Based on available research, there does not appear to be an ergogenic benefit in trained persons of all ages. More studies are needed to see if the results reported in previous studies translate to actual increases in skeletal muscle protein synthesis. This supplement might have

therapeutic effects in those with muscle-wasting disease (51, 102, 105).

Dehydroepiandrosterone

Dehydroepiandrosterone (DHEA) is classified as a prohormone. Prohormones are androgenic precursors that become enzymatically converted to testosterone derivatives once ingested and metabolized. Athletes take DHEA in an attempt to improve muscle strength and hypertrophy with fewer side effects than anabolic androgenic steroids. These are often marketed as legal alternatives to testosterone or steps away from testosterone synthesis. DHEA produces androstenedione and androstenediol, both precursors to testosterone synthesis. What the marketers of these supplements do not advertise is that DHEA is also a precursor to estrogen. Estrogen is found in higher levels in females than in males. Higher than normal levels in males may result in undesirable side effects including some female physical characteristics. Some users of DHEA will cycle the use of the compound or stack with other compounds (21, 42).

The limited research in athletes using DHEA, androstenedione, and androstenediol in attempts to improve muscle strength and hypertrophy do not show ergogenic effects. Most do not report a significant rise in testosterone; if such a rise occurred, it was short lived and not relevant, with levels quickly returning to baseline. DHEA, androstenedione, and androstenediol appear on the WADA list of prohibited substances both in and out of competition (21, 42).

COMMON SUPPLEMENTS MARKETED FOR FAT LOSS

Effective weight management requires balancing energy intake (not consuming more calories than burned) over time, but some individuals are looking for a quicker fix. Losing or maintaining weight with diet and exercise is time consuming and both physically and mentally hard for most people. Many supplements claim to ease this burden, promising that weight loss can be greatly improved with consumption of a simple product. In this section we look at the marketing claims made by some of the supplement manufacturers

Caffeine

Research studies reporting the effect of caffeine on weight or fat loss have generally been short term in nature. Another complication in this realm of literature is the fact that caffeine is often combined with other compounds or appears in multi-ingredient products, making it difficult to draw conclusions about caffeine itself. A few of these studies, ranging in length from 45 days to 6 months, reported significantly different weight loss with daily caffeine doses ranging from 192 to over 600 mg (5, 13). Data from a 12-year observational study reported men and women with increased caffeine intake had a weight gain difference of less than 0.5 kg compared to those with lower caffeine intakes (49).

Green Tea

Green tea is a popular beverage containing high levels of polyphenols. Approximately 70 to 80 percent of the polyphenols are catechins, predominately epigallocatechin gallate (EGCG). It is thought that the combination of the naturally occurring caffeine and EGCG might have stimulatory properties that enhance weight or fat loss (6, 9, 33).

Animal research shows green tea might have a role in enhancing fat loss by reducing food intake, reducing the absorption of dietary fat, suppressing or reducing the synthesis of fat, and increasing thermogenesis (energy burned). Human research on this topic is nonhomogeneous because of different doses, nonstandardization of doses in relation to body weight, use of the whole tea leaf rather than the extract, different EGCG content in supplements and brewed tea, other ingredients combined with EGCG (primarily caffeine), and subject compliance to green tea treatment. Given the mixed results in the scientific literature, evidence at this time is insufficient to say that green tea is an effective strategy for weight or fat loss for everyone. Studies show no significant effects on BMI, waist circumference, or body weight (9, 36). However, some studies have shown an increase in energy expenditure over 24 hours, and a few studies demonstrate a statistically significant effect on body weight or fat, though the values are clinically insignificant (6, 7, 9, 32, 33, 36). (This means that even though a difference is evident from a statistical and scientific standpoint, the difference might not be enough to cause noticeable changes.) A meta-analysis that combined the results from 15 randomized controlled trials lasting at least 12 weeks in length found that the combination of green tea catechins and caffeine resulted in small positive effects of green tea consumption on weight loss and weight maintenance (an approximate 1.3–1.4 kg greater weight loss compared to caffeine alone) (33). Other scientific reviews report that green tea catechins mixed with caffeine have positive effects on weight

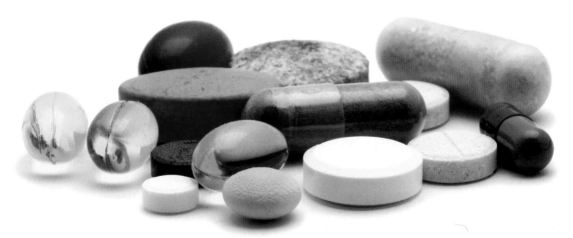

There are many weight loss supplements on the market today; however, there are no weight loss supplements that are both safe and effective.

loss, especially weight maintenance, following energy-restricted weight loss. Mechanisms may include sustained energy expenditure, increased fat oxidation, and preservation of lean body mass. However, it appears that habitual caffeine intake greater than 300 mg per day counteracts some of the effects (36).

If individuals or athletes enjoy the beverage, there is no reason to recommend its discontinuation. There are other health benefits of green tea, including the potential to support heart health (6, 7, 9, 32, 36, 58).

Garcinia Cambogia

Garcinia cambogia is a fruit native to southeastern Asia and is a popular cooking ingredient in southern India. Commercial garcinia cambogia weight-loss supplements contain between 20 and 60 percent hydroxycitric acid (HCA) and might contain other ingredients as well. HCA is found naturally in the rind of the fruit and can be isolated in its free form or synthesized in the laboratory. Both weight reduction and satiety have been reported with HCA consumption in rat studies. Some human trials report desired effects on BMI, body weight, and satiety, yet other studies did not concur. A meta-analysis on the topic concluded that HCA might be more effective for weight loss than placebo, but most of the studies were conducted short term on a small number of subjects. Clinical significance is still to be determined, and long-term effectiveness and safety is unknown (7, 23, 72).

Citrus Aurantium

Citrus aurantium is native to tropical Asia and found also in other tropical regions. Because the fruit tastes sour or bitter, it is also called "bitter orange." In 2004, the FDA issued a regulation prohibiting the sale of ephedra-containing dietary supplements in the United States. In response, supplement companies found a need for an alternative product to fill the void in weight-loss supplements. Citrus aurantium contains alkaloids that are adrenergic agonists and phytochemicals that are thought to work similarly to ephedra. A key alkaloid with potential weight-loss properties is synephrine, which is thought to decrease

food intake through reduced gastric motility and increased energy expenditure. Rodent studies have demonstrated reduced food intake with citrus aurantium or synephrine intake. Human studies show citrus aurantium can increase resting metabolic rate, but this doesn't translate to significant weight loss (57, 75, 76). While some limited research suggests that citrus aurantium is safe (75), other studies report side effects of hypertension, diarrhea, nausea, vomiting, cramps, headaches, insomnia, anxiety, and flu-like symptoms. One complication with reported side effects is that most dietary supplements contain many ingredients along with the citrus aurantium, so it is difficult to pinpoint the side effects to one ingredient (7, 57, 75, 76).

Conjugated Linolenic Acid

Conjugated linolenic acid (CLA) is a fatty acid found naturally in the milk and meat of cows, sheep, and goats and is considered an umbrella term for several different types of fats that are similar in chemical structure. There are about 20 different chemical configurations of CLA, called isomers, and each isomer may have a different physiological effect on the body. CLA contains double bonds that are most abundant in positions 9, 10, 11, and 12 along the carbon chain, and these numbers are used partially to describe the form. Forms of CLAs can be further named depending on whether the functional chemical group is on the same side of the carbon chain (called cis) or on the opposite side of the carbon chain (called trans). For example, one form of the supplement that you may see in a weight-loss product could be called the cis-12, trans-10 isomer.

Research in various animal models has demonstrated that CLA delivers promising results for body fat loss, but these results have not extended to studies on humans. Human studies report mixed results; those that did report positive effects on weight loss or body composition were unconvincing and not clinically important (i.e., the amount of weight lost was too small to matter much). Most of the studies used between 3 and 6 grams per day, a dosage that appears safe for consumption. Long-term safety and efficacy are still in question (23, 48). In human studies, supplementation with both isomers of CLA increased insulin resistance (insulin resistance can increase sugar build-up in the bloodstream, which can be dangerous and over time lead to type 2 diabetes). Randomized, double-blind, placebo-controlled studies show CLA supplementation has an adverse effect on insulin and glucose metabolism in adults with type 2 diabetes (52) and increases insulin resistance in obese men with metabolic syndrome (69). CLA increased insulin resistance and lipid peroxidation compared to placebo in obese men (69). Both DHA and flaxseed oil helped reduce or prevent CLA-induced insulin resistance in animal studies (39, 99). It is not clear if omega-3 fatty acids can attenuate CLA-induced insulin resistance in humans. When examining any scientific studies on the efficacy of CLA on weight or fat loss, it is important to pay attention to the isomer that was used in the study as different isomers may have different effects, especially in different species used in the research model.

Chromium Picolinate

Chromium is an essential trace element that plays a role in carbohydrate, protein, and fat metabolism. It is a cofactor required for insulin action and so is marketed for improving glucose metabolism and insulin resistance. Chromium picolinate, the form of chromium commonly found in dietary supplements, stimulates the neurotransmitters that play a role in food cravings, mood, and eating behavior. It is theorized that chromium may result in appetite suppression and increased thermogenesis (energy expenditure as well as improved insulin). Research studies investigated doses of chromium picolinate ranging from 200 to 1,000 µg taken daily for 6 weeks to 8 months by obese and overweight people (as defined by a BMI greater than or equal to 25) and, at best, those taking the supplement lost an average of 1.1 kg more than those taking a placebo, though there was no correlation between the amount of chromium taken and the amount of weight lost.

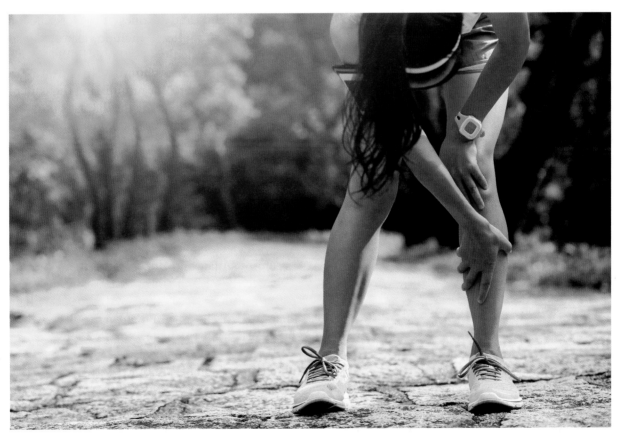

Some supplements may help alleviate joint pain as a result of years of repetitive motion.

These were short-term studies and are not considered good evidence of clinical significance. Overall, this supplement appears well tolerated, but reports of weakness, dizziness, headaches, nausea, and vomiting have been reported in clinical trials (23, 57, 60, 65, 81).

Chitosan and Glucomannan

Chitosan is a polysaccharide believed to bind with dietary fat in the GI tract and thus enhance weight loss. Research in mice has demonstrated reduced food intake with chitosan supplementation. Some human research studies have reported greater weight loss, but other studies report no effect of chitosan consumption on fecal fat excretion. These early trials have been criticized for their poor quality (38, 64). More recent research studies of better quality did not support a large weight-loss effect, and these authors concluded that weight loss from chitosan ingestion was clinically irrelevant. Side effects are not considered serious but include gas, bloating, GI upset, and possibly constipation (23, 38, 57).

Glucomannan is a water-soluble dietary fiber derived from konjac root (Amorphophallus konjac) that might act in the stomach and intestines by absorbing water. This increased bulk can provide a feeling of satiety and thus reduce energy intake (61). Most research studies used a dose between 2 and 4 grams per day. Examination of results from several published trials do not support statistically significant weight loss with supplementation. More studies are needed before conclusions can be made. As with chitosan, side effects can be uncomfortable, including GI stress with loose stools or diarrhea. Some tablets might be difficult to swallow, yet this has not been reported with capsule or powdered forms (57, 61, 103, 104).

COMMON SUPPLEMENTS FOR GENERAL HEALTH

Some supplements are clearly marketed toward a particular sport or type of activity, while others might have an appeal and application to a broader audience. Many of these supplements claim to improve physical health, and any benefits might also apply to the physically active adult or competitive athlete.

Glucosamine and Chondroitin

Osteoarthritis is a degenerative joint disease caused by wear and tear of cartilage tissue from excess body weight (one of the top causes), mechanical stress through repetitive motion (running up and down a field for years), and oxidative damage and inflammatory responses from the anabolic-catabolic balance of the joint, synovium, matrix, and chondrocytes (all parts of the working joint). While some people get this condition later in life as a result of age, many athletes and active individuals are at risk because of the volume of training that accompanies many sports (25). Many individuals seek pain medications, particularly nonsteroidal anti-inflammatory drugs (NSAIDs, such as ibuprofen or aspirin) to decrease their symptoms, but over time NSAIDs can lead to a number of side effects, including stomach pain and ulcers (that might lead to bleeding), heartburn, headaches, and dizziness. For those allergic to NSAIDs, side effects include rashes, throat swelling, and difficulty breathing (100).

Glucosamine and chondroitin sulfate are popular supplements for minimizing the pain of osteoarthritis and delaying the disease's progression. Glucosamine is a naturally occurring amino sugar found in meat, fish, and poultry and made by cartilage cells. It is used as a building block of the cartilage matrix. Chondroitin sulfate is a type of protein present in cartilage. Research on this topic examines outcomes of reduction in pain and decreased joint space narrowing (more narrow spaces mean less cartilage to cushion joints). Glucosamine sulfate and glucosamine hydrochloride help rebuild the cartilage matrix and decrease activity of an enzyme that damages tissue. Sulfate is a source of the essential nutrient sulfur, which is important for cartilage (35).

Current research suggests 1,500 mg a day of glucosamine sulfate combined with 500 mg a day of chondroitin might help with symptoms of pain and improve cartilage growth or maintenance at the joint (25).

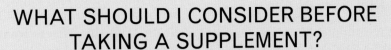

WHAT SHOULD I CONSIDER BEFORE TAKING A SUPPLEMENT?

There are many other factors to think about when deciding whether to take a supplement, or which one to take. Here are some questions to consider:

> Do you have a diagnosed nutrient deficiency? If so, you should be under the care of a qualified health care practitioner. A supplement may or may not be the answer. Sometimes a nutrient deficiency can be corrected through medical nutrition therapy.

> Do a product's claims sound too good to be true? Do they sound exaggerated or unrealistic? If so, research the product thoroughly before purchasing it.

> Are a product's claims only from testimonials? If so, use reason before believing these claims.

> Can you not find any data regarding a product's safety? Note that no news is not always good news. Lack of scientific evidence of harm does not mean the product is safe. It might mean only that no research is available.

Probiotics and Prebiotics

The human gut provides about 70 to 80 percent of our immune protection, acting as a physical barrier and interacting with gut-associated lymphoid tissue, which protects the body from invasion of foreign cells (45). It is normal to have bacteria in the gastrointestinal tract, called gut flora, and the goal in using probiotics is to modify the gut flora so that the number of beneficial bacteria increases while reducing the number of potentially harmful ones. Probiotics are live microorganisms, which when administered in adequate amounts should confer a health benefit. However, research is not clear on what constitutes adequate amounts, and the amount may be different for every individual. The most common species are Lactobacillus and Bifidobacterium. A probiotic should be nonpathogenic (contain only good, healthy bacteria, not harmful ones), be resistant to processing (gastric juices, bile), colonize intestinal epithelial tissue (increase the number of good bacteria in the gut), and provide measurable benefit. Probiotics are sold in many forms, including capsules, powders, and fermented dairy products (26, 67).

Research is evolving on the effectiveness of probiotics in the general population and use may be of interest among athletes. Specific species and strains can support immune health, vaginal health, incidence and duration of diarrhea in infants or adults, gut transit time (how fast food moves through the gut), and other functioning. A small number of studies report certain species and strains promote health in athletes and trained individuals. The most commonly reported benefits in this population include reduced incidence and duration of respiratory and GI illness during periods of heavy training load and stress. In reviewing the published research, a limiting factor is that different strains are used in the scientific literature, as well as differing durations of the supplementation. This makes it difficult to compare studies and make generalizations based on research findings (22, 67).

A prebiotic is an ingredient that targets the microbiota (bacteria) already present within the gut, acting as a "food" for the target microbes. Prebiotics are not digested until they reach the colon, where they become fermented. Foods containing prebiotics include yogurt, kefir, kombucha, raw sauerkraut, barley, bananas, oats, wheat, soy bean, asparagus, leeks, chicory, artichokes, garlic, and onions. Like probiotics, some research suggests prebiotic consumption might help athletes reduce their risk of developing respiratory and GI illnesses during periods of heavy training and psychological stress (22).

DRUGS COMMONLY USED IN SPORTS

While many dietary supplements are readily available and legal for use and purchase, other substances are not legal. In addition to illegal substances, some athletes use alcohol in attempts to improve performance outcomes. These products are not only potentially problematic for competition eligibility but also have negative impacts on overall health.

Stimulants

The most commonly used prohibited stimulant-based drugs are amphetamine and its derivatives, D-methamphetamine and methylphenidate. These drugs are used in medical settings for specific purposes, yet athletes turn to them for their purported ability to increase energy and concentration, and thereby enhance performance. They might also be used in some weight-class sports as a means of reducing body weight and fat. Prohibited stimulants tend to produce significant side effects in both the central nervous and cardiovascular systems. Use of amphetamines, or related compounds, even when prescribed by a doctor and taken as directed, can cause tremors, tachycardia, jitteriness, and insomnia, and more seriously, myocardial infarction, stroke, and even death. The side effects from methylphenidate include Raynaud phenomenon (feelings of numbness or cold), profuse perspiration, and reduced appetite. Combining stimulants with exercise, or exercise in the heat, can have additional effects that lead to heat illness or heat-illness-related death (30).

Anabolic Androgenic Steroids

In a medical setting, anabolic androgenic steroids (AAS) are used to treat clinical testosterone deficiency. In the world of competitive sports, athletes take these compounds in an attempt to gain skeletal muscle mass. In addition to the banned or prohibited status among sport organizations, many dangerous side effects are associated with their illegal use (i.e., not prescribed by a physician to treat a medical condition) (30), especially since the doses taken may be well beyond the therapeutic level prescribed to treat medical conditions. The most common undesirable side effects include gynecomastia (growth of breasts), testicular atrophy (reduction in

PUTTING IT INTO PERSPECTIVE

IS NATURAL ALWAYS SAFE?

Many people seek natural food and supplement products, assuming they are healthier than their counterparts and safe for consumption—and often this is the case. The FDA does not officially regulate the term "natural," yet in the eyes of the FDA, "natural" means that no artificial or synthetic ingredients have been added (91). However, natural does not guarantee safety. Natural products will be safe for many people, but they can have side effects and might interact with each other or with over-the-counter or prescription drugs. For example, vitamin K interferes with blood-thinning medications, and St. John's wort can speed the breakdown of many drugs (including antidepressants and birth control pills), thereby reducing their effectiveness (66).

In addition, some products labeled as natural might be contraindicated for people with certain diseases or conditions. For example, a joint health supplement may contain natural ingredients such as glucosamine that should be used with caution by people with diabetes or shellfish allergies, and high doses of caffeine can increase heart rate (66). Manufacturers of supplement products might not include warnings about potential adverse effects or list those persons who should not use the supplement. The general recommendation is not to take any supplement unless you are certain it will not aggravate a preexisting condition or interact adversely with any other medication or supplement you are already taking. Of course such certainty is hard to come by. If you feel the need to take a supplement with unknown contraindications or side effects, always start with small doses and be sure your physician and pharmacist know you are taking it.

testicle mass), and widespread acne, especially on the chest and back. More significant side effects affect the cardiovascular system, including increases in total cholesterol and LDL cholesterol and reductions in high-density lipoprotein cholesterol. Further, in some instances, illegal or unsupervised use of AAS use can lead to liver damage, accelerated puberty, and stunted growth in young people. Women have additional, sometimes irreversible, side effects of dysfunction in menses, male-pattern hair growth or alopecia, voice deepening, and clitoris enlargement. Some athletes will use multiple forms of AAS and a cycling pattern of use to minimize side effects. They might also use other drugs concurrently in attempt to counteract side effects. Athletes must fully understand the legal implications, competition eligibility issues, and most important, the many health risks associated with AAS use (30).

Human Growth Hormone

Human growth hormone (hGH) is naturally released in the body, with its highest secretion during the adolescent growth spurt. Deep sleep, heat stress, hypoglycemia, and exercise stimulate endogenous release. Human growth hormone in its natural form requires a prescription and is intended to treat a limited number of medical conditions, including short stature, Turner syndrome, Prader-Willi syndrome, muscle wasting from AIDS, and growth hormone deficiency. Prescription and distribution of this drug is tightly regulated. Taking hGH for nonlegitimate medical reasons (e.g., to enhance performance or for anti-aging benefits) while not under the supervision of a licensed physician or medical practitioner permitted to prescribe these substances might be illegal. Some athletes use hGH in an attempt to improve cardiorespiratory fitness, increase skeletal muscle mass, reduce fat mass, or recover more

quickly from injury. The side effects associated with hGH are numerous, including depression, fluid retention, and with long-term use, acromegaly (chronic elevated levels of hGH in the body). Symptoms of acromegaly include swelling and subsequent abnormal growth of the hands and feet; overgrowth of bone in the face (protruding of the brow and lower jaw, enlargement of the nasal bone, and spacing of the teeth); carpal tunnel syndrome; and enlargement of body organs, including the heart. Still other symptoms might include joint pain; coarse, oily skin; skin tags; enlarged lips, nose, and tongue; voice deepening; sleep apnea; excessive sweating and foul odor; fatigue and weakness; headaches; impaired vision; decreased libido; erectile dysfunction in men; and menstrual cycle abnormalities or breast discharge in women. Many of these symptoms develop with long-term use and elevated hGH levels. Currently, it remains unclear whether higher doses over a shorter time, as used by some athletes, would result in the same level of side effects (17, 30).

ALCOHOL USE

Athletes choose to use alcohol for a variety of reasons, from the perception of "taking the edge off" to social acceptance and team building. While prevalence of alcohol consumption is similar in the athletic and general populations, its use is especially popular in the college setting during weekend festivities and celebrations associated with team success. The NCAA has cited alcohol as the most abused drug in collegiate sport (4). Recent research suggests college athletes associate alcohol consumption with an enhanced sense of well-being and that social drinking helps build group identification (106).

While the research on the effects on performance of low to moderate alcohol intake preexercise or during exercise is inconclusive, detrimental effects on athletic performance have

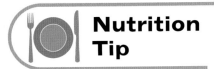

Nutrition Tip   The FDA and the National Institutes of Health's Office of Dietary Supplements provide research-based information about dietary supplements. If you are considering taking a supplement, visit the websites of these government organizations for basic information and useful tips.

been reported (11, 80). For example, alcohol might negatively affect metabolism, thermoregulation, motor skills, and mental concentration. Some of these negative effects might persist for hours after consumption. Alcohol likely impairs endurance performance through impairment of gluconeogenesis, glucose uptake, and glucose use. A recent study examined the effects of alcohol consumption on rates of skeletal muscle protein synthesis after an acute exercise bout and reported reduced rates even when the alcohol was coingested with protein (62). This would likely result in slowed recovery and repair and growth of tissue (4, 11, 16, 80).

Overconsumption of alcohol can lead to alcohol-related illness or death. This is of increasing concern among college students, as excess alcohol consumption can lead to undesirable consequences. It is estimated that over 1,800 college students die from alcohol-related unintentional injuries each year (56). A relation is also suspected between alcohol use and suicidal tendencies among students (46). In addition, alcohol-related physical and sexual assaults have affected over 690,000 and 97,000 college students, respectively. Approximately 25 percent of college students report suffering negative academic consequences related to drinking alcohol, such as missing classes, exams, papers, and falling behind (56).

Postexercise nutrient intake is critical for optimal recovery for athletes. While alcohol is not a nutrient, it does contain energy (approximately 7 kcal/g). Postexercise is the time when an athlete should be focusing on rehydration, adequate repletion of glycogen with carbohydrate sources, and maximizing skeletal muscle protein synthesis with dietary protein intake. If time after training is spent consuming alcohol instead of nutrients, recovery can be compromised (11, 62, 80).

SUMMARY

Dietary supplements are defined and regulated by the FDA, and advertising is regulated by the FTC. Supplements are regulated differently from food additives and drugs. FDA standards govern Supplement Facts labels and the claims that manufacturers are allowed to make about a product. Allowable claims can be categorized into three groups: nutrient content, health, and structure/function claims. Nutrient content claims refer to the amount of a given nutrient in a product, whereas health claims describe a relation between a nutrient and disease. Both of these types of claim are approved by the FDA. Structure/function claims are not approved by the FDA and require a disclaimer about the product.

Some sports organizations have lists of banned substances that are prohibited of participants; other sport groups do not impose such regulations. Several professional organizations or certification programs are available to help a person navigate this issue and the process of certifying products that are sold to the consumer. Some dietary supplements may enhance performance or body composition, and others do not. While there are hundreds of supplements on the market, it might be easiest to classify them into categories such as those for endurance sports, strength and muscle growth, and weight management. A greater quantity of research data is available for some supplements compared to others. For example, some science supports the use of caffeine as an ergogenic aid in endurance sports and creatine for strength-training gains. While research is always emerging in this field, not all supplements have the same amount of research to support use or refute claims.

Supplements presented in this chapter might perform as claimed, but that does not imply endorsement by this textbook. Athletes or others interested in using supplements should analyze the cost-to-benefit ratio and seek professional guidance when needed. The potential physiological benefits or performance gains of a product need to be weighed against potential disadvantages and should then be used only after evaluation for safety, efficacy, and compliance with relevant anti-doping codes and legal requirements. When supplements are used, the regimen should be fitted to the individual's needs and goals.

■ FOR REVIEW ⟩

1. Why do athletes choose to use dietary supplements?
2. How are dietary supplements regulated?
3. What are the three categories of claims used on dietary supplements, and how do they differ?
4. What are a few considerations when exploring the use of dietary supplements?
5. What is peer-reviewed scientific evidence?
6. Explain the seals used on supplement labels. What do they mean?
7. Which organizations provide information about banned substances?
8. For the following supplements, list the popular claim, purported mechanism of action for performance improvement, and the overall impression of safety and efficacy:
   - Caffeine
   - Sodium bicarbonate
   - Glycerol
   - Nitrate
   - Creatine
   - Beta-alanine
   - HMB
   - DHEA
   - Green tea
   - Garcinia cambogia
   - Citrus aurantium
   - CLA
   - Chromium picolinate
   - Chitosan
9. Why would athletes use pre- and probiotic supplements?
10. Describe the negative aspects of using stimulants, anabolic androgenic steroids, and alcohol in sport.

PART IV

APPLICATION OF NUTRITION FOR SPORT, EXERCISE, AND HEALTH

The final section of this book includes information on applying sports nutrition principles. This section covers ideal body weight and composition for health and athletic performance and presents different assessment methods to estimate body composition. Nutrition for aerobic training and sports (chapter 11) brings the information conveyed in chapter 2 full circle by giving specific examples of fueling for endurance sports. Chapter 12 covers the principles behind before, during, and postresistance exercise nutrition, as well as overall diet and how this impacts training gains. Supplements specific for resistance training are also covered. The following chapter outlines strategies to achieve optimal body composition, including decreasing fat and gaining muscle for recreational and competitive athletes. The principles behind these dietary strategies are also discussed. Finally, chapter 14 covers how to work with active individuals who fall into special populations and have unique nutrition needs.

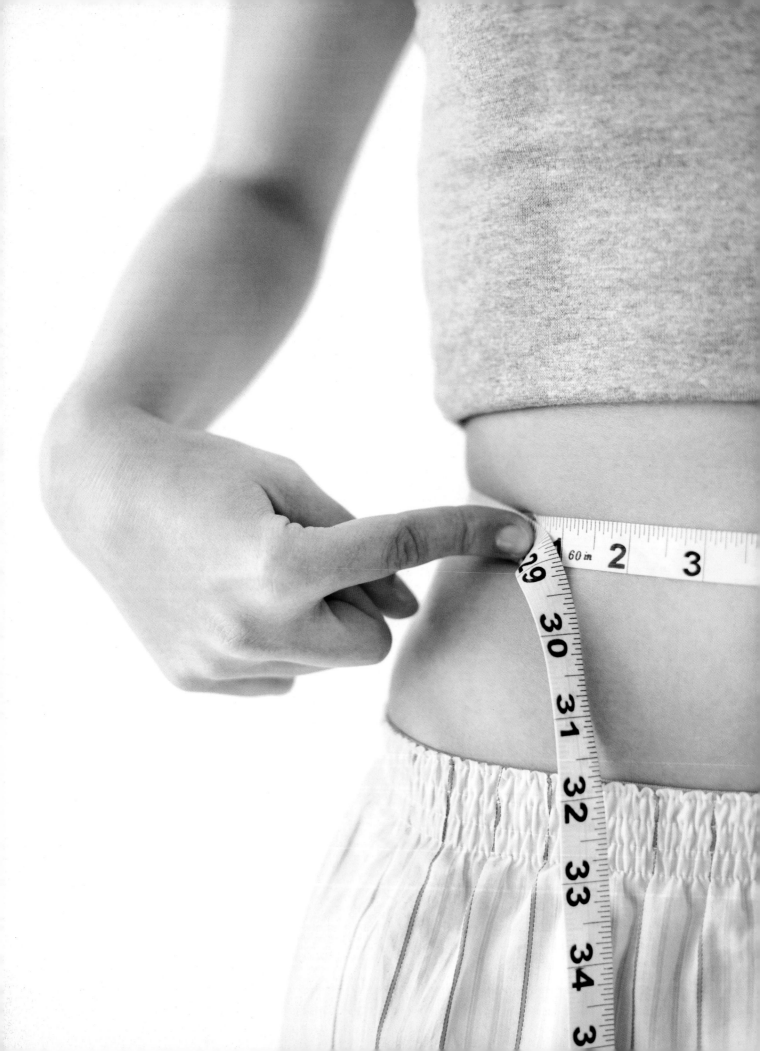

CHAPTER 10

Body Weight and Composition

▶ CHAPTER OBJECTIVES

After completing this chapter, you will be able to do the following:

> Explain the difference between body weight and body composition.

> Explain how body weight and body composition affect sports performance.

> Describe the compartments of the body as they pertain to body composition.

> Discuss the genetic and environmental factors that contribute to body composition.

> Discuss the principles behind the common methods of body composition assessment.

> Explain how to interpret body composition estimates.

Health organizations use different terms to describe the composition of the human body. Some terms refer to the absolute size of the body (e.g., body weight or mass), whereas other terms assess the body's composition, or relative amounts of muscle, fat, bone, and water in the body. It is important to distinguish between the size and composition of the body because they tend to have far different impacts on human health. Excess body weight, caused by high body fat, is dangerous. Lean body mass, which is comprised primarily of muscle, bone, and water, is healthier than adipose tissue, especially when present in large quantities in the body.

The conditions termed "overweight" and "obesity" increase a person's risk of morbidity from hypertension; dyslipidemia coronary heart disease; gallbladder disease; stroke; type 2 diabetes; sleep apnea; osteoarthritis; respiratory problems; and endometrial, breast, prostate, and colon cancers. In fact, the U.S. Centers for Disease Control and Prevention (CDC) has declared modern American culture to be "obesogenic" in nature, meaning that the normal "way of life" causes Americans to be fatter and heavier than ideal. The American culture promotes excessive intake of unhealthy, **energy-dense foods** and makes it very easy to be habitually physically inactive (5). Body weight that is higher than what is considered healthy for a given height is described as over-weight or obese (6). More specifically, **overweight** means that one weighs more on a scale than the healthy reference standard, whereas being obese means that one is carrying a higher percentage of body fat than what is desirable within the healthy reference standard. Sixty-nine percent of adults over 20 years of age are overweight, and 35 percent of these people are obese. Weight management is undeniably a challenge for many Americans, including sedentary, moderately active, and even competitive athletes (5, 6).

In 2013, the American Medical Association (AMA) presented a report classifying **obesity** as a disease and basing the diagnosis on having a body mass index (described later in the chapter) above $30 kg/m^2$ (3). Their position is that classifying obesity as a disease will help the way that medical professionals address it with their patients. Other professional groups have published arguments against classifying obesity as a disease because they believe that it is only a risk factor for other diseases and by diagnosing this in the large number of individuals who are obese could result in more health care costs from drugs and surgeries. Their position is that by labeling an obese person as having a diagnosed illness would promote a drug or surgical intervention rather than lifestyle change. Furthermore, there are imperfections in using body mass index to classify a person as obese (14, 27).

OBESITY AND INFLAMMATION

Chronic inflammation is an underlying factor in several diseases, including obesity. Fat tissue pumps out inflammatory compounds. There is a theory that as white adipose tissue (WAT) increases, it shifts from an anti-inflammatory or neutral tissue to one that is proinflammatory. WAT secretes proteins called adipokines. It is believed that normal-sized adipocytes secrete anti-inflammatory molecules, whereas full adipocytes (seen with weight gain) secrete proinflammatory molecules. As overweight and obesity increases over time, there may be a shift to an overall proinflammatory state (1). Overweight and obese individuals may also have altered gut flora, with more harmful bacteria and less beneficial bacteria as compared to those of normal weight. This condition might also contribute to higher levels of inflammation. Note that this is a new area of research. The current evidence suggests that it is the actual adipose tissue that contributes most to inflammation (1).

FACTORS CONTRIBUTING TO BODY WEIGHT AND COMPOSITION

Both genetic and environmental factors contribute to the accumulation of body fat. Humans are born with a tendency to store body fat in amounts that are predetermined by our genetic makeup. Genetics influence where fat is deposited on the body, as well as muscularity; this does not mean, however, that our ultimate body shape and size are completely outside our control. We have the ability to shape our environment by adopting healthy eating behaviors, exercising regularly, and engaging in activities of daily living. This can be difficult because, as consumers, we are inundated with an abundance of inexpensive, energy-dense foods and many jobs that, although mentally exhausting at times, demand little physical exertion. Successfully overcoming the temptation to be physically inactive and to overeat or choose unhealthy food requires a level of discipline that escapes many people. This is unfortunate because our food selections and level and type of physical training ultimately determine how close to our genetic potential we become. A tiny percent of the population has a genetic condition that makes it extremely challenging to achieve and maintain a body weight and composition that promotes health and well-being (29).

Genetic Factors

Genetics contribute to our height, weight, body fat distribution, and metabolism, regardless of our environment. Identical twins raised in different households have been found to have similar body weights to one another, while children of adopted parents have been shown to more closely resemble the body types of their biological parents than their adoptive parents. In addition to body weight and fat distribution, children also tend to inherit specific body types, such as being tall and thin or short and stout. This is important to remember when setting body composition-related goals because some ideals might be unattainable no matter how hard one trains or how disciplined they are about food choices. For example, a very tall and thin person might never be able to put on enough muscle mass to be a bodybuilder, nor may a very muscular, stocky person ever achieve extreme leanness and become an elite runner (29).

Another area of active research that suggests a genetic component to body weight and fatness is known as the **set point theory**, which proposes that the brain, hormones, and enzymes work together to regulate body weight and fat at a genetically predetermined level that solidifies sometime during young adulthood. This theory surmises that any attempt to voluntarily change body weight from the set point initiates a series of physiological and metabolic responses that ultimately result in no further loss of body fat, or a plateau. These responses may include storing fat more efficiently, decreasing metabolism, or stimulating appetite (29).

Environmental Factors

Environment plays a significant role in body weight regulation. Although genetic factors limit what can be accomplished, healthy behaviors and choices, such as choosing the correct foods and portion sizes and getting sufficient quantity and quality of exercise; activities of daily living; and learning behavioral modification and self-monitoring techniques certainly can help maximize genetic potential. Poor food choices are often learned behaviors that can become lifelong habits. Over time, new habits can be established by building on small, positive changes. Although athletes might seem more disciplined than the general population, they too struggle with food choices, as a result of many factors, including limitations in financial resources, lack of knowledge about nutrition, need for convenience, and preferences for certain foods (29).

BODY WEIGHT AND COMPOSITION CONCERNS IN ACTIVITY AND SPORT

Many competitive athletes are young and do not have long-term health consequences at the forefront of their minds. However, it is important for athletes to strike a balance between weight for optimal performance and for long-term health. Instead, immediate performance outcomes are often the focus. Similarly, some individuals are new to activities, such as cycling or running races, and want to commit to short-term goals that enable them to complete an event. Like the general public, some athletes also face the struggle of needing to decrease or maintain an ideal weight and body composition for optimal performance. Many athletes have **body image** concerns, especially those in sports in which they might be "judged" on aesthetics and performance, such as gymnastics, figure skating, and physique sports (including bodybuilding, bikini, and fitness competitions).

Most athletes who are concerned about weight management are either overweight or obese and want to reduce their body fat levels to conform to healthy values, or they are already normal weight, or even lean, and want to further reduce body fat and increase lean mass for either aesthetic or performance reasons. Body weight and composition are somewhat easily manipulated and thus tend to be target areas of change when considering certain sports or activities. Many active people place a huge emphasis on body weight, making the assumption that body weight is an absolute predictor of athletic performance. While weight and fat can certainly play a role in athletic success, no one weight or percent fat level is indicative of positive outcomes (28). It is important that athletes seeking weight or fat loss do so safely as to not jeopardize their health or physiological function. Fortunately, the well-established weight-management principles that hold for the general population also apply to athletes and active individuals (20).

It is not uncommon for many athletes to fluctuate in weight throughout a year, depending on whether they are in the off-season, training season, or competition period. For most athletes, the competition period is when body fat is the lowest, but this level might be hard to maintain throughout the other periods. Too much fluctuation is not the best situation for the athlete because it sometimes requires more extreme measures to obtain and maintain the ideal competition weight. Ideally, an athlete would have a healthy body weight that could be maintained for much of the year, with slight adjustments during increased training in preparation for competition. Extreme chronic dieting or repeatedly losing and gaining significant amounts of weight can be an indicator that the athlete is trying to achieve an unrealistic body weight (20).

Different sports and activities differ significantly in the body composition that might affect performance outcomes. For some sports or activities, skeletal muscle size and shape might be the target, while others might require a balance of strength and power for movement. Many sports have weight classes for competition and require competitors to achieve a delicate balance of the lowest possible body weight while maximizing skeletal mass and power (28).

On the opposite side of the spectrum, it is disadvantageous to be overweight or overfat in many sports because it is physiologically inefficient to carry the extra mass. In some sports, such as long-distance running and cycling, a lower body mass can contribute positively to

PUTTING IT INTO PERSPECTIVE

NEGATIVE CONSEQUENCES OF YO-YO DIETING

The term "yo-yo dieting" has been used to describe a situation in which a person goes on a diet to lose weight only to gain that same weight back. Such diets are often fads that call for eliminating key food groups in an attempt to reduce energy (calorie consumption). They usually promote quick weight loss, and many have a defined period of time. Once the individual completes the diet, the weight is gained back—sometimes even more weight returns than was originally lost. Lean body mass is often lost during these diets, yet primarily fat is gained back. Ultimately, such diets do not maintain a healthy body composition, nor do they teach lifelong healthy eating habits. Competitive athletes, and others, might succumb to such methods with the intention of losing weight for improved performance. However, losing weight in an unhealthy fashion can be detrimental to performance.

efficiency in energy expenditure and improved heat dissipation. For bodybuilders or those in physique competitions, low levels of body fat are required in that participants are judged on their aesthetic appearance. Some individuals, such as gymnasts and acrobatic performers, require a body composition that optimizes biomechanical movement. In contrast, being too thin or too lean might negatively affect both performance and long-term health. For most athletes, it is desirable to have a higher percentage of lean mass with a lower percentage of body fat. While some optimal body composition ranges are presented later in the chapter, there is no one ideal body fat target associated with optimal performance in any given sport or activity (28). Chapter 13 provides a detailed discussion on achieving optimal body composition.

Body Mass Index

Body weight is different from **body mass index (BMI)**. **Body weight** or **body mass** is how much a person weighs on a scale and is usually expressed in pounds or kilograms. With a calibrated scale, this can be measured with great accuracy. BMI was originally created to access population-based rates of obesity.

BMI uses both body weight and height to classify people into four subclasses: underweight, normal, overweight, and obese. See table 10.1 for the classification and table 10.2 to determine how to calculate BMI (4, 5, 6, 12). BMI correlates with body fatness in most people, but it is not an actual measure of body fat (10, 30), nor is it a measure of visceral fat, the kind of fat stored in the abdomen and covering internal organs, including the liver, pancreas, and intestines (25). BMI cannot distinguish between excess fat and muscle or bone mass. BMI can overestimate fatness in athletes with higher lean body mass and therefore shouldn't be used with this population (8, 17, 31). In thin children, BMI is a better measure of fat-free versus fat mass (9). Age, sex, ethnicity, and muscle mass affect the association between BMI and body fat in both children and adults. BMI can overestimate body fat in athletes and others with

Table 10.1 BMI Classification

BMI (kg/m²)	Classification
Below 18.5	Underweight
18.5–24.9	Normal or healthy
25.0–29.9	Overweight
30–34.9	Obesity class I
35.0–39.9	Obesity class II
≥40	Obesity class III (extremely obese)

Table 10.2 Determining BMI

Measurement units	Formula and sample calculation
Kilograms and meters (or centimeters)	*Formula:* weight (kg) / (height [m])]² With the metric system, the formula for BMI is weight in kilograms divided by height in meters, squared. Because height is commonly measured in centimeters, divide height in centimeters by 100 to obtain height in meters. *Example:* weight = 68 kg, height = 165 cm (1.65 m) *Calculation:* $68 \div (1.65)^2 = 24.98$
Pounds and inches	*Formula:* weight (lb.) / [height (in.)]² × 703 Calculate BMI by dividing weight in pounds by height in inches squared and multiplying by a conversion factor of 703. *Example:* weight = 150 lb., height = 5'5" (65 in.) *Calculation:* $[150 \div (65)^2] \times 703 = 24.96$

muscular builds and underestimate body fat in older persons or those who have lost muscle (21).

A BMI between 18.5 and 24.9 kg/m² is considered a normal or healthy body weight. BMI within this range is associated with the lowest risk of developing a chronic disease or death. Those classified as overweight might have an increased risk of disease and death, and those who are obese have the highest risk of developing a number of diseases, including cardiovascular diseases and type 2 diabetes. BMI is a useful initial screening tool to help identify individuals who might be overweight or obese. BMI is also used to track population-based rates of overweight and obesity. However, BMI should not be used in isolation to determine health, disease, or disease risk (21). A disadvantage in using BMI is that it does not specifically differentiate between body weight and amount of body fat. Thus, BMI overestimates fat in those with high muscle mass. For example, a very muscular male athlete with low body fat could have a BMI that classifies him as overweight or obese. His weight would be higher than expected for his height, though he is not overfat, and thus not at a higher risk for disease based on body composition. If the BMI is 25 kg/m² or greater, it is important to determine whether weight loss should be the goal. Since BMI is associated with increased risk of developing certain chronic diseases, perhaps current body fat levels along with any medical laboratory values can be an indicator as whether weight loss is warranted. If an athletic person with large, defined musculature has a high BMI value, then BMI may not be the best tool for estimating level of body fatness. In such situations, having body composition (percent body fat) measured might be of value, although these techniques require the assistance of a qualified exercise professional (6).

Body Fat Patterns

In addition to body weight, the amount and placement of body fat can influence health and performance. Levels of body fat can rise as a result of adipose cell **hyperplasia** (growing more fat cells) or by cell **hypertrophy** (growth of existing cells). Given a state of chronic positive energy balance, the ability to store body fat is limitless. Whether there is a stage in life at which hyperplasia predominates over hypertrophy is controversial, but most agree that both ultimately occur as a result of chronic positive energy balance (24).

People have different body shapes, characterized by three types: ectomorph, mesomorph, and endomorph. Individuals can either be predominately one of the three shapes or fall somewhere between two shapes. In addition to body shape, there are also differences in body fat patterning. Overweight individuals who carry a majority of their weight around the middle fall into the **android** type, or "apple shaped." Such a person tends to have both subcutaneous (just beneath the skin) and visceral (deep) body fat, with the amount in each area varying from person to person. This shape—specifically, the larger amount of visceral body fat—increases the risk of developing chronic diseases caused by a multitude of factors, one being fat surrounding vital organs. Those who carry weight in their hips, thighs, and

---

PUTTING IT INTO PERSPECTIVE

HOW TO ESTIMATE A DESIRED BODY WEIGHT FROM BMI

What if your BMI is higher than the healthy BMI range? First, you need to determine if the BMI is high because of excess body fat or because you're a very muscular person. If you feel excess body fat is the culprit, you can use your current BMI to calculate a desired weight to allow you to move to the healthy BMI range. Simply take your height in inches squared and multiply it by the desired BMI (e.g., 24). Then divide by 703.

Example: A person weighs 180 lb. and is 5'5" tall. Current BMI is 30. The desired BMI is 24. 4,225 × 24 = 101,400. 101,400 ÷ 703 = 144 lb.

buttocks are called **gynoid**, or "pear shaped." This fat is usually predominately subcutaneous and not associated with the same risk of developing chronic disease. While the android shape is more common in men and the gynoid in women, this is not always the case (11). See figure 10.1 for a visual demonstration of android versus gynoid obesity patterns.

Taking a measurement of waist circumference is one way to look more closely at body fat patterns. Waist measures of more than 35 inches (88.9 cm) for women or more than 40 inches (101.6 cm) for men classify people as being at increased risk for developing chronic disease. Use of both BMI and waist circumference can be helpful in determining risk of chronic disease or the need for a weight-management intervention (6).

Body Composition

Body composition refers to the components that make up the body. While there are a few body composition models in the scientific literature, the one most commonly discussed in sports nutrition is the four-compartment model. In this model, the body is compartmentalized into body fat and lean body mass (LBM), sometimes referred to as fat-free mass (FFM). Fat-free mass includes everything except body fat. Organs, muscle, tendons, ligaments, bones, and skin are all part of fat-free mass. While FFM contains no body lipids, LBM contains a small amount of essential body lipids. LBM is further compartmentalized into skeletal muscle mass, total body water, and bone mass.

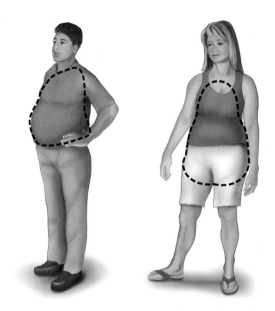

Figure 10.1 The android shape describes people who carry more body fat in their upper body, specifically the abdominal region. The gynoid shape describes people who carry more body fat in the lower part of their body, specifically the hips, buttocks, and thighs.

Any of these four components can change through diet or training interventions. Body water changes can occur very rapidly, while changes in bone mass take several months. Most athletes tend to focus on manipulating their body fat and skeletal muscle mass to achieve a body that is desirable for aesthetics, performance, or both (11).

PUTTING IT INTO PERSPECTIVE

HOW DO I MEASURE MY WAIST CIRCUMFERENCE?

> In a standing position, place the tape measure horizontally near your belly button, just above your hip bones.
> Measure at the narrowest portion of your waist.
> Make sure the tape is snug but not compressing the skin.
> Take the measurement once you comfortably exhale.
> For additional information on taking waist circumference, visit the Centers for Disease Control and Prevention website (6).

There are different types of body fat, some of which are considered essential, while the rest are considered storage. Essential body fat is a component of many tissues and must be maintained as not to compromise physiological function. Storage fat, however, results from a chronic positive energy balance (too many calories) and can be altered (lost) without a negative impact on physiological function; in fact, a loss will likely improve health if a person is overfat. Essential body fat is approximately 3 percent of body mass for men and 12 percent of body mass for women; body fat percentages lower than these are not optimal for health and physiological functioning. With the rise of obesity in our society, there are not good estimates for "average" body fat values in the current general population. For most healthy adults, the total body fat percentage is between 12 and 15 percent for young men and between 25 and 28 percent for young women (18). Further classification of body fat percentages are listed in table 10.3 (16, 18).

ESTIMATING BODY COMPOSITION

While many techniques give a body composition "value," note that all of these are just estimates. There is no way to measure body composition with 100 percent accuracy in a living human body. All methods used today are based on early research on cadavers (26). Cadaver analysis was used to develop statistically sound prediction equations for body composition, and included in these is a percent error. If a female athlete has her body composition assessed by one of the techniques with a 4 percent margin of error, and she is assessed to have 15 percent body fat, this means her body fat could be anywhere between 11 and 19 percent. While errors are unavoidable, they can be minimized with proper equipment and technique. For example, the equipment must be calibrated, and a standardized operating protocol must be used. If measuring before and after a program or intervention, the same equipment should be used, and in most cases the same operator should take the measurements. Valid and reliable equations should be used to calculate body composition. The athlete being tested might need to follow a protocol that involves being in the same state of feeding or fasting and at a consistent hydration level (not after exercise or sweating). For females, time in the menstrual cycle may need to be consistent, depending on the type and purpose of the measurement. When following protocols for each specific measure of body composition, several methods are useful for assessing baseline body composition level or examining change with training and intervention. Ideal body composition includes a range of values that is individually determined as appropriate for a given individual. Any normative body composition targets should be set as a range of values rather than one number that might be considered ideal (28).

Understanding Compartment Models

Two-, three-, or four-compartment models may be used to estimate body composition. A two-compartment model assumes the body is separated, or "compartmentalized," into fat and LBM.

Table 10.3 Classification of Body Fat Percentages

Males	Females	Classification
2	12	Essential
5–10	8–15	Athletic
11–14	16–23	Good
15–20	24–30	Acceptable
21–24	31–36	Overweight
>24	>36	Obese

Data from Jeukendrup 2010; Lohman and Going 1993.

This model, developed in the 1940s, was based on the inverse relation between body density and body fat. If one can measure body density, then one can estimate body fat from the developed prediction equations. This model has a few assumptions that apply to all individuals, and these assumptions may or may not be true. When estimating body fat from body density, it is assumed that the density of all fat tissue and all LBM tissue is the same for all individuals and that the proportions of the water, muscle, and bone of the LBM are constant within and between all persons. This model is useful for detecting changes in total body fat, though one cannot detect the individual components that comprise total LBM. If body fat decreases and LBM increases, one cannot determine if LBM changes were caused by muscle, bone, or water, so LBM and muscle might be over- or underestimated if there are significant shifts in water content caused by hyper- or hypohydration during measurement. Since bone mass changes can take 6 to 12 months, and are relatively minor, changes in bone do not have an appreciable effect on body composition measures (11).

Since the total body water (TBW) portion of the LBM can change both drastically and rapidly, to adjust for hydration status of an individual, a three-compartment body composition model was proposed in 1961 (26). In this model, the body can be separated into fat and LBM, with an independent assessment of TBW. The methods for assessing TBW with the greatest possible accuracy require a lab setting with radioisotopes where the hydrogen molecules are labeled. This requires the collection of saliva, urine, or blood and might also require a physician, depending on the isotope used and specimens collected. This method is expensive. While some bioelectrical impedance devices estimate TBW, they are not as accurate as isotope-dilution methods (11).

In a four-compartment model, measurements are made for body density (and hence body fat), TBW, and total body bone mineral. The remaining unmeasured component is assumed to be muscle mass. Like the three-compartment model, this model provides enhanced accuracy, but the measurement of more variables results in increased time and cost. Specialized equipment, laboratories, and personnel are needed, so this method is not as common as using the two-compartment model. While the three- and four-compartment models increase accuracy of body composition estimates, they are usually limited to a research setting in sophisticated laboratories. There is a six-compartment model, called the atomic-level model, which is used for validation of some of the common body composition models and techniques, but this model requires extensive research laboratories and is not used outside of the research setting (11).

Choosing a Method

Many factors can influence the choice of a body composition method. While everyone wants the one that is most accurate and convenient, it is not that simple. As mentioned, some methods require specialized equipment and skilled operators and can be quite expensive. Some of the simplest and inexpensive methods lack the desired accuracy. When considering a method, one must factor accuracy, cost, portability, ease of use, and subject comfort.

Recall that all body composition methods are estimates. In the methods described, mathematical equations are used to predict body composition values. The two key statistical methods used in body composition are correlation and regression. Correlation estimates the strength of a relation between two variables, while regression is used to predict one variable from another single or multiple variables. There are often population-specific equations that were developed on a narrow group of people with similar physical characteristics. Generalized equations were developed on a wider range of people and are better suited when used in settings where people might vary in age, gender, ethnicity, fatness, or athletic condition. It is important to know the research behind the published equation to ensure the best equation is used for the population being tested. This might require obtaining the original published article and understanding the application of it for those being measured. Many of the newer automated methods or workplace computer systems may have prediction equations built in and may or may not specify where that equation originated (11).

Using Body Composition Methods

Body composition assessment methods can be categorized as laboratory methods or field methods. Laboratory methods are found in sophisticated research settings. Though they tend to be expensive and sometimes require more in-depth techniques, these methods have the greatest accuracy. Some lab techniques also require additional levels of training, such as radiation safety training or a license to operate equipment. A few of the common techniques include hydrometry, hydrodensitometry, air displacement plethysmography, and dual-energy x-ray absorptiometry. These methods may provide some of the reference values for the derivation of equations used in the more common field methods. Field methods such as anthropometric skinfold thickness and bioelectrical impedance analysis are less accurate but are more convenient and not as expensive (11).

Hydrometry

Hydrometry is a measurement of TBW. In this method, the concentration of labeled isotopes of hydrogen or oxygen equilibrate with bodily fluids, and then samples from saliva, urine, or blood can be taken to estimate TBW. This method is costly, requires specialized lab equipment, trained personnel, and sometimes a physician. This method is not commonly used with athletes in field settings but has been used in research settings with both athletes and nonathletes (11).

Hydrodensitometry

Hydrodensitometry is also referred to as hydrostatic weighing or underwater weighing (UWW). Densitometry is the measurement of body density, and "hydro" means water. In this method, water is used to estimate the body density of an individual. A basic physics principle is applied here: body density = body mass/body volume.

Body mass or weight can be measured with great accuracy. Weighing a person underwater is used to estimate

body volume, and thus body density is derived. An established prediction equation is then used to calculate the percent body fat from the body density. Accuracy of the method will somewhat depend on using a proper prediction equation.

A specialized tank is required to weigh a person who is completely submerged in water. Some tanks use a hanging scale, and some of the better instruments have a scale on the bottom of the tank. The person being assessed must expel as much air as possible from the lungs.

The basic principle behind this technique involves buoyancy. Fat tissue is less dense than water, while LBM is denser than water. The more body fat a person has, the more buoyant they are (they float), and the less they weigh underwater. On the contrary, the leaner a person is, the less buoyant they are (they sink), and they will weigh more underwater. The other factor in the body

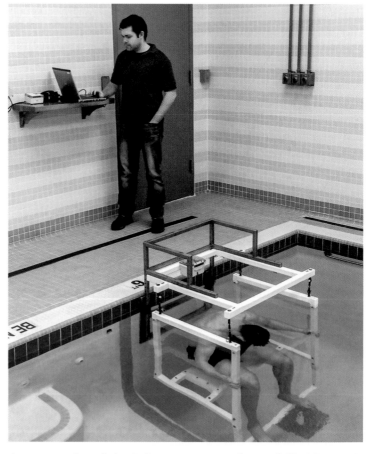

A person fearful of the water may have difficulty with hydrostatic weighing, while good swimmers can usually expel air while submerged.

that contributes to buoyancy is air in the lungs. A person is asked to expel that air while underwater, but completely emptying the lungs is not possible. The air that is left after the attempt to exhale is called residual lung volume. This value must also be measured and factored into the measurement.

One limitation of UWW is the variance in quality of tanks and equipment. A good, accurate system is quite expensive and requires technical skill to administer. While underwater weighing can be used on both lean and morbidly obese individuals (who are mobile), dimension of the tank itself can be the limiting factor. Even under the best of practices, the minimum **standard error of the estimate (SEE)** is ± 3.5 percent (2), and the minimal error published about this method demonstrates a 1 to 2 kg body fat error, or a little over 3 percent body fat in an average person. So, as described earlier, for a calculation resulting in a 15 percent body fat value, the range of possible accuracy would be 12 to 18 percent. If lower quality equipment or an inappropriate prediction equation is used, the error can greatly exceed this estimate (11). Taking the limitations into account, if this procedure is available, it can provide the athlete and his or her coaching staff information about a baseline percent body fat or changes in body fat with training and nutrition intervention.

Air Displacement Plethysmography

Similar to UWW, **air displacement plethysmography (ADP)** estimates body volume and thus body density. Instead of water displacement, air displacement is used. This procedure usually takes less than 10 minutes and requires the subject to sit quietly. The one discomforting factor of this method is that the person is completely enclosed in the machine (although light is available, and a window is usually provided). Like UWW, this equipment is quite expensive and usually limited to lab settings. It might not work well for very small individuals or children, and since the chamber size cannot be adjusted, some obese persons simply might not fit. If all conditions are ideal, the SEE is approximately ± 2.2 to 3.7 percent (2), which might still lead to an average 3 to 4 percent

error in the percent body fat (11). Additional research is needed to better establish the SEE, as the current values are not founded on an abundance of published data. Similar to UWW, if this procedure is available, it can provide athletes and coaches with information about a baseline percent body fat or changes in body fat with training and nutrition intervention.

Dual-Energy X-Ray Absorptiometry

Dual-energy x-ray absorptiometry (DEXA) was first developed to measure bone mineral density, but later it was found to quite accurately assess soft tissue composition (fat) at the same time. This method does require exposure to radiation, but the dose is relatively low and considered safe for most individuals (the dose is less than one-tenth the dose of a standard chest x-ray, and less than a day's exposure to natural radiation, including that from sunlight exposure). Despite the low dose, this method should not be used on pregnant women (23). In some states, urinary pregnancy tests are required. Subject comfort is relatively high in that the person must lie still on a table for approximately 10 minutes. The method is limited by the dimensions of the table and table weight capacity. A very tall person might exceed the dimensions of the table, thus compromising accuracy. Each machine also has a weight limit because of the sensitive x-ray tubes located within the table. Thus, overweight and obese or very large individuals might not be able to be tested. Other limitations are the great expense to purchase and provide service calls for required machine maintenance, the need of a trained operator, and state statutes. In many states, a specific license is required to operate the machine; in some states, a physician order or prescription is required. With an accurate machine and under ideal conditions, the SEE is ± 1.8 percent (2), and the percent body fat error is thought to be 1 to 2 percent (11). More research is needed to better establish the SEE, as its current values are not founded on sufficient published data. If we consider all methods of body composition assessment, DEXA has the lowest SEE (whereas skinfold thickness has the highest) (28).

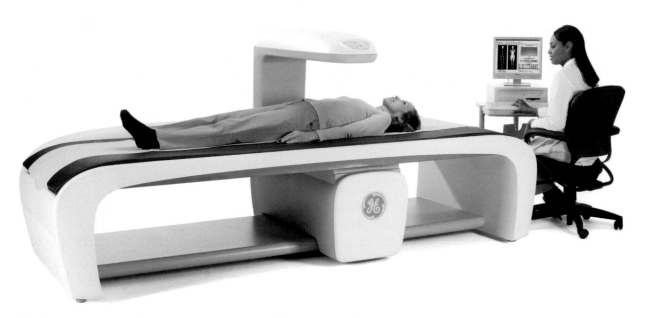

Dual-energy x-ray absorptiometry accurately measures bone mineral density and fat.

In addition to the relatively good accuracy, DEXA can provide valuable health information in terms of body composition and bone mineral density (BMD) that applies both to the recreational exerciser and the competitive athlete. BMD can be very useful, especially in younger athletes, in whom bone formation is still occurring. It is possible to see young female athletes with low BMD, especially in those sports where low body weight is preferred (22). In some of these weight-controlled sports, individuals use weight-control strategies that include eliminating food groups rich in calcium and vitamin D. Poor intake of calcium and vitamin D combined with low energy intake can result in reduced bone formation despite participation in exercise training. Even in women who are past the age of bone formation, knowing their value for BMD is critical. If the BMD is less than optimal, efforts and interventions can still be taken to prevent further BMD loss (22).

Skinfold Thickness

Skinfold thickness has been used in the field for many years and is still used today to estimate percent body fat. In this method, the thickness of a subcutaneous fat fold is measured with a device called a caliper. An assumption underlying the method is that subcutaneous fat is proportional to total body

fat. Subject comfort varies; for some, the pinch hurts for a few seconds, and for others, it is virtually painless. Subjects might feel self-conscious about having a person pinching their fat folds, so this method should always be done in a private setting. In this technique, skinfold thickness is measured, and prediction equations are used to first estimate body density and, from that, body fat. Over 100 different equations in the literature can be used for this purpose, so the operator must fully understand the equation used and its appropriateness for the population being measured. Some equations, called generalized equations, were developed on a nonhomogeneous population with varying characteristics (age, gender, body shape) (7, 15). Other equations are considered population specific, because they were developed on a homogeneous population of similar physical characteristics, and should not be used on individuals outside those parameters. When considering an equation for use, try to choose one that was developed using valid reference methods or multi-compartment models.

Once an equation is selected, you must determine through a review of the research literature which sites on the body to take skinfold thickness. Most equations require at least three sites but might include more. This procedure requires much precision, with careful attention to

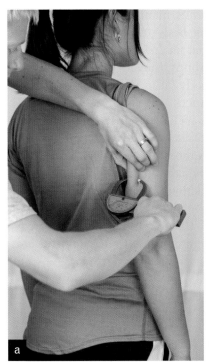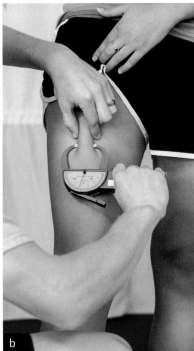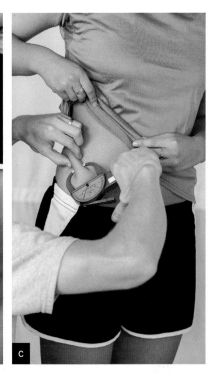

Many skinfold testing sites are used, including *(a)* triceps, *(b)* thigh, and *(c)* suprailiac.

anatomical landmarks and technique. Resources are available to learn about all possible sites and the exact landmarks and procedure to be used for each fold measurement (11, 19). Skinfold measurement technique takes practice with people of many different body types and shapes. Adhering carefully to the standardized procedures increases both the accuracy and consistency (reliability) of the measurements.

In addition to an appropriate equation, you will need a good skinfold caliper. Most of the valid equations use a high-quality metal caliper that produces a constant pressure throughout the measurement. Inexpensive (often plastic) calipers do not produce constant force throughout the measurement and tend to be much less accurate. Unlike some of the referenced methods, even a high-quality metal caliper can be purchased for less than a few hundred dollars and will last a long time with proper care.

Other factors to consider to improve accuracy when taking measurements include ensuring the skin is dry, allowing time after a workout for body fluid compartments to normalize (13, 19), and taking each measurement at least twice. If the first

measurements result is more than a 2-mm difference, a third (or fourth) measurement is required. It is best to rotate through all measurement sites and then repeat, instead of taking two or more sequential measurements from the same site (2). One limitation of skinfold measuring is the difficulty in measuring obese individuals. It can be challenging to identify anatomical locations, or to isolate one fold; sometimes the jaw of the caliper is not large enough. Also note that the accuracy of this method is extremely variable because of the vast choice of equations and the precision and skill required for success. Even in the best-case scenario, the SEE is approximately ± 3.5 percent (2), and is often significantly higher, depending on the equation used and operator skill (11). Also, standardization of skinfold sites, measurement techniques, and calipers all vary around the world. Still, all things considered, this method remains common because it is inexpensive, convenient, quick, and can be used on athletes by anyone trained in the proper protocol and technique, including team physicians, coaches, trainers, or even teammates. The comfort level of this method for athletes is relatively high.

Bioelectrical Impedance Analysis

Bioelectrical Impendence Analysis (BIA) is another popular method of estimating body composition, because of its ease of use, high subject comfort, and relative low cost. This method does not require great technician skill and can be easily used with all individuals, including those who are obese. In this technique, a harmless electrical current is passed through the body, and the impedance or resistance to that electrical current is measured. The principle behind this method is that LBM conducts electricity well, while body fat resists electricity. The higher the percent body fat, the higher the resistance value. Since LBM contains water, and water conducts electricity, hydration status can affect the reading. The subject should be in a state of euhydration for the most accurate measurement. Eating, drinking, exercise, and menstrual cycle stage must stay consistent when multiple measurements are taken.

Most research-quality machines measure the conduction through the whole body, requiring the placement of electrodes, and are more expensive than other devices. These devices usually give a value for resistance, and then the investigator can choose a prediction equation that ultimately predicts body fat. As with skinfold testing, many equations are available, so careful consideration is needed to increase accuracy. Other BIA machines may be considered lower-body analyzers (they look like a scale) or upper-body analyzers (they are hand-held devices). Since the machine is measuring the resistance to an electrical current, these devices may introduce more error. For example, someone with a gynoid fat pattern carries most of their body fat in the hips, buttocks, and thighs. If a hand-held device was used, the current is running primarily through the upper body and missing most of the body fat compartments. Similarly, an android–obese person carrying most of their fat in the upper abdominal region may get an inaccurate reading from a standing device because the electrical current is running primarily through the legs and lower body. These hand-held or standing devices are available at many major retailers, are less expensive, and are easy to use. Many have only one prediction equation and thus, no option for adjustments. An instant value is given for percent body fat. While these devices may be somewhat useful for estimating body fat in population groups, they might not be accurate for predicting body fat in individuals because of individual variances.

In a best-case scenario, when an effective analyzer and appropriate prediction equation is used, the SEE for this method is ± 3.5 to 5.0 percent, depending on the equipment and equation used for body fat prediction (2). If a lower-quality device is used, the error can be significantly higher. On the other hand, this is a relatively inexpensive method that is quite portable and can be used in obese persons with great comfort (11).

Interpreting Body Composition Results

As stated earlier, no method can measure body composition in a living human with 100 percent accuracy. In each method, assumptions are made that might not hold true in all individuals. Furthermore, no one method is better than the others in every case. Different methods measure different variables; for instance, hydrometry measures TBW; UWW and ADP measure body density; and DEXA measures bone mineral mass. Taken together, these methods can give a reasonably accurate value for body composition. When using a field method, you can increase accuracy as much as possible through proper equation selection, equipment, and technique. Even in the best of circumstances, errors can occur in any method of measurement. As discussed, if an individual is assessed at 20 percent body fat, and the method used has a 3 to 4 percent margin of error, the individual's actual percent body fat ranges from 16 to 24 percent. Such imprecision might not be an issue if assessments are being used primarily to track change over time, such as during nutrition and exercise intervention. If using the same technique and equipment, improvements over time can be assessed with accuracy. Most of the popular methods can be used in an initial assessment to help determine the overall health of the individual being measured and to help determine whether intervention is warranted (11).

Once an estimate of body fat is acquired, an individual might wish to reduce body fat. A desirable body weight can be calculated as a goal to obtain a certain percentage of body fat. This is the popular formula for this estimation:

Desirable body weight = LBM/(1 − desired percent body fat)

Example: A 180-pound male who has 20 percent body fat wants to reduce his fat to 15 percent:

180 lb. × 0.20 body fat = 36 lb. fat mass

180 lb. − 36 lb. fat mass = 144 lb. LBM

Desirable body weight = LBM /(1 − desired percent body fat)

144 / (1 − 0.15) = 144 / 0.85 = 169

SUMMARY

Body weight and composition is determined by a combination of genetic and environmental factors. While we cannot control our genetic makeup, we can control some of our environmental factors. A sound diet and personalized training program help us to maximize our genetic potential to achieve our goals. Body weight is a simple measurement of mass and does not take body compartment or tissues into account. Body composition is the proportion of the body that is fat in relation to lean body mass. Lean body mass can be further subdivided into skeletal muscle, water, and bone. These components of body composition can be estimated in various ways in both the research laboratory and field settings.

◼ FOR REVIEW ▶

1. Describe the components of body composition.
2. Explain the difference between overweight and obesity.
3. Describe the role of genetics in body weight and composition.
4. What is a desirable BMI?
5. What is a limitation to classifying an individual based on BMI?
6. Describe the different body fat patterns and the physiological differences.
7. Can percent body fat ever be too low? Explain your answer.
8. What is a limitation of using two-compartment models to measure body composition?
9. For each of the listed body composition assessment methods (hydrometry, hydrodensitometry, air displacement plethysmography, dual-energy x-ray absorptiometry, skinfold thickness, and bioelectrical impedance), list the physiological principle, strengths, limitations, and error of measurement.

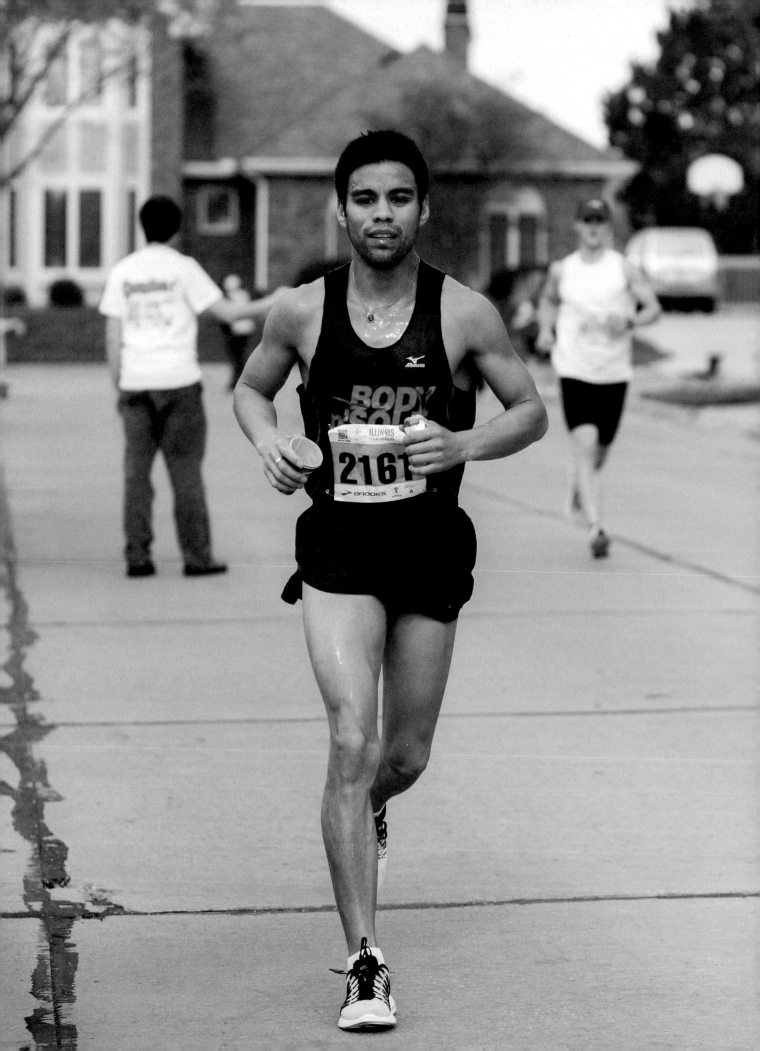

CHAPTER 11

Nutrition for Aerobic Endurance

▶ **CHAPTER OBJECTIVES**

After completing this chapter, you will be able to do the following:

> Identify the defining characteristics of endurance activities.

> Describe how ATP is produced from energy-yielding macronutrients during endurance activities.

> Identify nutrient requirements of endurance athletes, including preparation for, participation in, and recovery from competitive events.

> Explain how to select foods to meet nutrient requirements for endurance.

> Discuss unique challenges facing endurance athletes.

> Discuss how endurance training affects macronutrient metabolism.

Many sports and events—running, cycling, swimming, soccer, among others—are categorized as endurance activities because of the long duration they take to complete. While some of these events last less than an hour, others continue for many hours, or even days. Each endurance event has its own unique duration and environmental challenges, and thus its own set of nutrition requirements for energy-yielding macronutrients, micronutrients, and fluids (26).

ATP PRODUCTION DURING ENDURANCE ACTIVITIES

The continuous muscle contraction that is characteristic of endurance activities requires a near constant production of ATP at the skeletal muscle site, with stronger and faster movements necessitating greater ATP synthesis to meet the need for more energy. If ATP production cannot keep up with demand, movements will necessarily become slower or weaker (27). As discussed in chapter 2, ATP can be produced from several different systems working simultaneously inside the muscle, including

> the ATP-PC system,

> the partial oxidation of glucose (e.g., glycolysis),

> the complete oxidation of glucose,

> the complete oxidation of fatty acids, and

> the complete oxidation of amino acids.

The big question is which system is used to supply ATP during endurance exercise?

The answer lies in how quickly oxygen and substrate can be delivered to the working muscle. Metabolic systems are working together at any given time, and each system's contribution will depend on the ATP demand. At rest and lower-intensity activities ATP demand is low, and fat is the preferred fuel source. With increasing intensity of exercise, there is increased skeletal muscle ATP demand, and carbohydrate becomes the preferred source of fuel. The switch from predominantly fat to predominately carbohydrate is known as the crossover concept (6).

Ideally, the muscle will completely oxidize glucose and fatty acids to produce large quantities of

ATP with no metabolic by-products that contribute to fatigue (e.g., hydrogen ions produced from metabolism). In this ideal situation, glucose and fatty acids enter the muscle cell from the bloodstream, where they circulate in free form and are delivered to working muscle, along with plentiful oxygen. This perfect situation occurs when exercise intensity is relatively low (<50% $\dot{V}O_2$max, such as when walking) and will continue in this manner as long as there are sufficient free fatty acids (FFA) and glucose circulating in blood to meet the ATP demand. When exercise intensity becomes moderate or higher (>50% $\dot{V}O_2$max) the transport of substrates from the bloodstream into contracting muscle cells takes too long to match the demand for ATP, and as a result, begins the process of taking glucose and FFA from the limited supply of glycogen and triglycerides that are stored within the muscle itself. Glycogen stores can range from 70 to 500 grams, providing 280 to 2,000 kilocalories of energy (17, 18, 27), and intramuscular triglycerides compose of only a small portion of total fat stores in the body, approximating 1 to 2 percent (45, 58). The greater the exercise intensity, the greater the proportion of substrate that comes from intramuscular sources; at near maximal intensity, over 90 percent of substrate comes from within the muscle. Note that this relation between exercise intensity and glycogen use is critical for understanding the cause of substrate fatigue, discussed later in the chapter (5, 27, 42, 47).

Regardless of their origin (plasma or muscle), the combination of glucose and fatty acid oxidation provides roughly 95 to 98 percent of the total ATP produced during endurance exercise, with the remaining 2 to 5 percent coming from amino acids. This ratio remains consistent during exercise of all intensities, except during the later stages of very prolonged endurance exercise, when glycogen reserves are running low and amino acids from the breakdown of skeletal muscle can contribute up to 15 percent of total ATP production. Normally, amino acids are preserved for important functions related to growth, maintenance, and repair, but they are used in increasing amounts to produce ATP as glycogen levels in the body decline during lengthy exercise. Reliance on amino acids for fuel during endurance exercise can be reduced by the common practice of ingesting carbohydrate during activity. The relative percentages of glucose and fatty acids used during exercise depend primarily on exercise intensity, with higher intensities favoring greater glucose use and lower intensities favoring fat use (figure 11.1) (5, 6, 27, 42, 47).

The reason that carbohydrate use increases and fat use decreases with increasing exercise intensity is in part due to the amount of oxygen delivered to the muscle at higher intensities and also to the capacity of the muscle to use this oxygen to completely oxidize substrates. Moving faster or more forcefully activates the sympathetic nervous system, resulting in elevated heart rate, blood pressure, and respiration. The overall effect is to enhance oxygen delivery to the working muscle, thereby making it possible to fully oxidize FFA and glucose. If oxygen availability is plentiful and the muscle cell has the capacity to process the oxygen delivered to it, such as during low-intensity exercise (10–35% $\dot{V}O_2$max), then predominantly FFA will be used because the complete oxidation of FFA produces more ATP than does an equal amount of glucose. As exercise intensity increases to moderate and higher levels (>35% $\dot{V}O_2$max), oxygen uptake at the muscle becomes a limiting factor and begins to prevent some of the FFA and glucose from being completely oxidized; partial oxidation of glucose,

however, is unaffected by this shortage of oxygen. The result of all this is that glucose becomes the substrate of choice at intensities greater than approximately 35 percent $\dot{V}O_2$max and is virtually the sole ATP-producer at near maximal exercise. Moreover, the amount of glucose that is partially oxidized because of limited oxygen availability with high exercise intensity rises and contributes to a build-up of lactic acid and subsequent metabolic fatigue caused by the hydrogen ions. The fact that glucose can undergo partial oxidation to produce ATP and fatty acids cannot is just one reason that glucose is considered a more oxygen-efficient fuel than are fatty acids, meaning that glucose will produce more ATP per unit of oxygen than will the same amount of fatty acids (5, 6, 27, 42, 47).

ENERGY-YIELDING MACRONUTRIENT REQUIREMENTS OF ENDURANCE ATHLETES

Endurance athletes who can produce ATP at a rapid rate for long periods have a distinct advantage over their competitors who cannot do so as rapidly or for quite as long. These advantages come from physiological adaptations as a result of specific aerobic training. Exercising at high intensities might help you go faster, but it will surely result in progressive glycogen use over time, as glucose is pulled from intramuscular sources rather than from the blood. Fatigue resulting from glycogen depletion of skeletal muscles was discussed in chapter 3. Without glucose, virtually all voluntary muscle movements will eventually slow down or cease because of the inability to synthesize ATP from *any* source. Athletes experiencing substrate fatigue from lack of carbohydrate stores and the metabolic ability to use them will slow down, walk with a stagger, or fall. The rate of glycogen depletion can be blunted by maintaining a constant supply of glucose in the blood through intake of carbohydrate during exercise, but even this can only preserve a finite amount of muscle glycogen. In addition, maximizing the amount of glycogen in skeletal muscle before the event begins is another way to increase the amount of

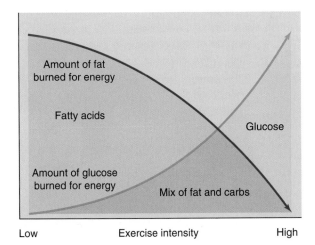

Figure 11.1 The switch from primarily fat for fuel to primarily carbohydrate as the preferred fuel with increasing exercise intensity is known as the crossover concept (6).

time the athlete can exercise before running out of glycogen. Finally, glycogen could be spared if more fatty acids were oxidized instead of glucose. The drawback to this is that oxidation of fatty acids require ample oxygen, which isn't as plentiful during intense exercise. So, there seems to be a cost to using fatty acids in place of glucose, and that cost is the inability to move as fast or as forcefully as possible. If finishing an endurance event is more important than finishing as fast as possible, then training the body to use more fatty acids than glucose might be a good idea. This concept, called training low, is when training in preparation for an event includes workouts in a state of lower glycogen stores and is discussed in greater detail later in the chapter. This section will provide recommendations for the consumption of energy-yielding macronutrients (fat, carbohydrate, protein) for optimal ATP production before, during, and after endurance events (5, 6, 16, 27, 47).

Habitual Intake of Energy-Yielding Macronutrients

Ideally, athletes and active individuals would consume a diet that promotes the following characteristics over a long period of time (e.g., decades):

> consistent healthy body weight ideal for their sport,

> overall health and well-being,

> prevention and management of disease, and

> optimal physical performance.

The first ideal requires that athletes consume energy in amounts that are consistent with what they expend. Consistently consuming less than adequate energy could have many drawbacks, depending on the total calorie deficit (amount of calories below average daily calorie needs) and foods consumed. These drawbacks might include nutrient deficiencies, loss of lean tissue

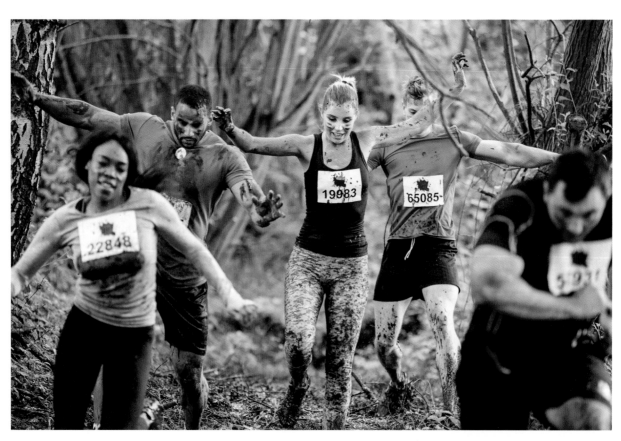

Team endurance sports like the Tough Mudder have grown in popularity.

(e.g., muscle, particularly if protein intake is not sufficient; see chapter 13), compromised immune and endocrine function, and impaired sport performance (26, 30, 31, 53).

Energy requirements of endurance athletes vary considerably but can be quite high for some sports (table 11.1). Recreational exercisers or novice athletes might require an additional 500 kilocalories a day to support their activity, while runners or cyclists training for a long-distance competitive event might need an additional 2,000 kilocalories a day, or more, to support their training.

DO YOU KNOW ?

Extreme glycogen depletion (insufficient glycogen to meet ATP demand) in those who regularly consume carbohydrates (as opposed to those who have adapted to a low-carbohydrate diet or ketogenic diet) results in the skeletal muscle's inability to generate ATP for contraction. This "bonking" or "hitting the wall" is characterized by the inability to move forward. Performance will be significantly altered until fuel once again becomes available.

Energy expenditure of ultraendurance athletes range from 5,000 to 10,000 kilocalories per day. Since scientific literature that provides solid estimates of energy expenditure for men and women in different sports is scarce, athletes must pay close attention to their energy balance. If endurance athletes are unintentionally losing weight, they should increase energy intake; if they are unintentionally gaining weight, they should reduce intake. Athletes with high energy expenditures often have trouble consuming adequate energy. To meet these energy demands, these individuals must often snack continuously throughout the day or consume bigger meals and be selective in choosing energy-dense foods (26).

Recall from chapter 3 that the DRI for carbohydrate for adults is 45 to 65 percent of total energy intake, with added sugar intake limited to 10 percent of energy or less each day (34). Since athletes' requirements do not always fit into these parameters, it is best to express carbohydrate recommendations in absolute quantities (e.g., grams or g/kg body weight), rather than as a percentage of total energy. General carbohydrate recommendations for athletes

Table 11.1 Energy Demands and Considerations for Different Sports

Energy demand	Sport	Special considerations
Relatively low energy expenditure	Baseball Golf	Careful carbohydrate supplementation, if any, should not lead to energy imbalance.
Generally high energy expenditure	Basketball Cycling Running Ice hockey Soccer Tennis Swimming Wrestling* Rowing*	Expenditure varies based on body size, training volume, and training or competition time. Expenditure tends to be greater at the collegiate and professional levels. Intake and expenditure must be individualized based on performance and body composition goals.
Generally high energy expenditure per kg body weight, but athletes may be small	Figure skating Gymnastics	Intake and expenditure must be individualized based on body composition goals. Body weight and composition are emphasized.
Highly variable	Weightlifting Track and field events Football Martial arts	Intake and expenditure must be individualized based on body composition goals.

*Body weight and body composition are of critical importance.

Based on Karpinski and Rosenbloom 2017.

PUTTING IT INTO PERSPECTIVE

CARBOHYDRATE AVAILABILITY VERSUS HIGH CARBOHYDRATE

The term "energy availability" refers to energy intake minus energy expenditure and has been used, especially for female athletes, to describe the dietary energy remaining for other body functions after exercise training. It can be argued that "carbohydrate availability" is a preferable way to think about carbohydrate needs in athletes. Intake alone may not be the best measure of physiological status. Carbohydrate availability takes into account the total daily intake and timing throughout the day and whether this intake meets the demand of exercise by adequately supplying glucose for the working skeletal muscle and central nervous system. Intake matched to or exceeding demands would be considered a state of high carbohydrate availability, whereas low carbohydrate availability would mean carbohydrate intake or stores are too limited to meet the demands of training (33, 53).

were summarized in chapter 3 (table 3.6), and sample daily carbohydrate gram targets based on body weights were provided in table 3.7.

The AMDR for fat is 20 to 35 percent of total energy intake. A valid habitual intake goal that falls within the AMDR range for most endurance athletes is 1.0 to 2.0 g/kg body weight, with the higher end of the range recommended for those participating in training regimens significantly increasing the total daily energy expenditure. Dietary fat recommendations are tricky because, in practice, endurance athletes need to estimate their carbohydrate and protein needs first, and then fill in the remaining kilocalories with fat. If an athlete desires to stay in a state of energy balance, it may turn out that fat intake falls at the lower end of the AMDR. Chronic fat intakes less than 20 percent of total kilocalories are discouraged for most athletes who do not have extreme energy expenditures, as smaller percentages might impair fat-soluble vitamin absorption and lead to less than optimal levels of essential fats, such as omega-3 fatty acids (53). Lower fat intakes should be reserved for acute periods of time in preparation for competition (34, 53).

Endurance training produces a great deal of microscopic injuries within muscle that must be repaired, as well as the need to replace proteins, particularly in the mitochondria, that tend to undergo significant turnover because of the repetitive stress of lengthy exercise. This process requires a balance between muscle protein syntheses and muscle protein breakdown. In addition to physical training, the anabolic process of muscle protein synthesis is also stimulated by dietary protein intake. For these reasons, athletes in general need 1.2 to 2.0 g/kg of dietary protein. Athletes with larger training volumes leading to extensive skeletal muscle adaptation, repair, and remodeling tend to benefit from consumption at the upper end of the range. Endurance athletes need more dietary protein than their sedentary counterparts, but they typically do not have the most extensive skeletal muscle protein turnover and thus can consume at the lower end of the range (53). Athletes on a lower-calorie diet need more protein to minimize muscle mass loss during weight loss (see chapters 12 and 13) (30).

Carbohydrate Loading

Maximizing glycogen reserves preceding an endurance event is a common strategy among athletes. The process of **carbohydrate loading**

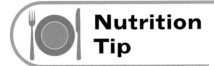

was introduced in 1967 and has been used for years in an attempt to super-compensate glycogen stores (4). The theory is that if one can deplete glycogen with exercise followed by repletion with a high-carbohydrate diet, then more glycogen will be stored than if one maintained an exercise routine and consumed a steady amount of carbohydrate. Carbohydrate loading appears to be an effective strategy for endurance events lasting 90 minutes or more if implemented at least 24 hours before an event (53). Athletes who benefit from this strategy include distance runners, road cyclists, cross-country skiers, and open-water swimmers. Research suggests performance can be improved by approximately 2 to 3 percent when glycogen stores are super compensated, as compared to normal stores (23). Note that since every gram of stored glycogen also retains 3 to 4 grams of water (23, 29), it is not uncommon for glycogen-loading protocols to induce up to a 2-kg gain in body weight, which actually may cause the athlete to feel "weighed down" prior to the event (23). Whether an athlete can perform well with the added body water weight is left to them to decide (4).

Carbohydrate loading can be approached in various ways, though all include a high-carbohydrate intake in the days leading up to an event to maximize glycogen stores (and thus to increase carbohydrate availability during the later stages of an event). Exercise-induced glycogen depletion is approximately 90 minutes instead of to exhaustion, and carbohydrate intake is at a moderate level of approximately 5 g/kg body weight. The repletion stage is followed by tapering (decreasing) exercise and increasing daily carbohydrate intake to approximately 10 g/kg body weight daily. Table 11.2 summarizes this strategy for carbohydrate loading, which is recommended for continuous endurance activity of 90 minutes or more (35, 46).

Other carbohydrate-loading strategies have been demonstrated as well. For example, one can consume a high-carbohydrate diet for 3 days in concert with tapering exercise the week before competition and complete rest the day before the event. The total diet should provide adequate energy and carbohydrate per day, approximately 8 to 10 g/kg body weight. This regimen should increase muscle glycogen stores 20 to 40 percent above starting levels (14). However, higher intakes

Table 11.2 Sample Carbohydrate Loading Protocol

Day	Task
1	Glycogen depletion 90 to 120 minutes of moderate- to high-intensity exercise at 75% $\dot{V}O_2$max Mixed diet with carbohydrate intake (4-5k g/kg)
2-3	40 to 60 minutes of low- to moderate-intensity exercise Moderate carbohydrate intake (4–5 g/kg)
4-5	20 minutes of light training Higher carbohydrate intake (8–10 g/kg)
6	Rest Higher carbohydrate intake (8–10 g/kg)
7	Event

Data from Sherman et al. 1981.

of 10 to 12 g/kg body weight of carbohydrate have been suggested for marathon runners, road-race cyclers, and some team games during the 36 to 48 hours prior to the event (7, 9). While carbohydrate loading appears to be effective for improving performance for some endurance athletes, the research data are mixed (50, 51, 60). Study protocols vary in energy intake, training status (fitness level), and gender of the research subjects (50, 51, 60). Thus a trial approach is recommended.

Additional research has suggested that it is possible to enhance glycogen levels without a depletion stage. Athletes can consume a high-carbohydrate diet (10–12 g/kg body weight) coupled with rest for as little as 36 to 48 hours before an endurance event. This provides more flexibility in methods to glycogen load. Carbohydrate intake before an event should include choices that are low in dietary fiber or residue in order to prevent excessive or untimely bowel movements. Athletes should experiment with intake during practice or training rather than wait until the week or day of the actual event. Athletes need to determine the optimal training, total carbohydrate intake, and food choices that best suits their goals (10, 35, 53).

Day of an Event

Precompetition intake the day of an event can be critical for optimal performance. Athletes should prepare for an event by consuming enough food to avoid hunger, provide adequate fuel and fluids, and top off glycogen stores, while minimizing potential for gastrointestinal (GI) distress. There is no one precompetition meal that best suits everyone; carbohydrate and other nutrient intake will vary depending on factors such as type of event, time of event, environmental conditions, physiological

training status of the athlete, stress of the athlete, and individual preferences. Ideally, many athletes prefer to begin an endurance event with full glycogen stores. Note, however, that other athletes might choose a different approach, which will be discussed later in the chapter (9). Further, some research suggests consuming carbohydrate just prior to an event might have additional benefits. Most research has been on endurance athletes whose sport involves continuous movement but might also apply to those in sports with intermittent high-intensity periods, such as soccer. Carbohydrate ingestion before an event will likely be beneficial for prolonged, sustained, or intermittent activities lasting an hour or longer and for those who have not eaten several hours before an event (9, 53). For events of shorter duration, adequate glycogen stores will likely be enough to supply the needed fuel for ATP synthesis.

The amount of carbohydrate recommended the day of an event depends on the amount of time preceding the start of the activity:

> If an event is 3 to 4 hours away, there is time to digest a full meal containing 3 to 4 g/kg body weight of carbohydrate. Aerobic endurance athletes who eat at least 4 hours before competition should include approximately 1 to 4 g/kg body weight of carbohydrate and 0.15 to 0.25 g/kg body weight of protein (52, 53).

> If the event is 2 hours away, the carbohydrate recommendation is reduced to 1 to 2 g/kg body weight (53).

> If an event is early in the morning, the athlete might have only about an hour to prepare and consume a meal. The carbohydrate recommendation is then 0.5 to 1 g/kg body weight (table 11.3) (10, 13, 53).

Table 11.3 Carbohydrate Recommendations Before an Endurance Event

Hours before event	Carbohydrate (g/kg BW)	Suggestions
3 to 4	3–4	Mixed energy-yielding macronutrient meal with carbohydrate beverage
2	1–2	Light meal or snack or carbohydrate beverage
1	0.5–1	Snack or carbohydrate beverage

BW = Body weight
Note: Low fiber or residue foods should be consumed.
Data from Burke et al. 2011; Cermak and van Loon 2013; Thomas, Erdman, and Burke 2016.

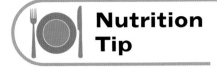

Nutrition Tip

Some athletes might decide to try a new food or strategy before an important event. This can have undesirable consequences, as the body might respond to one particular food or supplement differently from others. In addition, some athletes feel pressure or nervousness on an event or game day, which can affect digestive function. It is advisable to stick with foods and supplements used during preparation and to save new strategies and foods for practice days.

In order for this meal to be well tolerated by the athlete, it should have low-fiber carbohydrates and perhaps a little protein, depending on the intensity and duration of the event and personal preference. Since fluids are also important, consuming a carbohydrate-containing beverage along with the meal might be desirable if carbohydrate needs cannot be met through food alone. Fluid needs are discussed in chapter 8. Each athlete should experiment with intake amounts prior to competition. Generally, a small meal or snack with a beverage is sufficient, but all athletes are different and must determine what works best for them. Some athletes need to have a little solid food in the stomach, whereas others do not tolerate anything solid and prefer a beverage only. Precompetition jitters can affect how athletes respond to food and fluids, but this is difficult to replicate in practice and thus hard to prepare for (10, 13, 26).

Intake of Energy-Yielding Macronutrients During an Event

It appears that consuming carbohydrate immediately before and during exercise lasting longer than 60 minutes has a beneficial effect on endurance performance because it provides additional glucose to the working skeletal muscle, and thereby lessens the need for the muscle to tap into its glycogen reserves. The amount of carbohydrate recommended is a fairly wide range of 30 to 90 grams per hour and is meant to provide as much glucose as can be oxidized without causing GI distress (figure 11.2). The higher end of the range

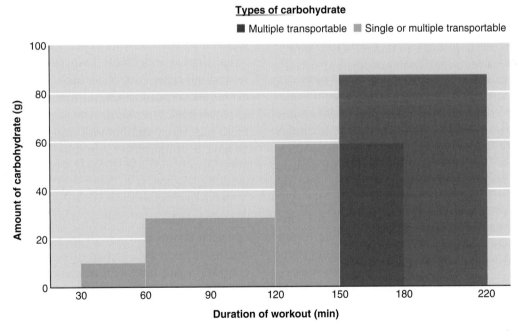

Figure 11.2 Both amount and type of carbohydrate is important to optimize endurance performance. More total carbohydrate and carbohydrate from different sources are needed with increased training time. The upper doses and types are most important for the elite endurance athlete wishing to maximize glucose oxidation. This is not applicable to the recreational athlete exercising for an hour a day.

(60 to 90 g/hour) is reserved for events lasting longer than 2.5 hours. Although individuals differ in their rate of glucose breakdown, little scientific evidence suggests that requirements differ based on body weight. It is for this reason that daily training and pre-event recommendations are in absolute terms (e.g., g/hour) instead of relative terms (e.g., g/kg body weight/hour) (10, 13, 21, 22, 53). Note that the research studies examining these higher rates of glucose use were conducted in controlled laboratory studies using cyclists. Whether these findings translate to all endurance athletes is yet to be determined.

In addition to considering the total amount of glucose ingested and used, it is also important to attend to the way different types of carbohydrates are broken down and used at different rates. The limiting factor in carbohydrate availability during activity is the intestinal absorption of glucose. Glucose requires one type of transport system to cross the small intestinal wall for absorption. This sodium-dependent transporter can absorb a maximum of 60 grams per hour of glucose. However, this is not the case when other forms of carbohydrate are simultaneously consumed. For example, fructose uses a completely different transporter (GLUT5) than glucose (GLUT4) and allows an opportunity to ultimately get more glucose to the working muscle (recall that fructose gets converted to glucose once absorbed) (figure 11.3) (13, 21, 22, 53).

When glucose is combined with fructose in an approximate 2-to-1 ratio, the carbohydrate mix can be absorbed at a higher rate of 90 grams per hour, because both transporters are working simultaneously. Think of it as having two doorways for the carbohydrate to get through rather than one—both doorways are open to welcome the carbohydrate at the same time: fructose enters through one doorway, and glu-

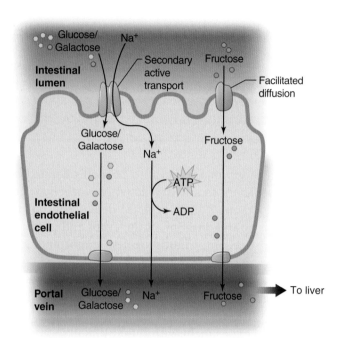

Figure 11.3 Because glucose and fructose use different mechanisms of transport into the intestinal cell, they are not competing for entry space, thus more total carbohydrate in the form of glucose can get into the body and to the working muscle.

cose enters through the other. Taking advantage of this concept allows an athlete to maximize the amount of total carbohydrate that can be delivered to working muscle, a concept that can be of great value during extremely long events (e.g., >2.5 hours) but not so much during relatively shorter events. Many products on the market contain both glucose (and glucose derivatives) and fructose (e.g., gels, bars, and liquids), and they all appear to have a similar effect, so individual preference and tolerance should be considered when choosing which to use (13, 21, 22, 53).

Most pre-event meals focus on carbohydrate content, without guidelines for fat. While some research shows that a high-fat preexercise meal results in increased plasma free fatty acid concentration and fatty acid oxidation, it is unclear whether this translates to an actual performance benefit in humans. Further, consuming large amounts of fat immediately before exercise can result in GI stress. For this reason, consuming a high-fat meal during the day of competition is not recommended, but small amounts of healthy

DO YOU KNOW ?

The limiting factor for using glucose as a fuel source is the absorption of dietary carbohydrate. Research shows that athletes who regularly consume carbohydrate can increase the absorptive capacity of the small intestine—called "training the gut." This should be practiced well before an important event (22)!

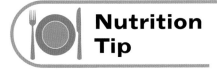

Nutrition Tip

The body can digest and use only so much carbohydrate at a time. Most sports drinks designed for endurance athletes are a 6 to 8 percent carbohydrate solution because solutions greater than that result in GI distress (13, 21, 22, 53). It might seem acceptable to consume juice or other sugary beverages, but most of these have a carbohydrate concentration well above 6 to 8 percent. While it is possible to dilute to the correct carbohydrate concentration, this is not a convenient process. Also, these beverages might not contain the correct forms of carbohydrate and might be missing needed electrolytes.

fats are not contraindicated, either (11, 53). More information on manipulation of dietary fat and carbohydrate in attempts of metabolic adaptations to benefit performance will be presented later in the chapter.

Research examining the effects of consuming protein during endurance events is limited. Some studies suggest that co-ingestion of carbohydrate and protein during endurance activities can promote overall protein accretion and increased time to exhaustion, but other research has not confirmed these findings. Further, critics of this work argue that time to exhaustion is not necessarily an indicator of improved performance because few events actually go to exhaustion, and that actual improvements in event finish time would be better to gauge. In studies that do assess race finish times, co-ingestion of carbohydrate with protein does not seem to improve finish time over consuming carbohydrate alone. Thus, there is little rationale at this time to routinely recommend the consumption of protein during endurance exercise (3, 59).

Macronutrient Intake After an Event

Optimizing glycogen repletion is important for athletes who have to train or compete hard on multiple occasions in the same day or on successive days. Glycogen stores replenish at a rate of about 5 to 7 percent per hour, with 20 to 24 hours needed to reestablish stores. Without purposefully modifying dietary patterns, glycogen

PUTTING IT INTO PERSPECTIVE

CONTINUOUS ENDURANCE SPORTS VERSUS ENDURANCE ACTIVITIES

Some matches in sports, such as tennis, can last for several hours and thereby qualify as endurance events, but they are never continuous in the way that long-distance running is, for example. Sports like tennis and soccer are characterized by high-intensity bouts of activity interspersed with shorter periods at lower intensity or relative rest. These sports not only require large amounts of carbohydrate for fuel, but also the ingested carbohydrate might improve motor skills, mood, force production, fatigue, and perceived exertion. While the research on carbohydrate intake in intermittent sports is not as abundant as it is for continuous endurance sports, carbohydrate intake during prolonged, intermittent activities is recommended for optimal performance. For events lasting 60 to 90 minutes, 60 grams per hour of carbohydrate will likely suffice. Carbohydrate intakes greater than 60 grams will likely be of benefit only if the event stretches to 2 to 3 hours, if the intensity of activity is high for a majority of the event, or if the athlete does not begin the event in a fed, glycogen-filled state and yet relies on glycogen for fuel (i.e., has not adapted to a low-carbohydrate diet and is competing in a lower-intensity event) (10, 13, 19, 48, 53).

will eventually replenish with normal eating and sufficient carbohydrate intake; however, this process might take some time and not maximize stores between bouts of activity. This is fine on the last day of an event when the athlete will be resting or taking time off, but it is not ideal for the athlete needing to train or perform again within 24 hours. Optimizing glycogen replacement is even more important if subsequent training or an event takes place within several hours of the first activity period, and in this case, it is wise to begin ingesting carbohydrate as soon after activity as possible (3, 10, 12, 20, 22, 53).

To replenish glycogen, the two factors needed most are glucose and insulin. Consuming carbohydrate-rich foods will provide the glucose and insulin response needed for glycogen synthesis. Muscle glycogen synthesis occurs in two stages, the first being insulin-independent and the second being insulin-dependent. During the first phase (30 to 60 minutes postexercise), it appears that glycogen depletion itself is a stimulus for glycogen re-synthesis. It is thought that depleted levels of glycogen and skeletal muscle contraction during exercise act as a stimulus for translocation of the GLUT4 protein to the muscle's cell membrane (figure 11.4). It appears that this enhanced glucose transport declines rapidly if carbohydrate is not consumed within an hour or 2 after exercise. In addition, lower levels of glycogen stimulate activity of the enzyme **glycogen synthase**, which is the key enzyme responsible for glycogen synthesis (3, 10, 12, 20, 22, 53).

The second phase of skeletal muscle glycogen synthesis, beginning 1 to 2 hours postexercise and lasting for up to 48 hours, is marked by a period of enhanced insulin sensitivity. Because this period is so dependent on carbohydrate intake and its subsequent glycemic response, it is most ripe for nutrition strategies aimed at maximizing glycogen synthesis. Based on the best available data, the recommendation for immediate carbohydrate intake postexercise ranges from 1.0 to 1.5 g/kg body weight, with 1.2 g/kg considered the optimal amount. A mixture of carbohydrate, namely glucose, glucose polymers, fructose, and if practical, galactose, appears to provide the best results. Some evidence suggests that fructose ingestion causes a more rapid replenishment of

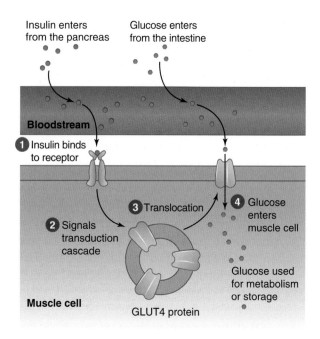

Figure 11.4 To replenish glycogen in the cells of the liver and skeletal muscle, both glucose and insulin are needed. Glucose comes from the ingestion of dietary carbohydrate, and insulin is secreted as a result of this intake.

liver glycogen compared to glucose; however, fructose alone does not optimally restore muscle glycogen (13). The recommended carbohydrate should be consumed immediately after exercise to maximize that enhanced metabolic window followed by repeated consumption at frequent intervals (e.g., every 15–30 minutes) for 4 to 6 hours or until the daily carbohydrate intake goal is achieved. Delaying carbohydrate intake for as little as 2 hours postexercise might cause the athlete to miss the window of opportunity and not maximize glycogen stores prior to the next event. Again, this is important for multiple-day or successive-day events, but not as important if there is no need to optimize glycogen stores between events (3, 10, 12, 20, 22, 53).

The type of carbohydrate might not be as important as the amount. It appears that glycogen can be replenished equally well with both liquid and solid carbohydrates, so the athlete's personal preference should be the primary determinant. It is also not clear whether the glycemic index of the carbohydrate makes much of a difference during the second phase of glycogen repletion. While it seems logical that high-glycemic index foods would induce an elevated insulin response and glycogen synthesis, this phenomenon has not been repeatedly demonstrated in the scientific literature. In fact, some data suggest that any form of carbohydrate, regardless of its glycemic index, ingested immediately postexercise will promote glycogen replenishment. More research is needed before we can recommend a definitive glycemic index pattern postexercise to maximize glycogen synthesis and stores (3, 10, 12, 15, 20, 22, 53).

It is clear that carbohydrate should be eaten immediately after an endurance event has ended, but what about the other energy-yielding macronutrients, fat and protein? Do they also have an effect on glycogen replenishment? This has been studied for several years, and thus far findings are not conclusive. In theory, protein or certain amino acids might enhance postprandial insulin secretion and thus glucose uptake and glycogen synthesis. However, the data suggest that this may occur only when carbohydrate intake immediately after exercise is less than the recommended amount. In fact, when consuming the recommended amount of 1.2 g/kg body weight carbohydrate, adding protein does not enhance glycogen repletion. Although protein may not have a valuable impact on glycogen repletion, it does play an important role in other processes involved with skeletal muscle growth and repair (see chapter 5) and should be included in the immediate postexercise meal for this reason alone (3, 38, 53).

FOOD SELECTION TO MEET NUTRIENT REQUIREMENTS

Whereas estimating nutrient requirements is a relatively straightforward process, actually selecting foods and beverages to meet daily nutrient requirements can be a challenge. Many athletes are unfamiliar with the process of researching the nutrient contents of various food products and then taking the next step of combining them in such a fashion that they meet their daily nutrient needs. Athletes wanting to consume a target amount of carbohydrate (e.g., 350 g) merely need to read the labels on all of the products they plan to eat that day and calculate the number of servings of each that in aggregate will provide the recommended amount of carbohydrate. For example, assume a male athlete wants to eat 1 cup of the product described by the label in figure 11.5. From the label, it is clear that one serving of the product equals 1/2-cup, so if 1 cup of the product is desired, that is equivalent to two servings (55, 56). Figure 11.6 provides a sample list of foods containing about 350 grams of carbohydrate.

It is also obvious from the label that one serving of the product provides 13 grams of carbohydrate, of which 3 grams each are in the forms of sugar and fiber. Since the athlete plans to eat two servings, he will consume 26 grams of total carbohydrate, 6 grams of sugar, and 6 grams of fiber. So, when looking at the big picture for the day, ingesting this product will contribute 26 of the 350 grams of carbohydrate allotted for the entire day, or 18 percent of the athlete's recommended daily intake. Further, the amount of sugar and fiber in the product also contribute to the amounts allowed for those nutrients. Note that sugar intake should be kept below 10 percent of the total energy consumed each day, and fiber should be limited

Nutrition Facts

8 servings per container

Serving size   1/2 cup (55g)

Amount per 1/2 cup

Calories   140

	% Daily Value*
Total Fat 8g	12%
Saturated Fat 1g	5%
Trans Fat 0g	
Cholesterol 0mg	0%
Sodium 160mg	7%
Total Carbohydrate 13g	4%
Dietary Fiber 3g	12%
Total Sugars 3g	
Added Sugars 3g	1%
Protein 3g	
Vitamin D 2mcg	10%
Calcium 260mg	20%
Iron 8mg	45%
Potassium 235mg	6%

* The % Daily Value (DV) tells you how much a nutrient in a serving of food contributes to a daily diet. 2,000 calories a day is used for general nutrition advice.

Figure 11.5 Based on this product's food label, 1 cup is two servings and contains a total of 26 grams of carbohydrate.

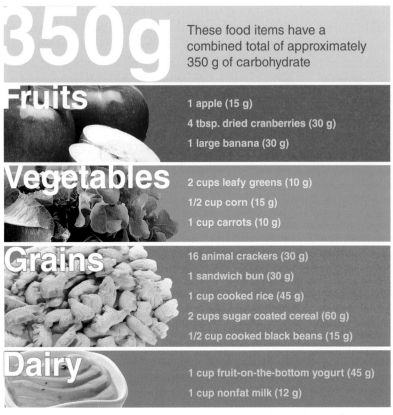

These food items have a combined total of approximately 350 g of carbohydrate

Fruits
- 1 apple (15 g)
- 4 tbsp. dried cranberries (30 g)
- 1 large banana (30 g)

Vegetables
- 2 cups leafy greens (10 g)
- 1/2 cup corn (15 g)
- 1 cup carrots (10 g)

Grains
- 16 animal crackers (30 g)
- 1 sandwich bun (30 g)
- 1 cup cooked rice (45 g)
- 2 cups sugar coated cereal (60 g)
- 1/2 cup cooked black beans (15 g)

Dairy
- 1 cup fruit-on-the-bottom yogurt (45 g)
- 1 cup nonfat milk (12 g)

Figure 11.6 These foods should be spread out throughout the day with consideration for training schedule and recovery.

Food labels work great for manufactured products, but what about foods that don't have labels, such as fruits and vegetables? In this case, we have a couple of choices. Many grocery stores will have food composition tables in the produce aisle for reference. Another option is to use a standard food composition table found in many general nutrition textbooks—but the most comprehensive one is provided by the USDA in the form of an extensive database of foods that is available to the general public and simple to access (http://ndb.nal.usda.gov) (57). Similar to the food labels on products, the USDA database provides total carbohydrate, fiber, sugar, fat, and protein contents per serving, but the database also provides much more nutrition information—probably much more than the typical athlete will need.

immediately before and during competition. In the current example, these calculations were done for just one product, but in a real situation they need to be done for every food product consumed throughout the day, aggregated, and then compared to the recommended daily requirements (54-56).

TYPES OF CARBOHYDRATE AND PERFORMANCE

Traditional sports drinks, gels, and other supplements marketed for endurance athletes usually contain a combination of glucose, sucrose, and maltodextrin (also known as a glucose polymer).

PUTTING IT INTO PERSPECTIVE

CAFFEINE AND GLYCOGEN REPLENISHMENT

Caffeine is often used as an ergogenic aid for enhanced endurance performance, but some evidence suggests that it might also be helpful during glycogen replenishment during recovery from exercise. While the mechanism is unclear, it appears that caffeine might increase insulin sensitivity during recovery period and also improve intestinal absorption of carbohydrate. Note that some individuals are sensitive to caffeine, and ingestion could result in undesirable side effects such as jitteriness or sleeplessness. All things considered, an athlete interested in caffeine as an ergogenic aid should consume the smallest dose that results in the desired effect in order to decrease the risk of undesirable side effects (3, 53).

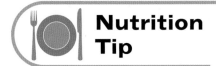

Nutrition Tip

Consider if the serving size on a food label is for a cooked or raw product. For example, oats most commonly report the serving size as dry oats, but when cooked, they become engorged with water, so that a cup of cooked oats has far fewer nutrients than a cup of dried oats.

Maltodextrin has the highest glycemic index of these sugars, but all are digested rapidly, providing a quick source of energy immediately before and during exercise. Ingesting these products result in an increased insulin level that facilitates the uptake of glucose into the muscle to be broken down for fuel (43).

Some athletes are concerned about glucose and insulin spikes and falls, as an inconsistent level of blood glucose can alter perception of fatigue and cause a negative impact on performance. A few new products have appeared on the market that claim to provide energy without the same amount of instability as glucose, sucrose, and maltodextrin, and without the same level of insulin needed for uptake. Carbohydrates with a higher molecular weight than glucose or maltodextrin are made in a laboratory and absorbed more slowly. These compounds were originally formulated for people with glycogen storage disease, and then extended for individuals with diabetes. In the sports nutrition community, the compounds are often referred to as superstarch or waxy maize. The theory and promotion behind their use as a sports supplement is that they do not provide a rapid rise in blood glucose, so effort, whether perceived or real, will be improved. Studies that consistently show favorable changes in blood glucose and insulin responses, glucose uptake and oxidation (use), glycogen re-synthesis, or absolute improved performance in the field are lacking. In reality, exercised muscles respond just fine to a rise in blood glucose, so the benefit of using these compounds remains questionable (25, 41, 43, 44, 49).

UNIQUE CHALLENGES FACING ENDURANCE ATHLETES

All sports have their own unique characteristics that often require participants to take certain measures to help them perform or tolerate the activity better. In this section we describe situations in which endurance athletes might want to take such measures.

Inability or Unwillingness to Consume Extra Carbohydrate During Activity

In many cases an athlete cannot or will not consume additional carbohydrate during an endurance activity. Consuming carbohydrate during activities less than 1 hour in duration is not warranted when the goal is to spare glycogen; however, there may be other reasons to justify this practice. Some studies show improved performance after subjects simply rinse their mouths with a carbohydrate-containing beverage and spit it out without swallowing, or "mouth rinsing." The exact mechanism is unknown, but it appears that the brain can detect the presence of carbohydrate or energy in the mouth, perhaps anticipate carbohydrate delivery into the body, and somehow that leads to improved performance. It appears that tasting carbohydrate is more stimulatory than other products because the same level of brain activity is not seen with nonnutritive sweeteners, so it is more than just perceived sweet taste that triggers the excitation in the brain. This finding can have practical applications, particularly for athletes who do not tolerate traditional sports beverages or who participate in weight-sensitive sports and cannot afford to consume excess calories (e.g., wrestlers, gymnasts). Perhaps this strategy would allow them to exercise at a greater intensity without fatigue, or a lower perception of fatigue without the unwanted energy (calories). While more research is needed, it remains prudent to ensure carbohydrate stores are adequate before exercise for athletes interested in using this strategy for an ergogenic effect (22, 24).

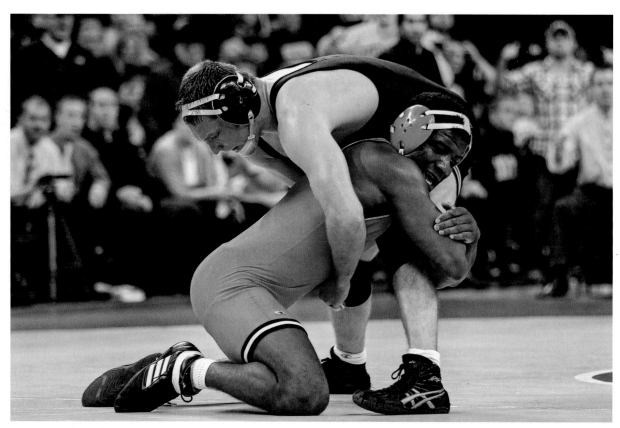

Wrestlers who must make weight need to monitor their food consumption prior to weigh-in.

Gastrointestinal Distress

Some endurance athletes have cited GI stress during training and competition, a condition that certainly can cause impaired performance. The severity of GI distress might vary from mild to severe, with the most common symptoms being nausea, vomiting, abdominal pain, and diarrhea. Discomfort and unwanted stops at a portable toilet can be the difference between winning and losing, or for less competitive athletes, between dropping out and finishing a race. The exact prevalence of GI distress in endurance athletes is not known, but studies report it to be up to 93 percent for any one symptom (37, 39, 40).

Nutrition intake can significantly affect symptoms of GI distress. The traditional culprits are fiber, fat, protein, concentrated carbohydrate solutions, fructose alone, or dehydration. For example, fiber, fat, and protein can delay gastric emptying, and consuming fructose alone or a high mixed-carbohydrate solution during higher-intensity exercise can cause fluid shifts in the GI tract that may cause GI distress and impaired performance. It is not clear whether the GI tract can be trained to better tolerate the food it receives; however, it is important to at least experiment with nutrition strategies during practice before implementing them in a competitive environment (37, 39, 40).

Desire to Enhance Fatty Acid Oxidation

Success or failure in most endurance activities depends physiologically on the ability to produce ATP at a rapid rate over a long duration, an endeavor that requires large storage reserves of glycogen and the capacity to effectively use fuel sources other than muscle glycogen, specifically

PUTTING IT INTO PERSPECTIVE

MINIMIZING GI DISTRESS FOR ATHLETES

The following strategies can be used to prevent or minimize GI distress in endurance athletes. However, if an athlete has a diagnosed medical condition, such as celiac disease, irritable bowel syndrome, or Crohn's disease, which requires medical nutrition therapy, then a referral should be made to a RDN familiar with these conditions.

> Avoid high-fiber foods during the day, or even days, before competition. On all other days, consuming a diet with adequate fiber will help keep the bowel regular.

> Avoid high-fructose foods, particularly drinks that are exclusively fructose; beverages containing both fructose and glucose might be better tolerated.

> Avoid dehydration by starting the event well hydrated and consuming fluids throughout the event.

> Do not ingest concentrated carbohydrate-containing beverages.

> Practice new nutrition strategies many times before implementing them during competition.

Reprinted from E.P. de Oliveira, R.C. Burini, and A. Jeukendrup, 2014, "Gastrointestinal complaints during exercise: Prevalence, etiology, and nutritional recommendations," *Sports Medicine* 44(suppl 1): S79–S85. This article is distributed under the terms of the Creative Commons Attribution License.

fatty acids. A protocol designed to train the body to preferentially oxidize fatty acids over glucose during exercise—called "training low, competing high"—has gained increased attention. The underlying theory behind this protocol is that by conducting training sessions in a somewhat glycogen-depleted state, the body will "learn" to prefer fatty acids over glucose as a fuel. Some protocols combine this with a lower-carbohydrate, higher-fat diet, often referred to as "fat loading," for a short period prior to the competitive event, before ultimately switching to a higher-carbohydrate diet right before the event. From a physiological standpoint, this protocol does appear to accomplish its mission; it can result in increased intramuscular triglyceride stores and elicits greater fat oxidation and decreased use of skeletal muscle glycogen during exercise. The problem is that in sporting events success is measured based on performance and not metabolic adaptations or source of fuel. At this time, there is no evidence of improved performance. More field-based research studies are needed in order to see if metabolic adaptations translate into improved performance. While training low might result in some physiological adaptations, it might also trigger undesirable side effects, such as fatigue during exercise and inability to train at high intensities, either of

which contributes to failure instead of success (1, 2, 8, 9, 16, 36, 53).

This topic has been controversial in the sports nutrition literature for some time. Some of the earlier studies, conducted prior to 2006, were used to argue the case for this protocol. These studies had different study designs that make comparison difficult, and the sample sizes and total number of studies were small. These studies concluded that a low-carbohydrate, high-fat (LCHF) diet resulted in fat being the preferential fuel source, and glycogen was spared. These studies did not match for or consider initial glycogen levels, so the conclusion is not fully accurate. Still, the observed increased use of fat as a fuel source (increased fatty acid oxidation) is worth further examination (9). The research studies conducted through 2006 did demonstrate some interesting findings, which are summarized here (9):

> Consuming a LCHF diet for as little as 5 days can cause skeletal muscle adaptations such as increased intramuscular triglyceride stores; increased activity of the enzyme hormone sensitive lipase, which facilitates fatty acid mobilization from storage; and enhanced cellular metabolic processes that ultimately allow an increased oxidation (use) of fat for fuel. As fat oxidation is increased, it appears that carbohydrate oxidation (breakdown

or use) is reduced and that this reduction is caused by changes in skeletal muscle glycogen utilization.

> Even after several days of using a LCHF diet and then switching to a higher-carbohydrate regimen, the enhanced fat utilization persists. These fat metabolism adaptations remain even if carbohydrate is introduced closer to an event.

> Despite the metabolic changes that appear to take place with consumption of an LCHF diet, the translation to an actual performance benefit is lacking. The studies had small sample sizes, and these changes might not apply to all individuals. People who don't respond well or tolerate carbohydrate during exercise would adapt better to this protocol than those who do well with carbohydrate loading and consumption of carbohydrates during exercise. Further, many of these protocols in the research studies were conducted on submaximal exercise in a glycogen-depleted state. This may not be what is happening in the field.

> Some athletes who consumed LCHF diets report a perception in improved training capacity and decreased perceived exertion and heart rate. LCHF consumption might actually impair performance in the field, particularly in activities of higher intensity or power requirement in which glycogen utilization is the preferred source of energy (9).

With the increased use of social media, support of this approach has increased based on anecdotal evidence. Because of the rise in popularity of the concept, and that absolute conclusions cannot be made based on the previous research, it is surprising that only a few additional studies have been completed and published on this topic. None have shown a performance benefit to the LCHF diet, and one of the studies did not impose a typ-ical carbohydrate restriction used in the LCHF protocol. More research needs to be completed that compares nonketogenic LCHF diets versus ketogenic LCHF diets. Some theorize that chronic carbohydrate restriction resulting in ketone production is beneficial because the body can adapt to use these ketones as a fuel source during exercise. This sounds nice in theory, but we have no data on the amount of energy that ketones can provide as an exercise substrate (9).

Until more research is available, it is important to think of the use of LCHF diets and exercise performance. The popular media and anecdotal promotion of this approach implies that it is based on evidence from and applicable to a wide range of athletes. In reality, it might be applicable only to ultraendurance athletes or those undergoing long periods of submaximal exercise, if it is beneficial at all. While general carbohydrate guidelines do exist for before, during, and after endurance activities, note that sports dietitians who are current in their practice work with their athletes to avoid unnecessary, excess carbohydrate intake and tailor recommendations for carbohydrate amount and type specific to the individual. Balance in all nutrition aspects of the diet is an important concept (9).

IMPACTS OF ENDURANCE TRAINING ON MACRONUTRIENT METABOLISM

Endurance training elicits numerous physiological adaptations that lead to enhanced performance, including improved delivery, uptake, and oxidation of glucose, larger skeletal muscle glycogen stores, greater oxygen uptake in working muscle, and a better ability to use lactate as a fuel source.

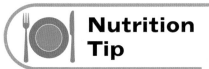 **Nutrition Tip** Sports nutrition guidelines are evidence-based and developed using the current available research. These guidelines are often suited for a wide range of individual athletes, but never replace the individualized approach that is likely necessary for optimal health and performance. Athletes might use these guidelines as a starting point during preparation and training, but they must learn what works best for them through trial and error. Sometimes an athlete might fall outside of an established guideline. The Certified Specialist in Sports Dietetics (CSSD) uses a modernized, periodized approach to meet the needs of individual athletes.

PUTTING IT INTO PERSPECTIVE

OVERTRAINING SYNDROME

Overtraining syndrome (OTS) is characterized by chronic inadequate energy intake coupled with long periods of low-carbohydrate intake and high-volume training. There can be an accompanied long-term performance decrement with or without physiological symptoms. Restoration of physiological function and performance can take several weeks to several months. The only "cure" for OTS is reduced training volume, or complete rest, along with consuming adequate energy, protein, carbohydrates, and fluids (13, 28, 32).

Trained skeletal muscle is also more sensitive to insulin and possesses a greater amount of GLUT4 proteins, thereby allowing enhanced glucose uptake and utilization. Endurance-trained individuals have larger left ventricle heart volumes, larger blood volume, increased capillary density, and greater myoglobin concentration, all of which contribute to greater oxygen delivery to the muscle, which when coupled with increased mitochondrial density and concentration of metabolic enzymes in muscle cells results in a greater ability to completely oxidize glucose and fatty acids.

SUMMARY

Endurance athletes participate in events that have demanding energy requirements that pose unique challenges to the body's main ATP-producing systems, particularly the ability to completely oxidize glucose for lengthy periods of time without fatigue. Carbohydrates are of primary importance for long-term ATP production, and numerous strategies exist to preserve muscle glycogen by delaying its utilization or increasing its content in muscle. Endurance athletes face distinct and demanding nutrient requirements for energy, fat, carbohydrates, and fluids, and the challenge of translating these requirements into actual food choices can be daunting. Fortunately, readily available tools that assist in the process of selecting foods, beverages, and supplements do exist, and these significantly help endurance athletes satisfy the unique nutrition requirements of their chosen activity.

■ FOR REVIEW ▶

1. Explain how carbohydrate and fat are used as fuel sources during exercise of varying intensities.

2. How can an athlete minimize fatigue during prolonged endurance exercise?

3. What are the carbohydrate recommendations before an endurance event? List for 1, 2, 3, and 4 hours pre-event. What types of carbohydrate are recommended at each time period?

4. What are the carbohydrate recommendations during exercise? Do the recommendations change with time and intensity?

5. What are the carbohydrate recommendations for recovery to maximize glycogen stores, including both quantity and timing?

6. Describe the role of glycemic index in making carbohydrate recommendations before, during, and after endurance exercise.

7. Many endurance-enhancing supplements are marketed specifically toward athletes. Can an endurance athlete obtain the same benefits from typical foods? Give examples.

8. Describe the theory behind "training low, competing high." Is this a widely recommended strategy? Why or why not?

9. List strategies for minimizing GI distress during endurance training.

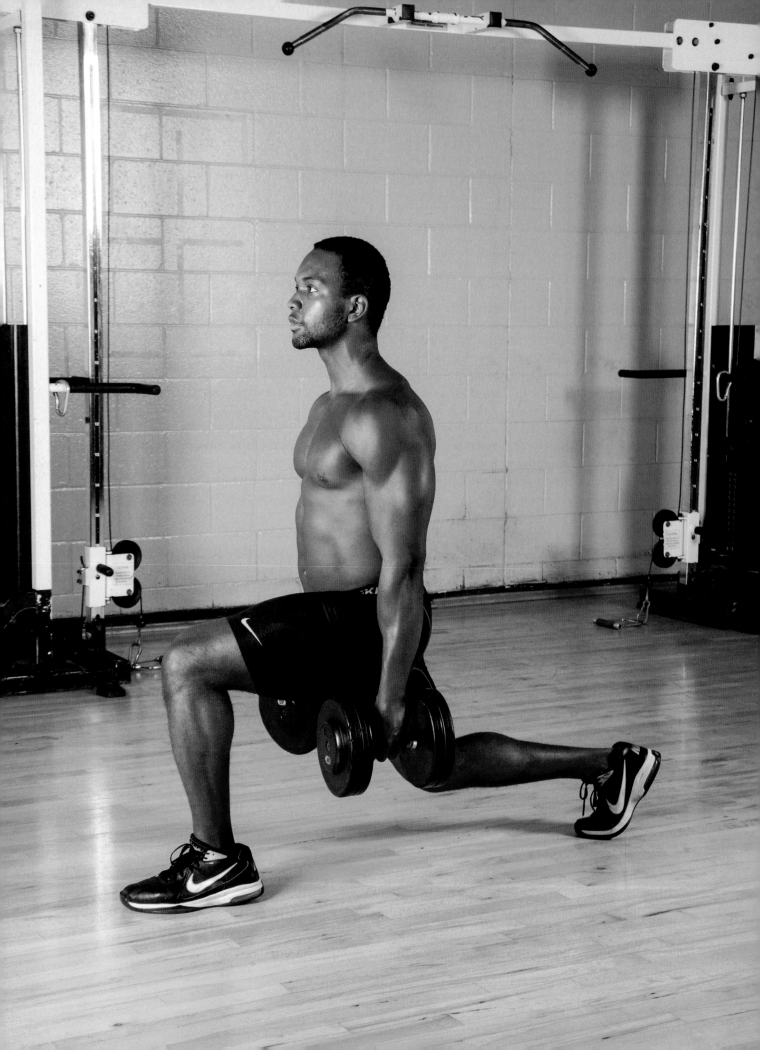

CHAPTER 12

Nutrition for Resistance Training

Many individuals include resistance training in their exercise program. In this chapter we discuss nutrition strategies to support resistance training by providing the energy (kilocalories) and nutrients needed to fuel muscle contraction, support muscle growth and repair, replace carbohydrate used during activity, and minimize muscle soreness. Although research continues to uncover how specific nutrients and supplements affect muscle functioning and acute and chronic training adaptations (gains made from a resistance-training program), inter-individual results from incorporating one or more of these strategies might vary considerably based on the training program one is following, genetic differences in response to training, training status (from untrained to highly trained), age, gender, overall diet, adaptation to one's diet, and possibly **nutrigenomics** (the interaction between nutrition and genes—a relatively new area of study).

Though an individual's overall diet, including consistent intake of kilocalories and certain nutrients, can have a profound effect on improvements made through resistance training, considerable research has focused on the timing of specific nutrients and how supplements during the preexercise, exercise, and postexercise periods influence performance, recovery, and changes in muscle mass, strength, and power over time.

DO YOU KNOW ?

Many people recognize the role of muscle mass in strength and athletic performance; however, muscle mass also has an important role in reducing risk of obesity, cardiovascular disease, type 2 diabetes, osteoporosis, and **sarcopenia**, the age-related loss of muscle mass and strength (130).

NUTRITION BEFORE RESISTANCE TRAINING

The main purpose of the preexercise meal, consumed within an hour or less before resistance training, is to hydrate the athlete, top off glycogen stores, and decrease hunger. In addition, adding protein to one's preexercise meal or snack might be advantageous if the athlete hasn't consumed protein for several hours prior, or if their daily protein needs are high and the preexercise meal represents an important opportunity to help them meet their daily protein needs. For instance, a 280-pound male athlete who is trying to gain 20 pounds will have substantial daily protein needs and might find it challenging to consume the quantity of food (including protein) necessary to gain weight, particularly if he is training for several hours a day (more time spent training means less available hours to eat).

Hydration

Staying hydrated is important for resistance training. Hypohydration compromises resistance-training performance and recovery (55, 56). However, methodological considerations in study design make it difficult to clearly distinguish the mechanism through which hypohydration affects strength, power, and high-intensity exercise. Cardiovascular strain such as decreases in maximal cardiac output and blood flow to muscle tissue (and thus a decline in the delivery of nutrients and metabolite removal) are plausible contributing factors (55, 57). The studies to date indicate dehydration of 3 to 4 percent body weight loss reduces muscle strength by approximately 2 percent, muscular power by approximately 3 percent, and high-intensity endurance activity (maximal repeated activities lasting >30 seconds but <2 minutes) by approximately 10 percent (55).

Hypohydration also impacts the hormonal response to exercise. In one resistance training study, increasing levels of hypohydration (from 2.5% of body weight to 5% of body weight) led to progressive increases in the stress hormones cortisol and norepinephrine, and a subsequent increase in blood glucose, presumably to cope with increased physiological demands (the stress response leads to greater energy availability). These results suggest hypohydration significantly enhances stress from resistance exercise, and could impair training adaptations. Over time, these changes could decrease training adaptations to resistance training if consistently performed in a hypohydrated state (57).

Given the impact of hypohydration on strength, power, and repetitive activity lasting more than 30 seconds but less than 2 minutes, athletes engaging in resistance-training sessions or participating in sports that require these variables, such as American football, soccer, wrestling, ice hockey, and rugby, should ensure they are adequately hydrated prior to training or competition. There are no specific pretraining guidelines for resistance exercise because any recommendations depend on hydration status prior to exercise.

Carbohydrate

Carbohydrate, from circulating blood sugar and muscle glycogen, is the primary source of fuel used during resistance training. In addition, maintaining adequate glycogen stores can help attenuate muscle breakdown during exercise and keep both the immune and nervous system functioning normally. Low carbohydrate intake can acutely suppress immune and central nervous system functioning (18, 67).

Consuming carbohydrate prior to training can help decrease muscular fatigue, particularly in fast-twitch muscle fibers, which tire quickly compared to slow-twitch muscle fibers; spare the use of protein as a source of energy; and perhaps also improve performance (44, 54, 67). This strategy is particularly important for athletes who exercise first thing in the morning after an overnight fast; those who haven't consumed enough carbohydrate in the time period since their last training session; and those who are lifting weights right after speed work, endurance exercise, or any other type of training that requires a significant amount of carbohydrate for energy. Like many aspects of nutrition, there is a caveat to the need for carbohydrate prior to resistance training. The body can adapt to sustained alterations in the intake of energy-yielding macronutrients (carbohydrate, protein, fat), and thus individuals on a low-carbohydrate diet might not experience any negative effects or performance decrements once adapted to this diet, provided their diet contains enough protein to build and repair muscle and energy to help spare protein losses (from protein breakdown in muscle as a source of energy). However, there is a paucity of data on this topic (83), so at this time low-carbohydrate diets are not recommended for those engaging in a resistance-training program.

In one study, six trained men were given either a carbohydrate supplement (1 g of carbohydrate per kg body mass before exercise and 0.17 g of carbohydrate per kg body mass every 6 minutes during the session) or a placebo sweetened with saccharin and aspartame (nonnutritive sweeteners). They performed a series of static contractions of the quadriceps at 50 percent maximum contraction with 40 seconds of rest between sets until muscle failure (i.e., they couldn't do anymore). Time to exhaustion and force output were significantly higher in the group receiving carbohydrate compared to the group consuming the placebo (123).

Carbohydrate loading is a technique endurance athletes have used for several decades to super-compensate glycogen stores and improve performance. In general, the athlete will taper their training program for a specified period of time—from a few days to weeks prior to an event—while consuming a higher-carbohydrate diet, generally between 8 and 10 grams of carbohydrate per kilogram body weight each day (48). Few studies have looked at the effect of carbohydrate loading on resistance exercise per-

> **DO YOU KNOW ?**
> Muscle breakdown increases when resistance training is performed on an empty (fasted) stomach (9, 92).

formance. However, in one study, healthy young men were randomized to receive either a moderate-carbohydrate diet (4.4 g of carbohydrate per kg body weight) or higher-carbohydrate diet (6.5 g of carbohydrate per kg body weight) for 4 days before a resistance exercise test, including 4 sets of 12 repetitions of maximal-effort jump squats with a load of 30 percent of 1 repetition maximum (1RM) and a 2-minute rest period between sets (48). Power performance didn't differ between groups, indicating a higher-carbohydrate diet did not enhance power-endurance performance over four sets of exercise. However, it isn't clear if an even greater intake of carbohydrate, reaching 8 to 10 grams per kilogram body weight, would have led to a performance difference or if the diet used would have made a difference over the course of several sets.

Bodybuilders might carbohydrate-load prior to competition to increase muscle size, a practice that makes sense physiologically (particularly if they consume a lower-carbohydrate diet for a few days, followed by carbohydrate loading), yet only one study to date has examined this practice. There was no change in muscle size following a low- versus high-carbohydrate diet; however, study subjects consumed the same amount of total energy during the period of low-carbohydrate intake (3 days of 10% energy from carbohydrate) as they did during the 3-day period of carbohydrate loading (80% energy from carbohydrate) (7). Thus it is possible that a difference might have been noted if they also increased total energy intake (50).

Protein and Amino Acids

Research shows that protein or essential amino acids (EAAs) consumed prior to resistance training will stimulate muscle protein synthesis (110, 111, 113), and prolonged supplementation can improve lean mass, body fat percentage, and muscle hypertrophy (21, 28). Protein can be taken pre- or postexercise to enhance acute muscle protein synthesis (91, 129).

NUTRITION DURING RESISTANCE TRAINING

During resistance training, carbohydrate and hydration are the most important nutrition considerations. Hormonal changes facilitate the delivery of glucose to muscle cells for energy, which affects the production of muscle force and rate of muscular contraction. Glycogen (via glycogenolysis) contributes a significant amount of energy used during resistance training (44). Decreases in glycogen can impair force production and strength while accentuating muscle weakness (44, 54). Studies examining glycogen use during resistance training found subjects used 13 percent of their glycogen stores after one set of 10 reps of biceps curls to 45 percent of their glycogen stores after a few sets of different exercises (43, 71, 72). Carbohydrate intake during resistance training can help maintain glycogen stores and might

enhance performance (43, 44). Carbohydrate needs during training depend on glycogen levels and carbohydrate intake over the course of the day before training.

Athletes who start training in a hypohydrated state should sip water or other fluids to prevent excessive hypohydration and subsequent decrements in strength. As mentioned in the previous section, maintaining adequate hydration status is important for performance in strength and power training and events.

Protein or amino acids can be consumed during training to increase muscle protein synthesis (24). In one study, protein ingestion during prolonged (>2 hours) resistance training led to a greater increase in acute muscle protein synthesis during exercise compared to a carbohydrate control (90). However, this strategy is probably not be necessary if protein is consumed before or after exercise.

NUTRITION AFTER RESISTANCE TRAINING

Hormones released during exercise prepare the body to use protein and carbohydrate. Athletes should take advantage of this time period after resistance training to replenish their glycogen stores and also provide high-quality protein that will deliver amino acids to muscle tissue to start the growth and repair process.

Replacing Glycogen

Carbohydrate intake after resistance training helps replace glycogen, facilitate recovery, and decrease muscle breakdown (9, 43, 92). After training, it is important to replace glycogen over the time period prior to the next training session for maximum strength and power (43). Athletes training or competing within several hours of the initial training session (two training sessions per day) should consume carbohydrate immediately after resistance training. During the first 45 minutes (approximately) after the completion of training, muscles rapidly soak up carbohydrate. After about 45 minutes, the rate of glycogen resynthesis decreases (53, 85). Individuals who have more than 8 hours between training sessions or those who do not train every day do not necessarily need to consume carbohydrate immediately after training in an effort to rapidly replace glycogen. Instead, they can fully replenish their carbohydrate stores over the period of time prior to their next bout of training if total daily dietary carbohydrate intake is adequate (84).

In a crossover study, men trained in a fasted state, performing knee-extension exercises until failure (exhaustion), and consumed either 1.5 grams of carbohydrate per kilogram body weight immediately after training and again 1 hour later or water at these same time points. The group consuming carbohydrate replaced glycogen stores to 91 percent of preexercise levels by 6 hours after training, whereas the group consuming water replaced muscle glycogen levels to 75 percent of preexercise levels (85).

Many factors affect the amount of carbohydrate needed to fully replenish glycogen stores, including glycogen levels prior to the start of training, the intensity and duration of resistance training, body weight, habitual carbohydrate consumption, and if carbohydrate was consumed before or during exercise.

Building and Repairing Muscle

A series of steps are involved in building and repairing muscle tissue, as shown in figure 12.1.

Two factors influence net **muscle protein balance**: muscle protein synthesis and muscle protein breakdown. Muscle protein synthesis must be greater than breakdown for growth to occur (41). Chronic net gains in the muscle protein pool lead to improvements in strength and hypertrophy over time. When muscle protein breakdown chronically exceeds muscle protein synthesis, a net loss occurs in the protein pool (muscle atrophy) over time (24, 91).

Muscle protein synthesis is suppressed during exercise. Resistance training increases both muscle protein synthesis and muscle protein breakdown. Though net muscle protein balance improves, it remains negative (catabolic state)

until protein or essential amino acids are consumed (9, 92). Blood flow to muscle increases after resistance training, enhancing the delivery of the amino acids from protein to muscle (9). The synergistic effect of resistance training combined with greater amino acid availability (from consuming protein or essential amino acids) leads to a greater increase in muscle protein synthesis compared to resistance exercise alone, leading to a net gain in muscle proteins (outweighing breakdown) post-exercise (9, 91, 92). Muscle protein breakdown after resistance training varies, with reported ranges from 31 to 51 percent (9, 92). Relatively small amounts of carbohydrate, between 30 and 100 grams, consumed after resistance training reduces muscle protein breakdown (14, 41). However, muscle protein synthesis is considered the most important part of this equation, making up more than 70 percent of improvements in net protein balance through resistance training, whereas muscle protein breakdown has a smaller contribution to net protein balance (41). Net muscle protein balance remains negative if carbohydrate alone is consumed without the addition of essential amino acids or protein (figure 12.2) (14, 41).

Type, amount, and timing of protein are the three most important factors to consider after resistance training to enhance muscle protein synthesis (129). The ideal type of protein is high in leucine and digested quickly, leading to a rapid rise in amino acids in the bloodstream (a "fast" protein). Faster proteins lead to a greater increase in acute muscle protein synthesis (over the 3-hour period postexercise) compared to proteins that are digested more slowly and thus lead to a slower release of amino acids into the bloodstream. Whey is a fast protein, soy a moderate-speed protein, and casein is digested slowly. In trained individuals, milk increased acute muscle protein synthesis to a greater extent

DO YOU KNOW ?

Muscle protein breakdown is a physiologically important process that helps remove damaged proteins. Think of this process as tearing down part of an old building and rebuilding it with newer, stronger materials. Though breakdown is essential, excess breakdown is not beneficial.

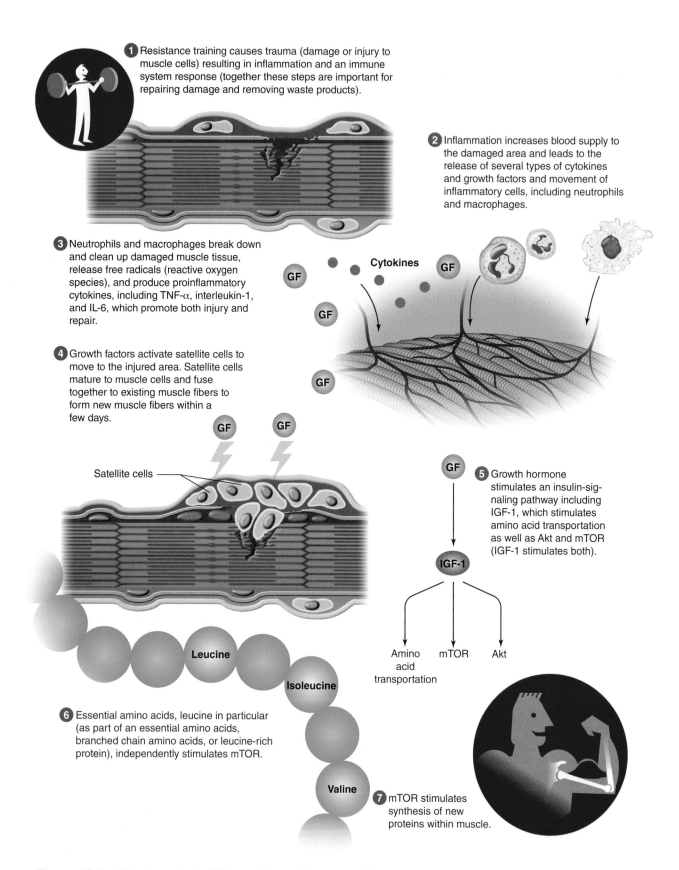

1 Resistance training causes trauma (damage or injury to muscle cells) resulting in inflammation and an immune system response (together these steps are important for repairing damage and removing waste products).

2 Inflammation increases blood supply to the damaged area and leads to the release of several types of cytokines and growth factors and movement of inflammatory cells, including neutrophils and macrophages.

3 Neutrophils and macrophages break down and clean up damaged muscle tissue, release free radicals (reactive oxygen species), and produce proinflammatory cytokines, including TNF-α, interleukin-1, and IL-6, which promote both injury and repair.

Cytokines

GF

4 Growth factors activate satellite cells to move to the injured area. Satellite cells mature to muscle cells and fuse together to existing muscle fibers to form new muscle fibers within a few days.

GF

Satellite cells

5 Growth hormone stimulates an insulin-signaling pathway including IGF-1, which stimulates amino acid transportation as well as Akt and mTOR (IGF-1 stimulates both).

IGF-1

Amino acid transportation   mTOR   Akt

Leucine

Isoleucine

6 Essential amino acids, leucine in particular (as part of an essential amino acids, branched chain amino acids, or leucine-rich protein), independently stimulates mTOR.

Valine

7 mTOR stimulates synthesis of new proteins within muscle.

Figure 12.1 The steps to building and repairing muscle tissue.

Based on Charge and Rudnicki 2004; Hamada et al. 2005; Tidball 2005; Tiidus 2008; Gran and Cameron-Smith 2011; Frost and Lang 2012.

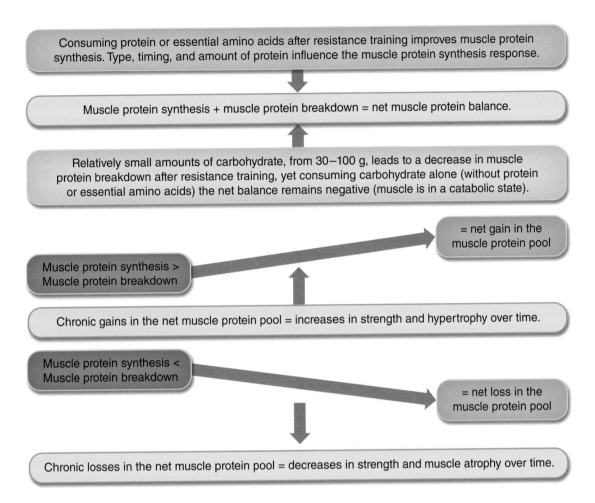

Consuming protein or essential amino acids after resistance training improves muscle protein synthesis. Type, timing, and amount of protein influence the muscle protein synthesis response.

Muscle protein synthesis + muscle protein breakdown = net muscle protein balance.

Relatively small amounts of carbohydrate, from 30–100 g, leads to a decrease in muscle protein breakdown after resistance training, yet consuming carbohydrate alone (without protein or essential amino acids) the net balance remains negative (muscle is in a catabolic state).

Muscle protein synthesis > Muscle protein breakdown

= net gain in the muscle protein pool

Chronic gains in the net muscle protein pool = increases in strength and hypertrophy over time.

Muscle protein synthesis < Muscle protein breakdown

= net loss in the muscle protein pool

Chronic losses in the net muscle protein pool = decreases in strength and muscle atrophy over time.

Figure 12.2   The muscle protein balance equation.

than soy; whey protein, compared to soy and casein, led to the greatest rise in acute muscle protein synthesis (over the 3-hour period postexercise, when protein is consumed); and soy resulted in a more significant increase than casein (47, 105, 127). While speed is important for an immediate increase in muscle protein synthesis, there is a benefit to blending proteins. Protein blends including a mix of fast and slow proteins such as whey, soy, and casein combined or milk (which contains approximately 80% casein and 20% whey) effectively stimulate muscle protein synthesis and lead to a more prolonged increase in muscle protein synthesis compared to the consumption of a fast protein alone (91, 95). In healthy, recreationally active men and women, a blend of whey, soy, and casein (25% whey, 25% soy, 50% casein, including a total of 1.8 g of leucine) led to a similar increase in muscle protein

synthesis over a 2-hour period after a bout of resistance training as whey protein matched for leucine content (1.9 g of leucine). Only the blend resulted in an increase in muscle protein synthesis 2 to 4 hours after exercise (95). Blending fast and slow proteins may be beneficial if a person waits several hours (3–5 or more) before eating again or exercises at night and consumes protein prior to sleeping.

The amino acid leucine triggers the initiation of muscle protein synthesis at meals and after exercise, though protein-derived amino acids are necessary for protein synthesis to continue running (126). In healthy young men, a relatively small amount of whey protein (6.25 g) combined with leucine (for a total of 3 g of leucine), or 6.25 grams whey combined with essential amino acids minus leucine (essential amino acids minus leucine for a total leucine content of 0.75 g in the whey plus essential amino acids) stimulated muscle protein synthesis during the 1- to 3-hour period after exercise to the same extent as 25 grams of whey protein (total leucine equals 3 g). However, muscle protein synthesis remained elevated above fasting levels in the 3- to 5-hour period after exercise after consuming 25 grams of whey compared to the whey plus leucine treatment and whey plus essential amino acids minus leucine treatments. This study suggests leucine or essential amino acids without leucine can be added to a small amount of protein to maximally stimulate acute muscle protein synthesis, though protein synthesis will continue to be elevated for a longer period of time if a greater amount of whey protein is consumed postexercise (27).

As noted in figure 12.3, research suggests younger adults need approximately 2 to 3 grams of leucine or 0.05 grams of leucine per kilogram body weight, whereas older adults might need 3 to 4 grams of leucine as part of an amino acid mix or protein postexercise to maximize muscle protein synthesis (79, 82, 112). Younger adults can meet this leucine threshold with 20 to 25 grams of high-quality protein (providing about 8.5–10 grams of essential amino acids), such as egg or whey. If opting for a protein source with less leucine per serving, more protein is necessary

to meet the leucine threshold of 2 to 3 grams. For instance, approximately 30 grams of soy protein contains approximately 2 grams of leucine. Older adults need more leucine and protein because of age-related decline in muscle sensitivity to amino acids (discussed later in the chapter). A minimum of 40 grams of protein is recommended for maximizing muscle protein synthesis after resistance training in this age group (3, 15, 76, 80, 91).

Total amount of lean body mass does not influence the amount of protein needed after resistance training. However, protein needs increase with greater amounts of muscle used during a resistance training bout. When more muscle is activated, more amino acids are taken up by muscle. Muscle protein synthesis was stimulated to a greater extent in resistance-trained men after ingestion of 40 grams compared to 20 grams of whey protein following a bout of whole-body resistance exercise (73). Depending on many factors, including a person's age, type of training, training load, type of protein consumed, total energy, and protein intake, it is possible that even higher amounts of protein can lead to a more robust acute muscle protein synthesis response.

For maximum muscle protein synthesis, the idea of an "anabolic window of opportunity" has been put forth. Many have suggested muscle

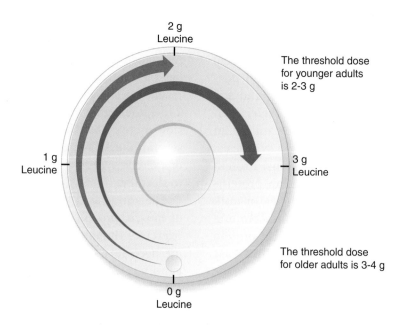

Figure 12.3 Leucine turns on muscle protein synthesis.

protein synthesis is greatest if protein is consumed within a specific period of time, typically 1 hour, after exercise. However, the exact time period for resistance-trained individuals is not clear, while consuming protein within a 3-hour window after resistance training does not appear to be important for untrained individuals, perhaps because of their later spike in muscle protein synthesis several hours after exercise (129).

Does Food Work as Well as Protein?

Eating a food-based source of protein, such as meat, enhances muscle protein synthesis after resistance training. However, current research is insufficient to determine if protein supplements lead to a greater impact on acute muscle protein synthesis, as well as strength and hypertrophy adaptations over time, compared to food-based sources of protein, or if they are equivalent (with all other factors being equal, including total energy intake and total protein intake).

Negro and colleagues (2014) reported healthy men who consumed 135 grams (4.7 oz.; 20 g of protein and >2 g of leucine) of tinned beef after resistance training over the course of an 8-week study increased muscular strength, though there was no difference compared to the placebo group. No significant differences in lean mass were found in either the food group or control group (78). While tinned beef is more rapidly digested than some other types of red meat, it is still considerably slower than fast proteins, such as whey (peak plasma EAA concentrations occurred at approximately 2 hours postconsumption; whey peaks at approximately 30 minutes) (89). The lack of significant differences between groups might not be caused by the speed of release of amino acids into the bloodstream from tinned beef but rather from the low total daily protein intake in both groups: 1 gram of protein per kilogram body weight per day (78).

In another study, middle-aged men (59 ± 2 years) who were habitually consuming "at or above the recommended dietary allowances for protein" (total daily average protein intake was measured by a 3-day dietary recall, yet the amount was not indicated in the article) were given protein prepackaged food, which provided 1 gram of protein per kilogram body weight per day and enough energy for weight maintenance, for the 2 days prior to the start of the study.

Subjects were randomly assigned to consume either 0 ounces, 2 ounces (12 g protein), 4 ounces (24 g protein), or 6 ounces (36 g of protein) of ground beef (15% fat) after unilateral resistance exercise of a randomly selected leg on an empty stomach (after an overnight fast). In middle-aged and elderly individuals, for both the rested (non-exercised leg) and exercised leg, 6 ounces of beef led to significantly greater increases in muscle protein synthesis compared to lower doses of beef (figure 12.4) (97).

Does Protein Timing Matter?

After exercise, an individual is in a catabolic state until food is consumed. The muscle protein synthesis response to amino acids postexercise decreases over time, which makes the time

PUTTING IT INTO PERSPECTIVE

ALCOHOL AND EXERCISE

If you want to get in a good lift before heading out to the bars to throw back a few beers, you might feel as if you are pumping up your muscles, but you have only wasted a training session. In men, alcohol consumed after exercise decreases the effect of dietary protein on muscle protein synthesis and impairs anabolic signaling. Alcohol does not have the same effect in women (36). Also, high doses of alcohol decrease testosterone in men, and long-term use decreases the androgen receptor, so even if you have a lot of testosterone circulating, there's a decrease in your body's ability to use testosterone.

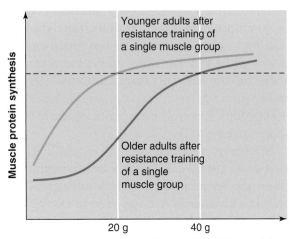

Figure 12.4   Muscle protein synthesis increases with greater protein intake up to approximately 20 to 25 grams of high-quality, high-leucine protein in younger adults and 40 grams of high-quality, high-leucine protein in older adults. Muscle protein breakdown decreases slightly with greater protein or amino acid intake.

period soon after resistance training particularly important for maximizing acute muscle protein synthesis in trained individuals (91). Protein timing might be more important for individuals exercising in a fasting state or those not consuming enough protein per day (in which case, either timing or the additional protein provided from the supplement makes the difference) (101). Timing protein intake soon after exercise is far less important in untrained individuals, possibly due to their later peak in muscle protein synthesis after exercise (77).

In a randomized, crossover study, 10 untrained and 10 trained men were put on a diet for weight maintenance (providing 1.5 g protein per kg body weight) for 11 days. Three hours after eating breakfast each day, they started their resistance-training session. They were given protein (0.3 g/kg body weight; 21.7 ± 1.3 g for trained, 19.3 ± 1.5 g for untrained) and carbohydrate (0.8 g/kg body weight; 57.9 ± 3.4 g for trained, 51.5 ± 4.0 g for untrained) either 5 minutes after the completion of training or 6 hours later, for 11 days (the first 8 days were used for acclimation and the last 3 days for data collection). The trained group had greater muscle protein accumulation when taking the supplement immediately postexercise as compared to 6 hours later, while the timing of protein intake did not affect the accumulation of muscle protein (as measured by whole-body protein metabolism; muscle protein synthesis represents approximately 30% of whole-body protein synthesis) in untrained men (27, 77). These results are consistent with previous research, which found untrained individuals reach peak muscle protein synthesis more than 4 hours after exercise and maintain this state for several hours (106).

Postexercise Protein Intake for Older Adults

Aging alters the anabolic response to protein intake. Although regular exercise improves an older person's response to protein intake (33), older adults need more protein (and more leucine) than younger adults after resistance training to maximize muscle protein synthesis. Studies suggest

PUTTING IT INTO PERSPECTIVE

STRENGTH-TRAINING GAINS

Strength increases during the first few months of resistance training are achieved not only through changes in muscle size but also through changes in neural adaptations, so novices might get stronger before they notice any appreciable increase in muscle size (37). Also, the same strength-training program can elicit a wide range of responses. Some individuals will show little to no gains, while others might have profound changes in muscle size and strength (51, 122, 124). The wide variability in response to a well-designed strength-training program might help explain some of the variability observed in response to nutrition interventions (52).

the elderly need approximately 40 grams of high-quality protein to maximize the acute rise in muscle protein synthesis after resistance training (88). Consuming protein in the time period immediately after exercise may be particularly important in the elderly who do not consume the RDA for protein. Though some studies have found that protein supplementation improves acute muscle protein synthesis in the elderly, a longer-term study (12 weeks) found that 10 grams of casein hydrolysate protein consumed before and after resistance training did not further improve strength or muscle mass compared to a placebo in healthy elderly individuals who habitually consumed adequate amounts of protein (1.1 g/kg body weight/day) (118).

DO YOU KNOW ❓

Invasive procedures are required to examine changes in muscle protein synthesis, so there are not enough studies in children to make a research-based recommendation for protein intake after resistance training in this age group (12, 13).

Impact of Concurrent Training

Concurrent training sessions are those performed back to back. For instance, a coach might choose to have athletes work on speed immediately followed by strength training, or vice versa. Some studies report interference—aerobic training interferes with resistance exercise performance. However, other studies show moderate-intensity endurance exercise does not impair acute bouts of resistance exercise, anabolic signaling, or the hypertrophy response (2, 19, 35, 69, 70). Physiological and molecular responses to concurrent training depend on the duration and type of exercise (running followed by upper-body lifting may not have any interference effects, while running or repetitive sprint activity followed by lower-body lifting will likely result in interference; cycling has less of an impact than running), whether the athlete is in a fed or fasted state, how trained the athlete is (and adaptation to concurrent training regiments), and sequence of concurrent training (29, 94).

Scant research has examined the impact of concurrent training and nutrition interventions compared to studies examining how pre-, during, and postworkout nutrition alters acute changes after a single training session (128). A concurrent training model seems to lead to greater acute increases in muscle protein synthesis in the fed state compared to resistance exercise alone (19, 35).

While it is difficult to determine optimal nutrition strategies because of the sheer number of variables, including different types of concurrent training programs, more general recommendations can be made based on both the research on concurrent training models, nutrition interventions used in single training studies (endurance, sprint performance, resistance training etc.), and proposed mechanisms responsible for exercise interference (5, 90).

Some athletes may want to perform endurance exercise in a glycogen-depleted state to promote greater adaptations in skeletal muscle. Immediately after endurance exercise they might also delay carbohydrate intake for the same reason. However, these strategies need to be carefully considered, as they can lead to skeletal muscle breakdown and decreases in energy, as well as resistance-training performance, particularly when used in a concurrent model where resistance training is performed immediately after endurance exercise (90). For peak training performance, athletes should consume enough carbohydrate after aerobic or high-intensity interval training and prior to strength training to refill their glycogen stores. In addition, over the course of prolonged concurrent sessions, the athlete may want to consider a small amount of dietary protein or BCAAs if their stomach can handle it) during aerobic or high-intensity interval training or prior to strength training in addition to a leucine-rich, fast protein soon after resistance training to maximize muscle protein synthesis.

HOW DAILY DIETARY INTAKE AFFECTS MUSCLE

Though pre-, during, and postexercise nutrient intake has received considerable attention, other factors are essential for optimal resistance-training performance including total daily

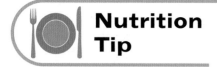

protein intake, per meal amount of protein, and intake of specific nutrients that support muscle functioning.

Studies in children and adolescents suggest these athletes also need more protein than their sedentary counterparts to meet the demands of growth and training. Though it isn't entirely clear how much protein they need per day, 1.2 to 2.0 grams of protein per kilogram body weight per day has been put forth as a general recommended range (13, 20). As the body ages, muscle mass tends to decrease as a result of sarcopenia. This is a major challenge, but exercise, particularly resistance training, and the consumption of an adequate amount of protein per meal and per day represent promising strategies to delay the onset and progression of sarcopenia. Older adults should aim for 1.1 to 1.5 grams of protein per kilogram body weight daily (80).

Meal Patterns and Muscle Growth

Resistance training can increase muscle sensitivity to amino acids for up to 48 hours after activity. As shown in figure 12.5, protein intake at any point during this 48-hour period has an additive effect (additive to resistance training) on muscle protein synthesis (91). Therefore, consuming regular meals containing an efficacious amount of protein can help maximize muscle protein synthesis. The recommendation for younger adults is 0.25 to 0.30 grams of protein per kg body weight or 30 grams of protein and 2 to 3 grams of leucine per meal, and for older adults, 30 to 40 grams of protein and 3 to 4 grams of leucine per meal (22, 64, 74, 81, 91).

In adults, the initiation of protein synthesis is regulated by leucine, which up-regulates the mTORC1 pathway that controls the synthesis of proteins in muscle (27, 61). A high-quality, leucine-rich protein should be a central part of each meal if the goal is to maintain or build muscle. See figure 12.6 for the leucine content of commonly consumed proteins. The anabolic effect (up-regulation in muscle protein synthesis) of a meal lasts approximately 3 to 5 hours, so regular meals evenly spaced apart might be best for maximizing muscle growth (4, 11, 27, 95).

The body does not store protein to stimulate muscle protein synthesis at a later time, though the gut can retain amino acids and release them later for incorporation into tissues, including muscle (33). However, the consumption of a very large amount of protein at one meal does not lead to greater acute muscle protein synthesis compared to a more

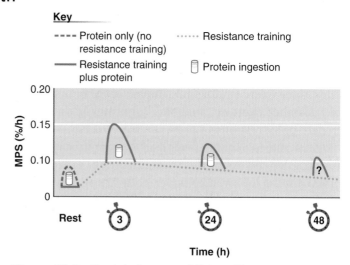

Figure 12.5 Protein has an additive effect to resistance training, enhancing muscle protein synthesis more than resistance training alone.

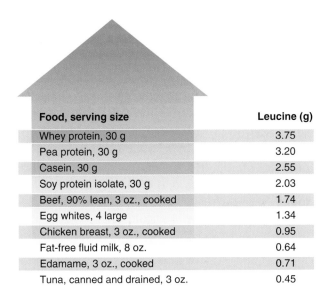

Food, serving size	Leucine (g)
Whey protein, 30 g	3.75
Pea protein, 30 g	3.20
Casein, 30 g	2.55
Soy protein isolate, 30 g	2.03
Beef, 90% lean, 3 oz., cooked	1.74
Egg whites, 4 large	1.34
Chicken breast, 3 oz., cooked	0.95
Fat-free fluid milk, 8 oz.	0.64
Edamame, 3 oz., cooked	0.71
Tuna, canned and drained, 3 oz.	0.45

Figure 12.6 Leucine content of common foods and supplements.

Data from Babault et al. 2015; Pennings et al. 2011; U.S. Department of Agriculture 2013.

modest amount of protein (104). In a 7-day crossover feeding study with a 30-day washout period (a period where they went back to their regular diet) between each trial, researchers examined how different patterns of protein intake affected muscle protein synthesis over a 24-hour period. Each of the two study diets provided enough energy for weight maintenance and 1.2 grams of protein per kilogram body weight per day (90 g of protein). Diet 1 provided an even distribution of protein intake: about 30 grams at breakfast, 30 grams at lunch, and 30 grams at dinner. Diet 2 provided a skewed distribution of protein intake set to mimic a typical American diet (a lower-protein breakfast with most protein consumed at dinner): about 10 grams at breakfast, 15 grams at lunch, and 65 grams at dinner (114). Carbohydrate content at each meal was held constant, while dietary fat content was manipulated to ensure total daily calorie intake remained similar on each diet and that carbohydrate, fat, and protein intake was not different between the diets. Consuming an even distribution of protein at each meal resulted in an approx-

imately 25 percent greater mixed muscle protein synthesis (contractile proteins make up a large part of this) over the 24-hour period, as measured on study day 1, compared to when protein intake was skewed. By day 7, when study subjects were habituated to the diet, a similar muscle protein synthetic response was observed. This study suggests an even distribution of approximately 30 grams of protein per meal leads to greater muscle protein synthesis compared to a skewed distribution that reflects a typical American diet, even after 7 days of habituation to the pattern of protein intake. It isn't clear from this study if higher per-meal doses of protein would have resulted in greater increases in acute muscle protein synthesis and greater improvements in muscle mass and strength over time (74, 98). It is possible that greater quantities of protein may lead to greater net protein gains (33). At this time, at least 30 grams of protein per meal is suggested for adults to fully stimulate muscle protein synthesis (64), while aged individuals might need more protein per meal (15, 80). Figure 12.7 shows examples of foods with 30 grams of protein.

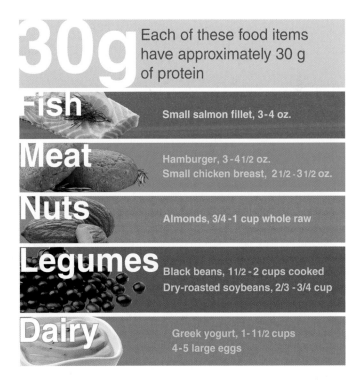

Figure 12.7 What does 30 grams of protein look like?

Increasing Muscle Protein Synthesis in Protein-Poor Meals

If 30 grams of protein at each meal seems like a lot of food, or if a higher-protein diet is contraindicated, another strategy might increase acute muscle protein synthesis to the same extent as a higher-protein meal. Leucine or EAAs can be added to meals to increase muscle protein synthesis while keeping dietary protein intake and total nitrogen load lower (27, 62, 96, 119). However, this strategy might not translate to the same long-term results as consuming adequate amounts of protein at each meal.

In a 2-week study, leucine added to meals low in EAAs improved acute muscle protein synthesis and anabolic signaling in older adults consuming just over the RDA for protein (0.81 ± 0.04 g protein per kg body weight per day) (22). However, a longer-term study found the addition of leucine to meals did not improve muscle mass, strength, or muscle quality in diabetic or healthy older adults who consumed enough protein throughout the day (66).

PUTTING IT INTO PERSPECTIVE

WHAT IS THE MAXIMUM AMOUNT OF PROTEIN YOUR BODY CAN DIGEST AND USE AT ONE TIME?

What is the ideal amount of protein per meal to maximize muscle protein synthesis and satiety (fullness) without wasting food or money? Current studies suggest 25 to 45 grams per meal might be best for maximizing muscle protein synthesis, though we do not know what the upper limit is beyond which protein synthesis will not continue increasing to any appreciable extent (68, 74, 75). The ideal amount of protein per meal varies among individuals based on age, training status, amount of energy consumed each day, amount of protein they consume each day, the quality and leucine (or EAA) content of the protein, other nutrients consumed at meal time in conjunction with protein, and health status (33, 40, 91, 100). Some researchers suggest there is a "muscle full" effect, a dose-dependent upper limit of muscle tissue saturation of amino acids, beyond which the amino acids are no longer used to increase muscle protein synthesis but instead are oxidized (4). However, no studies have actually examined the maximum amount of protein intake at a meal and how this relates to changes in muscle strength and mass over time (33). In addition, few studies have examined how consistently higher total daily protein intake (above the recommendations listed in this text) affects measures of resistance-training performance and lean body mass. No studies to date have separated the effect of higher protein intake from higher calorie intake on these variables (comparing diets with the same total amount of energy but considerably higher amounts of protein in one diet). One study in resistance-trained individuals found that 4.4 grams of protein per kilogram body weight per day along with more total energy each day did not lead to greater increases in lean body mass compared to 1.8 grams of protein per kilogram body weight per day and significantly fewer kilocalories per day (1).

HOW DIETING AFFECTS MUSCLE

A higher protein intake combined with resistance training can preserve muscle while on a lower-calorie diet. However, the overall calorie deficit and speed of weight loss are important factors influencing muscle loss when dieting. If the calorie deficit is small, higher amounts of dietary protein and resistance training can counter most of the breakdown in muscle proteins. When the size of the caloric deficit is large, protein alone cannot stop the loss of skeletal muscle mass completely (91).

Even short periods of energy restriction can decrease postmeal increases in muscle protein synthesis. One study found a 27 percent decline in postmeal muscle protein synthesis after 5 days on a reduced-calorie, yet higher-protein diet (30 kcal per kg fat-free mass and 1.4–1.6 g of protein per kg body weight), which shows that even when protein intake is twice the RDA, it isn't always enough to preserve muscle protein synthesis during times of major caloric restriction.

In another study, 39 adults were randomized to receive 0.8 grams of protein per kilogram body weight per day (the RDA for protein), 1.6 grams of protein per kilogram body weight per day (twice the RDA), or 2.4 grams of protein per kilogram body weight per day (three times the RDA). For the first 10 days of the study, they were placed on a diet for weight maintenance. After this period, subjects were put on a 21-day diet consuming 40 percent fewer kilocalories than they needed to maintain weight. All groups lost the same amount of weight regardless of dietary protein intake. However, the groups consuming two and three times the RDA for protein lost significantly more fat and less fat-free mass than the group consuming the RDA for protein. Also, the anabolic response to a protein-rich meal was significantly lower when subjects were given the RDA for protein on the lower-calorie diet compared to when they consumed the RDA for protein on the regular- weight maintenance diet. The anabolic response to a meal was not different between the weight maintenance and lower-calorie diet phases when subjects consumed two or three times the RDA. Combined, these results suggest consuming two to three times the RDA for protein while consuming significantly less energy preserved muscle mass during weight loss (86).

Low-Carbohydrate Diets and Resistance Training

Though carbohydrate is the main source of energy used during resistance training, research in endurance athletes shows the body can adapt to a lower-carbohydrate diet over time and increase reliance on fat stores for use during exercise (18, 49). However, no studies published in resistance-trained individuals examine how following a nonketogenic low-carbohydrate diet affects resistance training. The studies to date on low-carbohydrate diets show a very low-carbohydrate, high-protein diet (7% carbohydrate, 63% protein, 30% fat) and low-carbohydrate, moderate-protein diet (20% carbohydrate, 50% protein, 30% fat) led to greater total weight and fat mass losses (though not significant) compared to a high-carbohydrate, low-protein diet group (55% carbohydrate, 15% protein, 30% fat) in healthy obese women engaged in a circuit-training program (59).

> **DO YOU KNOW ?**
>
> It is more difficult to gain muscle when cutting kilocalories because lower-calorie diets decrease the intracellular signaling necessary for the synthesis of new proteins in muscle, and muscle tissue may be less sensitive to protein when calorie intake is insufficient (87).

Ketogenic Diets and Resistance Training

Ketogenic diets are very high-fat diets, containing approximately 80 to 90 percent of energy from fat, or 3 to 4 grams of fat for every 1 gram of protein and carbohydrate. Carbohydrate intake is kept low enough so the body goes into a state of nutritional ketosis, as determined by circulating

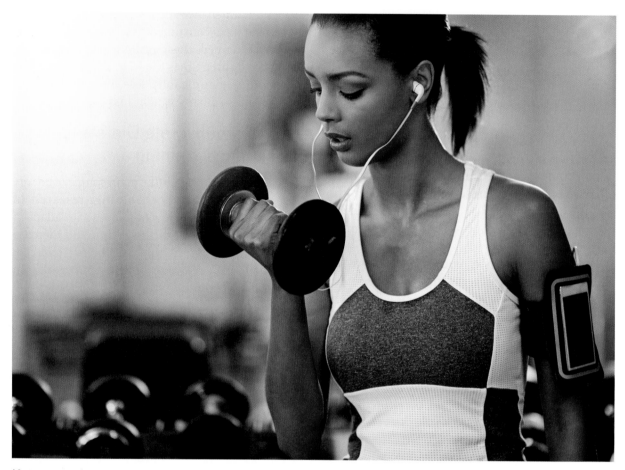

Ketogenic diets are not ideal for gaining muscle.

ketone levels reaching more than 0.5 mmol/L as measured through urine, blood, or breathe tests. Ketones are used as a source of energy when the body has insufficient glucose.

Ketogenic diets were originally designed to decrease the incidence and severity of seizures in epileptic patients, and they are very effective for this purpose. Now they are being studied as a potential therapy for minimizing the damaging effects resulting from traumatic brain injury.

> **DO YOU KNOW** ❓
>
> Nutritional ketosis should not be confused with ketoacidosis—the rapid production of specific ketone bodies leading to a life-threatening change in the body's acid-base buffering system in uncontrolled diabetics.

However, some athletes and active gym-goers are going "keto" to improve athletic performance or lose body fat. Proponents of ketogenic diets suggest an increased reliance on body fat as a source of fuel will lead to greater overall fat loss, fewer hunger pangs, and a decrease in mental and physical fatigue. Additionally, some suggest the likelihood of gastric distress is minimized because the athlete will not have to rely on carbohydrate during exercise and will consume fewer kilocalories, which will decrease the likelihood of stomach upset (93).

It takes at least 7 days for a person to reach nutritional ketosis, and 3 to 4 weeks to fully adapt to relying on ketones to fuel exercise. The diet is not ideal for resistance training because many of the signaling modules needed for muscle hypertrophy are reduced while following a ketogenic diet. In addition, protein intake must be kept fairly low in order to stay in a state of ketosis. A lower-protein diet can impair muscle gains. In one study subjects placed on a ketogenic diet while consuming less than 1.2 grams of protein per kilogram of ideal body weight per day lost muscle, and their athletic performance declined. The ketogenic diet is not beneficial for fat loss compared to consuming the same amount of energy from a lower-fat diet. NIH researchers admitted 17 overweight or obese men to a metabolic ward and placed them on a high-carbohydrate baseline diet for 4 weeks followed by 4 weeks on an isocaloric ketogenic diet. (This diet contained the same amount of energy as the high-carbohydrate diet.) The men lost weight and body fat on both diets. The ketogenic diet did not lead to greater fat loss as compared to the high-carbohydrate diet, and in fact body fat loss slowed during the ketogenic diet and subjects lost muscle (45).

Trading carbohydrate for fat seems like a huge benefit for athletes, particularly endurance athletes who train and compete for several hours at a time (120). In addition to using body fat, fat actually produces more energy (ATP) (83). However, fat is a slow source of fuel—the human body cannot access it quickly enough to sustain high-intensity exercise—so this diet is really only (potentially) applicable to ultrarunners and triathletes competing at a relatively moderate to slow pace. However, to date, there is no research to suggest either a ketogenic diet or a carbohydrate diet is superior to a higher carbohydrate diet for endurance performance.

Some individuals opt for a modified ketogenic diet, which is really a low-carbohydrate, as opposed to ketogenic, diet. A study in gymnasts found that a very low-carbohydrate (<30 g of carbohydrate per day), a so-called modified ketogenic diet (4.5% carbohydrate, 54.8% fat, and 40.7% protein, which equaled approximately 2.8 g of protein kg/day), for 30 days resulted in significant fat mass losses, while the gymnasts were able to maintain their lean body mass. In addition they also maintained power and strength while training 30 hours per week (83).

A ketogenic diet has some nutrition and cardiovascular drawbacks. Studies in epileptic children show soon after starting the diet, blood cholesterol levels rise and artery stiffness increases (30, 58). High total and LDL cholesterol are risk factors for cardiovascular disease, while artery stiffness decreases the ability of the arteries to expand to accommodate changes in pressure. Increased artery stiffness is an early sign of vascular damage and a risk factor for cardiovascular disease (23). After 6 to 12 months on the diet, or if a patient goes off the diet, blood cholesterol levels dropped back to normal, while artery stiffness returned to normal after 24 months on the diet (30, 58). A high-fat diet may also increase levels of harmful bacteria and decrease levels of beneficial bacteria in the gut (gut bacteria influences many aspects of health, including immune system and gastrointestinal tract functioning) (16). In addition, food choices are very limited, which makes it difficult to get enough calcium, vitamin D, potassium, and folate versus folic acid. Ketogenic may increase sodium needs due to electrolyte excretion. Potassium and sodium are critical for muscle functioning (including heart functioning), so a ketogenic diet should never be attempted without a physician's guidance. During the first few weeks on the diet, individuals might suffer headaches and feel fatigued, as if exercise requires more effort (125).

DO YOU KNOW ❓

A ketogenic diet is always low in carbohydrate, but a low-carbohydrate diet is not necessarily a ketogenic diet. The literature includes a wide variety of definitions for "low carbohydrate." A ketogenic diet is always high in fat, with 80 to 90 percent of energy coming from dietary fat.

NUTRIENTS THAT SUPPORT MUSCLE FUNCTIONING

Several nutrients are important for muscle functioning, including magnesium, vitamin D, and zinc. Low levels of magnesium can lead to muscle cell dysfunction and a decrease in muscle cell carbohydrate uptake, whereas magnesium deficiency can lead to muscle cramping, muscular twitching or spasms, muscular fatigue, numbness, and tingling (26, 39).

Vitamin D positively influences muscle strength, whereas a vitamin D deficiency leads to muscle weakness and pain (102). A systematic review and meta-analysis found vitamin D supplementation has a small but significant positive effect on muscle strength with no effect on muscle mass or muscle power. Supplementation was more effective in people 65 years of age or older, in addition to those who were deficient prior to the start of the study (8). Note that vitamin D supplementation also decreases risk of falls in the elderly (10, 65).

Low zinc status can lead to declines in muscle strength and power output, while correcting a zinc deficiency can improve muscle strength (17, 63, 117). All vitamins and minerals and their impact on athletic performance are discussed in chapters 6 and 7.

SPORT SUPPLEMENTS FOR RESISTANCE TRAINING

Creatine monohydrate is a supplement that increases body weight, strength, and muscle mass in healthy younger adults (31, 60, 107). In addition, a 2014 meta-analysis in older adults found creatine supplementation taken in combination with resistance training led to greater increases in lean body mass and some measures of strength, as well as significant improvements and functional performance compared to placebo (34).

Beta-hydroxy-beta-methylbutyrate (HMB) is a metabolite of leucine, although only 5 percent of leucine is converted to HMB during metabolism (116). HMB increases protein synthesis, though less effectively than leucine, and decreases muscle protein breakdown in an insulin-independent manner (126). However, studies on this supplement are mixed, and HMB might only be beneficial for the frail elderly who are unable to exercise or those on bedrest (32, 103, 121).

SUMMARY

Carbohydrate, from circulating blood sugar and muscle glycogen, is the main source of energy for resistance training. When carbohydrate stores are low, performance suffers, while immune and central nervous system functioning can be acutely suppressed. Adequate carbohydrate after exercise provides energy for the calorie-expensive process of muscle building and repair, helps decrease muscle breakdown, and replaces glycogen so the athlete has adequate energy for the next training session. In addition to carbohydrate, hydration status affects resistance-training performance by altering the hormonal and metabolic response to resistance exercise and making the heart work harder.

Protein isn't necessary for resistance-training performance, though it is essential for recovery and training adaptations. Both protein and essential amino acids consumed prior to or after resistance training will stimulate acute muscle protein synthesis. At least 20 to 40 grams of protein should be consumed after exercise, though more is likely preferable in some circumstances. Over time, a sound resistance-training program combined with postworkout protein and protein-rich meals spaced evenly throughout the day will improve strength and muscle hypertrophy in adults. Aging alters the anabolic response to protein intake; older adults benefit from greater amounts of protein postexercise and at mealtime.

▰▰ FOR REVIEW ⟫

1. Why do dieters need more protein each day? How much protein should they aim for?

2. Explain why a ketogenic diet is not beneficial for those engaging in a resistance-training program.

3. Why do older adults need more protein than younger adults after exercise?

4. How does alcohol affect training in men?

5. Describe the factors that influence an individual's protein needs.

6. What regulates protein synthesis in children?

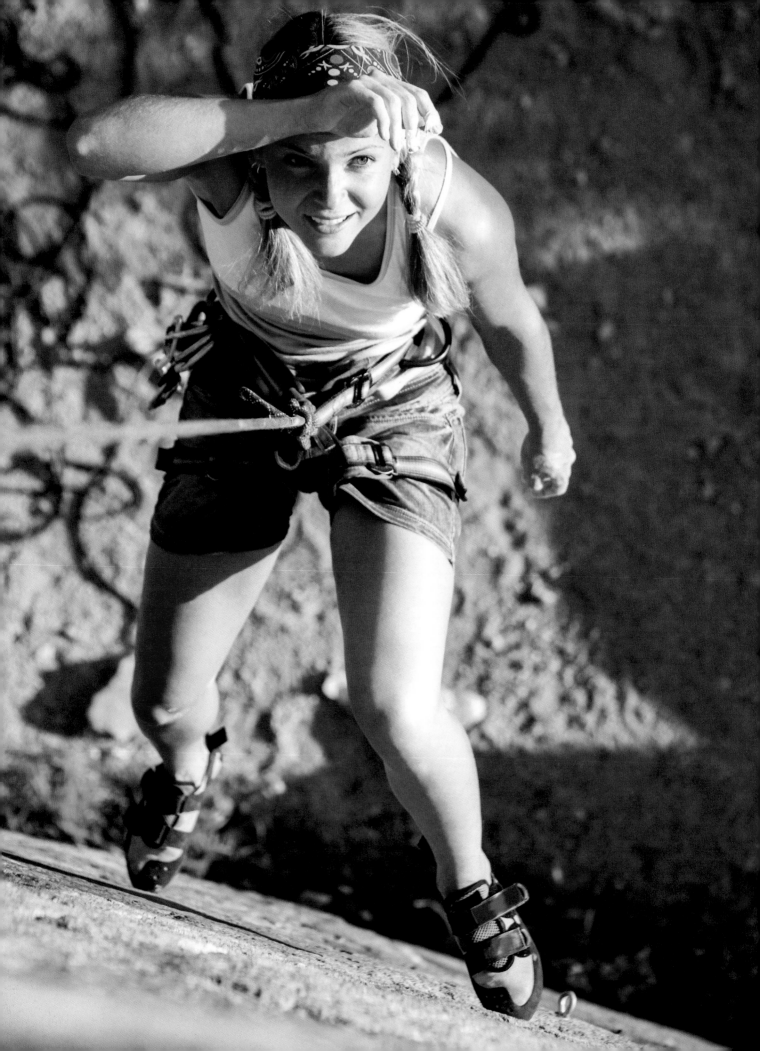

CHAPTER 13

Changing Weight and Body Composition

▶ CHAPTER OBJECTIVES

After completing this chapter, you will be able to do the following:

> Describe the health implications associated with excess body fat.

> Describe the health implications associated with very low body fat.

> List strategies an athlete can use to gain lean body mass.

> Discuss the key behind popular diets, and how they help people lose weight.

> Discuss how low energy (calorie) intake affects the ability to increase muscle hypertrophy.

> Discuss why higher protein intake is important during weight loss.

As you recall from chapter 10, body composition is the ratio between fat and fat-free mass. There is no universal definition for "optimal body composition," which is subjective (40). Also, what an athlete considers ideal might vary from what a coach or performance staff considers ideal. In order to manipulate body composition, fat and muscle are altered through training and nutrition. However, each individual's response to diet modifications and training varies, including how much body fat can be lost or muscle gained within a particular timeframe. Body composition goals may be adjusted over time based on how the body responds, health status (including injuries), and for athletes, how changes in body composition affect performance.

UNDERSTANDING BODY FAT

The two main types of body fat are essential body fat and storage fat. **Essential fat**, necessary for physiological functioning, is found in bone marrow, the heart, lungs, liver, spleen, kidneys, intestines, muscles, and fat-rich tissues of the central nervous system (78). Essential fat for men and women is approximately 3 percent and 12 percent body fat, respectively (78). In women, essential fat is higher because it includes fat in the breasts, hips, and pelvis for reproduction. **Storage fat** is energy accumulated for later use and found around internal organs (**visceral fat**) and directly below the skin (**subcutaneous fat**). Storage fat increases over time when excess energy (calories) is consumed, and decreases when more energy is burned than is consumed. Visceral fat wraps around organs like a blanket and contributes to inflammation (68). Higher levels of visceral fat are associated with higher risk for several chronic diseases (35, 44), whereas subcutaneous fat might help the body fend off disease and protect it during blunt force trauma, such as a car crash (36, 140).

DO YOU KNOW ?
It is possible to be within normal weight yet have high levels of visceral fat (126).

Health Implications of Excess Body Fat

Excess body fat, technically called adipose tissue, takes a toll on the entire body. Obesity increases risk of many health problems and diseases, including

> type 2 diabetes,
> heart disease,
> stroke,
> certain types of cancer,
> sleep apnea,
> osteoarthritis,
> fatty liver disease,
> kidney disease,
> depression,
> chronic inflammation,
> osteoarthritis, and
> complications during pregnancy, such as gestational diabetes; high blood pressure, which can affect the health of the mother and the baby; premature birth; stillborn birth; and neural tube defects.

Based on Arabin and Stupin 2014; Gregor and Hotamisligil 2011; Guffey, Fan, Singh, and Murphy 2013; Marshall and Spong 2012; Pi-Sunyer 2009; Polednak 2008; Roberts, Dive, and Renehan 2010.

Obesity also increases risk of **all-cause mortality** (death from all causes), cancer mortality, and cardiovascular mortality (103). More than 33 percent of adults and approximately 17 percent of children in the United States are obese (92).

It is best to measure body fat directly rather than relying on indirect measures such as BMI. BMI can incorrectly classify individuals with low body fat and high muscle mass as obese, while those with high body fat and low body weight can have a "normal" BMI even when they have an unhealthy amount of body fat. The various methods of measuring body fat were presented in chapter 10. Table 13.1 includes body fat ranges and their classification.

Excess fat around the waist is associated with increased risk of disease. The waist-to-hip ratio is used as a measure of higher waist circumference and reflects increased visceral fat better than BMI (figure 13.1) (31, 105).

Table 13.1 Body Fat Percentages for Males and Females and Their Classifications

Males	Females	Rating
5–10	8–15	Athletic
11–14	16–23	Good
15–20	24–30	Acceptable
21–24	31–36	Overweight
>24	>36	Obese

Note that these are rough estimates. The term athletic in this context refers to sports in which low body fat is an advantage.

Reprinted, by permission, from A. Jeukendrup and M. Gleeson, 2010, *Sport nutrition,* 2nd ed. (Champaign, IL: Human Kinetics), 316.

Blood Vessels, the Heart, and Kidneys

Obesity can increase blood lipids, including cholesterol and triglycerides (blood fats). Lipoproteins transport cholesterol through the body. **Low-density lipoprotein (LDL)** carries cholesterol from the liver to tissues, where it is used for a variety of functions, including incorporation as a structural component in cell membranes and the synthesis of steroid hormones. Though cholesterol is essential, high blood LDL can increase cholesterol build-up in arteries and is associated with increased risk for heart disease (52). **High-density lipoprotein (HDL)** carries cholesterol back to the liver for excretion or recycling, thus HDL is sometimes referred to as "good" cholesterol and is not associated with increased risk for heart

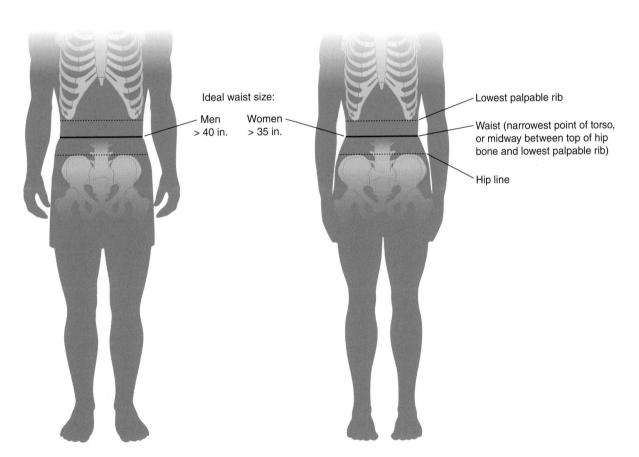

Figure 13.1 Measuring waist circumference.

Based on National Heart Lung and Blood Institute 1998.

disease. There are varying types or subclasses of LDL and HDL, each of which has different effects in the body. Triglycerides are not directly artery clogging, though high levels of triglycerides are associated with increased risk of cardiovascular disease (80, 90).

Excess body fat causes the heart to work harder to pump blood, as the heart must overcome resistance in blood vessels to deliver blood throughout the body. Over time, greater force of blood against artery walls leads to an increase in blood pressure (111), a condition called **hypertension**, which can damage and weaken artery walls. Plaque (composed of fat, cholesterol, calcium, and other substances) adheres more easily to damaged artery walls (figure 13.2). Plaque build-up, called **atherosclerosis**, decreases the diameter of arteries, narrowing the space blood travels through. Narrow artery walls decrease the flow of oxygenated blood to tissues and organs and increase risk of blood clots, which can block blood flow partially or completely (88). High blood pressure and atherosclerosis are risk factors for cardiovascular disease, diseases of the heart and blood vessels, and chronic kidney disease. Healthy kidneys help maintain blood pressure by regulating blood volume and electrolytes and through hormonal control. Damage to kidneys can impair kidney functioning, which may result in fluid build-up in blood vessels and an even greater increase in blood pressure (139).

Obesity, Insulin Resistance, and Type 2 Diabetes

Overweight and obesity can impair the body's ability to use insulin properly. High blood sugar can lead to greater plaque build-up in arteries and increase the amount of insulin released from the pancreas to decrease sugar in the blood. Insulin helps reduce blood sugar (typically referred to as blood glucose) in two ways:

> Insulin reduces glucose production in the liver (from stored glycogen), thereby helping reduce blood sugar.

> Insulin helps muscle, fat, and liver cells take up sugar (glucose) from the bloodstream, which lowers blood sugar.

After removing glucose from the bloodstream, insulin stimulates glucose storage in the form of glycogen in liver and muscle. Stored muscle glycogen is used for energy during exercise. Over time, high blood sugar decreases the body's ability to use insulin effectively, which can lead to insulin resistance (cells become resistant to the action of insulin) and type 2 diabetes (89). Ninety percent of those with type 2 diabetes are overweight or obese (143). Type 2 diabetes can damage many parts of the body, including nerves, kidneys, eyes, and skin, while also increasing risk of heart attack and stroke (32).

Normal artery   Narrowing of artery

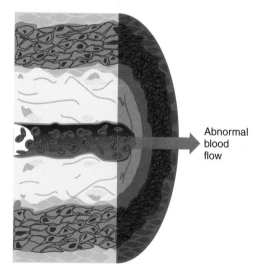

Normal blood flow

Abnormal blood flow

Figure 13.2 Plaque build-up in an artery.

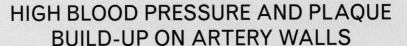

HIGH BLOOD PRESSURE AND PLAQUE BUILD-UP ON ARTERY WALLS

Atherosclerosis is similar to the build-up of dirt and debris inside a garden hose. When gunk builds up in a hose, you must turn up the water pressure to continue getting the same amount of water from the hose. Plaque build-up in arteries means the heart must work harder and generate more force to push blood through the body. That force damages artery walls.

Cancer and Other Health Consequences

Gaining weight increases the risk for several cancers, even if the weight gain doesn't result in overweight or obesity. Scientists believe this increased risk might be caused by several factors, including an increase in estrogen produced from fat; increased insulin and insulin-like growth factor-1 (IGF-1), which might fuel the development of some types of tumors; chronic inflammation (fat produces inflammatory compounds); and an increase in hormones produced in fat cells that might affect cell growth (28, 84, 106).

DO YOU KNOW ?

Smoking and exposure to second-hand smoke also damages artery walls.

Inflammation and excess fat around the neck might make the airway smaller, resulting in sleep apnea (113). Fat build-up in the liver can injure liver tissue, leading to damage, scarring (cirrhosis), and liver failure (97). Also, excess weight puts pressure on weight-bearing joints, increasing wear and tear of cartilage, the cushioning between joints, and risk for osteoarthritis (60).

Health Implications of Low Body Fat

When body fat gets too low, energy levels and one's tolerance for cold decreases. Athletic performance might also suffer. Body fat below essential fat can compromise health and be associated with **low energy availability**—energy intake insufficient to meet energy expenditure and physiological needs. Low energy availability can disrupt reproductive functioning, leading to irregular menstrual cycles or complete cessation of menstruation (147). Irregular menstruation and altered menstrual functioning can compromise bone health and might also increase risk of infertility (16).

PUTTING IT INTO PERSPECTIVE

ATHLETES AND OBESITY

Athletes are not immune to obesity and obesity-related health consequences. A study in 90 Division I college football players found that 21 percent were obese (all were linemen), as defined by 25 percent body fat or greater, as measured by BOD POD; 21 percent had insulin resistance (13 of the 19 players with insulin resistance were linemen); and 9 percent had metabolic syndrome (all linemen) (9).

DECREASING BODY FAT

An individual might want to decrease body fat for a variety of reasons, including lowering disease risk and improving health, body image, or athletic performance.

Studies examining weight loss show numerous approaches can be effective, as long as they create an energy deficit over time (144). However, losing weight too quickly can lead to a decrease in muscle mass, greater drop in metabolic rate (energy burned each day) than predicted by weight loss alone, and less energy available to train and get through each day (18, 34, 54, 133). Generally speaking, rapid weight loss should be avoided unless warranted for health reasons.

Determining a Healthy Weight Goal and Daily Energy Needs

The first step in determining a healthy body weight goal is weighing in a euhydrated state and measuring body composition (133). These measures can be used to determine how much body fat individuals should lose to put them within an optimal range for health or, for athletes, within a sport-specific body fat range.

PUTTING IT INTO PERSPECTIVE

CAN YOU BE FIT AND FAT?

The concept "fit and fat" suggests a high level of cardiovascular fitness attenuates some of the metabolic and cardiovascular disease risk factors associated with being overweight or obese (30). As a result, obese individuals who are fit may be healthier and live a longer life than normal-weight unfit individuals (146). Research lends some support to this theory: unfit individuals have twice the risk of death from all causes (all-cause mortality) as compared to overweight and obese fit individuals (6), demonstrating the powerful effect exercise has on health. Also, overweight and obesity does not affect everybody the same way, and where fat is located on the body affects health. Thus it is possible for two individuals with similar amounts of body fat, stored in different areas, to have very different risk profiles. As discussed in chapter 10, individuals who are "pear shaped" (gynoid), carrying more fat around their buttocks and thighs, have a lower risk for obesity-related chronic diseases than do those who are "apple shaped" (android), who carry more fat around the belly (which means more visceral fat). The pattern of body fat storage is largely determined by genetics.

The following factors are considered characteristics of those who are healthy and obese (119):

> A waist size of no more than 40 inches for a man or 35 inches for a woman
> Normal blood pressure, cholesterol, and blood sugar
> Normal insulin sensitivity
> Physically fit

Few people meet the criteria for fit and fat, probably because of low levels of physical activity; many who are overweight and obese aren't getting enough physical activity to move them into this category. Furthermore, "obesity is independently associated with reduced cardiovascular fitness" (30). Does this mean it is okay to be overfat as long as you are fit and meet the criteria listed above? Not necessarily. It is unclear if an individual who is considered fit and fat (or healthy and obese) will stay healthy and avoid unhealthy metabolic changes over time. In addition, these studies primarily examined metabolic health, and, unfortunately, overweight and obesity can have many other negative effects on health. Excess weight can lead to joint pain and damage and is the leading cause of osteoarthritis and sleep apnea; it is associated with increased risk of some types of cancer, as well as other negative health effects. Obese individuals should engage in an exercise program sufficient to improve cardiovascular fitness and help reduce body weight.

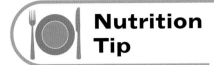

If you are competing in a sport, either recreationally or competitively, it is best to focus on weight loss during the off-season or in the base phase of training. If you are working on weight loss in-season or before competition, cut calories as little as possible to preserve muscle mass, prevent a large drop in RMR, and minimize training and performance decrements.

Next, energy needs can be estimated by using one of the following equations.

Harris-Benedict Equation

Men BMR = 66.5 + (13.8 × weight [kg]) + (5 × height [cm]) – (6.8 × age [yr])

Female BMR = 655.1 + (9.6 × weight) + (1.9 × height [cm]) – (4.7 × age [yr])

Cunningham Equation

RMR = 500 + (22 × lean body mass [kg])

Mifflin-St. Jeor Equation

Men RMR = (10 × weight [kg]) + (6.25 × height [cm]) – (4.92 × age [yr]) + 5

Women RMR = (10 x weight [kg] + (6.25 x height [cm]) – (4.92 x age [yr]) – 161

All of these equations take body weight into account, and some also consider age, height, and lean body mass to predict **basal metabolic rate (BMR)** or **resting metabolic rate (RMR)**. BMR measures the amount of calories burned at rest in a comfortable temperature at least 12 hours after activity and 10 to 12 hours after eating. RMR is measured at least 3 to 4 hours after activity or strenuous activity. The Cunningham equation considers lean body mass and is thus more applicable to athletes and other active individuals (127). BMR or RMR can be multiplied by an activity factor or METs (metabolic equivalents) can be added to estimate total daily energy needs to maintain weight. Table 13.2 shows common activity factor values. Subtract the desired daily caloric deficit from total calories per day for weight loss. METs are an estimate of energy expenditure during activity (1, 46). When considering number of calories burned each day, be sure to account for activities of daily living (nonathletic activities such as walking, gardening, playing with the kids, etc.) as well as energy burned through restlessness (fidgeting and constant movement) (66). Some individuals are extremely active outside of their training or athletic endeavors, whereas others tend to be sedentary when not training (128).

Weight loss isn't simple math, and people don't lose weight in a linear fashion. In 1958, a physician discovered that 1 pound of fat stores approximately 3,500 calories (145). This discovery resulted in thousands of textbooks, articles,

PUTTING IT INTO PERSPECTIVE

DETERMINING IF WEIGHT GOALS ARE REALISTIC

A realistic weight goal

> takes weight history, history of family, body weight and shape, and past history of eating disorders, obesity, and disordered eating into account;
> does not compromise health or increase risk of injuries;
> promotes sound eating habits and supports training and performance;
> meets the needs for growth, development, and reproductive functioning; and
> can be maintained without extreme weight control practices or constant dieting (75).

Table 13.2 Activity Factor

Activity	Multiply BMR by
Sedentary	1.2
Light activity (sitting, standing, some walking)	1.375
Moderate activity (exercise 3–5 days/week)	1.55
Very active (heavy training 6–7 days/week)	1.725
Extremely active (tough exercise or a physically demanding job)	1.9

websites, and weight-loss programs inaccurately predicting weight loss by dividing 3,500 by the daily calorie deficit to get the number of days it would take to lose a pound. For instance, many would assume subtracting 500 calories per day from the amount of calories necessary to maintain weight would lead to a 1-pound weight loss in 7 days. However, this simple math equation is inaccurate because it makes many assumptions: that we need the exact same amount of calories each day to be in a state of energy balance; that calories burned each day through physical activity and activities of daily living remains constant from day to day; that we can calculate exactly how many calories we are eating; that we consistently adhere to the diet; and that our bodies do not adapt to dieting and weight loss. Metabolism decreases with weight loss, providing one explanation for less than expected weight-loss results (14). However, decreased adherence to a particular diet might be the primary factor slowing the rate of weight loss or leading to a plateau in weight (42, 43, 125).

Validated weight-loss calculators can be used to predict the approximate amount of time it will take to lose weight. These calculators take metabolic slowing through weight loss into account. They are easy to find online. One weight loss calculator is titled "Weight Loss Predictor" and was created by Pennington Biomedical Research Center. A second one is the "Body Weight Planner" by the USDA.

Energy-Yielding Macronutrient Requirements for Weight Loss

Many people lose muscle when dieting, which contributes to, yet doesn't fully account for, the drop in metabolic rate that occurs with dieting. Several factors affect the amount of muscle mass lost, including activity (type, frequency, and duration); speed of weight loss; total protein intake; total daily energy deficit; gender; baseline level of body fat; and possibly individual differences in hormonal response to dieting. During dieting, muscle mass losses are relatively smaller in obese individuals as compared to those of "normal" weight (49).

A lower-calorie diet that does not contain enough protein will lead to significant muscle loss (55, 98, 99). During weight loss, protein needs are higher to preserve muscle tissue (19, 47, 85). A protein intake of at least 1.2 grams per kilogram body weight (0.55 g of protein per lb. body weight) is recommended to maintain muscle during dieting, though more protein, 1.8 to 2.7 grams of protein per kilogram body weight per day (or approximately 2.3–3.1 g protein per kilogram fat-free mass per day), might be preferable for attenuating the loss of muscle (86). Protein needs depend on many factors, including the amount of the caloric deficit, type of proteins consumed, and training program (type, duration, intensity, and frequency).

DO YOU KNOW ?

A caloric deficit of 500 to 1,000 calories below estimated daily energy needs is generally recommended for weight loss (86, 115). However, individuals with lower energy needs (women, older adults) in addition to growing children and teens should minimize their total caloric deficit to ensure they are getting enough nutrients for good health (more calories equals more opportunities to consume nutrients) and for growth, development, and reproductive functioning.

PUTTING IT INTO PERSPECTIVE

PREVENTING A WEIGHT-LOSS PLATEAU

Even if muscle mass is preserved, losing weight typically leads to a drop in metabolism. Some research shows this drop is greater than predicted (18, 24, 54, 121, 142), whereas other studies suggest the drop is relatively small (measured at 50 to 100 calories per day in one study) (77). Reasons for this decrease in metabolism, often referred to as metabolic adaptation, aren't entirely clear, though it is correlated to the degree of energy deficit (the greater the energy decrease, the greater the drop in metabolism) and changes in circulating leptin (54, 61). Leptin, a hormone secreted by fat cells, helps regulate body weight and energy balance (148). Also, fewer calories are necessary to carry less body weight. We burn less energy (fewer calories), even during activities of daily living, such as raking leaves (assuming our intensity level is the same), at a lower weight than we do at a higher weight. To account for metabolic adaptation, dieters must adjust energy intake over time to continue losing weight or to maintain their new body weight. The greater the weight lost from dieting, the greater the decrease in metabolism, which dieters must account for to maintain their new weight. Rapid and massive weight loss seems to lead to the greatest drop in metabolic rate. Weight regain after weight loss is quite common—and complex. Adjusting energy intake for weight maintenance likely slows the process of regaining lost weight.

In addition to meeting recommended guidelines for total daily protein intake, per-meal protein dose matters. The exact amount of protein needed at each meal to maximally stimulate muscle building likely depends on several variables, including the type of protein consumed, total daily energy intake, body weight, and training program. At mealtime, a minimum of 25 to 30 grams of protein containing 2 to 3 grams of leucine for younger adults and at least 3 grams of leucine for older adults is recommended to maximally stimulate muscle protein synthesis (74). Those who are dieting should also consume a minimum of 20 to 30 grams of a high-quality, fast-digesting protein such as whey (when a vegetarian protein is consumed, eat a minimum of 30 grams). Older adults should have at least 30 grams and possibly closer to 40 grams after resistance-training sessions.

In addition to protein, an adequate amount of carbohydrate must be consumed if a training program includes high-intensity exercise. Carbohydrate is the primary source of fuel used during high-intensity exercise because the body can readily access and use it for energy. Fat is a slow source of energy, which means the body cannot access and use fat quickly enough to sustain high-intensity training (71). If the body lacks an adequate supply of carbohydrate for use as energy, intensity will drop.

Popular Diets and Approaches to Dieting

A variety of dietary approaches can lead to weight loss. These might include counting calories,

DO YOU KNOW ?

Losing weight quickly increases the likelihood of losing muscle during weight loss (18, 34).

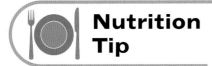

Nutrition Tip

A RDN trained in sports nutrition can help athletes and active individuals identify a realistic weight goal and create a plan to meet this goal without the use of extreme diets and unsafe weight-loss practices (56, 123).

PUTTING IT INTO PERSPECTIVE

HOW CAN I FEEL FULL WHEN DIETING?

Satiation and satiety help limit overall food intake. **Satiation** is the satisfaction of appetite during a meal, which helps us determine when to stop eating. Satiety is the feeling of fullness after a meal, which affects when we decide to eat again. Satiety decreases over time after eating (23). Several factors influence satiation, including sensory feedback, expectations of feeling full, gastric distension caused by the volume of food consumed, and hormonal feedback to the brain; all of these factors help to regulate the amount, duration, and frequency of food consumption (13, 21, 136). Foods that are higher in volume, such as whole fruits and vegetables, broth-based soups, and whipped shakes can increase satiation.

Protein increases satiety in a dose-dependent manner (the more protein consumed at one time, the more full we feel, though it isn't clear what the upper limit is, beyond which feelings of fullness are not increased). Per-meal doses of at least 30 grams are recommended (95). However, habitual consumption of a high-protein diet might decrease protein's impact on satiety over time (69). A high-protein breakfast, particularly, appears to be important for improving satiety during the day. Choosing solid as opposed to liquid sources of calories can also enhance satiety (64, 65). Fiber improves satiety, the degree to which depends on the type of fiber consumed. Beta-glucan (from oats and barley), lupin kernel fiber, whole-grain rye, rye bran, and a mixed diet of fiber-containing foods (grains, legumes, vegetables, and fruits) might be best for enhancing satiety (100).

Increases in satiety do not necessarily correspond to a decrease in food intake over the course of a day, as multiple factors affect a person's desire to eat, including the sight or smell of food, habit, and emotional state (we eat when we are bored or stressed, for instance).

cutting down on one macronutrient (as in a low-fat diet or low-carbohydrate diet), watching portion sizes, taking a nondiet approach, excluding certain foods or food groups, and intermittent fasting or eating only within a certain window of time (e.g., daytime hours between 8 and 5).

Low-fat and low-carbohydrate diets are often compared for effectiveness, yet research indicates that both approaches work. A meta-analysis of 48 randomized controlled clinical trials examining the effectiveness of popular weight-loss diets—including Atkins, Zone, South Beach (low carbohydrate), LEARN, Jenny Craig, Nutrisystem, Weight Watchers (moderate approaches), Ornish, and Rosemary Conley —for overweight and obese adults (BMI >25) found most lower-calorie diets result in weight loss as long as participants stay on the diet. Additionally,

DO YOU KNOW ❓

Behavior therapy and support improves weight-loss results and enhances weight maintenance after weight loss.

low-fat and low-carbohydrate diets resulted in the greatest weight loss, though these differences were minor in comparison to the rest of the diets (55). Research reviews examining popular diets have come to the same conclusion: Most are equally effective, and evidence is insufficient to recommend one particular dietary approach for all people (53, 110, 131).

Does the Type of Food You Eat Matter?

When individuals are cutting calories, they have fewer opportunities to get the vitamins, minerals, fiber, and protein necessary for optimal health. This means they must make their calories count by focusing on nutrient-rich foods. They might also want to choose foods with no (or little) processing, as well. The research is limited, but emerging evidence suggests the body expends more energy digesting foods that are less processed, or absorbs fewer calories from the food during digestion, as compared to highly processed foods.

DOES CARBOHYDRATE MAKE YOU FAT?

REFLECTION TIME

Carbohydrate does not make you fat. However, if you consume more energy than you burn, you will gain weight. Well-designed metabolic ward studies (study subjects are held at the research institution, and all food is provided; food intake and physical activity are strictly measured and observed) show obese adults lose more body fat when they reduce dietary fat intake rather than cutting down on carbohydrate (41).

Studies examining intake of whole almonds, pistachios, walnuts, and peanuts suggest incomplete energy absorption from fat. Study subjects absorbed 5 to 21 percent fewer calories than the nuts contained (percentages differed based on the nut). Fewer calories were absorbed from the nuts due to incomplete breakdown of the cell walls within the food (4, 91, 120). In addition, some research shows less dietary fat (and so less calories) is absorbed from peanuts as compared to peanut oil, peanut butter, and peanut flour (130).

In a crossover study in healthy women, study subjects were provided either a sandwich with cheddar cheese on multigrain bread or processed cheese on white bread. Meals contained the same amount of protein, carbohydrate, fat, and calories. Calorie expenditure was significantly greater after the whole food as compared to the processed meal (137 ± 14.1 calories vs. 73.1 ± 10.2 calories), suggesting more energy is expended during the

digestion of less-processed foods as compared to highly processed foods (5).

Training for Losing Body Fat

Training programs can be tailored to increase calories burned and therefore help with weight loss. Two components make up the total amount of energy burned as a result of exercise:

1. Energy burned during exercise.
2. **Excess postexercise oxygen consumption (EPOC)**—the energy burned after exercise.

Resistance training is critical for up-regulating muscle protein synthesis when dieting (3, 85, 121) to help ensure muscle mass is maintained (or improved) during weight loss. In addition to burning calories during resistance training and in the time period after training, through excess postexercise oxygen consumption, the body requires

PUTTING IT INTO PERSPECTIVE

HOW DO I KNOW WHAT DIET IS BEST FOR ME?

No one diet works for everyone. Research shows the ability to adhere to a diet is the most important factor that predicts successful weight loss, while lack of adherence is one of the biggest barriers to long-term success (55, 73). Individuals should choose a diet or plan they can adhere to, one that presents the fewest number of challenges and allows them to maintain their health and level of exercise. Instead of following a rigid approach to losing weight, maintaining some flexibility to alter the approach as needed or to switch diets might improve adherence (55). For instance, a person can start by counting calories and then transition to portion sizes and mindful eating. Mindful eating helps people get in touch with their physiological hunger and satiety cues. In addition, mindful eating helps people examine when they are eating due to stress, boredom, habit, and for other reasons not related to hunger. Once a person identifies why they are eating (e.g., if they are really hungry or using food to cope with something else in life) in addition to their eating cues (i.e., time of day, sight of the vending machine, etc.), they can work on better habits so they do not habitually turn to food when they are not truly hungry.

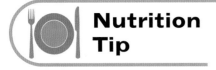

energy (calories) to repair training-induced microscopic damage in muscle while laying down new proteins in muscle. Resistance-training programs designed for weight loss focus on recruiting a greater amount of muscle mass in each session to maximize the amount of calories burned during the session and afterward (excess postexercise oxygen consumption) (138). For example, a program might include more squats instead of calf raises or leg extensions. In addition to focusing on recruiting more muscle mass in each training session, performing supersets (completing two sets of different exercises back to back before resting, such as a set of squats immediately followed by deadlifts prior to resting) increases total calories burned during and after exercise (57).

In addition to resistance training, incorporating aerobic exercise into a training program can enhance total energy burned during the day. Steady-state (constant intensity) aerobic work sessions can be intermixed with high-intensity interval training (HIIT) to increase total energy burned. Although several studies have suggested HIIT training, which involves repeated bouts of high-intensity exercise followed by low-intensity exercise, increases energy burned during exercise and excess postexercise energy consumption to a greater extent than steady-state exercise (11, 37, 48, 58), a systematic review and meta-analysis, including 31 studies, found HIIT training doesn't lead to greater weight loss than steady-state exercise when matched for total calories burned. However, HIIT does lead to greater calories burned in a shorter period, so a person can get more results for a shorter time commitment (http://onlinelibrary.wiley.com/doi/10.1111/obr.12536/abstract). Note that HIIT training can be difficult for individuals who are very overweight or who have chronic health conditions or injuries.

A sound training program is an essential component for altering body composition in favor of less fat and more muscle, but overall daily activity is important as well. Research shows many people compensate for increases in exercise by being less active the rest of the day. They decrease their activities of daily living, so they burn fewer calories during the rest of the day when they are not working out (128). Activities of daily living include walking to class, cleaning, mowing the lawn, gardening, and washing the car (26, 66).

Training can increase the total amount of calories burned in various ways, but the best exercise for weight loss is the one that an individual will stick with over time, both during the weight-loss period and afterward, for weight maintenance.

Several strategies can be used to help an individual cut calories and thereby lose weight. Research-based nutrition and exercise strategies are shown in figure 13.3.

PUTTING IT INTO PERSPECTIVE

WILL BUILDING MUSCLE TURN ME INTO A CALORIE-BURNING MACHINE?

Muscle tissue burns significantly more calories at rest than fat tissue. Though this difference is statistically significant, it might not translate to a very meaningful difference in calories burned over a short period. One pound of muscle burns 5.9 calories per day at rest (RMR), whereas each pound of fat burns 2.0 calories per day at rest (RMR). So if you gain 5 pounds of muscle, you'll burn approximately 20 more calories each day (141).

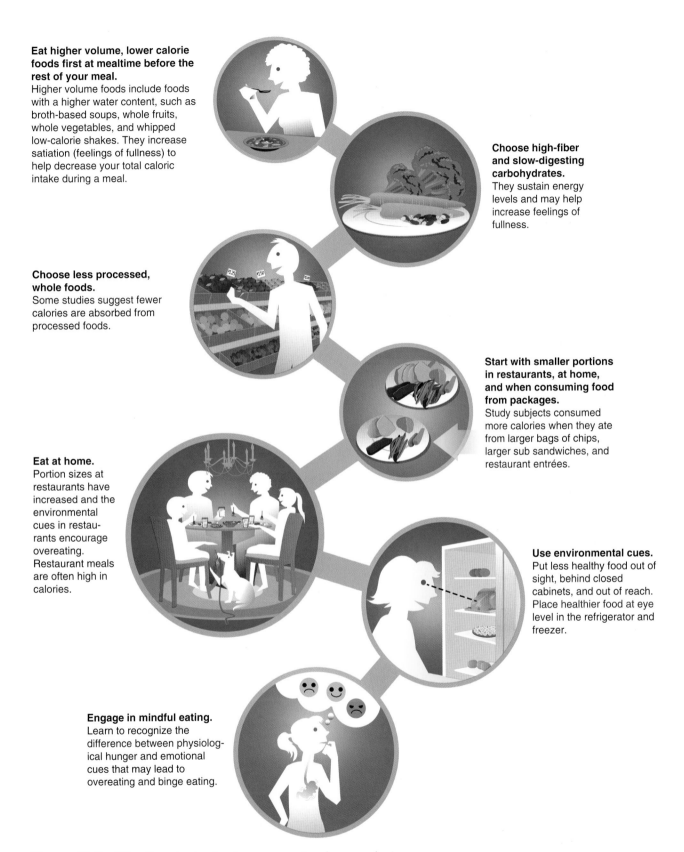

Eat higher volume, lower calorie foods first at mealtime before the rest of your meal.
Higher volume foods include foods with a higher water content, such as broth-based soups, whole fruits, whole vegetables, and whipped low-calorie shakes. They increase satiation (feelings of fullness) to help decrease your total caloric intake during a meal.

Choose high-fiber and slow-digesting carbohydrates.
They sustain energy levels and may help increase feelings of fullness.

Choose less processed, whole foods.
Some studies suggest fewer calories are absorbed from processed foods.

Start with smaller portions in restaurants, at home, and when consuming food from packages.
Study subjects consumed more calories when they ate from larger bags of chips, larger sub sandwiches, and restaurant entrées.

Eat at home.
Portion sizes at restaurants have increased and the environmental cues in restaurants encourage overeating. Restaurant meals are often high in calories.

Use environmental cues.
Put less healthy food out of sight, behind closed cabinets, and out of reach. Place healthier food at eye level in the refrigerator and freezer.

Engage in mindful eating.
Learn to recognize the difference between physiological hunger and emotional cues that may lead to overeating and binge eating.

Figure 13.3 Effective strategies for consuming fewer calories.

Sport-Specific Weight and Body Fat Goals

Average body fat levels for men and women in the United States are approximately 22 to 28 percent for men and 32 to 40 percent for women (67). Athletes will likely be higher or lower than these ranges. Obesity, even for the active individual or athlete, comes with health consequences. Note also that extremely low body fat, defined as below essential body fat levels—less than 5 percent for men and 12 percent for women—can impair immune system and endocrine functioning (129).

Three categories of sports are most commonly associated with lower body fat (75, 123):

1. Sports in which carrying a lower body weight is advantageous such as endurance athletes, ski jumping, and jockeys
2. Weight-class sports such as wrestling and judo
3. Aesthetic sports such as gymnastics and figure skating.

All athletes who must meet weight-class goals should be monitored for use of extreme weight-loss practices that are harmful to health and increase injury risk (122). Athletes who are still growing should also be closely monitored, as severe energy restriction can interfere with growth and development (75).

A wide range of body fat values has been reported in elite athletes, making it difficult to determine ideal ranges for each sport. See table 13.3 for general ranges. Note that body fat measurement techniques and instruments and equations used vary widely among athletes.

GAINING MUSCLE MASS

Improving muscle mass can help prevent injuries, slow sarcopenia (the age-related decline in muscle mass) and possibly improve athletic performance. Some individuals also choose to gain muscle mass for aesthetic reasons. Several factors influence the ability to increase muscle size (hypertrophy) and strength, including genetics, current training, previous history of training, and nutrition. The most important modifiable factor necessary for muscle hypertrophy is a well-designed, periodized resistance-training program. A sound diet can improve results obtained from a training program. For muscle hypertrophy, it is important to consume enough total calories and protein. Sufficient calories are necessary to provide both the energy to train and the energy necessary for the synthesis of new proteins in muscle.

> **DO YOU KNOW ?**
>
> Studies show that changing your diet will lead to greater weight loss than changing your exercise program (22, 114, 116). However, dieting alone (without exercising) leads to greater decreases in muscle mass compared to combining diet with exercise, particularly with anaerobic exercise (e.g., resistance training) (125).

Energy Needs

Energy needs for weight gain can be estimated by calculating RMR and calories expended through activity, and then adding calories on top of this number. The majority of extra calories should come from protein and carbohydrate. At least 44 to

Table 13.3 Body Fat Percentage in Athletes

Sport	Males	Females	Sport	Males	Females
Baseball	12–15%	12–15%	Rowing	6–14%	12–18%
Basketball	6–12%	20–27%	Shot putting	16–20%	20–28%
Bodybuilding	5–8%	10–15%	Cross-country skiing	7–12%	16–22%
Cycling	5–15%	15–20%	Sprinting	8–10%	12–20%
American football (backs)	9–12%	No data	Soccer	10–18%	13–18%
American football (linemen)	15–19%	No data	Swimming	9–12%	14–24%
Gymnastics	5–12%	10–16%	Tennis	12–16%	16–24%
High jumping and long jumping	7–12%	10–18%	Triathlon	5–12%	10–15%
Ice and field hockey	8–15%	12–18%	Volleyball	11–14%	16–25%
Marathon running	5–11%	10–15%	Weightlifting	9–16%	No data
Racquetball	8–13%	15–22%	Wrestling	5–16%	No data

Reprinted, by permission, from A. Jeukendrup and M. Gleeson, 2010, *Sport nutrition*, 2nd ed. (Champaign, IL: Human Kinetics), 316.

50 calories per kilogram body weight is suggested for weight gain (118).

In well-designed overfeeding studies, participants are given meals to help determine the effect of varying calorie and energy-yielding macronutrient intake on weight, fat, and muscle mass. In these studies, consuming more of the extra calories from protein led to a greater increase in lean body mass. A 10- to 12-week overfeeding study in normal and overweight participants provided 39.4 percent more calories each day than needed for weight maintenance and either 6, 15, or 26 percent of the extra calories as protein. All groups increased body fat, though overfeeding protein led to greater lean body mass gains and an increase in energy expenditure (12). In another study, participants were overfed for 8 weeks and given a diet containing 5, 15, or 25 percent protein. Those given 15 or 25 percent protein stored 45 percent of the extra calories consumed as muscle mass, while those on the low-protein diet stored 95 percent of extra calories as fat (33). While protein is important for weight gain, there are individual differences in weight gained (fat mass and muscle mass) when calorie intake is increased. Individuals with more fat-free mass may gain less weight when overfed compared to those with less fat-free mass. Plus, the amount of calories burned each day increases when overfed, as discussed earlier in the chapter. Thus weight gain cannot be accurately predicted based on the amount of extra calories consumed (10). In other words, adding an extra 3,500 calories per week will not lead to exactly 1 pound of weight gained.

A study in lean and obese men overfed (50% more than calorie needs to maintain weight) carbohydrate or fat found carbohydrate overfeeding led to an increase in total calories burned and 75 to 85 percent of excess calories stored as fat, while overfeeding fat had minimal impact on total calories burned and led to 90 to 95 percent of excess calories stored as fat (51).

Protein Needs

As noted in chapter 12, it is not entirely clear exactly how much protein is optimal for building muscle; the total amount of protein that should be consumed depends on a person's health status, total calorie intake, and training program. The type of protein consumed might also influence optimal protein intake for hypertrophy; vegetarian proteins may need to be consumed in higher amounts and combined to get all essential amino acids in each serving. To maximize muscle hypertrophy, a total daily protein intake of approximately 1.2 to 2.0 grams per kilogram body weight is recommended (8, 15).

In addition to total daily protein intake, consuming a high-quality, fast protein, one that is quickly digested and leads to a rapid rise in amino acids in the bloodstream, soon after resistance training will up-regulate muscle protein synthesis better than resistance training alone. The exact time period after training during which one should consume protein isn't entirely clear, though for individuals who are resistance-trained (not novices) it is preferable to consume protein sooner, within about 1 hour, rather than later. This strategy may be most important for those who train in a fasted state (83, 112). If using this strategy, one should consume a minimum of 20 to 25 grams of high-quality protein containing at least 2 grams of leucine per serving (82). If choosing a vegetarian protein source, select at least 30 grams of a variety of proteins, covering all essential amino acids and including at least 2 grams of leucine. Older adults need at least 40 grams of a protein containing at least 3 grams of leucine after exercise to maximally stimulate acute muscle protein synthesis (82, 101).

Resistance training increases muscle protein synthesis for at least 48 hours after training, so regular meals with at least 25 to 30 grams of protein, providing at least 2 grams of leucine for younger adults and 3 grams of leucine for older adults, will maximally stimulate acute muscle protein synthesis at each meal (17, 63, 96).

Carbohydrate Needs

Carbohydrate is the body's primary source of energy for resistance training; when carbohydrate availability is low, training intensity will drop. Carbohydrate also helps decrease muscle breakdown after a workout and, like the other energy-yielding macronutrients (protein and fat), carbohydrate contributes to total daily caloric needs.

Though fat is the primary source of fuel during moderate-intensity activity (30–65% of $\dot{V}O_2$ max), as intensity increases, carbohydrate use also increases, with muscle glycogen becoming an important source of energy (132, 137) (recall the crossover concept, shown in figure 11.1). The maximum rate of ATP production from fat is 0.4 mmol/minute, while the maximum rate of ATP re-synthesis from stored muscle glycogen is 1.0 to 2.3 mmol/minute (7). Thus, ATP is not produced fast enough from stored fat to meet the demand for energy during high-intensity activity (117). Resistance training with low glycogen leads to a decrease in the rate of ATP production (as the body must rely on a slower production of ATP), fatigue, and a decrease in power output (29, 93, 94). Studies examining different weightlifting protocols reiterate the importance of muscle glycogen; participants used 24 to 45 percent of their glycogen stores after a few sets (72).

Sports Supplements

Protein and creatine are the two most effective supplements for increasing muscle mass. Supplementation with a high-quality protein that provides at least 2 grams of leucine per serving for younger adults and at least 3 grams of leucine per serving for older adults provides a convenient and effective way to consume protein soon after finishing a workout to increase acute muscle protein synthesis. There is not enough research to date to compare food sources of protein such as chicken and fish, to supplemental forms of protein.

Supplementing with creatine monohydrate may increase in body weight, strength, and muscle

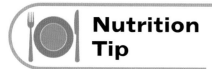

Nutrition Tip

When consuming more calories each day, your metabolism will increase, so over time your weight gain might start to plateau and an even greater increase in calories will be needed to continue gaining weight.

mass in healthy younger adults and older adults (20, 25, 59). However, individual responses will vary with creatine supplementation. Some people are considered nonresponders, meaning they do not see any changes in strength or muscle mass (124).

LOSING FAT AND GAINING MUSCLE AT THE SAME TIME

In addition to the risk of losing muscle while losing weight, it is more difficult to gain muscle when cutting calories because lower- calorie diets decrease the intracellular signaling necessary for the synthesis of new proteins in muscle, and muscle tissue might be less sensitive to protein when a person is dieting (99).

Despite these challenges, it is possible to lose body fat and preserve, or even gain, muscle at the same time by combining a higher-protein diet with an intense resistance-training program (70, 81, 102). For example, 31 overweight or obese postmenopausal women were put on a reduced-calorie diet of 1,400 calories per day (with 15%, 65%, and 30% calories from protein, carbohydrate, and fat, respectively) and randomized to receive either 25 grams of carbohydrate (maltodextrin) or a whey protein supplement twice a day for the 6-month study period. The group receiving the additional protein lost 3.9 percent more weight than the carbohydrate group and preserved more muscle mass (81).

In another intervention study, young, overweight, recreationally active men (prior to the study they exercised once or twice a week) were placed on an intense 4-week diet and exercise program. Their diet contained 40 percent fewer calories each day than necessary for weight maintenance (providing a total of 15 calories per pound of lean body mass). Half of the men were randomly selected to receive a higher protein diet (2.4 g of protein per kg body weight; 1.09 g of protein per lb. body weight; 35% protein, 50% carbohydrate, and 15% fat). The rest of the men were placed on a lower-protein diet (1.2 g of protein per kg body weight; 0.55 g of protein per lb. body weight; 15% protein, 50% carbohydrate, and 35% fat). Though this diet was lower in protein, it provided 50 percent more protein than

the RDA for protein (0.8 g/kg body weight per day). Both groups were given enough carbohydrate to sustain a higher-intensity training program. All meals were prepared and provided to participants during the study, which helped control for calories and energy-yielding macronutrients consumed. In addition to their meals, participants were given dairy shakes during the day and immediately postexercise (the lower-protein group was given lower-protein shakes with carbohydrate in them; the higher-protein group received more protein in their shakes). Supervised workouts consisted of full-body resistance circuit training three times per week, high-intensity interval training twice per week, and a time trial. In addition to their structured exercise program, all participants were instructed to accumulate at least 10,000 steps per day, as monitored by a pedometer worn on their hip.

Both the lower-protein and higher-protein groups lost weight, with no significant difference between groups. Men in the higher-protein group gained 2.64 pounds of muscle and lost 10.56 pounds of body fat, while men in the control group gained very little muscle (0.22 lb.) and lost 7.7 pounds of fat. Both groups improved all but one measure of strength in addition to aerobic and anaerobic capacity. There were no differences between groups in strength, power, aerobic fitness, or performance at the end of the study. In this study, a higher-protein, reduced-calorie diet combined with a high-intensity circuit-training program including interval training and sprints helped participants build muscle. In addition to their total protein intake, participants in the

> **DO YOU KNOW ?**
>
> It is important to keep in mind that altering fat or muscle mass will not necessarily result in improvements in athletic performance or body image. Simply gaining muscle mass does not automatically translate to improvement on a field or court, in a pool, or on a track. Also, shedding body fat or gaining muscle will not necessarily improve a person's body image; plus, some individuals may be striving for what is unachievable and therefore never be satisfied with how they look.

higher-protein group also consumed more protein per meal (approximately 49 g per meal) than those in the lower protein group (approximately 22 g per meal) (70).

Dieters who want to gain muscle while losing fat may want to consider consuming more than 2 grams of protein per kilogram body weight (120). Protein intake should be spaced out evenly throughout the day (regular meals containing at least 25–30 g of protein).

SUMMARY

Overweight and obesity result in many health consequences that can be reversed with weight loss. For athletes, decreasing body fat may also be driven by weight requirements of their sport or position, aesthetic demands, performance goals, decreasing risk of injuries, and joint pain. Losing body weight, especially when done quickly and without adequate dietary protein, can lead to a substantial decrease in muscle mass. To prevent muscle mass losses when cutting calories, one must consume more total protein and engage in resistance training. However, rapid weight loss can also lead to a more substantial drop in metabolism, so this approach is not recommended unless needed for rapid reversal of obesity-related health consequences. Weight loss is often less than predicted from nutrition and exercise interventions because many people tend to decrease their daily activity once they increase their exercise, adherence to diets drops over time, and metabolism drops with weight loss.

Gaining muscle can improve quality of life in older adults and those who are disabled by helping them perform typical daily tasks, such as lifting their groceries or opening a can of food. For athletes, gaining muscle can decrease risk of injuries and improve strength and power. Greater intake of both calories and protein, as well as an effective resistance-training program, is necessary for muscle hypertrophy. It is possible to gain muscle

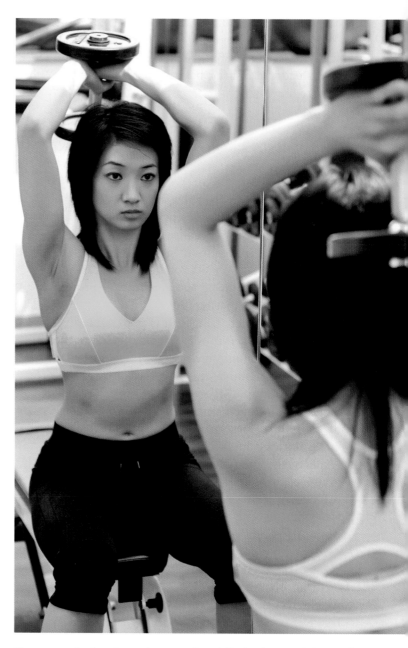

If you are trying to gain muscle while losing weight at the same time, keep in mind the diet and training information provided in this chapter to help you achieve your goals.

and lose fat at the same time. Doing this requires fewer calories, more protein per day, and a well-designed training program. Like weight loss, individual results from following a hypertrophy program or program designed for fat loss and hypertrophy at the same time will vary among individuals.

▮▮ FOR REVIEW ▶▮▮▮▮▮▮▮▮▮▮▮▮▮▮▮▮▮▮▮▮▮▮▮▮▮▮▮▮▮▮▮▶

1. Why do protein needs increase on a reduced-calorie diet?
2. Describe the health implications that can result from body fat below essential fat levels.
3. Describe the health implications resulting from and associated with excess body fat.
4. Why is carbohydrate essential for high-intensity training?
5. What is low energy availability, and how does it affect health?
6. Why don't people lose weight in a linear fashion? Why don't they lose as much as they predict they would have?
7. What makes popular diets effective?

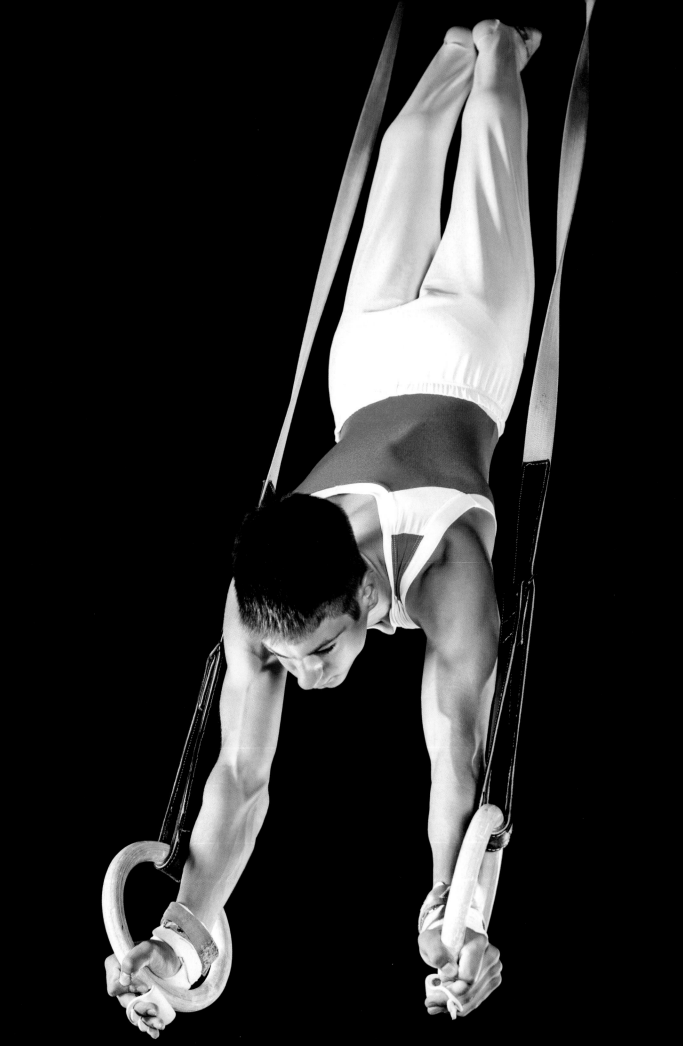

CHAPTER 14

Nutrition Concerns for Special Populations

> **CHAPTER OBJECTIVES**
>
> After completing this chapter, you will be able to do the following:
>
> - Discuss the most important nutrition concerns for child and adolescent populations.
> - Discuss the special nutrition needs of masters-level athletes and active older adults.
> - Describe special nutrition concerns for athletes with diabetes.
> - Identify special considerations for athletes who are pregnant.
> - Describe special nutrition concerns for vegetarian athletes.
> - Discuss nutrition challenges associated with disordered eating and eating disorders in physical activity and sport.

Many athletes and other active individuals face distinct dietary challenges that differ from those of the majority. These differences often have implications for health and exercise performance and might require an individualized approach to meeting nutrition needs. Concerns about the needs of distinct groups, or special populations, differ across the life stages. Nutrition needs of the child athlete, for example, are quite different from those of the masters athlete. When trying to ensure a proper diet that meets all nutrition needs, the considerations of some individuals, such as vegetarians, diabetics, or those with eating disorders, might be far different from those we have discussed in earlier chapters. In this chapter we focus on nutrition for physically active youth, including young athletes; athletes who compete at a masters level; physically active seniors; physically active individuals and athletes who are pregnant, diabetic, or vegetarian; and physically active individuals and athletes who have eating disorders.

CHILDREN AND ADOLESCENTS

More opportunities than ever before exist for children and adolescents to participate in sports, and children are participating in competitive sporting activities at younger ages. Over 38 million children in the United States participate in team sports, the majority of them during high school (53). Other trends include increased female participation in sports, increased participation in **extreme sports**, earlier specialization, and year-round training. Some children and adolescents participate in long, intense training several times a week, often without sufficient recovery because of their busy schedules. Such situations call for nutrition plans that meet all needs for growth and development, promote health, enhance athletic performance, and aid in injury prevention. However, during periods of rapid growth with accompanying high-energy needs, many children and adolescents, including athletes, fall well short of meeting the standard guidelines for nutrition. Common meal patterns are often low in fruits, vegetables, calcium-rich foods, and micronutrients. Excessive saturated fat, sodium, and sugar

are consumed. Unsafe weight-loss practices, disordered eating, and clinically defined eating disorders are of extreme concern in the young, as they can have significantly negative impacts on growth and development.

Children and Prepubescent Adolescents Are Not Small Adults

Both benefits and drawbacks are associated with youth participation in sport. While some of these can also be observed in adults, others are unique to this life stage and can be more significant, with lasting impacts into adulthood. Exercise associated with youth sport improves physical fitness, reduces body fat, and decreases risk of chronic disease. Youth participation in sport also enhances bone health, decreases the likelihood of depression and anxiety, improves self-esteem, improves academic achievement, and provides overall improvements in emotional well-being. Risks for both acute physical injury and overuse injury are heightened in the young. Children tend to injure themselves at different anatomic structures than adults. Their bones are weaker than their tendons and ligaments, putting them at risk for fractures throughout the bone and growth plate. Some adolescent athletes have decreased flexibility, coordination, and balance, which can increase injury risk while also affecting sport performance, stress, anxiety, and self-esteem. Quick return to sport without appropriate rehabilitation can result in chronic pain, repeated injury, and impaired functioning (38, 50).

In addition to an immature skeleton, children and adolescents have distinct physiological differences that affect energy expenditure, fuel (substrate) utilization, and thermoregulation during exercise. Along with increased demands for energy and many nutrients—as a result of rapid anatomical, physiological, and metabolic changes—children have an immature anaerobic metabolic system prior to the onset of puberty, which might affect their ability to perform well in high-intensity exercise. Children rely more on fat oxidation and are thus less likely to achieve high rates of ATP generation via the anaerobic pathway.

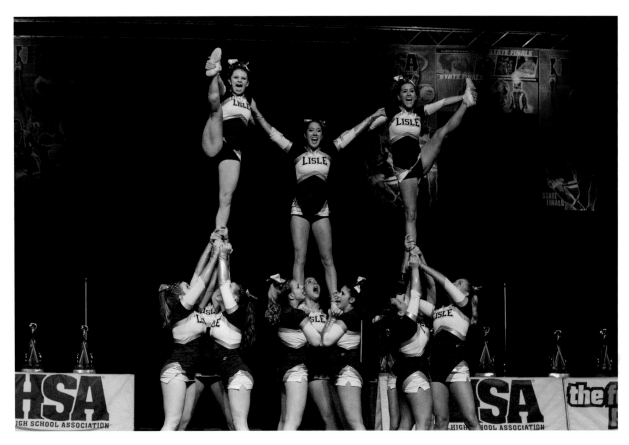

Young athletes require practical guidelines and adult support to meet the nutrition demands for their life stage and sport.

Children should be cautiously introduced to strenuous activity. Along with limited muscle **glycolytic** activity, children also have lower muscle strength related to reduced anaerobic capacity and experience minimal muscle fiber growth in response to exercise. Given the obvious need to avoid child exploitation, not much research data is available on young athletes, and what is available is fraught with small sample sizes and study designs that address the research question only indirectly. An example of this is applying research findings from studies conducted in adults to children.

Children should not be thought of as "mini-adults," and neither should they be grouped collectively when considering their physical development. Many factors, including genetics and environment, affect the individual onset of maturation and must be considered during nutrition planning. Both physiological and psychological differences affect youth's dietary patterns, as well as their perception and receptivity to nutrition information. Many young athletes are most interested in performance, with little thought given to the impact of lifestyle choices on long-term health. Consciously or otherwise, they depend on the adults in their lives for guidance. Like their nonathletic peers, young athletes are impressionable and are often up-to-date with popular trends. Strategic use of infographics and media links can be powerful educational tools.

Some adolescent athletes may be curious if dietary supplements will help their performance and give them an edge over their competition, particularly if they have witnessed a teammate's or other athlete's success after taking a supplement. As future professionals interested in working with young athletes, it is important and beneficial to talk with them about the benefits and risks of various ergogenic aids, as well as discussing the benefits of natural aids (e.g., carbohydrate, protein, and fat) and what it means to live a healthy lifestyle. Discouraging the use of unproven or dangerous dietary supplements can help balance a young athlete's "win at all costs" mentality. Steering young athletes early in the direction of optimal nutrition and harnessing the benefits of whole foods will not deter all of them from experimenting with dangerous and illegal supplements, but it will make a difference and yield long-term benefits for many.

Growth and Development in Childhood

Childhood growth can be erratic and is slow compared to adolescence growth. These variable growth patterns result in considerable fluctuations in dietary energy needs. During periods of rapid growth, children might experience unexpected periods of lethargy, poor coordination, and movement inefficiency. Training load itself can be a concern with youth, as available information on the effect of intense exercise on growth in children is sparse. In many cases, once training load decreases, "catch-up" growth can occur, but an imbalance in energy intake and expenditure (not enough calories to meet the demands of growth and training) can have long-term effects on both performance and health. Chronic low **energy availability** can lead to short stature,

delayed puberty, menstrual irregularities, poor bone health, and increased risk of injury. Along with monitoring energy intake and training volume, professionals working with prepubescent athletes should monitor growth via body mass trends and anthropometric variables and not rely solely on growth charts.

Growth charts are used to assess height and weight for age in children. The guidelines below are used to determine weight category for age.

> - Underweight: <5th percentile
> - Normal weight: 5th to <85th percentile
> - Overweight: 85 to <95th percentile
> - Obese: ≥95th percentile

Growth and Development in Adolescence

The period of adolescence is a nutritionally vulnerable time of life influenced by peer pressure, desire for increased autonomy, and significant physical, cognitive, emotional, and social changes. Growth patterns in adolescence are strongly related to genetics but can be influenced by many factors, including energy balance (energy intake and expenditure). Growth spurts tend to occur around 10 to 12 years of age for females and roughly 2 years later for males (figure

---

PUTTING IT INTO PERSPECTIVE

ENERGY AVAILABILITY

Energy availability equals dietary intake minus exercise energy expenditure (normalized to fat-free mass [FFM]). Energy availability is the amount of energy available to the body to perform all other functions after the energy cost of exercise is subtracted.

Example:

Female is 62 kg (136.4 lb.)

2,600 kcal − 600 kcal = 2,000 kcal

2,000 kcal/62 kg = 32.3 kcal/kg

Having an energy availability below 30 kcal/kg is associated with impairments of a variety of body functions. Energy availability of 45 kcal/kg FFM per day was found to be associated with energy balance and optimal health (76), but more research is needed.

14.1). Key body composition changes begin to emerge during this period. Females begin to develop greater fat mass, whereas males begin to acquire more lean body mass and blood volume. Because of these changes, males may seem more advanced than females on the playing field, since these physiological changes support power and performance. As a cumulative result of adolescent growth spurts, adolescents accrue an estimated 15 percent of their final adult height and 45 percent of maximal skeletal mass during their adolescent years. From a measurement standpoint, this translates into roughly 10 inches (25 cm) and 53 pounds (24 kg) for females and 11 inches (27 cm) and 70 pounds (31 kg) for males.

As shown in Figure 14.2, the appearance of secondary sexual characteristics is a key indicator of pubertal age. For example, a 13-year-old boy who is actively going through puberty has aspects of energy metabolism and muscle physiology that are more advanced than a 15-year-old boy who has not started puberty. In this scenario, the 13-year- old likely has greater glycolytic potential in strength and power sports, is better suited for experiencing muscle metabolic adaptations

to training, and has greater capacity to recover from heavy exercise because of the hormonal environment supported by puberty.

Energy Needs

Determining energy needs for children and adolescents is an inexact science in which many of the best estimates for calculating energy needs are extrapolated from adult data. However, relying on data derived from adults is a flawed approach because children are less metabolically efficient than adults. For instance, energy needs for children during walking and running activities in sport may be as much as 30 percent higher compared to adults. Methodology used to predict daily energy needs are further complicated when children compensate for bouts of strenuous physical activity by becoming more sedentary with other physical activities (i.e., less walking, more sitting).

It can be difficult for active adolescents to support optimal growth and development with adequate energy intake while also meeting the increased energy demands of their sport. Time

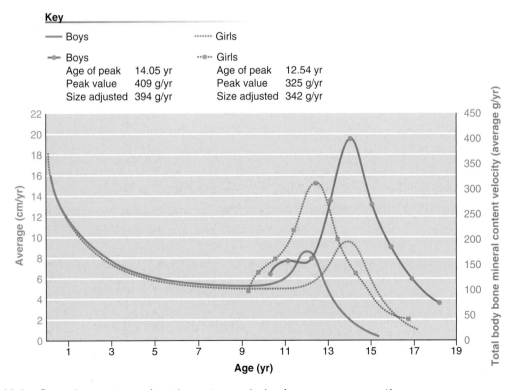

Figure 14.1 Growth spurts are key times to maximize bone mass accretion.

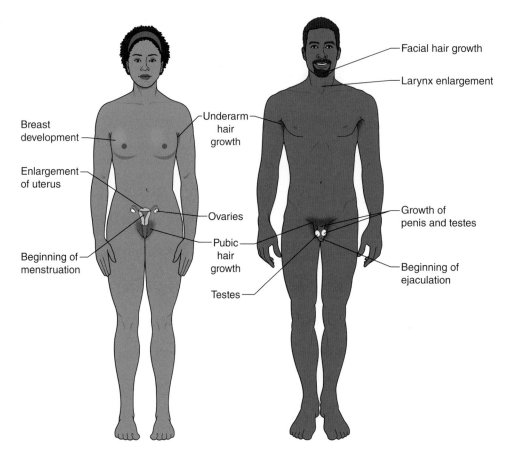

Figure 14.2 Secondary sexual characteristics in females and males.

constraints, travel, and sport-specific eating attitudes can make it challenging to meet energy needs. In addition, high rates of childhood obesity can make energy intake recommendations and strategies to meet them less than clear. Child and adolescent athletes desiring to "bulk up" could gain excess fat resulting in reduced speed, endurance, agility, work efficiency, and acclimation to heat, while also potentially increasing their risk of developing obesity. In 2011 to 2014, approximately 17 percent of 2- to 19-year-olds were obese (56).

Child and adolescent athletes who are overweight or obese should be encouraged to exercise and follow strategies that promote healthy eating. In this age group, a focus on promoting weight loss is not always recommended. Unless comorbidities are present and weight loss is recommended and monitored by a primary care provider, most professionals agree that promoting weight maintenance and healthy lifestyle changes

while waiting for height to increase will lead to a lower BMI and is considered a healthier strategy (52). Strategies to encourage healthy eating include the following (54):

> Choose smaller portions of foods and drinks.
> Place healthy foods and drinks within easy reach.
> Keep less healthy foods out of sight.
> Cut down on fast food.
> Cut down on distractions while eating (TV, phones, the computer, etc.).
> Don't tell children to "clean their plate."
> Don't reward children's good behavior with food.

Nutrition Needs

In addition to meeting their energy needs for growth, development, and activity, children and teens need to meet their energy-yielding macronutrient (carbohydrate, protein, fat) needs for health and sport. Specific recommendations in other areas of the diet are also warranted to support performance, health, and overall diet quality. Many recommendations are unique to this age group and are described below.

Carbohydrate

Carbohydrate needs for optimal athletic performance and recovery are listed in table 14.1. In sporting activities lasting longer than 1 hour or at greater than 70 percent $\dot{V}O_2$max, children and adolescents may be limited by sparse carbohydrate stores and thus rely more on exogenous carbohydrate sources (those they consume before and during activity) and less on glycogen to fuel performance. Strength training in youth can enhance glycolytic activity, but maximal adaptation is not appreciated until sometime during adolescence when the limited glycolytic activity from childhood is resolved. A diet containing a minimum of 50 percent of energy needs as carbohydrate is recommended. To help meet carbohydrate needs, young athletes can consume carbohydrates in sports foods (drinks, gels, bars) during training and competition (66). To improve diet quality, child and adolescent athletes would benefit from expanding their palate by consuming a variety of carbohydrate-rich foods, including whole grains, dairy, vegetables, and fruits that provide a wide range of micronutrients, phytonutrients, and fiber.

Protein

For child and adolescent athletes, protein needs are higher than for nonactive peers, but research suggests that additional needs (above sport amounts) are not required to support growth and development. The g/kg body weight recommendations available for adults are considered applicable in adolescence, with an upper limit of 1.7 grams of protein per day per kilogram body weight (78). Concerns for inadequate protein intake arise with chronic energy restriction, and these concerns are exacerbated if chronic energy restriction is combined with intense physical training. This combination could alter protein metabolism and impair growth and maturation. Child and teen athletes can improve the quality of their diet by making better choices of protein foods to consume. Some children have been found to be more reluctant to add animal-based protein foods to their diet and prefer foods higher in carbohydrate and fat. In adolescence, the quality of protein consumed

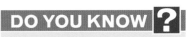

DO YOU KNOW ?
Sugar-sweetened beverages, such as soda, rank among the top five energy sources consumed for people over 2 years of age (80).

Table 14.1 Carbohydrate Intake Guidelines for the Adolescent Athlete

RECOVERY GUIDELINES	
Immediate recovery (0-4 hr)	1–1.2 g/kg/hr up to 4 hours, then resume daily needs
Daily recovery (low intensity or skill based)	3–5 g/kg/d
EXERCISE PROGRAM GUIDELINES	
Moderate exercise (1 hr/d)	5–7 g/kg/d
Endurance (training 1–3 hr/d)	6–10 g/kg/d
Extreme exercise (training 4–5 hr/d)	8–12 g/kg/d
DURING SPORT GUIDELINES	
Short duration (0-75 min)	Not required or small amount
Medium or long duration (75 min–2.5 hr)	30–60 g/hr

Based on Debrow et al. 2014.

could be improved via leaner sources dense with nutrients.

Fat

In recommendations for fat consumption, the minimal absolute grams of fat have not changed much over the years in adults, and there is limited research in children and adolescents. Although younger athletes rely more on aerobic metabolism, no evidence currently exists to support a performance benefit from higher fat intake. The most prudent advice for fat intake aligns with following the acceptable macronutrient distribution range (AMDR) of 20 to 35 percent of total energy consumed. For overweight or obese child and teen athletes, mild reductions in dietary fat (within the AMDR range) are a prudent weight-management strategy. As far as quality of food sources that supply fat to the diet in this age group, fat intake is strongly associated with increased consumption of cheese, poultry, and snack foods. Many child and teen athletes may not know how to fill the void by reducing such foods as chips, cookies, cakes, and do not realize "crispy," "pan fried," and "creamed" are food descriptors associated with increased fat content. This might contribute to intakes above 10 percent of total calories from saturated fatty acids and might increase the consumption of trans fatty acids.

Fluids

Compared to adults, children have a greater surface area to mass ratio because of their smaller body and muscle mass, which may result in greater heat absorption. Children also generate more heat, have a higher sweat threshold, a lower sweat capacity, and take longer to acclimate to hot environments. Many of these physiological observations begin to resolve during adolescence. Hydration for young athletes is discussed in chapter 8.

It is particularly important for young athletes to begin practice and competition well hydrated. Urine color should be clear or light yellow at the initiation of exercise. Structured hydration protocols for adolescents can be found elsewhere (18) and describe the effects of sweat rates, sport dynamics, availability of fluids, environmental factors, level of fitness, duration, intensity, and fluid preferences on hydration status.

Micronutrients

Research suggests active children and adolescents have greater vitamin and mineral intake than their nonactive peers, and exercise does not appear to increase needs. However, this does not mean that micronutrient deficiency is not an issue, as many adolescents fall short in their consumption of three major micronutrients: iron, calcium, and vitamin D. The RDAs for each of these nutrients, consequences of deficiency, and strategies for increasing consumption are discussed in chapters 5 and 6.

DO YOU KNOW ?

Unsafe hypohydration and dehydration practices to lose weight that are commonly practiced in sport include fluid restriction, spitting, use of laxatives and diuretics, rubber suits, steam baths, and saunas.

DO YOU KNOW ?

About half of the world's children aged 6 months to 5 years have at least one micronutrient deficiency. Most micronutrients cannot be made within the body and must be acquired through the diet. Thus children and adolescents should be eating well-chosen diets that include a variety of fruits and vegetables, grains, protein, and dairy, as well as other fortified foods in order to prevent micronutrient deficiencies.

Ergogenic Aids and Dietary Supplements

Some adolescent athletes become vulnerable to the lure of dietary supplements because they are influenced by their peers, sport heroes, and the media. Lay publications, manufacturer claims, and the use of supplements by famous athletes may add to the allure for some adolescent athletes. As a future professional in nutrition or athletics (or both), you must stay abreast of the trends in this area. As described in chapter 9, recommendations for athletes in this age group regarding supplement use are available. Read position statements and other reputable research on the dietary supplement practices of athletes in this age group to ensure you are prepared to work with young athletes in the future.

MASTERS ATHLETES

Aging brings unique opportunities and experiences. From the standpoint of athletic performance, aging can be detrimental because of its effects on all physiological functions. However, exercise is widely accepted as essential for preventing chronic disease and slowing the loss of physical function associated with aging. Further, given what we know about the importance of physical activity and exercise throughout the lifespan, it is not a surprise that more people are staying involved in exercise and competitive sport in their 50s and beyond. The term "masters athlete" is not universally defined by age and varies by sporting activity; however, most masters champions are in their 40s and beyond. Masters-level events are gaining popularity at the local, national, and international level. Many recommendations for masters athletes are extrapolated from recommendations for younger athletes and nutrition needs for the aging, as outlined by the DRIs (33).

Exercise as an Essential Lifestyle Behavior in Aging

The world's population in 2040 is estimated to include 1.3 billion people with 14% of the population over the age of 65. This estimation is roughly double the approximate 506 million people over 65 in 2008 (81). Regular physical activity and exercise is essential for keeping the aging population in better health. Exercise is essential for slowing the losses of cardiorespiratory and cardiovascular function, muscle function, and bone mineral density, while helping to control changes in body mass and cognitive function and preventing insulin resistance.

Cardiovascular and Metabolic Health

Aging athletes who continue to perform endurance exercise retain greater aerobic capacity than their sedentary age-matched peers (69). Although a decrease in $\dot{V}O_2max$ with aging that begins at about the age of 30 is inevitable, those who begin and maintain endurance exercise can improve their fitness level. Several factors are thought to contribute to this age-related decline in $\dot{V}O_2max$, including social factors such as limited time, commitment to

Masters athletes compete across several age categories.

career and family, and less time spent exercising. Physiological changes also contribute and have been explained by changes to exercise economy and lactate thresholds (75). Despite some losses in aerobic performance, one of the benefits of exercise in aging is its effect on maintaining healthy lipid profiles that put masters athletes at lower risk of metabolic and cardiovascular disease (63).

In addition to promoting optimal lipid profiles and cardiovascular health, exercise during aging augments overall metabolic health by decreasing risk of insulin resistance. Skeletal muscle helps use blood glucose, and exercise helps improve both insulin signaling and noninsulin-dependent glucose uptake induced by muscle contraction. In the absence of exercise during aging, it is common for fasting blood glucose levels to rise because of insulin resistance. If unresolved, a series of events may take place involving weight gain, increased inflammation, and increased likelihood of developing type 2 diabetes mellitus. The benefit of regular exercise in staving off diabetes cannot be overstated; the effect appears to be independent of age and instead more likely associated with decreasing risk of obesity (11).

Musculoskeletal Health

Strong bones and muscles are essential to maintaining normal physical functioning and independent living during aging. Usually starting sometime in our 40s, a slow, progressive decline begins in muscle mass (62). Muscle mass declines 3 to 8 percent each decade, while strength declines approximately 1.5 percent per year and accelerates to 3 percent per year after age 60, while powerful, fast-acting muscle fibers convert to slower muscle fibers (39, 57, 84). Sarcopenia increases one's risk of falling, a major cause of head injuries, broken bones, and hospitalization in the elderly (34, 41, 42, 68). Though muscle loss cannot be completely stopped during aging, it can be blunted through resistance training and eating a well-balanced diet that supports muscle tissue (13). It is never too late to start a resistance-training program; years of evidence suggests muscle strength can be improved at any age, and this functional benefit can improve gait speed and balance with aging (10). Resistance training also expresses its beneficial effects on bone mass. This is especially important for aging women, who begin to lose bone much earlier than men because of lost estrogen with menopause. Estrogen is important for bone mass accretion.

In addition to resistance training, any exercise has a positive effect on muscle and bone, and these effects can be maximized through high-impact exercise (87). High-impact exercise results in greater stimulation of muscle and mechanical stress on bone, which helps produce stronger tissue. It is through this type of exercise that masters athletes tend to be stronger and have better bone health compared to sedentary counterparts. When examining bone health, even when exercise provides moderate impact, bone health can be improved. These benefits

PUTTING IT INTO PERSPECTIVE

PREVENTING OSTEOPOROSIS

Osteoporosis is a silent and increasingly common disease characterized by weak, porous bones. Bone density and quality of bones are reduced during the disease process, and bones commonly become fragile, leading to increased risk of fractures. A simple fall or slip for a person with osteoporosis can lead to a catastrophic bone fracture that can limit physical mobility, contribute additional weakness to muscles and bones, and spark significant functional decline. While this disease is most associated with aging, it has been identified in younger people. It can be prevented during young adulthood through weight-bearing exercises, a diet with adequate energy intake, and adequate vitamin D and calcium. For the college student, this can be as simple as taking up weight training or dancing while avoiding extreme weight loss practices and consuming more calcium-rich foods.

have been documented in physically active adults who were 65 years of age and older and showed greater bone mineral content from both swimming and running compared to nonactive controls (82).

Body Weight

Obesity is currently estimated to affect approximately one-third of the adult population, which puts this disease in epidemic status. Overweight, a prerequisite to obesity, is also of concern, with physical inactivity serving as a major risk factor. Masters athletes are also at risk of weight gain, but exercise is one effective strategy for lessening age-related weight gain. It is well established that regular exercise is essential for maintaining a healthy weight, especially after achieving a weight loss (74). The absolute amount of exercise needed to prevent weight gain has been studied and has informed recent physical activity guidelines (19). It appears that research subjects who average 60 minutes of moderate physical activity per day gain the least amount of weight (35).

In summary, engaging in regular, moderate-intensity physical activity can prevent overweight and obesity. This level of physical activity is consistent with the level for most masters athletes.

Cognitive Function

Exercise during aging has multiple positive effects on systemic health, body system function, prevention of weight gain, metabolic disease, and possibly, cognitive function. Masters athletes have greater white matter integrity in areas of the brain related to motor control, visuospatial function, and working memory (79). Recent studies have found that cognitive performance and cerebral blood flow are strongly associated with cardiorespiratory fitness and that the benefits of healthy heart function leading to brain function improvements can be modified by fitness (37).

Energy Needs

The calculation and estimation of energy needs for aging athletes is an inexact science, with many of the same limitations encountered in other life-stage groups. Many energy prediction equations do include an age variable that is incorporated into the calculation to reduce the number of calories required for total energy expenditure (TEE). This is based on the premise that aging is directly associated with reduced metabolic activity. While this association is real, reductions in metabolic rate are more likely caused by a reduction of total muscle mass than age and a reduced BMR. An experienced masters-level athlete likely has a higher metabolic rate than an age-matched individual who is sedentary.

As discussed in chapter 2, TEE is comprised of basal metabolic rate (BMR), **thermic effect of food (TEF)**, and physical activity. All of these factors have been independently shown to decrease with age, but physical activity is clearly the most variable. While many equations to predict TEE are commonly used in practice, if a masters athlete has recent body composition data, the preferred method is to use the Cunningham equation. This equation uses fat-free mass as a variable and has been shown to estimate RMR more accurately than other equations (77).

Nutrition Needs

We know little thus far about the specific nutrition needs of masters-level athletes because data is limited for this population. However, to date, there is good evidence on the physiological benefits of exercise in aging, sports nutrition recommendations for adults, and important data on physiological outcomes of diet and exercise interventions in older recreational athletes. These data are currently being used to extrapolate nutrient recommendations for masters-level athletes. The following sections will describe energy, macronutrient, micronutrient, and hydration recommendations for aging athletes.

Macronutrients

Sport nutrition guidelines continue to call for an individualized and periodized approach to carbohydrate and protein needs based on training load, and intensity. Carbohydrate needs for training are not age-specific but depend on training and competition demands. A diet consisting of high-carbohydrate, nutrient-dense foods such as whole-grain breads and cereals, fruits and vegetables, and low-fat dairy foods provide quality carbohydrate to meet the masters athlete's needs. Protein is essential throughout the lifespan, helping promote muscle and connective tissue recovery from exercise, while also supporting bone health, and assisting in the support of metabolic adaptation. Protein sometimes becomes the "forgotten nutrient" that is essential for bone health. As with carbohydrate, protein needs should be based on training intensity and volume of both endurance and resistance exercises. General guidelines for the intake of energy-yielding macronutrients for masters athletes are provided in table 14.2.

Micronutrients

It is generally accepted that as more energy is consumed, more micronutrients are also consumed. Since athletes of all ages tend to consume more energy than their sedentary counterparts, many athletes also consume more micronutrients. When these athletes also focus on consuming fortified foods and many sports foods that contain added micronutrients, they might feel even more assured they are meeting their micronutrient needs. However, some studies report that athletes are coming up short on key micronutrients, which could have a negative effect on health and performance. Review chapters 6 and 7 for further discussion.

The need for some micronutrients (vitamin D, vitamin B_6, vitamin B_{12}, and calcium) increases beyond the age of 50, while the need for iron and chromium decreases (30). When examining studies that report on nutrient intake in aging athletes, the most cited micronutrients of concern, because of limited intake, were vitamin D, calcium, and vitamin B_{12}. While both vitamin D and calcium are tied to bone health, it is now also clear that both support muscle function and immunity—two important findings for masters athletes. Aging athletes should aim for 1,000 to 1,200 mg of calcium per day from calcium-rich foods. If supplements are used, aging athletes should consider using a form that has high bioavailability, such as calcium citrate. For vitamin D, controversy continues over the amount needed in the blood (as 25[OH]D) to signify sufficiency to promote health and athletic performance. Although hotly debated, the IOM defines deficiency when serum 25(OH)D falls below 20 ng/ml (64). Using this definition, it has been estimated that 20 to 100 percent of community-dwelling elderly are vitamin D deficient if not on a vitamin D supplement (28). In the older population, it has been found that vitamin D levels were associated with poor physical performance when subjects were matched by age and gender over a 3-year period (86). Poor vitamin D status is a real concern in aging, and it should be emphasized that consuming natural food sources of vitamin D is not a reliable way to prevent or reverse a deficiency (28). For this reason, a three-pronged approach to improve and maintain vitamin D status is advisable: consumption of vitamin D-rich foods, responsible midday sun exposure, and vitamin D supplementation as needed.

Table 14.2 Energy-Yielding Macronutrient Recommendations for Masters Athletes

	Carbohydrate		Protein	Fat	
AMDR	45–65% of daily calories		10–35% of daily calories	20–35% of daily calories	
General sports nutrition guidelines	Light exercise (low intensity)	3–5 g/kg/d	1.2–2.0 g/kg	Total fat	20–25%
	Moderate (1 hr/d)	5–7 g/kg/d			
	High (1–3 hr/d)	6–10 g/kg/d		Saturated fat	<10%
	Very high (>4–5 hr/d)	8–12 g/kg/d			

Data from Institute of Medicine 2005; Thomas, Erdman, and Burke 2016.

PUTTING IT INTO PERSPECTIVE

NEGATIVE CONSEQUENCES ASSOCIATED WITH DEHYDRATION

Body fluid deficits that cause a 2 percent or higher drop in weight can impair aerobic performance and cognitive function (1, 65). Dehydration can decrease speed, strength, stamina, and recovery time. It can also raise perceived effort of exertion and lead to an increased body temperature and increased risk for injury. In some scenarios, the heat stress associated with dehydration can contribute to an increased risk of life-threatening exertional heat illness (i.e., heatstroke).

Fluids

Aging elicits many physiological changes that create challenges in determining hydration needs for masters athletes. With aging comes a decreased response to thirst, and the thirst mechanism related to the sensation of thirst is slower to respond both when additional fluid is needed and when fluid needs are met. Further, alcohol and several medications can contribute to a compromised hydration status that might be risky during physical exercise. Masters athletes should not rely solely on thirst to meet fluid needs and should adopt a drinking strategy to maintain adequate fluid intake. See chapter 8 for guidelines on fluid consumption.

INDIVIDUALS WITH DIABETES AND METABOLIC SYNDROME

According to the American Diabetes Association, in 2012, 29.1 million Americans, or 9.3 percent of the population, had **type 2 diabetes mellitus**. Of this staggering number, 21.0 million were estimated to be diagnosed, and 8.1 million undiagnosed. Almost 1.5 million Americans are diagnosed with diabetes every year. At this rate, over the next 25 years, the number of Americans with diagnosed and undiagnosed diabetes could nearly double. Many athletes are now playing sports with metabolic diseases such as diabetes, and dietary plans must be designed to meet their metabolic demands and energy needs. Diabetes affects carbohydrate availability and its use by body cells, so specific dietary, exercise, and medication considerations are necessary for athletes with diabetes. With a proper management plan

in place, athletes with diabetes can perform just as well as their peers, as evidenced by the 2000 Olympics, where two athletes with diabetes won gold medals in swimming.

Diabetes is generally characterized by high blood glucose levels caused by either a lack of insulin or the body's inability to use insulin efficiently. In **type 1 diabetes mellitus** (figure 14.3), **hyperglycemia** results from the pancreas not making insulin and requires insulin injection to normalize blood glucose levels. The loss of insulin production is a result of an autoimmune insult on the pancreas and presents with a quick onset, typically in childhood. In contrast, in type 2 diabetes mellitus (figure 14.4)—the most common form of diabetes, representing approximately 90 percent of all diabetes diagnoses—insulin resistance is the dominant mechanism.

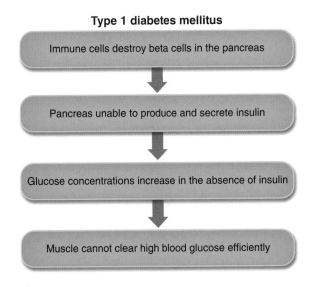

Type 1 diabetes mellitus

Immune cells destroy beta cells in the pancreas

Pancreas unable to produce and secrete insulin

Glucose concentrations increase in the absence of insulin

Muscle cannot clear high blood glucose efficiently

Figure 14.3 Type 1 diabetes.

Type 2 diabetes mellitus

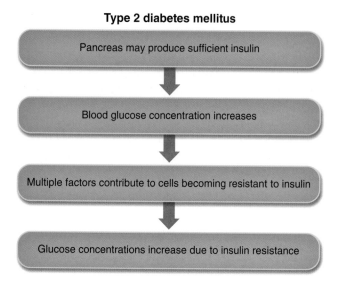

Pancreas may produce sufficient insulin

Blood glucose concentration increases

Multiple factors contribute to cells becoming resistant to insulin

Glucose concentrations increase due to insulin resistance

Figure 14.4 Type 2 diabetes.

Insulin resistance, a precursor to type 2 diabetes, is the body's inability to respond to and use the insulin it produces. Obesity, high levels of fat in the blood, and a diet high in saturated fat are contributing factors to insulin resistance.

When insulin resistance begins, the pancreas will make extra insulin to make up for it. Over time, the pancreas is not able to keep up and cannot make enough insulin to keep blood glucose levels within normal limits. The pancreas wears down and might stop making insulin because of the constant glucose stimulus it receives. Type 2 diabetes mellitus is treated with lifestyle changes, oral medications, and in some cases insulin.

Type 2 diabetes is associated with **metabolic syndrome** and can lead to permanent organ damage. This syndrome is characterized by high blood pressure, high blood sugar levels, excess body fat around the waist, and abnormal cholesterol levels. When these factors are present together, they increase the risk of heart disease, stroke, and diabetes. Type 2 diabetes is a major cause of morbidity and mortality worldwide and strongly associated with inactivity, obesity, and family history (16). Over 90 percent of those with type 2 diabetes are overweight or obese.

While type 2 diabetes is typically diagnosed later in life, the rise in obesity and physical inactivity in youth has increased the prevalence of type 2 diabetes in children and teens.

The glucose in the blood stream that has limited capacity to enter cells begins to accumulate in the blood at concentrations higher than normal. Chronic hyperglycemia from diabetes can cause a host of problems due to a change of viscosity of the blood that the added glucose creates and can affect the interaction of glucose with red blood cells as well as small blood vessels in many body tissues.

The poor absorption and disposal of glucose by the body's cells occurs as a result of a series of defective events and creates severe alterations to normal energy metabolism. A major component of cellular glucose uptake relies on the action of cellular glucose transporters. These transporters are a large family of proteins that reside in the cell and, upon receiving a signal, will translocate to the outer membrane to allow glucose to enter the cell. Without receiving a proper signal, glucose uptake is impaired and can result in mild to severe rises in blood glucose, depending on the severity of the signal impairment. The signal required to initiate glucose transporter movement comes from insulin. This peptide hormone is

PUTTING IT INTO PERSPECTIVE

METABOLIC SYNDROME IN ATHLETES

Aggressive lifestyle changes can delay or even prevent the development of serious health problems and help prevent the cluster of conditions associated with metabolic syndrome. Athletes are well positioned to delay the onset of or decrease the severity of metabolic syndrome with frequent exercise and weight control. While lack of exercise is a strong predictive factor for both diabetes and metabolic syndrome, there is concern about athletes with ongoing interest in weight gain (such as American football linemen). These athletes might become obese, placing them at greater risk for metabolic syndrome when their playing days are over (76).

secreted from the pancreas in response to very small rises in blood glucose after consuming a meal. Insulin normally binds to receptors on the surface membrane of cells. The docking of insulin to its receptor creates a cascade of intracellular signaling events that stimulate glucose transporter translocation to the cell surface. Normally this activity results in normal glucose uptake and a decrease in blood glucose levels. In diabetes, there can be a disruption in insulin release by the pancreas and a decreased response, or insulin resistance of the cells to any insulin that is secreted.

As introduced earlier, complications of diabetes are rooted in two major concerns: cellular starvation, due to the lack of glucose, and hyperglycemia. When the cells are deprived of glucose, the body is fooled into thinking that cells are starving and therefore initiates a series of events that unfortunately does more harm than good. The liver is signaled to release its stored glucose in hopes of providing more fuel for starved cells; however, this only results in higher blood glucose concentrations. Once blood glucose concentrations get high enough, the kidneys start to respond by filtering the excess glucose into the urine as a means to help manage hyperglycemia. The problem with this response is that it creates additional urine, leading to excessive urination, known as **polyuria**. This increases thirst and creates a symptom known as **polydipsia**. Because of these series of events, many people with untreated type 2 diabetes also experience increased hunger, known as **polyphagia**, which can further contribute to hyperglycemia. While some form of these bodily symptoms may develop in an effort to address the issue of cell starvation, other signals are amplified in response to the ineffectiveness of the previous strategies. Figure 14.5 summarizes the series of events that lead to these metabolic abnormalities and the body symptoms that result.

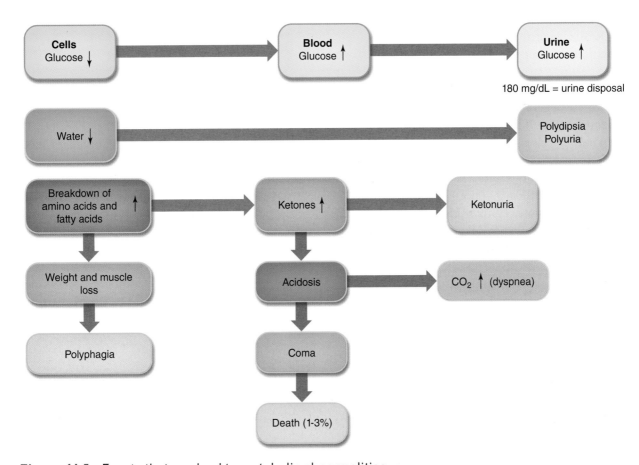

Figure 14.5 Events that can lead to metabolic abnormalities.

As the body recognizes that previous attempts to fuel cells have limited effectiveness, it will then turn to using protein and fat as fuel. The body will increase skeletal muscle protein catabolism in order to use amino acids as substrates for gluconeogenesis, as discussed in chapter 2. Fat utilization will also increase in hopes that fat will meet the ATP demands of the cell. Collectively, the end result of increased protein and fat utilization is body weight loss, muscle wasting, and muscle weakness. While the loss of valuable protein to glucose production has limited impact on solving the metabolic dilemma at hand, increased attempts to use more fat as a fuel source creates additional problems. Without an adequate supply of intracellular glucose, fat cannot be completely oxidized, and intermediate products of fat metabolism can build up, forming ketone bodies. If left unchecked, a significant rise in ketone bodies can lead to a condition known as **ketoacidosis**, which can result in acidification of blood and body fluids that may be life threatening and result in a coma.

The treatment regimen for diabetes depends on the type of diabetes diagnosed. Type 1 diabetes mellitus is typically met with a treatment regimen that involves insulin injections, combined with regular exercise and a healthy diet to control blood sugar levels. For type 2 diabetes mellitus, cells are not responsive to insulin, resulting in perturbations in glucose uptake. Treatment depends on multiple factors, including average blood glucose levels and amount of endogenous insulin production. Some people with type 2 diabetes mellitus can control their blood glucose levels through healthy eating and physical activity. In addition to diet, exercise, and lifestyle changes, medications to lower levels of blood glucose are often prescribed to enhance cellular sensitivity to insulin, allowing glucose to be transported more effectively into the cells for energy. Some of the signs and symptoms of diabetes and clinical parameters used to diagnose diabetes appear in table 14.3.

DO YOU KNOW ?

One of the most easily observed characteristics of ketoacidosis is fruity-smelling breath. This is caused by acetone (a ketone) being produced by organs that are starved of glucose in response to the body's hyperglycemic state. This is one way in which a friend or family member may be able to detect ketoacidosis with just a simple observation.

Symptoms of Type 1 Diabetes

> Polyuria
> Polydipsia
> Polyphagia
> Unusual weight loss
> Extreme fatigue and irritability

Symptoms of Type 2 Diabetes

> Any of the type 1 symptoms
> Frequent infections
> Blurred vision
> Cuts or bruises that are slow to heal
> Tingling or numbness in the hands or feet

Athletes diagnosed with type 2 diabetes mellitus must understand the effect exercise and competition have on their blood glucose levels. To effectively understand and manage this effect, frequent self-monitoring of glucose before and after exercise is necessary to avoid abnormally low levels of blood sugar called **hypoglycemia**. Since muscle contraction provides an additional

Table 14.3 Diagnosing Criteria for Diabetes

Diagnosing diabetes	Normal	Prediabetes	Diabetes
Glycohemoglobin test (A1C)	Less than 5.7%	5.7–6.4%	6.5% or higher
Fasting plasma glucose (FPG)	Less than 100 mg/dl	100–125 mg/dl	126 mg/dl or higher
Oral glucose tolerance test (OGTT)	Less than 140 mg/dl	140–199 mg/dl	200 mg/dl or higher

Based on American Diabetes Association, 2016, "Classification and diagnosis of diabetes," *Diabetes Care* 39(suppl 1): S1-S22.

stimulus for glucose intake, and medications are also usually taken to create the same effect, the two stimuli together can sometimes create too much glucose uptake, which limits glucose availability to the central nervous system. The effect of exercise on glucose uptake is strong and can continue for several hours after exercise, with a prolonged impact on blood glucose levels. While this is thought to be very helpful for preventing hyperglycemia, this can be a negative consequence for an athlete with high training demands who is not properly fueled. Monitoring of blood glucose for several hours after exercise may be necessary to monitor for hypoglycemia.

Athletes with type 1 diabetes must be more cautious than athletes with type 2 diabetes. These athletes are presented with a number of challenges in achieving tight blood glucose controls that support athletic performance and devising food and insulin regimens that must adapt quickly to an unpredictable sporting environment. Insulin must be injected at the right times at the right amounts, matched to physical activity level, and paired with carbohydrate intake. Additionally, the mode of exercise that determines whether an activity is more anaerobic or aerobic in nature must be considered because of their different effects on blood sugar management. Aerobic exercise may not cause insulin levels to fall, resulting in a higher risk of hypoglycemia. Furthermore, exercise will increase insulin sensitivity for several hours and may further increase hypoglycemia risk. Anaerobic exercises tend to cause a release of hormones that promote the spilling of additional glucose into the blood that may not be accounted for once

DO YOU KNOW ❓

Because of the direct effect chronic hyperglycemia has on body tissues, other chronic diseases may develop. Tissues that have very small blood vessels and are vital to the function of a particular organ system are particularly susceptible to chronic high blood glucose levels. The most common complications occur with the eyes, kidneys, nerves, and heart, and may ultimately result in blindness, kidney dysfunction, heart disease, and nerve degeneration.

insulin is already dosed, resulting in a greater risk of hyperglycemia. In order to train and compete safely and effectively, type 1 diabetes athletes must possess good self-management skills to be able to adjust the timing and dose of insulin injections. Proper control of blood glucose will facilitate safe participation in sport and minimize medical complications.

Blood Sugar Management Strategies

Monitoring of glucose levels prior to, during, and after exercise is essential to determining whether an athlete needs to make changes in diet, exercise program, or medication regimen. Maintaining a blood glucose of 70 to 110 mg/dl on a regular basis is the foundation of controlling diabetes. Portable blood glucose testing devices take a small sample of blood from capillaries at the tips of the fingers, which is placed on a chemically treated test strip and inserted into the testing device. The device provides a quick digital readout of the blood glucose level and is usually tested several times throughout the day. The most important times for testing in the athlete is prior to exercise, immediately after exercise, and several hours after exercise. Decisions on whether to start training or competing or make adjustments to carbohydrate intake or insulin are based on preexercise monitoring of blood glucose. If glucose concentrations from the capillary blood test are greater than 250 mg/dl, the athlete should do a urine test for the presence of ketone production in the body. This test is completed by using a different type of chemically treated test strip that interacts with a small amount of urine to change color if ketones are present. Athletes with type 1 diabetes and insulin-dependent type 2 diabetes are more prone to ketone production and should not exercise with a combination of hyperglycemia and urine ketones because of an elevated risk of ketoacidosis. Table 14.4 provides specific considerations for the initiation of exercise related to blood glucose concentrations for both hypo- and hyperglycemia and the presence of urine ketones. When hypoglycemia is present prior to exercise, an athlete must make time to consume carbohydrate and adjust insulin dosage

Table 14.4 Glucose Level Considerations When Initiating Exercise

Preexercise glucose level	Recommendation made by qualified professionals
<100 mg/dl	Ingest additional carbohydrates prior to initiating exercise: 15–40 g carbohydrates (or more) depending on actual glucose level and athlete's typical response to added carbohydrates.
>250 mg/dl	Test urine for ketones.
>250 mg/dl, with ketones present	Do not exercise. Make insulin or medication adjustments and then retest glucose and ketones.
>250 mg/dl, without ketones present	Exercise can be initiated.
>300 mg/dl, without ketones present	Exercise with caution.

as necessary and should not exercise until hypoglycemia is resolved. The amount of carbohydrate required to help glucose levels rebound to above 100 mg/dl will vary but generally is between 15 and 40 grams. One cup of 100 percent orange juice provides approximately 30 grams of carbohydrate to increase blood sugar concentrations.

Many athletes with diabetes become accustomed to their training and competition cycles and develop a good feel for what adjustments are needed for blood sugar control. However, they should keep in mind that any changes to their training cycle may make their normal regimen inadequate for proper blood sugar control. For instance, any exercise lasting greater than 60 minutes in duration requires additional focus on blood glucose testing. Further, anytime the type, intensity, or duration of exercise is modified, the athlete should expect the need for closer monitoring of glucose concentrations and more adjustments.

General Nutrition Recommendations

For athletes with diabetes, the foundation of a healthy diet closely resembles the diet recommendations for the general population. The 2015 Dietary Guidelines for Americans along with the MyPlate food guidance system should form the basis of the foods that make up the diet. Carbohydrate remains the predominant energy for fueling exercise and should make up the bulk of the diet. The acceptable macronutrient distribution range (AMDR) provides general guidelines for each energy-yielding macronutrient in terms of the

percent of total energy that should be consumed, and dosing the daily amount of carbohydrates needed depending on daily activity demand relative to body mass (g/kg body weight) is the most practical approach to get started. With these tools, the diabetic athlete can begin to build a healthy diet based on cultural food preferences and training–nutrition periodization concepts discussed in other chapters of this text.

All carbohydrate foods can fit into a diabetic athlete's diet, but the bulk of the carbohydrates chosen should be nutrient dense, provide fiber, and originate from a variety of food groups. The goal for carbohydrate intake should be to balance intake throughout the day, to support fueling needs of activity, and to support stable blood sugar levels to minimize hypo- and hyperglycemia. Foods high in sugar should be minimized and should not regularly replace nutrient-dense carbohydrate choices.

Protein and fat make up the remaining energy needs of the diabetic athlete's diet. The specific requirements for each generally fall in line with the AMDR recommendations and guidelines set forth by the Dietary Guidelines. Additionally, protein needs for recovery and optimal muscle adaptation to training and fat intake guidelines to promote cardiovascular health are similar to those for nondiabetic athletes and the general population. Adjustments in macronutrient composition of the diet may be necessary following consultation with a physician, a **Certified Diabetes Educator (CDE)**, or a Registered Dietitian Nutritionist (RDN) to personalize recommendations not only to meet the demands of the sport but also to promote euglycemia between the recommended range of 70 to 100 mg/dl and cardiovascular health. Most of the day-to-day monitoring and adjustments to the diet are based on the goal of eating at approximately the same time each day while maintaining consistent intake of carbohydrate throughout the day through meals and snacks.

Specific Nutrition Recommendations

Athletes with type 1 diabetes mellitus should be knowledgeable about estimating the amount of carbohydrate consumed in each meal in order to match insulin requirements. The key consideration regarding carbohydrate intake during meals is the *quantity* of carbohydrate consumed and not so much the type of carbohydrate or a rigid schedule for carbohydrate intake. These athletes must self-monitor blood glucose levels regularly in order to learn what affects their blood glucose level.

In preparation for training or competition, it is vital that enough carbohydrate is available to the body before, during, and postexercise. Likewise, the amount of insulin administered must be tailored to how much carbohydrate has been consumed (1, 25) and adjusted depending on the type, intensity, and time of the exercise. For type 1 diabetes athletes, the glycemic index of foods has not been of much value for athletes with diabetes, and thus the total amount of carbohydrates ingested and the timing of ingestion are the most important variables. Since excessive carbohydrate intake in the days prior to an event can adversely affect blood sugar control, the practice of carbohydrate loading is often not advised (25).

Carbohydrates should be readily available to consume for exercise or competition lasting more than 30 minutes. Target carbohydrate consumption goals are generally 20 to 30 grams consumed every 30 to 60 minutes of endurance exercise. Depending on food preferences and the sport or activity, this can be accomplished by drinking most 8-ounce sports drinks, one sports gel, 4 ounces of 100 percent fruit juice mixed with 4 ounces of water, or a cereal–fruit breakfast bar. Athletes with type 1 diabetes participating in explosive, anaerobic events typically do not need additional carbohydrate during the event. During

exercise, athletes with type 1 diabetes should be well versed in picking up on the early symptoms of hypoglycemia and recognize that prolonged exertion might make identifying hypoglycemia difficult. If hypoglycemia is evident, immediate access to rapid-acting carbohydrate must be administered to increase circulating glucose levels.

The postexercise goal for type 1 diabetes athletes is to replenish glycogen stores and prevent hypoglycemia in the postexercise period when insulin sensitivity is enhanced. Carbohydrate intake recommendations for exercise recovery is similar to that for nondiabetic athletes—approximately 1.0 to 1.2 g/kg per hour until normal meals to meet fueling needs resume (76).

Specific nutrition recommendations for athletes with type 2 diabetes mellitus are often based on blood glucose response to exercise and adherence to an exercise program. When the etiology of type 2 diabetes mellitus is considered, the value of exercise as the cornerstone of blood sugar control cannot be overstated. Exercise improves insulin sensitivity and through an insulin-independent mechanism, primes the muscle for increasing the peripheral uptake of glucose. In fact, exercise has other benefits through promoting carbohydrate oxidation and glycogen storage, metabolic adaptations to burn more fuel more efficiently at higher intensities that can support fat loss and weight maintenance with improved body composition (60, 61). Just 20 to 30 minutes of any exercise improves insulin sensitivity, and a single bout of endurance exercise can affect insulin sensitivity for 24 to 72 hours (60). The effects of regular resistance exercise are also impressive. Resistance exercise increases muscle mass, which increases the size of the number one organ responsible for glucose uptake and disposal. Bigger engines can burn more energy! A goal for type 2 diabetes athletes is to manage energy intake to promote slow weight loss and to exercise regularly to promote insulin sensitivity.

Once an exercise program is initiated, the diet should be modified to reduce energy intake. Over time, these two strategies will work together to reduce fat mass and improve insulin sensitivity. Immediately prior to exercise, no additional carbohydrate should be consumed, since the goal is to promote weight loss. During exercise, additional carbohydrate should be avoided (as long as there are no signs of hypoglycemia) in order to preserve the energy deficit created by the adoption of a healthier diet and to avoid sabotaging progress in weight loss. If carbohydrate must be consumed, a keen awareness of carbohydrate density is important, again to prevent excessive energy intake. During the postexercise timeframe, insulin sensitivity is improved and energy use is amplified, so individuals with type 2 diabetes mellitus are advised not to immediately consume carbohydrate and instead wait until their next regular meal (36).

Preventing Diabetes Emergencies in Sport

The first step in preventing hypo- and hyperglycemic emergencies in athletes with diabetes is for athletes to have a track record of consistently managing their diabetes well. Consistent euglycemia coupled with good hemoglobin A1C scores and confidence in the interplay between their training, diet, and medication is essential for building a foundation to reduce emergency risk. Beyond these guidelines, those with diabetes at the greatest risk are those who require insulin. Athletes on oral medications are at a lower risk, while athletes with type 2 diabetes controlled solely with diet and exercise have minimal risk. Hyperglycemia can occur as a result of insulin deficiency during exercise coupled with the actions of other hormones released during exercise that mobilize more glucose into the bloodstream from liver glycogen stores. Maintaining euglycemia prior to exercise and keeping injectable insulin readily available are important

> ### DO YOU KNOW ?
>
> The symptoms of hypoglycemia are individualized and do not normally appear until blood glucose levels reach 70 mg/dl or less. Athletes must know their own signs of hypoglycemia. These include shakiness, nervousness, sweating, irritability, confusion, rapid heartbeat, dizziness, hunger, fatigue, headaches, lack of coordination, and perhaps other symptoms.

strategies to prevent this emergency. If too much insulin is present during exercise or postexercise recovery, excessive amounts of blood glucose can be taken up by muscle tissue and the liver will stop releasing glucose, resulting in hypoglycemia. Consuming carbohydrate during exercise and exercise recovery and monitoring blood glucose levels for multiple hours postexercise is the best prevention strategy. Additional strategies to prepare for hypoglycemic emergencies include having a food bag on hand with glucose tablets and fruit juice, and making sure friends, family, teammates, and sporting staff are aware of the location of the food bag and how to notice the signs and symptoms of hypo- and hyperglycemia so they are prepared to act appropriately.

PREGNANT WOMEN

Following physician screening for contraindications to exercise, well-chosen exercise programs can safely be incorporated to promote the health of the developing fetus and mother. While some women may elect to maintain most of their pre-pregnancy exercise intensity and volume, others strive to remain active but reduce their training load and avoid athletic competition. Guidelines for exercise during pregnancy and the postpartum period can be found elsewhere (3).

Combining exercise with pregnancy creates unique nutrition challenges. Exercise alone increases energy needs and an elevated demand for many nutrients. When pregnancy is added to the equation, energy demands increase again in order to promote the healthy growth of the fetus. In addition to the increase in energy needs, macronutrient and micronutrient demands also increase and can be areas of concern for the mother and baby if the diet is not appropriately planned or well chosen.

Physiological Changes Lead to Diet Recommendations

An active lifestyle during pregnancy is linked to several benefits, including an increase in maternal metabolic and cardiopulmonary reserve, normal glucose tolerance, improved psychological well-being, and beneficial fetal and placental adaptations. Physical activity can help manage weight gain for pregnant athletes and nonathletes. As exercise commences, it is important to understand the normal metabolic changes that affect nutrition needs. During pregnancy, the major tenants are making sure nutrient intake is adequate to meet pregnancy demands while also emphasizing an active lifestyle. An unhealthy diet and sedentary lifestyle during pregnancy can tip the balance of normal metabolic changes and lead to high or uncontrolled glucose, excessive weight gain, and **gestational diabetes mellitus (GDM)**. You have probably heard people say that pregnant women need to "eat for two," but this is far from the truth. While energy needs are only marginally increased during pregnancy, nutrient needs increase substantially. The message should not be "eat for two" but "eat twice as healthy."

Several physiological changes affect exercise capacity and performance during pregnancy. These changes in turn have an effect on nutrition needs. The cardiovascular system is remodeled by ovarian and placental hormones in early gestation to accommodate the increasing blood volume that comes with pregnancy. Other cardiovascular changes include an increase in resting **cardiac output** during the first trimester and a remodeling of the thoracic cage and diaphragm to a higher position in order to accommodate placental and fetal growth. Symptoms of shortness of breath are common and are caused in part by these mechanical alterations and also by increased sensitivity to carbon dioxide in the blood stream. Thermoregulation steadily improves throughout gestation, with a downward shift in the temperature at which sweating is initiated. This results in quicker heat loss and is important because of heat generation by the fetus and fetal dependence on maternal temperature regulation. Metabolic changes support using the mother's blood glucose as a primary energy source for growth of fetus and placenta. To accommodate a greater demand for blood glucose, gluconeogenic pathways in the liver are up-regulated and there is increased insulin production in the pancreas to assist glucose uptake for the fetus. In the peripheral tissue, there is an increase in skeletal muscle insulin resistance and fat stores to make more fat available via lipolysis. While

these metabolic changes are considered normal, they can be a significant concern if a mother is living an unhealthy lifestyle that promotes these changes independent of pregnancy. For instance, a mother who remains sedentary during pregnancy and consumes a diet that promotes excessive weight gain might also be promoting insulin resistance. This lifestyle, combined with normal metabolic adaptations to ensure a developing fetus has adequate access to glucose, may tip the healthy balance to GDM. Other factors also play a role in the risk for developing GDM, including overweight status prior to pregnancy, family history of GDM, specific ethnicities and ancestry, and pregnancy after the age of 35.

Healthy Weight Gain

Unless directed otherwise by a physician, pregnancy is not the time to be concerned with or initiate efforts to lose weight. However, pregnant women must also avoid consuming more energy than necessary. The number of daily calories a pregnant woman needs during pregnancy depends on a host of factors, including her pre-pregnancy BMI, the rate of body weight change during gestation, age, and level of physical activity. Unfortunately, many women start off pregnancy overweight or obese. Others gain more weight than is healthy during their pregnancy. Obesity during pregnancy is a risk factor for both mother and child (in-utero, at delivery, and later in life), with some risks including gestational diabetes, gestational hypertension (high blood pressure), Cesarean delivery (C-section), birth defects, and even fetal death. If a woman is obese during pregnancy, this increases the chance her child will be obese later in life; and if the mother retains most of the weight gain acquired during pregnancy, she is at greater risk of developing type 2 diabetes mellitus and obesity later in life. Overweight women who retain previous pregnancy weight also tend to start their next pregnancy with a higher early rate of weight gain, which is strongly associated with weight retention at 6 and 12 months postpartum (21). All this considered, recommendations have been published by the Institute of Medicine to provide guidelines for total weight gain and the rate of weight gain recommended for the second and third trimester of pregnancy (table 14.5). The amount of weight gained depends on pre-pregnancy weight. Research shows that the risk of problems during pregnancy and delivery is lowest when weight gain is kept within a healthy range. The weight recommendations in the table are presented as a range to guide professionals in giving individualized advice (2). These recommendations serve as a healthy guide during pregnancy and can certainly guide planning of energy intake and energy expenditure to manage healthy weight gain. This information is valuable because exceeding weight gain recommendations is thought to contribute to fat reserves and weight retention and increases risk of GDM, pregnancy induced hypertension, and a difficult labor and birth. Proper diet and exercise can go a long way in managing weight gain, preventing GDM, and promoting a healthy pregnancy. While diet guidelines are addressed in the subsequent section, physical activity guidelines are important to remember. The current recommendation for pregnant women is 30 minutes of moderate exercise on most, if not all, days of the week following a discussion with a doctor before starting or continuing any exercise routine.

Nutrient Needs

Maternal energy needs during pregnancy are a moving target based on the stage of pregnancy and the level of physical activity. In general, pregnant women need between 2,200 calories and 2,900 calories a day. Metabolic rate increases 15 percent during the second and third trimesters of pregnancy without a significant change during the first trimester. This increase during the latter

two-thirds of pregnancy is thought to support the growth of the fetus, placenta, and maternal tissues (32). When translating these metabolic changes into energy needs, it is generally recommended that during the first trimester no additional energy beyond resting energy expenditure (REE) that is adjusted for physical activity is required to support pregnancy. Exceptions are generally recommended for expectant mothers classified as underweight by BMI at the onset of pregnancy. These expectant mothers would benefit from additional energy (calories) to support growth and weight gain. During the second and third trimester, additional calories required to support weight gain have been translated as approximately +340 to 360 kcals and +450 kcals during the second and third trimesters, respectively.

DO YOU KNOW ?
Additional energy needs during the second and third trimesters of pregnancy can easily be met by eating one extra snack per day. This is clearly not "eating for two!"

Simple, common-sense strategies can be employed to prevent excess energy consumption. Extra calories can be avoided by cutting down on foods high in fat and avoiding added sugars. Practical advice includes replacing all sugar-sweetened beverages and fried foods with healthy options such as low-fat milk and yogurt, whole fruit, vegetables, and grains. Note that there is not a specific energy estimation equation for pregnancy, and absolute energy needs will vary with exercise during pregnancy by the type of physical activity and the total energy expended. Along with focusing on diet quality, **nutrient density** of foods and meals chosen, and

Table 14.5 BMI and Weight Gain for Second and Third Trimesters

Pre-pregnancy BMI	Total weight (lb.)	Recommended rate for 2nd and 3rd trimesters (lb./wk)
BMI ≤18.5	28–40	1 (1–1.3)
BMI 18.5–24.9	25–35	1 (0.8–1)
BMI 25–29.9	15–25	0.6 (0.5–0.7)
BMI ≥30	11–20	0.5 (0.4–0.6)

PUTTING IT INTO PERSPECTIVE

NUTRITION FOR MULTIPLE BABIES

Women can healthily gain up to twice as much weight (depending on their pre-pregnancy BMI) when carrying twins compared to carrying a single child. Increased appetite leaves mothers of twins at risk for excessive weight gain during pregnancy, especially during the early months.
Increased complications with twin pregnancies include

> anemia—twice as likely to occur in women who are pregnant with twins than with a single baby, and

> hypertension—more than three times as likely to occur in women who are pregnant with twins than with a single baby.

strategically consuming multiple small meals that can help with nausea and heart burn, the most accurate assessment of weight progress is to monitor weight gain while being aware of the weight-gain guidelines based on pre-pregnancy BMI.

While supporting a healthy rate of weight gain with proper energy intake is the cornerstone of nutrition recommendations, note that carbohydrate, protein, and fat demands are best met as part of a well-chosen diet built on food variety and nutrient density. Pregnant athletes who maintain their training should not only strive to meet DRI recommendations for the carbohydrate, protein, and fat but also consider periodizing their macronutrient choices based on the mode and volume of training to support the energy expenditure of exercise while also supporting healthy weight gain. For example, the RDA for carbohydrate in adult women increases from 130 grams per day to 175 grams per day during pregnancy. When exercise training or an active lifestyle is added to pregnancy, carbohydrate needs can be significantly higher to support increased energy expenditure. The most practical way to determine carbohydrate needs for exercise during pregnancy is to first understand that additional carbohydrate is often needed, particularly pre- and postexercise. By assessing fatigue during exercise, and monitoring the rate of weight gain, carbohydrate needs can be adjusted accordingly. Note that carbohydrate is the primary source of energy for both mother and fetus, so it should be the predominate macronutrient fuel source

(50–65% of total energy consumed). Carbohydrate foods are also a great vehicle for providing fiber in the diet to aid in preventing hemorrhoids and constipation. According to the Institute of Medicine, the RDA and adequate intake (AI) of fiber for a pregnancy between the ages of 18 and 50 is 28 grams per day (31).

For protein, general pregnancy guidelines recommend an additional 20 to 25 grams per day during the second half of pregnancy above what was consumed during the pre-pregnancy period. This recommendation is based on the needs of pregnant women who are primarily sedentary. So pregnant women who participate in regular exercise should use the 20- to 25-gram recommendation as a baseline and might require additional protein during times of increased training duration or intensity. As exercise frequency and intensity decline during the third trimester, energy, carbohydrate, and protein needs might be only slightly elevated beyond sedentary pregnancy needs.

Assuming that energy intake demands are met as part of a well-chosen diet, macronutrient intake is usually directly associated with caloric intake and allow for all macronutrient demands to be met (table 14.6). This principle may not be the case if an expectant mother excludes certain food groups from the diet, develops an aversion for a wide range of healthy foods, or begins to follow a fad diet. In these scenarios, protein intake becomes an area of concern. Inadequate protein intake can be harmful for the mother and the baby. Low protein intake can negatively affect a mother's ability to recover from exercise, as well

Table 14.6 Macronutrient Needs for the Nonpregnant, Pregnant, and Pregnant Athlete

Energy-yielding macronutrients	Nonpregnant adult athlete	Pregnancy	Pregnancy plus exercise
Protein	46 g/d	66–71 g/d	71 g/d minimum
Carbohydrates (fiber)	130 (25) g/d	175 (28) g/d	175 (28) g/d minimum; needs increase to support exercise
Fats	20–35 (% daily calories)	20–35 (% daily calories)	20–35 (% daily calories)

Data from Institute of Medicine 2005.

as her normal adaptation to pregnancy. If low protein intake is coupled with low energy intake, body proteins will preferentially be oxidized for fuel and can lead to reduced fitness, lowered immune response, altered fetal development, and increased fatigue.

The metabolic adaptations resulting from exercise combined with pregnancy increase the need for some micronutrients. Meeting energy demands with a sound diet can help an active female meet her micronutrient needs during pregnancy. Pregnant athletes who are not gaining weight, consume poorly chosen diets, or eliminate one or more food groups might be consuming suboptimal amounts of micronutrients.

B Vitamins

An important function of B vitamins is their role in supporting metabolic pathways for energy production. The need for several of the B vitamins—thiamin, riboflavin, niacin—increases during pregnancy. Most B vitamin needs can easily be met by consuming enough energy to gain weight during pregnancy and choosing a wide range of nutrient-dense and fortified foods. The B vitamin of greatest interest during pregnancy is folate (and the synthetic form of folate known as folic acid). Folate deficiency can lead to serious effects on both the mother

DO YOU KNOW ?

Folate is important for proper DNA synthesis, red blood cell production, and nervous system development. All females of child-bearing age should ensure they are not deficient in folate if they have even a slight chance of becoming pregnant.

and her developing fetus. For the mother, megaloblastic anemia can result, causing fatigue and weakness that can contribute to an underlying etiology of depression, irritability, and poor sleep.

For the fetus, folate plays an important role in cell division and the development of the fetal nervous system. The most important stages of neural tube formation occur within the first month of conception, usually before a woman knows she is pregnant. In many cases, weeks of cell division have already taken place when a woman learns she is pregnant, and any defects that have occurred might be too late to address effectively, even if a healthy diet is adopted immediately. Note that folic acid supplementation is recommended for all women of child-bearing age to help prevent the risk of folate deficiency and to counter the folate depletion effect of alcohol consumption.

Other Vitamins of Concern

The combined physiological stress of pregnancy and exercise increases the need for both vitamin C and vitamin A. Fortunately, there is an overlap of foods that are good sources of most vitamins during pregnancy. Vitamin C is a water-soluble vitamin with requirements that increase from 75 mg to 80 to 85 mg during pregnancy to support collagen formation, hormone synthesis, proper immune function, and iron absorption and to increase antioxidant activity (22), all functions important for the pregnant athlete. Note that the increased need for vitamin C to serve as an antioxidant can easily be met through the diet—antioxidant supplementation has not been shown to enhance athletic performance and may

PUTTING IT INTO PERSPECTIVE

WHERE DOES ALL THE WEIGHT GO?

What accounts for the weight gained during pregnancy (48)?

> Baby: 7 to 8 pounds
> Larger breasts: 2 pounds
> Larger uterus: 2 pounds
> Placenta: 1.5 pounds

> Amniotic fluid: 2 pounds
> Increased blood volume: 3 to 4 pounds
> Fat stores: 6 to 8 pounds

be harmful (59). Pregnant athletes wanting to increase their antioxidant intake should focus on healthy dietary choices instead of relying on antioxidant supplementation.

Vitamin A assists in cell differentiation and proper immune function. Requirements increase from 700 to 770 micrograms (µg) during pregnancy (23). Despite this increase, mothers should seek to increase their vitamin A primarily from plant sources and avoid dietary supplements that contain retinol, unless otherwise directed by a physician. Supplemental forms of retinol can become toxic and unhealthy for the developing fetus (6).

The RDA for vitamin D for pregnant females is 15 micrograms per day of calciferol. Vitamin D deficiency during pregnancy is associated with medical complications such as gestational diabetes. Additionally, vitamin D deficiency can have negative fetal consequences, including low birth weight, neonatal rickets, asthma, or type 1 diabetes (8). Folate and vitamins A, C, and D deserve focus during pregnancy. Increased consumption of these nutrients should begin prior to pregnancy and continue until delivery.

Iron

Iron status can become compromised at the onset of pregnancy due to anatomical and physiological changes that result in expansion of blood volume and increased oxidative tissue demand. In active females, iron status can also be compromised because of increased iron losses with exercise. This is of significant concern, as iron is involved in fetal development and growth and red blood cell production. Iron needs during pregnancy are 27 mg per day (30), a level difficult to obtain without careful diet planning or supplementation. A focus on iron-rich foods should be the first strategy employed to meet iron needs.

VEGETARIAN POPULATIONS

The popularity of vegetarian diets has increased from 2.3 percent in 1998 (67). Vegetarian diets vary in the exact foods that are allowed and disallowed (table 14.7). It has been estimated that approximately 3.3 percent of the American population chooses not to consume meat, fish, or poultry (49, 76). About half of this percentage also do not eat any forms of animal food, including eggs and dairy products. Note that the definitions in table 14.7 are not all-inclusive, as new descriptors and definitions of vegetarian eating styles are described elsewhere (24). People choose vegetarian diets for many reasons—from ethnic, religious, moral, or philosophical beliefs to health promotion, food aversions, or financial constraints (76). Vegetarian diets can be nutritionally adequate when well chosen (i.e., includes an abundance of fruits, vegetables, whole grains, nuts, soy products, fiber, phytochemicals, and antioxidants) (49). This appears to hold true for vegetarian athletes as well, again as long as the diet is well chosen. Note, however, that some athletes adopt a vegetarian diet to disguise disordered eating (15, 26). The more limited the vegetarian diet, the greater challenge it is to consume an optimal intake of several nutrients. Vegetarians can benefit from

Table 14.7 Types and Characteristics of Vegetarian Diets

Types of vegetarian diets	Diet characteristics
Vegan	Avoids all animal products and animal-derived foods.
Ovo-vegetarian	Allows eggs but no other animal products.
Lacto-vegetarian	Allows milk and milk products.
Lacto-ovo vegetarian	Allows milk, dairy products, and eggs but no other animal proteins.
Semi-vegetarian	Allows some animal-derived foods. Red meat is often the primary animal food not allowed.
Pesco-vegetarian	Allows seafood but no other animal products.
Ovo-pesco vegetarian	Allows seafood and eggs but no other animal products.
Lacto-ovo-pesco vegetarian	Allows dairy products, seafood, and eggs but no other animal products.

comprehensive dietary evaluation and intervention from a sports dietitian to ensure their diets are nutritionally sound to support training, competition demands, and performance.

The amount of food required to meet the nutrient demands of vegetarians depends on the foods consumed and the energy needs of the athlete. Generally, for all vegetarians, foods rich in iron, calcium, zinc, and protein should be included daily; fortified foods and dietary supplements can be helpful in some scenarios. Vegetarians who consume milk, eggs, cheese, and yogurt can meet their nutrient needs more easily.

Effects on Exercise and Athletic Performance

Research is limited on the long-term effect of vegetarianism on athletic performance (47). At this time, vegetarian meal patterns are thought to be neither beneficial nor detrimental to athletic performance (83) but can be appropriate for athletes if well chosen (49, 76). Studies are needed to examine elite athletes who habitually consume vegetarian diets. The effect of vegetarian diets on promoting or maintaining changes in athlete body composition also needs to be explored because the achievement of the body composition associated with optimal performance is now recognized as a challenging but important goal (76). Some athletes following a vegetarian diet have been found to have a higher

percentage of body fat than their nonvegetarian peers (27).

Effects on Health

While data does not support a performance benefit as a result of following vegetarian diet patterns, several reported health-related outcomes are associated with these diet plans. Vegetarian diets have been shown to be lower in saturated fat, while providing higher levels of carbohydrates, fiber, magnesium, potassium, carotenoids, and flavonoids (49, 76). Vegetarians have also been reported to have lower death rates from heart disease and associated risk factors such as hypertension and high cholesterol. Vegetarian diets are also endorsed by the American Cancer Association (40) and are associated with a lower risk of prostate and colon cancer (49).

Health benefits associated with a vegetarian diet are multifactorial and likely a result of both what an individual is and is not eating. Increased consumption of phytonutrients, antioxidants, and dietary nitrate are likely key in promoting overall health and might help athletes avoid some of the oxidative stress and immunosuppression effects seen with heavy training (24).

Nutrition Needs

Nutrient concerns for vegetarian athletes can include inadequate intake of energy, protein,

Recommended daily servings

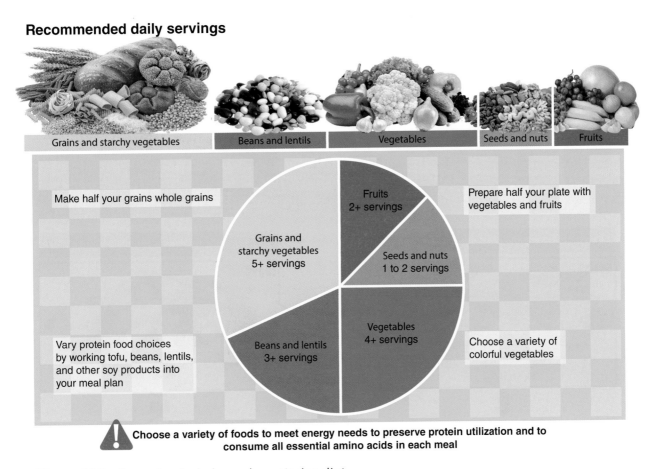

Grains and starchy vegetables | Beans and lentils | Vegetables | Seeds and nuts | Fruits

Make half your grains whole grains

Grains and starchy vegetables
5+ servings

Fruits
2+ servings

Seeds and nuts
1 to 2 servings

Prepare half your plate with vegetables and fruits

Vegetables
4+ servings

Beans and lentils
3+ servings

Vary protein food choices by working tofu, beans, lentils, and other soy products into your meal plan

Choose a variety of colorful vegetables

Choose a variety of foods to meet energy needs to preserve protein utilization and to consume all essential amino acids in each meal

Figure 14.6 Example of a balanced vegetarian diet.

fat, and omega-3 fatty acids (figure 14.6) (49). For active individuals, a vegetarian diet might provide insufficient energy to maintain weight and fuel performance. Often the solution to this problem is to consume higher-energy foods such as nuts, beans, corn, starchy vegetables like peas and potatoes, avocados, dried fruits, and 100 percent fruit juices.

While vegetarian athletes who include some animal products should be able to easily meet protein needs, vegans should be very aware of protein content of plant foods and consider this in their meal planning. One of the key tenants of vegan diet planning is to choose a variety of foods to meet energy needs to preserve protein utilization and to consume all essential amino acids in each meal. Fortunately, combining complementary protein foods at every meal is no longer thought to be necessary (88). However, complementary foods should be a foundation of the diet plan, along with plant sources that contain all nine

essential amino acids. These excellent sources of protein include soybeans, quinoa, and tofu. See figure 14.7 for examples of complementary protein foods.

While usually not deficient in dietary protein, vegetarian athletes often consume less protein than their nonvegetarian counterparts. Because plant proteins have a lower bioavailability, it has been suggested that vegetarians increase their protein intake by 10 percent (15). However, the target total daily protein range of 1.2 to 2.0 grams per kilogram body weight is the same as the range for nonvegetarians (76). Meeting daily protein needs to support athletic performance is important, as is supporting muscle protein synthesis by providing an even spread of protein intake across the day and consuming enough energy to support growth and maintenance of lean tissue. Vegetarian athletes should also be reminded that muscle protein synthesis occurs via stimulation of the protein synthetic machinery in response to

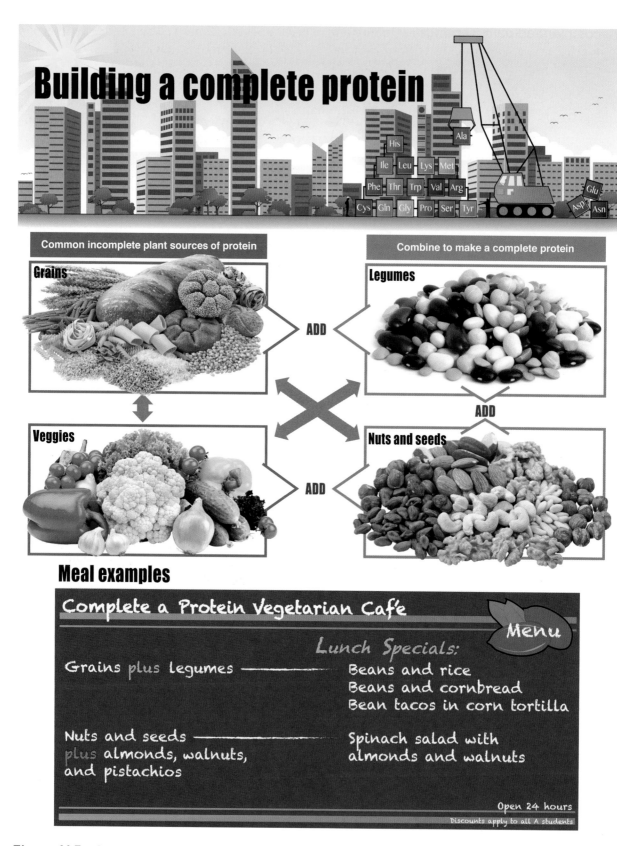

Figure 14.7 Complete protein meals.

a rise in leucine concentrations in combination with other essential amino acids from food for incorporation into new proteins (12). In addition to consuming a variety of high-quality plant protein sources, physically active vegetarians should also consume plant foods rich in leucine, such as soybeans, nuts, seeds, and legumes. Studies are still needed to determine the effectiveness of concentrated vegetable protein supplements in stimulating the muscle protein synthesis machinery following various modes of exercise.

Micronutrients

Depending on the extent of dietary limitations, micronutrient concerns for vegetarianism may include iron, zinc, calcium, iodine, vitamin D, and vitamin B_{12} (49, 76). Being a physically active vegetarian is a risk factor for low iron status, mainly because of the low bioavailability of non-heme plant sources. Physically active vegetarians should thus be regularly screened and aim for an iron intake greater that the RDA (i.e., >18 mg for women and >8mg for men) (14, 20). Females might be at greater risk because iron requirements for female athletes can increase up to 70 percent the EAR (17). Because of the decreased bioavailability of non-heme sources, iron intakes for vegetarians have been recommended as 1.8 higher than for nonvegetarians.

Iron deficiency in all athletes can occur with or without anemia and impair athletic performance by decreasing muscle function and limiting work capacity (20, 43). Even in the absence of anemia, a compromised iron status has been shown to negatively affect endurance competition times (17).

Athletes with clinically diagnosed iron deficiency should follow medical advice that usually includes oral iron supplementation (58), dietary interventions, and follow-up appointments with their care provider. Reversing iron-deficiency anemia can take 3 to 6 months; this delayed response continues to allow for side effects that affect health and performance during the treatment timeframe. This highlights the importance of monitoring iron intake from the diet and adopting eating strategies that promote an increased intake of food sources of well-absorbed iron (76). Athletes concerned about iron status or who have iron deficiency without anemia (e.g., low ferritin without IDA) should adopt eating strategies that promote an increased intake of food sources rich in iron by choosing food sources containing well-absorbed iron (e.g., heme iron and non-heme iron combined with vitamin C foods) as the first line of defense in their plan to promote optimal iron status.

Vegans are also at risk of developing a vitamin B_{12} deficiency because this nutrient is not found in plant foods. Since B_{12} is found in virtually all animal products, vegetarians following less limited plans that allow for animal products such as dairy should have no trouble getting enough B_{12}. Vegans must rely on an additional source of B_{12}, including fortified milk alternatives such as soy milk, fortified breakfast cereal, and fortified yeast products. If these food products cannot be consumed regularly, a supplemental form of B_{12} is recommended.

It has been estimated that 50 percent of female distance runners consume less than the RDA for zinc, which makes zinc a mineral of concern for

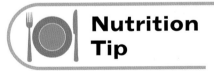

Nutrition Tip You can maximize iron bioavailability in a vegetarian diet in several ways. Good sources of non-heme iron such as spinach can provide more absorbable iron by combining spinach with fresh citrus vinaigrette or a fresh squeeze of lemon. Iron bioavailability in green leafy vegetables can also be improved by blanching them in boiling water for 5 to 10 seconds. Cooking vegetarian dishes in cast-iron skillets increases the iron content of food, especially if the food is acidic, such as tomato sauce.

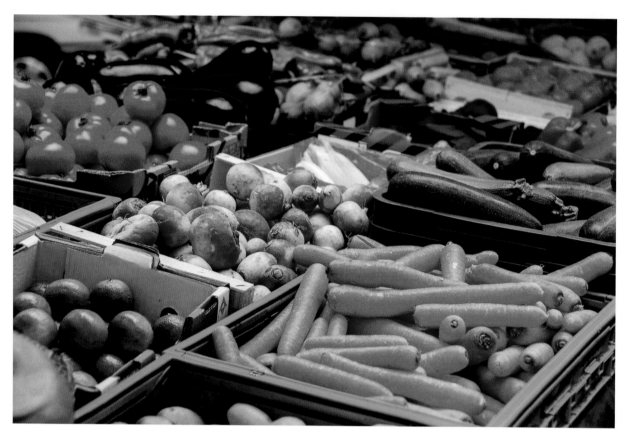

A balanced vegetarian or vegan meal is about more than vegetables. Use the guidelines from this chapter to ensure you're consuming a balanced diet that suits your needs.

vegetarian athletes, particularly if a diet is poorly chosen with low energy intake. Studies have shown that zinc intake and zinc status is highly variable in vegetarian athletes, which is partly explained by GI absorption inhibitors such as phytate and fiber that are abundant in vegetarian diets (29). As with other minerals in the vegetarian diet, zinc-rich foods should be included when planning meals.

Vegetarians who consume dairy take advantage of the most bioavailable source of calcium in the U.S. diet. Vegans, on the other hand, tend to have lower calcium intakes than nonvegetarians and lacto-ovo vegetarians and often fall below the RDA (49). Vegetarian athletes might have an increased risk of lower bone mineral density and stress fractures (85). Foods rich in calcium should be a focus in vegetarian meal planning. In some cases calcium supplementation is required to meet needs, especially if a vegetarian athlete is restricting energy intake. Calcium needs increase

to 1,500 mg per day to optimize bone health in athletes with low energy availability or menstrual dysfunction (51).

Other Concerns

Vegetarian diets might also be low in creatine and carnosine, which can be problematic for athletes who rely on strength, power, and anaerobic performance (9). Dietary creatine is found in animal flesh, and vegetarians have been shown to have a lower body creatine pool than nonvegetarians (9, 44). In both vegetarians and nonvegetarians about 1 gram of creatine is synthesized per day from endogenous body amino acids. Those who consume meat obtain approximately 1 gram per day of additional creatine. Vegetarians who supplement with creatine tend to have a greater increase in strength and lean body mass accretion and muscle creatine concentrations, as well as improved work performance (9). Another interesting finding is that a lacto-ovo vegetarian diet does not preserve muscle creatine levels, indicating that dairy products and eggs are not a replacement for meat when attempting to maintain body stores of creatine (45). It appears clear that vegetarian athletes who rely heavily on strength and power performance can benefit from short-term creatine supplementation. While anecdotal reports of side effects of creatine supplementation exist, there are no confirmed concerns regarding short-term use. The long-term effects of creatine supplementation are not well described in the scientific literature.

INDIVIDUALS WITH DISORDERED EATING AND EATING DISORDERS

Reports of eating behavior problems have become increasingly prevalent in the past decade, both for the athletes and the general population. Athletes face unique challenges; they must deal with the common sociocultural influences and also the pressure of fitting in and competing at a high level alongside peers and competitors. Many athletes are susceptible to a strong sense of pressure to look and perform a certain way, which might be compounded by coaches, trainers, and family members who have a strong opinion about the shape and size of body required to excel. For some, rigorous training and competition can spark threats to health and well-being that might produce negative health outcomes. An obsession with obtaining a particular body composition can trigger short- and long-term health problems for both male and female athletes that stem from low energy availability, disordered eating behaviors, and clinically defined eating disorders.

Disordered Eating Spectrum

Disordered eating behaviors develop in athletes when they continue to strive for an "ideal" at the expense of health and performance goals, leading to eating disturbances that can cause diagnosable eating disorders. Those who participate in weight-sensitive sports have the highest risk of developing disordered eating patterns. According to a position statement from the International Olympic Committee Medical Commission, these sports can be classified into three main groups (71):

1. Gravitational sports where moving the body against gravity is key to performance (e.g., long-distance running, mountain bike cycling, jumping sports)
2. Weight-class sports such as boxing, martial arts, wrestling, lightweight rowing, and weightlifting
3. Aesthetically judged sports such as figure skating, diving, and gymnastics.

Disordered eating occurs across a spectrum, starting with eating and exercise behaviors that are appropriate in the short term, such as energy restriction at certain training periods to "lean-up" or "make weight." Disordered eating practices often involve a preoccupation with body weight and shape, food restriction, dieting, binge eating, vomiting, or abuse of diuretics, laxatives, and diet pills (73). In contrast, eating disorders are spectral disorders: they exist on a continuum of severity, have a specific clinical diagnosis, and often become more severe the longer they are present.

Normal eating patterns for athletes might include the occasional use of weight-loss methods that are typically very short in duration, but for some, this can be coupled with strong body dissatisfaction. For some susceptible athletes, these behaviors—often a traditional part of their sport culture—can progress to chronic dieting and frequent weight fluctuation; fasting; passive (e.g., sauna or hot baths) or active dehydration (e.g., exercise with sweat suits) or both; and purging, such as use of laxatives, diuretics, vomiting, and diet pills. These behaviors might occur with or without excessive training (74). These athletes often feel fat on a daily basis, and their disordered eating behaviors can advance to become a clinically defined eating disorder, in which athletes succumb to extreme dieting, body image distortion, abnormal eating behaviors, and decreases in health and athletic performance (73). Failure to meet all criteria for anorexia nervosa or bulimia nervosa should not deter early and comprehensive intervention, as early recognition and intervention can prevent further development of a clinically defined eating disorder (55). Even in the absence of a clinically defined eating disorder, restrictive and purging behaviors are of concern because of their effect on energy availability.

Prevalence, Etiology, and Types

The prevalence of disordered eating in athletes is almost impossible to estimate. Prevalence of clinically defined eating disorders remains difficult to determine because many athletes do not seek diagnosis and treatment. Research on the topic of eating disorder prevalence is limited, with few studies in females, limited research in males, and poor study designs. A large study in Norway compared groups of Olympic athletes to a control group and found that athletes had approximately a three times higher incidence rate of eating disorders (13.5%) compared to nonathlete controls (70). The presence of eating disorders is not restricted to female athletes, as male athletes are susceptible as well. Eating disorders exist in recreational, high school, and collegiate sports and among personal trainers. It is not uncommon for these diseases to coexist with other psychological comorbidities such as anxiety, depression, substance use, and obsessive compulsive tendencies.

Eating disorders go beyond weight dissatisfaction and involve more than abnormal eating patterns and pathogenic weight control behaviors. An eating disorder is not about food per se but is a mental illness. The best way to understand the significance of an eating disorder diagnosis is to recognize that eating disorders are underpinned by a psychological pathology with serious nutrition and medical concerns.

Eating disorders were once viewed as disorders of choice, meaning the person afflicted could easily reverse their condition if they would just eat. This viewpoint did not foster providing guidance to families, and the concept of a genetic etiology was viewed as absurd. Over time etiological theory advanced from "choice" to family dysfunction, to complex interactions among genetics, neurobiology, personality characteristics, and environmental factors. It is now thought that over half of the variance associated with developing

an eating disorder can be attributed to genetics and that stressful environments can exacerbate eating disorders, but that families are not causative in eating disorder etiology. While genetic factors seem to be emerging as the cornerstone for eating disorder etiology, the overall cause is considered multifactorial, with interacting psychological, neurobiological, genetic, cultural, and social factors. A current prevailing theory is that neurophysiologic and genetic components might set the stage for eating disorder development that could be triggered by weight loss and might be the reason many psychological symptoms resolve with physical restoration. So when athletes face a sport culture that provides pressure to reduce weight and body fat, support for disordered eating is generated and often maintained. Psychosocial factors identified as contributing factors, which may occur alongside a backdrop of genetic predisposition, include a history of being teased, abuse, low self-esteem, and predisposing psychiatric diagnoses. Personality characteristics that help to cultivate eating disorders, once developed, include anxiety, perfectionism, low self-directedness, rigidity, emotional avoidance and isolation, and an obsessive evaluation of shape and weight control.

Eating disorders are defined by very specific physical and mental criteria, as outlined by the American Psychiatric Association's *Diagnostic and Statistical Manual of Mental Disorders*, 5th edition (*DSM-5*) (4). The *DSM-5* has recently designated four categories of eating disorders:

> Anorexia nervosa
> Bulimia nervosa
> Binge eating disorder
> Other specified feeding or eating disorders

Anorexia Nervosa

An anorexia nervosa diagnosis requires three criteria, including the restriction of energy intake below what is required to maintain weight that leads to a significantly low body weight in the context of age, sex, developmental trajectory, and physical health.

A "significantly low body weight" in adults is defined as a weight that is less than minimally normal. A second requirement for diagnosis is an intense fear of gaining weight or becoming fat, or persistent behavior that interferes with weight gain, even when at a significantly low weight. The final requirement is a disturbance in the way in which one's body weight or shape is experienced, undue influence of body weight or shape on self-evaluation, or persistent lack of recognition of the seriousness of one's current low body weight.

The physical effects of anorexia nervosa are shown in figure 14.8. Athletes who meet all the requirements for anorexia nervosa are further classified into one of two subtypes:

> Restricting type: During the last 3 months, the athlete has not engaged in recurrent episodes of binge eating or **purging behavior**.

> Binge-eating or purging type: During the last 3 months, the athlete has engaged in episodes of binge eating or purging behavior.

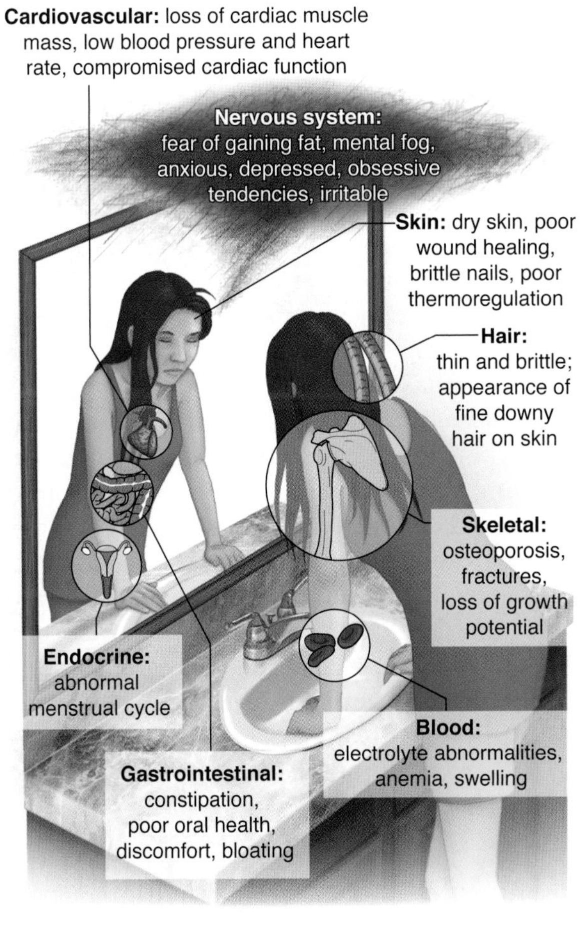

Figure 14.8 Physical effects of anorexia nervosa.

Bulimia Nervosa

A bulimia nervosa diagnosis has four specific criteria, characterized by

> recurrent episodes of binge eating once a week over 3 or more months, and

> recurrent inappropriate compensatory behavior to prevent weight gain, such as self-induced vomiting; misuse of laxatives, diuretics, or other medications; fasting; or excessive exercise.

These first 2 criteria must occur, on average, at least once a week for 3 months. Athletes must also present with

> a self-evaluation that is unduly influenced by body shape and weight, and

> symptoms that indicate the disturbance does not occur exclusively during episodes of anorexia nervosa.

Binge Eating Disorder

The distinct diagnosis of binge eating disorder is newer to the *DSM-5* and is intended to increase awareness of the substantial differences with the all-too-common phenomenon of overeating. binge eating disorder is "not just the occasional second helping of food"; rather, the disorder includes feeling out of control during the eating episode and feeling distressed about the eating pattern. Binge eating is defined by consuming an amount of food that is definitely larger than most people would eat in a similar period of time under similar circumstances marked by feelings of lack of control during the eating episode. For an athlete to receive a binge eating disorder diagnosis, key criteria must be met, including recurrent episodes of binge eating that are associated with three or more of the following:

> Eating much more rapidly than normal
> Eating until feeling uncomfortably full
> Eating large amounts of food when not feeling physically hungry
> Eating alone because of embarrassment by how much one is eating
> Feeling disgusted with oneself, depressed, or guilty after eating

Three additional criteria must also be met:

> Binge eating is accompanied by a marked level of distress.

> The binge eating occurs, on average, at least once a week for 3 months.

> The binge eating is not associated with the recurrent use of inappropriate compensatory behavior and does not occur exclusively during the course of bulimia nervosa or anorexia nervosa.

While disproportionately more females than males develop anorexia and bulimia, with binge eating disorder the ratio is less disparate, with an approximate of a 3-to-2 female-to-male ratio. While overeating is a challenge for many Americans, a recurrent binge-eating pathology is much less common, far more severe, and associated with significant physical and psychological problems.

Other Specified Feeding or Eating Disorders

At one time, the most frequent eating disorder diagnosis among athletes was eating disorder not otherwise specified (EDNOS). This was because relatively few patients met the strict criteria for the diagnosis of bulimia nervosa or anorexia nervosa. Those who develop disordered eating behaviors who advance to an eating disorder clinical diagnosis most often meet the criteria for a newly defined diagnosis called "other specified feeding or eating disorders (OSFED) (46, 72). Generally, OSFED is defined as a feeding or eating disorder that causes significant distress or impairment but does not meet the criteria for another feeding or eating disorder. OSFED is a new addition to eating disorder diagnoses found in the recently published *DSM-5*. The diagnosis of OSFED is still very serious, with patients having significant concerns about eating and body image and health risks similar to those of the other eating disorders. For example, an athlete who shows almost all of the symptoms of anorexia nervosa but who has retained a normal body mass index can be diagnosed with OSFED.

According to the *DSM-5*, OSFED has five subtypes that are atypical of other eating disorder diagnoses:

1. Atypical anorexia nervosa—restrictive behaviors without meeting low weight criteria

2. Bulimia nervosa—lower frequency or limited duration of binging and purging

3. Binge eating disorder at a lower frequency or limited duration

4. Purging disorder—recurrent purging of calories through self-induced vomiting, misuse of laxatives and diuretics, or excessive exercising without binge-eating behaviors

5. Night eating syndrome—recurrent episodes of night eating, as manifested by eating after awakening from sleep or by excessive food consumption after the evening meal

In the OSFED eating disorder category is also the diagnosis of unspecified feeding or eating disorder. This category serves as a preliminary diagnosis when insufficient information is available to make a specific diagnosis. Symptoms may include any of the disordered eating patterns that cause significant distress or impairment.

Impact of Disordered Eating on Health and Performance

Several sports have been identified as having an increased likelihood of harboring athletes who have an unhealthy body image and eating disorders. These sports tend to be those that place emphasis on an ideal body type, push for low body weights, or emphasize lean body shape. Further, sports that require revealing clothing, such as diving, can support body image issues and disordered eating patterns. Note that although some sports are more associated with eating disorders than others, individuals in any sport can develop an eating disorder. Also, athletes might show signs of short-term disordered eating patterns without developing a clinically defined eating disorder.

Health Concerns

Before we look at health concerns associated with disordered eating and eating disorder, note that these eating patterns occur along a continuum and may affect different athletes in different ways. This includes an athlete with an eating disorder who may appear normal and physically healthy while maintaining their training load and volume. On the other hand, an athlete with disordered patterns or OSFED may have health problems as significant as some cases of anorexia or bulimia nervosa. Initial weight changes might not affect health in ways that can be observed by peers. Behavioral changes such as social withdrawal, teammate conflict, reduced self-esteem or self-confidence, a loss of competitiveness, or an onset of depression and anxiety are not unusual.

Historically, the concept of low energy availability and its effect on health emerged (76) from the study of the female athlete triad (often shortened to triad) (figure 14.9). The triad is formed by the interconversion of three clinical conditions typically observed in young female athletes: disordered eating, menstrual irregularities, and low bone mineral content or density. Each of these three components occurs along a continuum, and at any one time each component could independently present as being mild, moderate, or severe. For instance, a female athlete with a disordered eating pattern might not meet the criteria for an eating disorder but might restrict energy intake enough to produce low energy availability during heavy training. The occurrence of **oligomenorrhea** or **amenorrhea** is believed to be induced by some degree of low energy availability and is detrimental to bone mineral density when female athletes present with low energy availability and dysmenorrheic tendencies. Female athletes with dysmenorrhea have been found to have low bone mineral density in the lumbar spine, hip, and whole body (5). Obtaining a history of disordered eating behaviors is valuable because the effects of low energy availability on bone are cumulative (7).

Our understanding of the triad has evolved into a broader understanding of the concerns associated with any movement along the spectra away from optimal energy availability, menstrual status, and bone health (38). It is now known that other physiological consequences can result from one of the components of the triad in active females, such as endocrine, gastrointestinal, renal, neuropsychiatric, musculoskeletal, or cardiovascular dysfunction (76). Further, this long list of physiological concerns also affects the

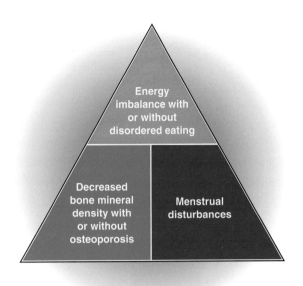

Figure 14.9 Female athlete triad.

health of male athletes, leading to an extension of the triad termed the relative energy deficiency in sport (RED-S). RED-S encompasses several physiological complications observed in males and females involved in sport who consume energy intakes that are insufficient to meet the needs for optimal body function once the energy cost of exercise has been removed (51). Health and performance consequences of RED-S are shown in figures 14.10 and 14.11.

Performance Problems

Exercise performance might not always be altered by disordered eating or in the early stages of an eating disorder; however, as an eating disorder advances in severity, the downfall of performance is inevitable. In some cases this will present as a physical injury that sidelines the athlete from training and competition. In other cases, the onset of performance decline is more gradual and might be a direct result of nutrition deficiencies, low energy intake, or the direct physical stress of purging behaviors.

A significant and chronic reduction in energy intake directly leads to reduced carbohydrate intake, which creates a greater reliance on body proteins to meet energy demands of the sport. This will ultimately reduce muscle mass, decrease

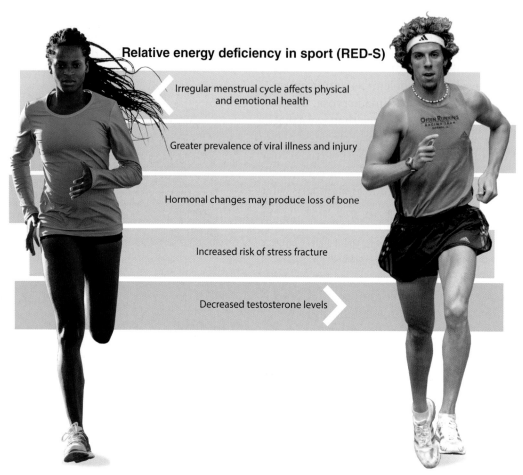

Relative energy deficiency in sport (RED-S)

Irregular menstrual cycle affects physical and emotional health

Greater prevalence of viral illness and injury

Hormonal changes may produce loss of bone

Increased risk of stress fracture

Decreased testosterone levels

Figure 14.10 Body systems affected by RED-S.

performance, and increase risk of injury. Energy intake is also strongly linked to micronutrient intake, so active individuals with an eating disorder will be at greater risk of inadequate consumption of calcium, iron, and other important nutrients. To simplify, the direct effect of inadequate nutrition on performance with eating disorders is most associated with low energy availability.

Low energy availability can occur from calorie restriction, excessive energy expenditure from exercise, or a combination of the two. Individuals with an eating disorder and low energy availability will lack the energy necessary to sustain high levels of exercise intensity and might also experience significant bone loss and iron depletion that impairs performance. Low energy

PUTTING IT INTO PERSPECTIVE

HELP FOR EATING DISORDERS

Athletes are at increased pressure to perform and have their body shaped in a specific way. Their appearance is analyzed as well as their athletic performance. These pressures could trigger an eating disorder or disordered eating in the athlete. If you know someone with an eating disorder or disordered eating, contact the Helpline at 800-931-2237 or seek online resources at www.nationaleatingdisorders.org.

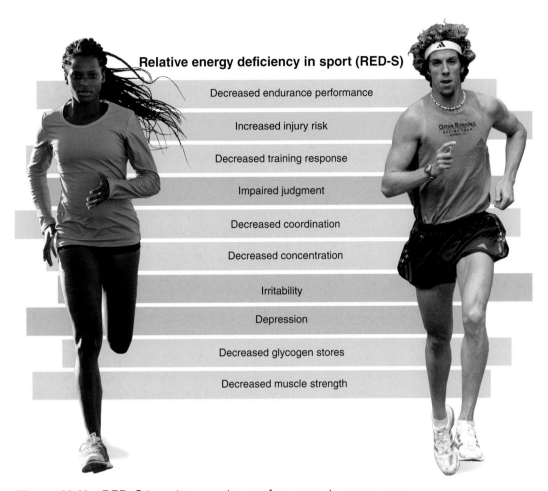

Relative energy deficiency in sport (RED-S)

Decreased endurance performance

Increased injury risk

Decreased training response

Impaired judgment

Decreased coordination

Decreased concentration

Irritability

Depression

Decreased glycogen stores

Decreased muscle strength

Figure 14.11 RED-S impairs exercise performance in many ways.

availability also disrupts normal hormonal responses, which can negatively influence adaptation to training and, for females, promote menstrual dysfunction. Other direct effects of low energy availability in eating disorder that negatively impact performance include decreased endurance, impaired judgment, decreased coordination, decreased concentration, irritability, depression, decreased glycogen stores, and decreased muscle strength (51). Similar to other aspects of disordered eating and eating disorder medical complications, impairments of health and performance occur across a continuum of reductions in energy availability and do not occur at one specific energy availability, value or threshold. Note that low energy availability is not synonymous with negative energy balance or weight loss, as chronic low energy availability might reset and lower the athlete's metabolic rate in such a way that low energy intake does not result in weight loss. It is clear that low energy availability in male and female athletes can compromise athletic performance in both the short and long term (76).

Prevention and Management

As with most medical conditions, the best defense against eating disorders is prevention. Education is the driving force behind prevention and can be used to prevent an unhealthy relationship with food, medical problems, and poor performance. To be able to identify athletes at risk sooner rather than later requires basic knowledge of the signs and symptoms of disordered eating. Physical, medical, psychological, and behavioral characteristics of the eating disorder spectrum are provided in table 14.8. Prevention of eating disorders occurs on

Table 14.8 The Three Prevention Levels of Eating Disorders

Prevention category	Goals	Targeted intervention
Primary	Protect individuals from pre-disposing risk factors	Education and instruction • Begins as early as puberty • Focus is on healthy eating and lifestyle patterns and positive self-image
Secondary	Early identification of those at risk, low energy availability, and the provision of early treatment	Screening and measurement • Eating disorders inventory (EDI) • Eating attitudes test (EAT) • *DSM-5*
Tertiary	Treatment of clinically defined eating disorders	Multidisciplinary interventions • Medical, psychological, nutritional care

Based on Maughan 2013.

three levels: primary, secondary, and tertiary. Each level is distinctly designed to prevent development and progression to the next level in order to keep the clinical condition from becoming chronic and debilitating.

SUMMARY

This chapter has addressed many of the nutrition concerns in excercise, physical activity, and sport that are seen at different life stages (child, adolescent, masters, pregnant), in the vegetarian lifestyle, and in pathological conditions including diabetes mellitus, metabolic syndrome, disordered eating, and eating disorders. For the child and adolescent, the importance of understanding their key physiological differences as compared to adults was emphasized. Nutrition recommendations were presented for this life-stage group. Energy expenditure, substrate utilization, and thermoregulation during exercise are all physiologically different in children. Adolescents have increased requirements for energy and many nutrients as a result of rapid anatomical, physiological, and metabolic changes. It is clear that in terms of their nutrition needs, children and adolescents should not be considered as small adults. At the other end of the lifespan, masters athletes have their own unique nutrition challenges. In aging, a stronger focus is placed on the physiological benefits of exercise and how nutrition can augment these effects. Unfortunately, data are insufficient on the specific nutrition needs of masters athletes, but we have good evidence of the importance of hydration, protein intake, and several key micronutrients.

Disease processes and lifestyle choices can also create unique nutrition concerns. Diabetes mellitus provides unique challenges for athletes and the peers and staff who work with them. A good understanding of the physiological processes involved in blood glucose response to exercise, diet, and medication is necessary to promote exercise performance and long-term health and safety. Knowledgeable and careful planning of dietary strategies that work in parallel with medication regimens to promote euglycemia before, during, and postexercise can support successful exercise and competition.

The vegetarian lifestyle can effectively support exercise and athletic performance. However, vegetarian and vegan female athletes are at increased risk for nonanemic iron deficiency, which may limit endurance performance. Vegans should follow a carefully chosen diet to obtain adequate intakes of iron, calcium, zinc, and vitamin B_{12}. If selected properly, vegetarian and nonvegetarian diets are fully capable of providing all the nutrients necessary for the physically active individual.

The diagnosis of an eating disorder is not easy. Athletes and nonathletes alike can exhibit disordered eating patterns, even if they don't meet the threshold for an eating disorder diagnosis. Conversely, it is important to recognize that not every athlete with a low body weight who occasionally exhibits disordered eating behavior has an eating disorder. An eating disorder diagnosis must encompass an identified psychological pathology associated with intense fear of gaining weight or of becoming fat, along with persistent behaviors that interfere with normal weight gain. Participation in exercise, sport, and pursuing a well-chosen diet are generally healthy behaviors for all athletes but menstrual status, nutrition behaviors, energy availability, and exercise volume should also be assessed. Education on the prevalence, etiology, and clinical manifestations associated with eating disorders should be widespread in environments that are likely to cultivate such disorders, including many sports settings and situations.

◼◼ FOR REVIEW ⟫

1. Describe how a child's anaerobic energy system is different from an adult's.

2. What is much more important than chronological age when evaluating a young athlete's nutrition needs and potential for athletic improvement?

3. What is the best strategy to prevent osteoporosis?

4. Which four micronutrients are needed at increased levels beyond the age of 50?

5. Explain the key differences between type 1 and type 2 diabetes mellitus.

6. For athletes with type 1 diabetes mellitus, what is the carbohydrate consumption goal during prolonged competition lasting 2 hours?

7. Why are vegans at an increased risk for anemia?

8. List some of the benefits of a vegetarian diet. What nutrients are of most concern for the vegetarian athlete?

9. Explain the difference between disordered eating and eating disorders.

10. What is meant by "energy availability"? How is this related to "RED-S"?

acetyl-CoA—An important molecule in the metabolism of carbohydrates, fats, and protein. Acetyl-CoA provides carbon atoms to the TCA cycle for energy production.

active transport—Movement of molecules across a cell membrane from a region typically of lower concentration to a region of higher concentration.

adenosine diphosphate (ADP)—Composed of adenosine and two phosphate groups; during glycolysis, ADP loses a phosphate group and energy is released.

adenosine monophosphate (AMP)—Composed of adenosine and one phosphate group; involved in energy metabolism.

adenosine triphosphate (ATP)—A molecule that stores the potential energy used to power many cellular activities. Composed of adenosine and three phosphate groups, ATP is created in cells from the breakdown of foods and is used when the cell needs energy to do something active, such as when a muscle cell contracts.

adipocytes—Fat cells.

adipose tissue—The cells that synthesize and store fat, predominantly found in subcutaneous locations but also surrounding vital organs, serving to protect them from physical damage.

aerobic capacity—A measure of fitness demonstrating the maximal amount of oxygen that can be used by active muscles during physical activity.

aerobic physical activity—Exercise involving large muscle groups moved in a rhythmic manner for an extended amount of time. Swimming, biking, and running are examples. Also termed endurance activity or aerobic exercise.

aerobic system—One of the body's energy systems; it has a large capacity to generate ATP but requires oxygen to function efficiently.

air displacement plethysmography (ADP)—A method to estimate body volume and thus body density. Instead of water displacement, air displacement is used. BOD POD is an example.

albumin—A simple form of protein that is soluble in water, such as that found in egg white, milk, and (in particular) blood serum, in which this protein serves as a transporter (carrying hormones, fatty acids, and more).

all-cause mortality—Death from all causes.

alpha bond—Connects two monosaccharides together within a disaccharide or polysaccharide. These bonds are digested readily in the human digestive system.

alpha-linolenic acid (ALA)—An omega-3 fatty acid found in plants, including flaxseeds and walnuts. ALA is an essential fat, the human body cannot make it, so it must be consumed in the diet.

amenorrhea—The abnormal absence of menstruation; missing three or more menstrual periods in a row.

amylopectin—The branched chain form of starch representing about 75 percent of the total carbohydrate in plants.

amylose—The straight chain form of starch; amylose is composed of hundreds to thousands of glucose molecules and represents about 25 percent of the total carbohydrate in plants.

anabolism—Metabolic processes involving the synthesis of new molecules.

anaerobic activity—Intense activity performed without relying on oxygen over a short period of time. Sprinting is an example.

anaerobic system—An important energy system of the body that does not require oxygen. This system can produce ATP faster than the aerobic system but is limited by carbohydrate availability and lactate production.

android—A body fat pattern representing accumulation of fat primarily in the abdominal region; often referred to as the "apple shape."

anemia—A general term used to describe a deficiency of red blood cells or decreased capacity of red blood cells to carry oxygen.

angiogenesis—The growth of new blood vessels.

antibodies—Proteins that make up our immune system and protect us from foreign pathogens or substances perceived as threats (food allergies for instance).

antioxidants—Compounds that protect plants from pests and disease and, in some cases, protect cells in the human body from damage caused by free radicals.

atherosclerosis—A disease characterized by plaque build-up in arteries that decreases the diameter of arteries, narrowing the space for blood to travel through. Atherosclerosis can increase risk for heart attack, stroke, and death.

ATP synthase—A protein complex in the ETC that is responsible for regenerating ATP from ADP and inorganic phosphate.

banned substances control group (BSCG)—A group that tests supplements for banned substances and provides 3rd party certification.

basal metabolic rate (BMR)—A measure of energy expenditure accounting for basic metabolic demands (living) during rest. BMR is measured in a temperate environment after a 10 to 12 hour fast and a refrainment from exercise for 10 to 12 hours.

beta bond—Connects two monosaccharides together within a disaccharide or polysaccharide. Carbohydrates with beta bonds cannot be digested in the human digestive tract.

beta cells—Insulin-producing cells within the pancreas.

bile—Substance synthesized by liver, stored in gall bladder, and secreted into the small intestine to help digest dietary fat. A primary constituent of bile is cholesterol.

bioelectrical impedance analysis (BIA)—A method for estimating body composition based on the resistance (impedance) of an electrical current running through the body.

bioenergetics—The study of the transformation of energy in living organisms.

body composition—The composition of the body that is fat mass compared to fat-free mass (lean body mass). Body composition can be further divided out into fat, muscle, water, and bone (a four-compartment model of measuring body composition).

body image—A subjective view of one's own body.

body mass index (BMI)—A person's weight in kilograms (kg) divided by height in meters squared.

body weight or body mass—How much a person weighs on a scale; usually expressed in pounds or kilograms.

branched chain amino acids (BCAAs)—Nonaromatic amino acids with a branch (a central carbon atom bound to three or more carbon atoms). There are three BCAAs, and all are proteinogenic: leucine, isoleucine, and valine.

calcitriol (1,25-dihydroxyvitamin D)—The active form of vitamin D in the body. Calcitriol is a steroid hormone that promotes calcium absorption, helps maintain blood calcium and phosphorus levels for normal bone mineralization, and has important physiological effects on cell growth, muscle, and immune system functioning while also reducing inflammation.

calorimetry—The act of measuring energy expenditure by observing changes in thermodynamic variables.

carbohydrate—An organic compound containing the elements carbon, hydrogen, and water. Carbohydrate is a major energy macronutrient in the human diet. The smallest carbohydrates are monosaccharides such as glucose, fructose, and galactose; the largest are polysaccharides such as starch and fiber.

carbohydrate loading—A nutrition strategy designed to avoid glycogen depletion during endurance activities by maximizing the storage of glycogen in muscles and liver through the consumption of a high carbohydrate diet for a few days prior to an event.

carbohydrate-electrolyte beverages (CEB)—Scientific term used to describe a family of beverages that contain a carbohydrate (sugar) source and electrolytes, primarily sodium.

carboxyl group—A weak acid group on a molecule characterized by having a carbonyl and hydroxyl group attached to the same terminal carbon atom.

cardiac output—The amount of blood the heart pumps in 1 minute and equal to the product of the stroke volume and heart rate.

carnitine shuttle—Shuttle located in the mitochondria that is responsible for transferring long-chain fatty acids across the inner mitochondrial membrane to proceed toward beta-oxidation.

catabolism—The breakdown of molecules to generate usable energy.

celiac disease—An autoimmune digestive disease, leading to an abnormal immune response when the protein gluten is ingested.

cell membrane—The outer covering of a cell that controls the exchange of materials between the cell and its environment.

certified diabetes educator (CDE)—Health professional who possesses comprehensive knowledge of and experience in prediabetes, diabetes prevention, and management. A CDE educates individuals with diabetes and helps the medical team and patient with the management of the condition.

cheilosis—Inflammation and cracking of the lips at the corners of the mouth.

chelated—Attached to another compound; chelated minerals are often attached to an amino acid.

chemical digestion—The breakdown of food in the mouth, stomach, and intestines through the use of acids and enzyme-catalyzed reactions.

chemical energy—Energy released from food during metabolic processing.

chemiosmotic coupling—The continuous flow of hydrogen ions through the ETC protein channels driven by an electrochemical gradient that produces proton motive force to drive ATP synthase.

cholecystokinin (CCK)—Peptide hormone of the gastrointestinal system responsible for stimulating the digestion of fat and protein.

cholesterol—A lipid-like substance found in all cells in the body and is incorporated into many hormones, vitamins, and substances used to help digest food. Cholesterol moves in the bloodstream in transport vesicles called lipoproteins. Cholesterol is a component of all animal tissues and found only in animal-based foods including eggs, red meat, poultry, cheese, and milk. In the human body cholesterol is a structural component of cell membranes, helps repair and form new cells, and is necessary for synthesizing steroid hormones (such as testosterone, androgen, and estrogen) and bile acids.

chylomicron—Lipoprotein particles that transport dietary lipids from the intestines to other locations in the body; they consist primarily of triglycerides but also contain phospholipids, cholesterol, and other proteins.

chyme—The semi-fluid, pulpy acidic mass that passes from the stomach to the small intestine, consisting of gastric juices and partly digested food.

cis configuration—Unsaturated fatty acids with hydrogen ions on the same side of the double bond.

coenzyme A—Derived from pantothenic acid, a B-vitamin, and functions in metabolic reactions.

collagen—The main structural protein found in human connective tissue, including tendons, ligaments, and cartilage.

colon—The part of the digestive tract that extends from the end of the small intestine to the anus. It absorbs water, minerals, and vitamins from the intestinal contents and eliminates undigested material during defecation. Also called the large intestine.

complex carbohydrates—Plant and grain foods, such as peas, beans, breads, and vegetables, containing abundant strands of polysaccharide carbohydrates. Complex carbohydrates also have vitamins, minerals, and fiber important to human health.

concurrent training—Two training sessions performed back to back. For instance, speed training immediately followed by strength training or vice versa.

Cori cycle—Metabolic pathway in which lactate produced by the anaerobic energy system in muscle cells moves to the liver and is converted to glucose, which then returns to the muscles and serves as a fuel source.

crossover concept—Describes fat and carbohydrate utilization as fuel sources during exercise. The crossover occurs when carbohydrate utilization exceeds fat utilization and the point at which this happens is determined by your aerobic fitness.

current good manufacturing practices (GMPs)—Manufacturing processes established and enforced by the U.S. Food and Drug Administration (FDA). GMPs provide for systems and processes ensuring proper design, monitoring, and control of manufacturing processes and facilities.

cytoplasm—The entire contents of a cell except for the nucleus.

cytosol—A component of the cytoplasm where a variety of metabolic reactions occur.

daily value (DV)—An indicator of how much of one serving of a particular food contributes to a person's nutritional needs; based on a 2,000 kilocalorie diet.

dehydration—The process of losing body water.

denature—A process through which proteins lose the quaternary structure, tertiary structure, and secondary structure because of exposure to a stimulus that changes protein structure. Common examples include strong acid (such as HCL in the stomach) and heat (cooking).

deoxyribonucleic acid (DNA)—A molecule that carries the genetic instructions used in the growth, development, functioning, and reproduction of all known living organisms.

dietary fat—The kind of fat found in foods and beverages.

dietary fiber—Material in plants, mostly non-starch polysaccharides, that is not digested by human digestive enzymes and instead passes through the digestive tract relatively unchanged before being eliminated.

dietary reference intakes (DRIs)—Reference values for macro- and micronutrients aimed at preventing or reducing the risk of chronic disease and promoting optimal health.

dietary supplement—A product taken by mouth that contains a "dietary ingredient" intended to supplement the diet. The "dietary ingredients" in these products may include vitamins, minerals, herbs or other botanicals, amino acids, or substances such as enzymes, organ tissues, glandulars, and metabolites. Dietary supplements can also be extracts or concentrates and may be found in many forms such as tablets, capsules, softgels, gelcaps, liquids, or powders.

digestion—The breakdown of food into its constituent parts using mechanical and chemical methods.

digestive elimination—The elimination of undigested food content and waste products from the digestive tract.

digestive tract—A term for the entire gastrointestinal tract from the mouth to the anus.

direct calorimetry—Measures heat production by the body, using carbon dioxide, oxygen, and temperature measurements to determine energy expenditure.

disaccharide—Sugars composed of two monosaccharide units. In the human diet, the most common disaccharides are maltose, lactose, and sucrose.

diverticulitis—Inflammation or infection of the small pouches, called diverticula, that bulge outward from the center of the colon (large intestine).

diverticulosis—A condition in which the large intestine contains small pouches, called diverticula, that bulge outward from the center of the colon. Diverticula themselves are not problematic and people having diverticulosis are often asymptomatic.

docosahexaenoic acid (DHA)—An omega-3 fatty acid. DHA is the major fat found in the brain and important for brain development and function. DHA is necessary for the production of compounds that help reduce inflammation in the brain stemming from reduced blood flow.

dual-energy x-ray absorptiometry (DEXA)—A laboratory method used to measure bone mineral density and soft tissue composition (percent body fat).

duodenum—The first part of the small intestine immediately beyond the stomach, leading to the jejunum.

dyslipidemia—Total cholesterol or triglyceride levels above the reference standard, or levels of high-density lipoprotein (HDL) cholesterol below a reference standard.

eccentric contractions—A movement where the skeletal muscle is lengthening. The downward phase of a bicep curl is an example.

eicosanoids—The physiologically active substances that are primarily derived from arachidonic acid; they are involved in intracellular signaling.

eicosapentaenoic acid (EPA)—An omega-3 fatty acid. EPA is a precursor to a group of eicosanoids that may be protective against heart attacks and strokes. EPA helps decrease inflammation by inhibiting the production of proinflammatory compounds.

electrolytes—Minerals that conduct electricity in the body. Electrolytes affect fluid balance, muscle pH, and muscle functioning. Sodium, chloride, potassium, calcium, magnesium, and phosphorus are electrolytes.

electron transport chain (ETC)—A series of protein complexes that transfers electrons from electron donors as a result of oxidation and reduction reactions while also transferring hydrogen ions within the mitochondria.

endoplasmic reticulum—A type of organelle in eukaryotic cells that is involved in protein synthesis.

endurance training—A regimen of physical activities designed to improve exercise endurance.

energy availability—The amount of energy available for body functions after the calories used during exercise is subtracted from the energy consumed in the diet.

energy-dense food—A food that has a high amount of energy (kilocalories) per gram or portion of the food item.

energy-yielding macronutrients—Nutrients that supply the body with energy; carbohydrates, fats, and proteins are the energy-yielding macronutrients. (Other macronutrients include water and lipids.)

enrichment—The addition of vitamins and minerals lost during food processing.

enterocytes—Epithelial cells found in the small intestine that contain digestive enzymes and microvilli on its surface.

enterokinases—Enzymes produced by cells of the duodenum and involved in human digestive processes; secreted from intestinal glands following the entry of ingested food passing from the stomach.

enzymes—Protein-containing biological catalysts that accelerate or catalyze chemical reactions.

ergogenic—A term commonly used in sport as something intended to enhance physical performance or recovery from training.

essential amino acids—Amino acids that cannot be made by the human body and must be consumed in the diet.

essential fat—The amount of fat necessary for physiological functioning. Essential fat is found in bone marrow, the heart, lungs, liver, spleen, kidneys, intestines, muscles, and fat-rich tissues of the central nervous system.

euglycemia—A normal concentration of glucose in the circulating blood.

euhydration—Normal state of body water content.

excess postexercise oxygen consumption (EPOC)—Calories burned after exercise has finished.

exercise physiology—The study of the body's responses to exercise, from acute bouts to chronic adaptations with repeated activity and long-term training.

extreme sports—Any sport perceived as having a high level of inherent danger.

FADH$_2$—The reduced form of FAD used for metabolic reactions and derived from the B-vitamin riboflavin.

fat-free mass (FFM)—Lean body mass defined as the total amount of nonfat body mass.

fat soluble—Vitamins stored in the body's fat tissues and more easily absorbed when consumed with dietary fat. Vitamins A, D, E, and K are fat soluble.

fatty acid—A molecule consisting of a long chain of carbon and hydrogen atoms connected to a single acid group at its end. The long carbon chain can be any length, but the ones found in the human diet tend to have between 12 and 22 carbon atoms.

Federal Trade Commission (FTC)—The FTC protects American consumers by preventing fraud, deception, and unfair business practices and ensuring competition in the marketplace.

feedback inhibition—A control mechanism that catalyzes a reaction to produce a specific compound that can reduce the rate of a metabolic reaction when the compound reaches high concentrations.

female athlete triad (triad)—Syndrome of three interrelated conditions that exist on a continuum of severity, including energy deficiency with or without disordered eating, menstrual disturbances/amenorrhea, and bone loss/osteoporosis; often shortened to simply "triad."

fermentation—Anaerobic breakdown of sugars by microorganisms in the gut.

fiber—A blanket term that describes the indigestible parts of plants.

food—The plants and animals humans ingest.

fortification—The addition of nutrients to improve the nutrition content of a food or beverage.

free radicals—Reactive oxygen and nitrogen species generated in the body through metabolism as well as exposure to various physiological conditions or disease states.

fructose—A monosaccharide carbohydrate found in many plant foods and some nutritive sweeteners.

galactose—A monosaccharide found in milk, usually bound to glucose as a disaccharide called lactose.

generally recognized as safe (GRAS)—A designation by the FDA that the substance intentionally added to a food is generally considered safe by experts under the intended conditions of use.

gestational diabetes mellitus (GDM)—High blood glucose levels during pregnancy in women who have never had diabetes. Diagnosis and management are important to protect the mother and baby's health.

glucagon—Hormone secreted by the alpha islet cells of the pancreas in response to hypoglycemia. It increases blood glucose concentration by stimulating glycogenolysis in the liver.

gluconeogenesis—Synthesis of glucose from noncarbohydrate sources in the liver and kidneys whenever the supply of carbohydrate is insufficient to meet the body's immediate requirements.

glucose—A monosaccharide found in plants primarily in the form of starch and also found in some nutritive sweeteners.

GLUT4—A protein found in cells that helps transport glucose across the cell membrane into the cytoplasm.

gluten—A protein found in foods made from wheat and other grains. Barley and rye contain proteins related to gluten (though all of these proteins are typically referred to as gluten).

glycemic—Foods that cause blood glucose levels to rise.

glycemic index—A ranking of carbohydrates according to how quickly they are digested and absorbed, and therefore raise blood glucose levels in the 2-hour time period after a meal, compared to the same amount (by weight in grams) of a reference food, typically white bread or glucose, which is given a GI of 100.

glycemic load—An indicator of the glycemic impact of a food that takes into consideration both the glycemic index and carbohydrate content, in grams, of the food. Glycemic load is computed as the product of a food's glycemic index and its total available carbohydrate content: glycemic load = [GI × carbohydrate (g)]/100].

glycemic response—Change in blood glucose after consuming food.

glycogen—A branched polymer of glucose monosaccharides that serves as the storage form of carbohydrate in the liver and muscles of animals and humans.

glycogenesis—The synthesis of glycogen from glucose subunits.

glycogenolysis—Cleaving of individual glucose molecules from the ends of glycogen, primarily in liver and skeletal muscle; the metabolic breakdown of glycogen to glucose.

glycogen synthase—Key enzyme responsible for glycogen synthesis in liver and skeletal muscle.

glycolysis—Aerobic or anaerobic process that converts glucose into pyruvate and 2 ATP.

glycolytic—Involving glycolysis.

gynoid—A body fat pattern typically representing accumulation of body fat in the lower half of the body, with more fat deposited in the hips, buttocks, and thighs. This pattern is often referred to as the "pear shape."

health claims—Describes the relationship between a food, food component supplement ingredient, and decreased risk of a disease or health-related condition.

high-density lipoprotein (HDL)—Carries cholesterol back to the liver for excretion or recycling; HDL is sometimes referred to as "good" cholesterol and is not associated with an increased risk for heart disease.

high-fructose corn syrup (HFCS)—A manufactured nutritive sweetener commonly added to food to improve palatability and shelf-life. HFCS is similar in sweetness to table sugar and contains roughly the same amount of fructose as glucose.

homeostasis—A state of balance or equilibrium.

hormones—Chemical messengers secreted directly into the blood to interact with organs and tissues of the body to exert their functions. There are many types of hormones, some of which are complex protein structures.

hydrodensitometry—In this reference method, water is used to estimate the body density and body fat of an individual. Also called hydrostatic weighing or underwater weighing (UWW).

hydrometry—A laboratory measurement of total body water (TBW).

hydroxyapatite—The storage form of calcium and phosphate in bones and teeth.

hypercalcemia—High blood calcium.

hyperglycemia—An abnormally high concentration of glucose in the circulating blood.

hyperhydration—Overhydration.

hyperphosphatemia—High blood phosphate.

hyperplasia—Growth of more cells.

hypertension—Long-term medical condition in which the blood pressure in the arteries is persistently elevated. Hypertension damages and weakens artery walls.

hypertrophy—Growth of existing cells.

hypoglycemia—An abnormally low concentration of glucose in the circulating blood.

hypohydration—The uncompensated loss of body water.

hyponatremia—Dangerously low blood sodium.

hypophosphatemia—Low blood phosphate.

indirect calorimetry—General energy expenditure measurement technique involving the measurement of oxygen and carbon dioxide gas exchange.

inflammation—The body's normal acute response to injury or attack from foreign invaders, involving localized heat, swelling, and pain. Ideally, inflammation is limited to what is required to counteract the present threat, but many chronic conditions are believed to be related to chronic inflammation.

informed-choice—A quality assurance program designed for sports nutrition products and their manufacturers and suppliers.

insensible perspiration—Fluid that evaporates through pores in the skin by sweat glands before the body recognizes it as moisture on the skin.

insoluble fiber—Portion of dietary fiber that is not soluble in water and adds bulk to the stool for easier elimination.

insulin—Hormone secreted by the beta islet cells of the pancreas in response to hyperglycemia (high blood sugar). Insulin promotes glucose uptake and storage, amino acid uptake, protein synthesis, and lipid synthesis and fat storage.

insulin-dependent glucose transport (IDGT)—Process of transporting glucose into a cell that requires the involvement of insulin.

insulin resistance—A condition in which cells fail to respond to the normal actions of insulin.

interesterified fats—Fats that have had fatty acids rearranged, chemically or enzymatically, along the glycerol backbone.

interstitial—Refers to a space between two structures or objects that are normally closely spaced.

intravascular—Occurring within a vessel or vessels of an animal or plant, especially within a blood vessel or blood vascular system.

isotopes—Element variations that have the same proton number but different neutron numbers.

ketoacidosis—A metabolic state associated with high concentrations of ketone bodies, formed by the breakdown of fatty acids and the deamination of amino acids. This is associated with a pathological metabolic state where the body fails to adequately regulate ketone production, causing an accumulation of ketoacids and resulting in a decrease in the pH of the blood. In extreme cases, ketoacidosis can be fatal and is most common in untreated type 1 diabetes mellitus. Ketoacidosis should not be confused with ketone production and subsequent ketosis resulting from a ketogenic diet. Ketones produced from a ketogenic diet are managed by the body and do not result in ketoacidosis.

kilocalorie—The same thing as a calorie. A unit of energy also called a kcal, large calorie. Refers to the amount of heat it takes to raise the temperature of one kilogram of water by one degree Celsius.

lactase—An enzyme that catalyzes the breakdown of lactose to glucose and galactose.

lactate—The molecule that remains when one hydrogen ion disassociates itself from a lactic acid molecule. Lactate serves as a fuel source that can be oxidized directly by many cells in the body, including brain, heart, and skeletal muscle. Lactate can also be converted back to pyruvate and glucose and oxidized in those forms.

lactate dehydrogenase (LDH)—The enzyme that catalyzes the reaction from pyruvate to lactate.

lactic acid—A substance produced when pyruvate, the end-product of glycolysis, binds with two additional hydrogen ions. Normally, one of the hydrogen ions immediately disassociates itself from the molecule and causes its surrounding environment to become more acidic.

lactose—A disaccharide containing glucose and galactose. Commonly known as "milk sugar" because it is present in many dairy products.

lactose intolerance—A condition marked by incomplete digestion of lactose. Consumption of dairy products such as milk and dairy products may lead to symptoms including diarrhea, gas, and bloating.

large intestine—The colon. The part of the digestive tract that extends from the end of the small intestine to the anus. It absorbs water, minerals, and vitamins from the intestinal contents and eliminates undigested material during defecation.

lean body mass (LBM)—The percentage of the body that is not fat. In a four-compartment model, LBM is comprised of water, skeletal muscle, and bone.

linoleic acid (LA)—An omega-6 fatty acid that is an essential fat. The human body cannot make it, so it must be consumed in the diet.

lipids—A category of macronutrients that are insoluble in water and have various biological functions in the body. There are three main types of lipids: triglycerides, sterols, and phospholipids.

lipogenesis—The metabolic process by which excess acetyl-CoA is converted into body fat.

lipoprotein—Any group of soluble proteins that combine with and transport fat or other lipids in the blood plasma.

liver—Glandular organ that has many functions in the body related to digestion and metabolism, including bile synthesis and secretion, gluconeogenesis, glycogen synthesis and storage, lipolysis, and transamination.

low-density lipoprotein (LDL)—A transport protein. LDL carries cholesterol from the liver to tissues.

low energy availability—Energy intake that is insufficient to meet energy expenditure and physiological needs. Low energy availability can disrupt reproductive functioning, leading to irregular menstrual cycles or complete cessation of menstruation.

luminal brush border—Microvilli-covered surface of simple epithelium where nutrient absorption takes place. The microvilli that constitute the brush border have enzymes for digestion anchored into their plasma membrane as integral membrane proteins. These enzymes are found near transporters that allow absorption of the digested nutrients.

macronutrients—Nutrients required in the diet in larger amounts: carbohydrate, protein, fat, water, and lipids.

maltase—An enzyme that catalyzes the breakdown of maltose to glucose.

maltose—A disaccharide containing two glucose molecules. Maltose does not occur naturally in foods but rather during the enzymatic breakdown of starch during digestion.

mechanical digestion—Involves physically breaking the food into smaller pieces. Mechanical digestion begins in the mouth as food is chewed and continues in the stomach as it churns.

medical nutrition therapy (MNT)—An evidence-based application of the Nutrition Care Process, usually including nutrition assessment, nutrition diagnosis, nutrition intervention, and nutrition monitoring and evaluation that typically results in the prevention, delay, or management of diseases or conditions.

medium chain triglycerides (MCTs)—A type of fat made up of a shorter carbon chain that allows it to bypass complex digestion and absorption processes and instead be absorbed directly into the blood.

messenger RNA (mRNA)—The form of RNA in which genetic information transcribed from DNA as a sequence of bases is transferred to a ribosome.

metabolic syndrome—The name for a group of risk factors that raises your risk for heart disease and other health problems, such as diabetes and stroke. The risk factors include abdominal obesity, high triglycerides, low HDL cholesterol, hypertension, and high fasting blood sugar.

metabolism—A collection of chemical reactions for bodily processes that consist of anabolic or catabolic reactions.

micronutrients—Nutrients required in small amounts, including vitamins and minerals.

microvilli—Folds and projections on enterocytes that serve to increase the surface area for the digestion and transport of nutrients from inside the intestine into the enterocyte.

mitochondria—The powerhouse of a cell where ATP production and respiration occurs.

modeling—The process through which new bone is formed at one site inside the bone and old bone removed from another site outside the bone. Modeling occurs during childhood and adolescence and shapes bone.

monounsaturated fatty acids (MUFA)—A type of unsaturated fatty acid that contains one double bond.

mouth—Initial part of digestive tract. Mechanical digestion from chewing and chemical digestion from the action of salivary amylase occurs in the mouth.

muscle protein balance—The difference between skeletal muscle protein synthesis (MPS) and breakdown (MPB).

muscular endurance—The ability to perform repeated skeletal muscle contractions or to hold a contraction over a period of time.

muscular flexibility—The ability to move through the joints range of motion.

muscular power—Rate at which the work (contraction) is performed.

muscular strength—The maximal force that a skeletal muscle or group of muscles can produce.

myocyte—Muscle cell.

NADH (nicotinamide adenine dinucleotide)—The reduced form of NAD used for metabolic reactions. A key component of NADH is the B vitamin niacin.

NADPH (nicotinamide adenine dinucleotide phosphate)—A reduced form of NADP that is formed in the pentose phosphate pathway and used in anabolic reactions.

National Center for Drug Free Sport (Drug Free Sport)—A premier provider of drug-use prevention services for many athletic organizations; delivers strategic alternatives to traditional drug-use prevention programs.

nonessential amino acids—Amino acids that can be synthesized by the human body.

nonexercise activity thermogenesis (NEAT)—The energy expended by the body for all activities not including exercise, sleeping, or eating.

nonglycemic—Foods that do not cause blood glucose levels to rise.

nonnutritive sweeteners (NNS)—Sweeteners that do not contain significant energy.

NSF—National Sanitation Foundation, newly named NSF International. NSF provides third-party certification, which is an independent analysis of a manufacturer's product with standards for safety, quality, and performance.

nucleus—Present in eukaryotic cells; the control center of the cell that contains genetic material.

nutrient absorption—The process of absorbing or assimilating digested substances into cells through diffusion or osmosis.

nutrient content claim—Statement about the level of a nutrient in a product. These are approved and regulated by the FDA and can be used on both foods and dietary supplements.

nutrient density—A measure of the number of nutrients contained in food compared to the amount of energy it provides. Foods considered nutrient dense provide a lot of vitamins and minerals with relatively little energy (calories).

nutrients—Specific substances that elicit a biochemical or physiological function in the body.

nutrigenomics—The interaction between nutrition and genes.

nutrition periodization—A principle in which nutritional guidelines are adjusted depending on the state of training.

nutrition—The study of how food supplies nutrients to the body and influences health and life.

nutritive sweeteners—Sweeteners that also contain energy.

obesity—A disease in which abnormal or excessive fat accumulation might impair health. There are grades of obesity.

oligomenorrhea—Light or infrequent menstrual periods occurring in women of childbearing age; often defined as a woman who regularly goes more than 35 days without menstruating.

oligopeptide—Molecules containing a relatively small number of amino acids.

oligosaccharide—Carbohydrates composed of 3 to 10 monosaccharide units.

oral glucose tolerance test (OGTT)—A screening test for diabetes mellitus, in which plasma glucose levels are measured in an individual after consuming an oral glucose load. An OGTT reveals type 2 diabetes mellitus or impaired glucose tolerance when plasma glucose levels exceed defined thresholds after consuming the glucose load.

organelles—Found in eukaryotic cells; they have specialized functions within a cell (e.g., nucleus, chloroplast, mitochondria, etc.).

osmolarity—The concentration of solutes, particularly sodium, in the blood.

osmosis—Movement of water across a cell membrane, from a region of low concentration of solutes to one of higher concentration.

osteoporosis—A disease characterized by low bone mass and structural deterioration of bone tissue leading to fragile bones and greater risk of fractures of the hip, spine, and wrist.

overload—Gradual increase of stress placed on the body during training.

overreaching—Excessive exercise volume that results in short-term performance decrement.

overtraining—A compendium of symptoms referred to as the overtraining syndrome (OTS). This condition is more serious than overreaching with long-term performance impairment that can take several weeks or months to achieve recovery.

overweight—Weighing more than desirable for optimal health.

oxaloacetate—A four-carbon compound that combines with acetyl-CoA to initiate the TCA cycle to form citrate. It is also involved in gluconeogenesis, the urea cycle, amino acid synthesis, and fatty acid synthesis.

oxidative decarboxylation—Forms carbon dioxide from the splitting of a carbon-carbon bond.

oxidative phosphorylation—The use of the aerobic energy system to use macronutrient fuel sources (carbohydrate, protein, fat) to phosphorylate ADP to form ATP.

oxidative stress—An imbalance between the production of free radicals and the body's antioxidant defenses.

pancreas—Glandular organ that secretes enzymes for the digestion of carbohydrates, proteins, and fats; also secretes the hormones glucagon and insulin that regulate the metabolism of carbohydrates, proteins, and fats.

pancreatic amylase—An enzyme secreted from the pancreas into the small intestine during digestion that catalyzes the breakdown of starch into sugars.

peak bone mass—Maximum bone strength and density.

pepsin—A protease enzyme that breaks down food proteins into smaller peptides. Produced in the stomach, pepsin is one of the main digestive enzymes in the digestive systems of humans.

pepsinogen—The proenzyme of pepsin, made and released by chief cells in the stomach wall.

peptide bonds—Chemical attachment formed between two molecules, usually involving two amino acids. A carboxyl group of one molecule reacts with an amino group of another molecule releasing a molecule of water.

phosphocreatine (PCr)—A fuel substrate that can rapidly donate its phosphorous group to ADP to form ATP.

phospholipids—Structural components of cell membranes and lipoproteins. Phospholipids are necessary for the absorption, transport, and storage of lipids and aid in the digestion and absorption of dietary fat.

phosphorylate—To add or introduce a phosphate group to a molecule or compound.

photosynthesis—As it relates specifically to human nutrition, photosynthesis is the process through which plants use energy from the sun to convert carbon dioxide and water into glucose plus oxygen.

physical activity level (PAL)—A factor used to express daily physical activity, typically used to estimate an individual's total energy expenditure. PAL is often used in combination with the basal metabolic rate to compute the amount of food energy an individual needs to consume in order to maintain a particular lifestyle.

polydipsia—Excessive thirst or excess drinking often associated with uncontrolled diabetes mellitus.

polypeptide—Chains of amino acids linked by a peptide bond that serve as components of proteins.

polyphagia—Excessive hunger or increased appetite that may be caused by medical disorders such as diabetes mellitus.

polysaccharide—Carbohydrate composed of long chains of monosaccharides linked by glycosidic bonds (e.g., cellulose, starch, and glycogen).

polyunsaturated fatty acids (PUFA)—A type of unsaturated fatty acid that contains more than one double bond. Polyunsaturated fatty acids are identified based on the location of their first double bond. Omega-3 and omega-6 fatty acids are examples.

polyuria—Excessive or abnormally large production or passage of urine; often associated with uncontrolled diabetes mellitus.

portal vein—A blood vessel that carries blood from the gastrointestinal tract, gallbladder, pancreas, and spleen to the liver.

postprandial hypoglycemia—Low blood sugar that occurs soon after consuming a meal, usually containing carbohydrate. Also called reactive hypoglycemia.

preformed vitamin A—The active form of vitamin A in the body; preformed vitamin A is found in animal liver, whole milk, and some fortified foods.

principle of detraining—Involves the loss of physiological training responses when exercise is discontinued.

principle of individuality—An exercise principle stating that we are somewhat limited by our genetic potential and that people respond in different ways to exercise.

principle of periodization—Schedules training for a particular sport or event into smaller periods of time or blocks with specific training goals in each.

principle of progressive overload—In order to see improvements in performance, the system being trained must have continuous demands placed upon it.

principle of specificity—The training routine must induce a physical stress specific to the system needed for performance enhancements.

proenzyme—A biologically inactive protein that is metabolized into an active enzyme.

proprietary blends—A list of ingredients that are part of a product formula specific to a particular dietary supplement manufacturer. The names and quantities of the individual ingredients in the blend are not disclosed.

protease activation cascade—A series of enzymatic events that lead to the activation of several digestive enzymes.

proteases—An enzyme that breaks down proteins and peptides.

proteinogenic—Amino acids that are precursors to proteins and are incorporated into proteins during translation.

proton motive force—The electrochemical force generated by the electron transport chain that drives ATP synthase to create ATP.

provitamin A carotenoids—Dark-colored pigments found in some vegetables, oily fruits, and red palm oil. Provitamin A carotenoids include beta-carotene, alpha-carotene, and beta-cryptoxanthin and must be converted to the active form of vitamin A in the body.

purging behavior—Self-induced vomiting or misuse of laxatives, diuretics, or enemas with psychiatric underpinnings.

pyrophosphate—The free phosphate group used to form ADP and ATP; sometimes referred to as inorganic phosphate.

pyruvate dehydrogenase complex (PDC)—A formation of three enzymes that act to convert pyruvate to acetyl-CoA.

quackery—An unproven or unsupported intervention usually promoted for the purpose of financial gain.

reactants—Substances that take part in and undergo changes during a reaction.

reactive hypoglycemia—Low blood sugar that occurs soon after consuming a meal, usually containing carbohydrate. Also called postprandial hypoglycemia.

refined carbohydrate—Plant foods that have been processed to remove portions of the whole grain, usually to make the final product more palatable.

registered dietitian nutritionist (RDN or RD)—A credential issued by the Commission on Dietetic Registration of the Academy of Nutrition and Dietetics to individuals who have expertise in food, nutrition, and dietetics. Education, supervised practice experience, and passing of a national exam is required.

relative energy deficiency in sport (RED-S)—A syndrome of impaired physiological function including, but not limited to, metabolic rate, menstrual function, bone health, immunity, protein synthesis, and cardiovascular health. Encompasses a cluster of health complications that occur in males and females when energy intake may be sufficient to fuel physical activity but is not sufficient to maintain the health of many body systems.

resorption—Bone breakdown.

resting energy expenditure (REE)—The amount of energy from food calories required during resting conditions of the body.

resting metabolic rate (RMR)—The amount of energy, usually expressed in kilocalories, required for a 24-hour period by the body during resting conditions. It is closely related to, but not identical to, basal metabolic rate (BMR). RMR tends to be slightly higher than BMR.

reversibility—The reversal of metabolic and physical benefits achieved from training when an individual stops training.

rhabdomyolysis—Serious skeletal muscle injury.

ribonucleic acid (RNA)—Molecule that plays various biological roles in coding, decoding, regulation, and expression of genes.

rule of five—A guideline used to help select whole grains and cereals that are deemed healthy. Rule is to select those grains having 5 grams or more of fiber and less than 5 grams of sugar per serving.

salivary amylase—An enzyme found in human saliva that catalyzes the breakdown of starch into sugars.

sarcopenia—Age related loss of muscle mass and strength.

satiation—The physiological satisfaction of appetite during a meal; satiation helps determine when to stop eating.

satiety—The sensation of fullness or absence of hunger after a meal.

saturated fatty acids—Fatty acids that have only single bonds between adjacent carbon atoms, so they can stack tightly on top of one another. Fats containing more saturated fatty acids are solid at room temperature.

secretin—Digestive hormone secreted by the wall of the duodenum; influences the environment of the duodenum by regulating secretions in the stomach, pancreas, and liver.

set point theory—A theory that any attempt to voluntarily change body weight from an established weight in adulthood initiates a series of physiological and metabolic responses that ultimately result in no further loss of body fat, or a plateau. These responses might include storing fat more efficiently, decreasing metabolism, or stimulating appetite.

simple carbohydrate—A monosaccharide; simple sugar.

simple sugar—A monosaccharide.

skinfold thickness—A method for estimating body composition based on the thickness of a fold of skin and underlying subcutaneous fat. The measurement is made using calipers.

small intestine—The part of the intestine that runs between the stomach and the large intestine and where the majority of digestion and absorption of food takes place.

soluble fiber—Portion of dietary fiber that is soluble in water to form a gel-like substance in the stool.

specificity—Targeting a specific energy system to initiate the desired effect of physical training.

sport nutrition—A specialty discipline that examines the role of nutrition in exercise metabolism and the translation to nutrient guidelines for optimal training, performance, and recovery from exercise.

standard error of estimate (SEE)—A measure of the accuracy of predictions using statistical regression lines.

starch—The form of polysaccharide carbohydrate stored in most plants, which makes it the principal carbohydrate of the human diet.

stearidonic acid (SDA)—An omega-3 fatty acid found in some seed oils; some fish, including sardines and herring; algae; and GMO (genetically modified organisms) soybeans.

sterols—A type of lipid with a multiple ring structure. Cholesterol is the most well-recognized sterol.

storage fat—Fat found around the internal organs (visceral fat) and directly below the skin (subcutaneous fat).

stroke volume—Most generally associated with the left ventricle; measured through the amount of blood ejected from the left ventricle from one contraction.

structure/function claim—States how a product, nutrient, or ingredient intends to affect the normal structure or function within the body or how it acts to maintain a particular structure or function. These claims cannot explicitly or implicitly link or associate the claimed effect of the nutrient, component, or dietary ingredient to a specific disease or state of health leading to a disease.

subcutaneous fat—A type of storage fat found directly below the skin.

substrate fatigue—A theory that attributes fatigue during long-duration exercise to skeletal muscle glycogen depletion.

sucrase—An enzyme that catalyzes the breakdown of sucrose to glucose and fructose.

sucrose—A disaccharide containing glucose and fructose. Commonly known as table sugar.

thermic effect of activity (TEA)—Energy expenditure to support the demands of physical activity.

thermic effect of feeding (TEF)—Energy expenditure from food absorption, metabolism, and storage of food ingestion accounting for no more than 10 percent of total daily energy expenditure.

thrifty gene—A hypothesis speculating that humans slow their metabolism and store more body fat during times of food scarcity.

total energy expenditure (TEE)—The sum of all energy expended over a set period of time (usually 24 hours).

trans fatty acids—Fatty acids that have hydrogen molecules on opposite sides of the double bond. Trans fatty acids are harmful for heart health.

transfer RNA (tRNA)—RNA consisting of folded molecules that transport amino acids from the cytoplasm of a cell to a ribosome.

tricarboxylic acid (TCA) cycle—Aerobic pathway also known as Krebs cycle or citric acid cycle; uses acetyl-CoA in a series of reactions to create carbon dioxide and ATP.

triglycerides—Lipids composed of one glycerol molecule and three fatty acid molecules that serve as the main constituent of body fat in humans and animals. Cooking oils, butter, animal fat, nuts, seeds, avocado, and olives are significant sources of triglycerides in the diet.

trypsin—A protease important in protein digestion by serving to break (cleave) peptide chains. A proenzyme of trypsin, trypsinogen, is produced in the pancreas and found in pancreatic juice.

type 1 diabetes mellitus—A condition in which the pancreas no longer produces enough insulin so glucose in the blood cannot be absorbed into cells of the body.

type 2 diabetes mellitus—A condition in which the body does not make or use insulin effectively. Left untreated blood sugar remains high.

unsaturated fatty acids—Fatty acids with kinks in their double bonds so they do not stack neatly on top of one another; fats containing more unsaturated fatty acids, as opposed to saturated fatty acids, are liquid at room temperature.

urea cycle—A cycle of biochemical reactions occurring in many animals that produces urea from ammonia (NH_3).

U.S. Anti-Doping Agency (USADA)—The national anti-doping organization for Olympic, Paralympic, Pan American, and Parapan American sport with a mission to "Preserve the integrity of competition—Inspire true sport—Protect the rights of U.S. athletes" and the vision "to be the guardian of the values and life lessons learned through true sport."

U.S. Food and Drug Administration (FDA)—The Consumer Protection Agency of the U.S. Government that monitors all products classified as foods sold in the United States.

U.S. Pharmacopeial Convention (USP)—A scientific, worldwide, nonprofit organization that sets standards for the identity, strength, quality, and purity of medicines, food ingredients, and dietary supplements manufactured and distributed for sale.

$\dot{V}O_2$max—A measure of the maximum volume of oxygen that an athlete can use, measured in milliliters per kilogram of body weight per minute.

villi, intestinal—Projections on the mucous membrane of the small intestine that increases its surface area, thus facilitating absorption of nutrients.

visceral fat—A type of storage fat found wrapped around the internal organs.

vitamins—Compounds necessary for metabolism, proper growth and development, vision, organ and immune functioning, energy production, muscle contraction and relaxation, oxygen transport, building and maintaining bone and cartilage, building and repairing muscle tissue, and protecting the body's cells from damage.

wellness—A multidimensional concept that includes spiritual, emotional, social, and occupational health as well as physical health.

whole grain—Grain that has been minimally refined or processed; usually eaten in its whole native state.

Chapter 1

1. Academy of Nutrition and Dietetics. Commission on Dietetic Registration of the Academy of Nutrition and Dietetics. 2016. https://www.cdrnet.org. Accessed January 5, 2016.

2. Academy of Nutrition and Dietetics. RDNs and Medical Nutrition Therapy Services. 2016. www.eatright.org/resource/food/resources/learn-more-about-rdns/rdns-and-medical-nutrition-therapy-services. Accessed September 7, 2016.

3. Academy of Nutrition and Dietetics. Sports, Cardiovascular, and Wellness Nutrition. 2016. www.scandpg.org. Accessed September 7, 2016.

4. Andreasen, CH, Stender-Petersen, KL, Mogensen, MS, Torekov, SS, Wegner, L, Andersen, G, Nielsen, AL, Albrechtsen, A, Borch-Johnsen, K, Rasmussen, SS, Clausen, JO, Sandbaek, A, Lauritzen, T, Hansen, L, Jorgensen, T, Pedersen, O, and Hansen, T. Low physical activity accentuates the effect of the FTO rs9939609 polymorphism on body fat accumulation. *Diabetes* 57:95-101, 2008.

5. Cauchi, S, Stutzmann, F, Cavalcanti-Proenca, C, Durand, E, Pouta, A, Hartikainen, AL, Marre, M, Vol, S, Tammelin, T, Laitinen, J, Gonzalez-Izquierdo, A, Blakemore, AI, Elliott, P, Meyre, D, Balkau, B, Jarvelin, MR, and Froguel, P. Combined effects of MC4R and FTO common genetic variants on obesity in European general populations. *J Mol Med (Berl)* 87:537-546, 2009.

6. Centers for Disease Control and Prevention. Control of infectious diseases. *MMWR Morb Mortal Wkly Rep* 48:621-629, 1999.

7. Churchward-Venne, TA, Tieland, M, Verdijk, LB, Leenders, M, Dirks, ML, de Groot, LC, and van Loon, LJ. There are no nonresponders to resistance-type exercise training in older men and women. *J Am Med Dir Assoc* 16:400-411, 2015.

8. Coyle, EF, Martin, WH, 3rd, Sinacore, DR, Joyner, MJ, Hagberg, JM, and Holloszy, JO. Time course of loss of adaptations after stopping prolonged intense endurance training. *J Appl Physiol Respir Environ Exerc Physiol* 57:1857-1864, 1984.

9. Dina, C, Meyre, D, Gallina, S, Durand, E, Korner, A, Jacobson, P, Carlsson, LM, Kiess, W, Vatin, V, Lecoeur, C, Delplanque, J, Vaillant, E, Pattou, F, Ruiz, J, Weill, J, Levy-Marchal, C, Horber, F, Potoczna, N, Hercberg, S, Le Stunff, C, Bougneres, P, Kovacs, P, Marre, M, Balkau, B, Cauchi, S, Chevre, JC, and Froguel, P. Variation in FTO contributes to childhood obesity and severe adult obesity. *Nat Genet* 39:724-726, 2007.

10. Fleg, JL, Morrell, CH, Bos, AG, Brant, LJ, Talbot, LA, Wright, JG, and Lakatta, EG. Accelerated longitudinal decline of aerobic capacity in healthy older adults. *Circulation* 112:674-682, 2005.

11. Frayling, TM, Timpson, NJ, Weedon, MN, Zeggini, E, Freathy, RM, Lindgren, CM, Perry, JR, Elliott, KS, Lango, H, Rayner, NW, Shields, B, Harries, LW, Barrett, JC, Ellard, S, Groves, CJ, Knight, B, Patch, AM, Ness, AR, Ebrahim, S, Lawlor, DA, Ring, SM, Ben-Shlomo, Y, Jarvelin, MR, Sovio, U, Bennett, AJ, Melzer, D, Ferrucci, L, Loos, RJ, Barroso, I, Wareham, NJ, Karpe, F, Owen, KR, Cardon, LR, Walker, M, Hitman, GA, Palmer, CN, Doney, AS, Morris, AD, Smith, GD, Hattersley, AT, and McCarthy, MI. A common variant in the FTO gene is associated with body mass index and predisposes to childhood and adult obesity. *Science* 316:889-894, 2007.

12. Gormley, SE, Swain, DP, High, R, Spina, RJ, Dowling, EA, Kotipalli, US, and Gandrakota, R. Effect of intensity of aerobic training on $\dot{V}O_2max$. *Med Sci Sports Exerc* 40:1336-1343, 2008.

13. Gray, GE, and Gray, LK. Evidence-based medicine: Applications in dietetic practice. *J Am Diet Assoc* 102:1263-1272, 2002.

14. Gullberg, B, Johnell, O, and Kanis, JA. World-wide projections for hip fracture. *Osteoporos Int* 7:407-413, 1997.

15. Henry, YM, Fatayerji, D, and Eastell, R. Attainment of peak bone mass at the lumbar spine, femoral neck and radius in men and women: Relative contributions of bone size and volumetric bone mineral density. *Osteoporosis International* 15:263-273, 2004.

16. Hu, F. *Obesity Epidemiology.* New York, NY: Oxford University Press, 2008.

17. Institute for Credentialing Excellence. NCCA Accredited Certification Programs. 2016. www.credentialingexcellence.org/p/cm/ld/fid=121. Accessed August 12, 2015.

18. Institute of Medicine. *Dietary Reference Intakes for Energy, Carbohydrate, Fiber, Fat, Fatty Acids, Cholesterol, Protein, and Amino Acids (Macronutrients).* Washington, DC: National Academies Press, 2005.

19. Issurin, VB. New horizons for the methodology and physiology of training periodization. *Sports Med* 40:189-206, 2010.

20. Kenney, WL, Wilmore, JH, and Costill, DL. *Physiology of Sport and Exercise.* Champaign, IL: Human Kinetics, 2015.

21. Kruskall, L, Manore, M, Eikhoff-Shemek, J, and Ehrman, J. Understanding the scope of practice among registered dietitian nutritionists and exercise professionals. *ACSMs Health Fit J* 21:23-32, 2017.

22. Leenders, M, Verdijk, LB, van der Hoeven, L, van Kranenburg, J, Nilwik, R, and van Loon, LJ. Elderly men and women benefit equally from prolonged resistance-type exercise training. *J Gerontol A Biol Sci Med Sci* 68:769-779, 2013.

23. Lemmer, JT, Hurlbut, DE, Martel, GF, Tracy, BL, Ivey, FM, Metter, EJ, Fozard, JL, Fleg, JL, and Hurley, BF. Age and gender responses to strength training and detraining. *Med Sci Sports Exerc* 32:1505-1512, 2000.

24. Lukaski, HC. Vitamin and mineral status: Effects on physical performance. *Nutrition* 20:632-644, 2004.

25. Manore, MM. Weight management for athletes and active individuals: A brief review. *Sports Med* 45 Suppl 1:83-92, 2015.

26. Meeusen, R, Duclos, M, Foster, C, Fry, A, Gleeson, M, Nieman, D, Raglin, J, Rietjens, G, Steinacker, J, and Urhausen, A. Prevention, diagnosis, and treatment of the overtraining syndrome: Joint consensus statement of the European College of Sports Medicine and the American College of Sports Medicine. *Med Sci Sports Exerc* 45:186-205, 2013.

27. National Academy of Sciences. Dietary Reference Intakes: Guiding Principles for Nutrition Labeling and Fortification. Washington, DC, 2003.

28. National Academy of Sciences. Dietary Reference Intakes for Water, Potassium, Sodium, Chloride, and Sulfate. Washington, DC, 2005.

29. Neufer, PD. The effect of detraining and reduced training on the physiological adaptations to aerobic exercise training. *Sports Med* 8:302-320, 1989.

30. Office of the Federal Register. Title 21: Food and drugs, Part 101—Food labeling. In *Electronic Code of Federal Regulations.* Washington, DC: U.S. Government Publishing Office. www.ecfr.gov/cgi-bin/retrieveECFR?gp=1&SID=4bf49f997b04dcacdfbd637d-b9aa5839&ty=HTML&h=L&mc=true&n=pt21.2.101&r=PART.

31. Ogden, CL, Carroll, MD, Kit, BK, and Flegal, KM. Prevalence of childhood and adult obesity in the United States, 2011-2012. *JAMA* 311:806-814, 2014.

32. Paddon-Jones, D, and Rasmussen, BB. Dietary protein recommendations and the prevention of sarcopenia: Protein, amino acid metabolism and therapy. *Current Opinion in Clinical Nutrition and Metabolic Care* 12:86-90, 2009.

33. Petrella, RJ, Lattanzio, CN, Shapiro, S, and Overend, T. Improving aerobic fitness in older adults: Effects of a physician-based exercise counseling and prescription program. *Can Fam Physician* 56:e191-e200, 2010.

34. Phillips, SM. Dietary protein requirements and adaptive advantages in athletes. *Br J Nutr* 108 Suppl 2:S158-167, 2012.

35. Phillips, SM. A brief review of higher dietary protein diets in weight loss: A focus on athletes. *Sports Med* 44:149-153, 2014.

36. Poole, DC, Wilkerson, DP, and Jones, AM. Validity of criteria for establishing maximal O2 uptake during ramp exercise tests. *Eur J Appl Physiol* 102:403-410, 2008.

37. Qi, Q, Chu, AY, Kang, JH, Huang, J, Rose, LM, Jensen, MK, Liang, L, Curhan, GC, Pasquale, LR, Wiggs, JL, De Vivo, I, Chan, AT, Choi, HK, Tamimi, RM, Ridker, PM, Hunter, DJ, Willett, WC, Rimm, EB, Chasman, DI, Hu, FB, and Qi, L. Fried food consumption, genetic risk, and body mass index: Gene-diet interaction analysis in three US cohort studies. *Br Med J* 348, 2014.

38. Riebl, SK, and Davy, BM. The hydration equation: Update on water balance and cognitive performance. *ACSMs Health Fit J* 17:21-28, 2013.

39. Ruiz, JR, Labayen, I, Ortega, FB, Legry, V, Moreno, LA, Dallongeville, J, Martinez-Gomez, D, Bokor, S, Manios, Y, Ciarapica, D, Gottrand, F, De Henauw, S, Molnar, D, Sjostrom, M, and Meirhaeghe, A. Attenuation of the effect of the FTO rs9939609 polymorphism on total and central body fat by physical activity in adolescents: The HELENA study. *Arch Pediatr Adolesc Med* 164:328-333, 2010.

40. Santoro, N, Perrone, L, Cirillo, G, Raimondo, P, Amato, A, Coppola, F, Santarpia, M, D'Aniello, A, and Miraglia Del Giudice, E. Weight loss in obese children carrying the proopiomelanocortin R236G variant. *J Endocrinol Invest* 29:226-230, 2006.

41. Schoenfeld, BJ, Pope, ZK, Benik, FM, Hester, GM, Sellers, J, Nooner, JL, Schnaiter, JA, Bond-Williams, KE, Carter, AS, Ross, CL, Just, BL, Henselmans, M, and Krieger, JW. Longer inter-set rest periods enhance muscle strength and hypertrophy in resistance-trained men. *J Strength Cond Res* 30:1805-1812, 2016.

42. Scribbans, TD, Vecsey, S, Hankinson, PB, Foster, WS, and Gurd, BJ. The effect of training intensity on VO(2)max in young healthy adults: A meta-regression and meta-analysis. *Int J Exerc Sci* 9:230-247, 2016.

43. Thomas, DT, Erdman, KA, and Burke, LM. Position of the Academy of Nutrition and Dietetics, Dietitians of Canada, and the American College of Sports Medicine: Nutrition and athletic performance. *J Acad Nutr Diet* 116:501-528, 2016.

44. Thompson, JL, Manore, MM, and Vaughan, LA. *The Science of Nutrition.* Upper Saddle River, NJ: Pearson Education, 2017.

45. U.S. Department of Agriculture. USDA Choose MyPlate. www.choosemyplate.gov. Accessed Web Page, 2016.

46. U.S. Department of Agriculture. Dietary Reference Intakes. 2016. https://fnic.nal.usda.gov/dietary-guidance/dietary-reference-intakes. Accessed September 5, 2016.

47. U.S. Department of Agriculture. USDA Food Composition Database. 2016. https://ndb.nal.usda.gov. Accessed September 7, 2016.

48. U.S. Department of Agriculture and U.S. Department of Health and Human Services. *Dietary Guidelines for Americans, 2015-2020.* Washington, DC: U.S. Department of Health and Human Services, 2016.

49. U.S. Department of Agriculture and U.S. Department of Health and Human Services. The Dietary Guidelines for Americans: What It Is, What It Is Not. In *Dietary Guidelines for Americans, 2015-2020.* U.S. Department of Health and Human Services, 2016. https://health.gov/dietaryguidelines/2015/guidelines/introduction/dietary-guidelines-for-americans/.

50. U.S. Department of Health and Human Services. *2008 Physical Activity Guidelines for Americans.* U.S. Department of Health and Human Services, 2008.

51. U.S. Food and Drug Administration. Food Labeling Guide. www.fda.gov/food/guidanceregulation/guidancedocumentsregulatoryinformation/labelingnutrition/ucm2006828.htm.

52. U.S. Food and Drug Administration. Changes to the Nutrition Facts Label. 2016. www.fda.gov/Food/GuidanceRegulation/GuidanceDocumentsRegulatoryInformation/LabelingNutrition/ucm385663.htm. Accessed September 7, 2016.

53. U.S. Food and Drug Administration. Guidance for Industry: A Food Labeling Guide (Appendix A: Definitions of Nutrient Content Claims). 2016. www.fda.gov/Food/GuidanceRegulation/GuidanceDocumentsRegulatoryInformation/LabelingNutrition/ucm064911.htm. Accessed January 7, 2016.

54. U.S. Food and Drug Administration. Guidance for Industry: A Food Labeling Guide (Appendix C: Health Claims). 2016. www.fda.gov/Food/GuidanceRegulation/GuidanceDocumentsRegulatoryInformation/LabelingNutrition/ucm064919.htm. Accessed January 7, 2016.

55. U.S. Food and Drug Administration. How to Understand and Use the Nutrition Facts Label. 2016. www.fda.gov/Food/IngredientsPackagingLabeling/LabelingNutrition/ucm274593.htm#overview. Accessed February 16, 2016.

56. U.S. Food and Drug Administration. Label Claims for Conventional Foods and Dietary Supplements. 2016. www.fda.gov/Food/IngredientsPackagingLabeling/LabelingNutrition/ucm111447.htm. Accessed January 5, 2016.

57. U.S. Food and Drug Admistration. Food Labeling Guide. 2016. www.fda.gov/Food/GuidanceRegulation/GuidanceDocumentsRegulatoryInformation/LabelingNutrition/ucm2006828.htm. Accessed September 7, 2016.

58. U.S. National Library of Medicine. Definitions of Health Terms: Nutrition. 2016. https://www.nlm.nih.gov/medlineplus/definitions/nutritiondefinitions.html. Accessed February 16, 2016.

59. Ward, BW, Schiller, JS, and Goodman, RA. Multiple chronic conditions among US adults: A 2012 update. *Prev Chronic Dis* 11:E62, 2014.

60. Xi, B, Chandak, GR, Shen, Y, Wang, Q, and Zhou, D. Association between common polymorphism near the MC4R gene and obesity risk: A systematic review and meta-analysis. *PLoS One* 7:e45731, 2012.

61. Xiang, L, Wu, H, Pan, A, Patel, B, Xiang, G, Qi, L, Kaplan, RC, Hu, F, Wylie-Rosett, J, and Qi, Q. FTO genotype and weight loss in diet and lifestyle interventions: A systematic review and meta-analysis. *Am J Clin Nutr* 103:1162-1170, 2016.

Chapter 2

1. Ainsworth, BE, Haskell, WL, Whitt, MC, Irwin, ML, Swartz, AM, Strath, SJ, O'Brien, WL, Bassett, DR, Jr., Schmitz, KH, Emplaincourt, PO, Jacobs, DR, Jr., and Leon, AS. Compendium of physical activities: An update of activity codes and MET intensities. *Med Sci Sports Exerc* 32:S498-S504, 2000.

2. Barnes, MJ. Alcohol: Impact on sports performance and recovery in male athletes. *Sports Med* 44:909-919, 2014.

3. Berg, JM, Tymoczko, JL, and Stryer, L. *Biochemistry*. New York: W.H. Freeman, 2012.

4. Buford, TW, Kreider, RB, Stout, JR, Greenwood, M, Campbell, B, Spano, M, Ziegenfuss, T, Lopez, H, Landis, J, and Antonio, J. International Society of Sports Nutrition position stand: Creatine supplementation and exercise. *J Int Soc Sports Nutr* 4:6, 2007.

5. Burke, DG, Chilibeck, PD, Parise, G, Candow, DG, Mahoney, D, and Tarnopolsky, M. Effect of creatine and weight training on muscle creatine and performance in vegetarians. *Med Sci Sports Exerc* 35:1946-1955, 2003.

6. Burke, LM, Collier, GR, Broad, EM, Davis, PG, Martin, DT, Sanigorski, AJ, and Hargreaves, M. Effect of alcohol intake on muscle glycogen storage after prolonged exercise. *J Appl Physiol* 95:983-990, 2003.

7. Burke, LM, and Read, RS. A study of dietary patterns of elite Australian football players. *Can J Sport Sci* 13:15-19, 1988.

8. Campbell, MK. *Biochemistry*. Philadelphia: Saunders, 1999.

9. Cooper, R, Naclerio, F, Allgrove, J, and Jimenez, A. Creatine supplementation with specific view to exercise/sports performance: An update. *J Int Soc Sports Nutr* 9:33, 2012.

10. Cunningham, JJ. A reanalysis of the factors influencing basal metabolic rate in normal adults. *Am J Clin Nutr* 33:2372-2374, 1980.

11. Deakin, V. Energy requirements of the athlete: Assessment and evidence of energy efficiency. In *Clinical Sports Nutrition*. Burke, L, Deakin, V, eds. Sydney, Australia: McGraw Hill Australia, 2015, pp. 27-53.

12. Gerich, JE, Meyer, C, Woerle, HJ, and Stumvoll, M. Renal gluconeogenesis: Its importance in human glucose homeostasis. *Diabetes Care* 24:382-391, 2001.

13. Guebels, CP, Kam, LC, Maddalozzo, GF, and Manore, MM. Active women before/after an intervention designed to restore menstrual function: Resting metabolic rate and comparison of four methods to quantify energy expenditure and energy availability. *Int J Sport Nutr Exerc Metab* 24:37-46, 2014.

14. Hobson, RM, and Maughan, RJ. Hydration status and the diuretic action of a small dose of alcohol. *Alcohol Alcohol* 45:366-373, 2010.

15. Insel, PM. *Nutrition*. Burlington, MA: Jones & Bartlett Learning, 2014.

16. Joy, E, De Souza, MJ, Nattiv, A, Misra, M, Williams, NI, Mallinson, RJ, Gibbs, JC, Olmsted, M, Goolsby, M, Matheson, G, Barrack, M, Burke, L, Drinkwater, B, Lebrun, C, Loucks, AB, Mountjoy, M, Nichols, J, and Borgen, JS. 2014 female athlete triad coalition consensus statement on treatment and return to play of the female athlete triad. *Curr Sports Med Rep* 13:219-232, 2014.

17. Koeth, RA, Wang, Z, Levison, BS, Buffa, JA, Org, E, Sheehy, BT, Britt, EB, Fu, X, Wu, Y, Li, L, Smith, JD, DiDonato, JA, Chen, J, Li, H, Wu, GD, Lewis, JD, Warrier, M, Brown, JM, Krauss, RM, Tang, WH, Bushman, FD, Lusis, AJ, and Hazen, SL. Intestinal microbiota metabolism of L-carnitine, a nutrient in red meat, promotes atherosclerosis. *Nat Med* 19:576-585, 2013.

18. Lee, JM, Kim, Y, and Welk, GJ. Validity of consumer-based physical activity monitors. *Med Sci Sports Exerc* 46:1840-1848, 2014.

19. Loucks, AB. Energy balance and energy availability. In *The Encyclopaedia of Sports Medicine*. John Wiley & Sons Ltd, 2013, pp. 72-87.

20. Lourenco, S, Oliveira, A, and Lopes, C. The effect of current and lifetime alcohol consumption on overall and central obesity. *Eur J Clin Nutr* 66:813-818, 2012.

21. Manini, TM. Energy expenditure and aging. *Ageing Res Rev* 9:1-11, 2010.

22. Manore, MM, and Thompson, JL. Energy requirements of the athlete: Assessment and evidence of energy efficiency. In *Clinical Sports Nutrition*. Burke, L, Deakin, V, eds. Sydney, Australia: McGraw Hill Australia, 2015, pp. 114-139.

23. Mountjoy, M, Sundgot-Borgen, J, Burke, L, Carter, S, Constantini, N, Lebrun, C, Meyer, N, Sherman, R, Steffen, K, Budgett, R, and Ljungqvist, A. The IOC consensus statement: Beyond the female athlete triad—Relative energy deficiency in sport (RED-S). *Br J Sports Med* 48:491-497, 2014.

24. Parr, EB, Camera, DM, Areta, JL, Burke, LM, Phillips, SM, Hawley, JA, and Coffey, VG. Alcohol ingestion impairs maximal post-exercise rates of myofibrillar protein synthesis following a single bout of concurrent training. *PLoS One* 9:e88384, 2014.

25. Pooyandjoo, M, Nouhi, M, Shab-Bidar, S, Djafarian, K, and Olyaeemanesh, A. The effect of (L-)carnitine on weight loss in adults: A systematic review and meta-analysis of randomized controlled trials. *Obes Rev* 17:970-976, 2016.

26. Roza, AM, and Shizgal, HM. The Harris Benedict equation reevaluated: Resting energy requirements and the body cell mass. *Am J Clin Nutr* 40:168-182, 1984.

27. Slootmaker, SM, Chinapaw, MJ, Seidell, JC, van Mechelen, W, and Schuit, AJ. Accelerometers and Internet for physical activity promotion in youth? Feasibility and effectiveness of a minimal intervention [ISRCTN93896459]. *Prev Med* 51:31-36, 2010.

28. Spriet, LL. New insights into the interaction of carbohydrate and fat metabolism during exercise. *Sports Med* 44 Suppl 1:S87-96, 2014.

29. St-Onge, MP, and Gallagher, D. Body composition changes with aging: The cause or the result of alterations in metabolic rate and macronutrient oxidation? *Nutrition* 26:152-155, 2010.

30. Stipanuk, MH. *Biochemical and Physiological Aspects of Human Nutrition.* Philadelphia: W.B. Saunders, 2000.

31. Stryer, L. *Biochemistry.* New York: W.H. Freeman, 1995.

32. Thomas, DT, Erdman, KA, and Burke, LM. American College of Sports Medicine joint position statement: Nutrition and athletic performance. *Med Sci Sports Exerc* 48:543-568, 2016.

33. U.S. Department of Agriculture and U.S. Department of Health & Human Services. *Dietary Guidelines for Americans, 2015-2020.* Wise Age Books, 2015.

34. Verster, JC. The alcohol hangover—A puzzling phenomenon. *Alcohol Alcohol* 43:124-126, 2008.

35. von Loeffelholz, C. The role of non-exercise activity thermogenesis in human obesity. In *Endotext.* De Groot, LJ, Chrousos, G, Dungan, K, Feingold, KR, Grossman, A, Hershman, JM, Koch, C, Korbonits, M, McLachlan, R, New, M, Purnell, J, Rebar, R, Singer, F, Vinik, A, eds. South Dartmouth, MA: MDText.com, 2000.

36. Westerterp, KR. Reliable assessment of physical activity in disease: An update on activity monitors. *Curr Opin Clin Nutr Metab Care* 17:401-406, 2014.

37. Widmaier, EP, Raff, H, and Strang, KT. *Vander's Human Physiology: The Mechanisms of Body Function.* Boston: McGraw-Hill, 2006.

Chapter 3

1. Academy of Nutrition and Dietetics and American Diabetes Association. Choose Your Foods: Food Lists for Weight Management. Chicago, IL, and Alexandria, VA: Academy of Nutrition and Dietetics and American Diabetes Association, 2014.

2. American Institute for Cancer Research. Get the Facts on Fiber 2016. www.aicr.org/reduce-your-cancer-risk/diet/elements_fiber.html?referrer=https://www.google.com. Accessed September 20, 2016.

3. Astrup, A, Raben, A, and Geiker, N. The role of higher protein diets in weight control and obesity-related comorbidities. *Int J Obes (Lond)* 39:721-726, 2015.

4. Atkinson, F, Foster-Powell, K, and Brand-Miller, J. International tables of glycemic index and glycemic load values: 2008. *Diabetes Care* 31:2281-2283, 2008.

5. Bennett, CB, Chilibeck, PD, Barss, T, Vatanparast, H, Vandenberg, A, and Zello, GA. Metabolism and performance during extended high-intensity intermittent exercise after consumption of low- and high-glycaemic index pre-exercise meals. *Br J Nutr* 108 Suppl 1:S81-S90, 2012.

6. Burke, L, Collier, G, and Hargreaves, M. Glycemic index: A new tool in sports nutrition. *Int J Sport Nutr Exerc Metab* 8:401-415, 1998.

7. Burke, LM, Hawley, JA, Wong, SHS, and Jeukendrup, AE. Carbohydrates for training and competition. *J Sports Sci* 29:S17-S27, 2011.

8. Burton-Freeman, B. Dietary fiber and energy regulation. *J Nutr* 130:272s-275s, 2000.

9. Cahill Jr, GF. Starvation in man. *Clin Endocrinol Metab* 5:397-415, 1976.

10. Chiu, C, Liu, S, Willett, W, Wolever, T, Brand-Miller, J, Barclay, A, and Taylor, A. Informing food choices and health outcomes by use of the dietary glycemic index. *Nutr Rev* 69:231-242, 2011.

11. Chiu, YT, and Stewart, ML. Effect of variety and cooking method on resistant starch content of white rice and subsequent postprandial glucose response and appetite in humans. *Asia Pac J Clin Nutr* 22:372-379, 2013.

12. Clark, MJ, and Slavin, JL. The effect of fiber on satiety and food intake: A systematic review. *J Am Coll Nutr* 32:200-211, 2013.

13. Cleveland Clinic. Lactose Intolerance. 2016. http://my.clevelandclinic.org/health/diseases_conditions/hic_Lactose_Intolerance. Accessed September 20, 2016.

14. Cummings, J, and Stephen, A. Carbohydrate terminology and classification. *European Journal of Clinical Nutrition* 61:S5-S18, 2007.

15. Fitch, C, and Keim, KS. Position of the Academy of Nutrition and Dietetics: Use of nutritive and nonnutritive sweeteners. *J Acad Nutr Diet* 112:739-758, 2012.

16. FoodInsight. Background on Carbohydrates & Sugars. 2016. www.foodinsight.org/Background_on_Carbohydrates_Sugars.

17. Foster-Powell, K, Holt, S, and Brand-Miller, J. International table of glycemic index and glycemic load values. *Am J Clin Nutr* 76:5-56, 2002.

18. Harvard Medical School. Simple changes in diet can protect you against friendly fire. *Harvard Heart Letter* 2007. www.health.harvard.edu/family-health-guide/what-you-eat-can-fuel-or-cool-inflammation-a-key-driver-of-heart-disease-diabetes-and-other-chronic-conditions.

19. Hermansen, K, Rasmussen, O, Gregersen, S, and Larsen, S. Influence of ripeness of banana on the blood glucose and insulin response in type 2 diabetic subjects. *Diabet Med* 9:739-743, 1992.

20. Hu, FB. Resolved: There is sufficient scientific evidence that decreasing sugar-sweetened beverage consumption will reduce the prevalence of obesity and obesity-related diseases. *Obes Rev* 14:606-619, 2013.

21. Immonen, K, Ruusunen, M, Hissa, K, and Puolanne, E. Bovine muscle glycogen concentration in relation to finishing diet, slaughter and ultimate pH. *Meat Sci* 55:25-31, 2000.

22. Institute of Medicine. *Dietary Reference Intakes for Energy, Carbohydrate, Fiber, Fat, Fatty Acids, Cholesterol, Protein, and Amino Acids (Macronutrients).* Washington, DC: National Academies Press, 2005.

23. Ivy, JL. Muscle glycogen synthesis before and after exercise. *Sports Med* 11:6-19, 1991.

24. Jensen, J, Rustad, PI, Kolnes, AJ, and Lai, Y-C. The role of skeletal muscle glycogen breakdown for regulation of insulin sensitivity by exercise. *Front Physiol* 2:112, 2011.

25. Karpinski, C, and Rosenbloom, C. *Sports Nutrition: A Handbook for Professionals.* 6th ed. Chicago, IL: Academy of Nutrition and Dietetics, 2017.

26. Kenney, WL, Wilmore, JH, and Costill, DL. *Physiology of Sport and Exercise.* 6th ed. Champaign, IL: Human Kinetics, 2015.

27. Kreitzman, SN, Coxon, AY, and Szaz, KF. Glycogen storage: Illusions of easy weight loss, excessive weight regain, and distortions in estimates of body composition. *Am J Clin Nutr* 56:292s-293s, 1992.

28. Marmy-Conus, N, Fabris, S, Proietto, J, and Hargreaves, M. Preexercise glucose ingestion and glucose kinetics during exercise. *J Appl Physiol* 81:853-857, 1996.

29. Marsh, A, Eslick, EM, and Eslick, GD. Does a diet low in FODMAPs reduce symptoms associated with functional gastrointestinal disorders? A comprehensive systematic review and meta-analysis. *Eur J Nutr* 55:897-906, 2016.

30. Massougbodji, J, Le Bodo, Y, Fratu, R, and De Wals, P. Reviews examining sugar-sweetened beverages and body weight: Correlates of their quality and conclusions. *Am J Clin Nutr* 99:1096-1104, 2014.

31. McArdle, WD, Katch, FI, and Katch, VL. Macronutrient metabolism in exercise and training. In *Sports and Exercise Nutrition.* 4th ed. Baltimore, MD: Wolters Kluwer, 2013, pp. 167-178.

32. Monro, J, and Shaw, M. Glycemic impact, glycemic glucose equivalents, glycemic index, and glycemic load: Definitions, distinctions, and implications. *Am J Clin Nutr* 87:237S-243S, 2008.

33. National Institutes of Health. Glucose test. *Medline Plus.* www.nlm.nih.gov/medlineplus/ency/article/003482.htm.

34. National Institutes of Health. Glucose tolerance test. *Medline Plus.* www.nlm.nih.gov/medlineplus/ency/article/003466.htm.

35. Ross, CA, Caballero, B, Cousins, RJ, Tucker, KL, and Ziegler, TR. *Modern Nutrition in Health and Disease.* 11th ed. Baltimore, MD: Lippincott Williams & Wilkins, 2014.

36. Slavin, JL. Position of the American Dietetic Association: Health implications of dietary fiber. *J Am Diet Assoc* 108:1716-1731, 2008.

37. Tarnopolsky, MA, Gibala, M, Jeukendrup, AE, and Phillips, SM. Nutritional needs of elite endurance athletes. Part I: Carbohydrate and fluid requirements. *Eur J Sport Sci* 5:3-14, 2005.

38. Te Morenga, L, Mallard, S, and Mann, J. Dietary sugars and body weight: Systematic review and meta-analyses of randomised controlled trials and cohort studies. *BMJ* 346:e7492, 2013.

39. Thomas, DT, Erdman, KA, and Burke, LM. Position of the Academy of Nutrition and Dietetics, Dietitians of Canada, and the American College of Sports Medicine: Nutrition and athletic performance. *J Acad Nutr Diet* 116:501-528, 2016.

40. Thompson, JL, Manore, MM, and Vaughan, LA. *The Science of Nutrition.* Upper Saddle River, NJ: Pearson Education, 2017.

41. U.S. Department of Agriculture. Dietary Reference Intakes: Macronutrients. https://fnic.nal.usda.gov/sites/fnic.nal.usda.gov/files/uploads/macronutrients.pdf. Accessed February 17, 2017.

42. U.S. Department of Agriculture. USDA Choose MyPlate. www.choosemyplate.gov. Accessed Web Page, 2016.

43. U.S. Department of Agriculture. USDA National Nutrient Database for Standard Reference, Release 26. www.ars.usda.gov/ba/bhnrc/ndl. Accessed February 17, 2017.

44. U.S. Department of Agriculture. Dietary Guidelines for Americans, 2015-2020. 2015. https://health.gov/dietaryguidelines/2015/guidelines.

45. U.S. Food and Drug Administration. Additional Information About High-Intensity Sweeteners Permitted for Use in Food in the United States. www.fda.gov/Food/IngredientsPackagingLabeling/FoodAdditivesIngredients/ucm397725.htm#Advantame.

46. U.S. Food and Drug Administration. Food Labeling Guide. www.fda.gov/food/guidanceregulation/guidancedocumentsregulatoryinformation/labelingnutrition/ucm2006828.htm.

47. U.S. Food and Drug Administration. Guidance for Industry: Questions and Answers on FDA's Fortification Policy. www.fda.gov/Food/GuidanceRegulation/GuidanceDocumentsRegulatoryInformation/ucm470756.htm. Accessed September 6, 2016.

48. U.S. Food and Drug Administration. High Intensity Sweeteners. www.fda.gov/Food/IngredientsPackagingLabeling/FoodAdditivesIngredients/ucm397716.htm.

49. U.S. Food and Drug Administration. How Sweet It Is: All About Sugar Substitutes. 2014. www.fda.gov/ForConsumers/ConsumerUpdates/ucm397711.htm.

50. U.S. Food and Drug Administration. CFR—Code of Federal Regulations Title 21. 2016. www.accessdata.fda.gov/scripts/cdrh/cfdocs/cfcfr/CFRSearch.cfm?fr=137.165. Accessed September 6, 2017.

51. U.S. Food and Drug Administration. "Natural" on Food Labeling. 2016. www.fda.gov/Food/GuidanceRegulation/GuidanceDocumentsRegulatoryInformation/LabelingNutrition/ucm456090.htm. Accessed September 20, 2016.

52. Zijlstra, N, de Wijk, RA, Mars, M, Stafleu, A, and de Graaf, C. Effect of bite size and oral processing time of a semisolid food on satiation. *Am J Clin Nutr* 90:269-275, 2009.

Chapter 4

1. Adlof, RO, Duval, S, and Emken, EA. Biosynthesis of conjugated linoleic acid in humans. *Lipids* 35:131-135, 2000.

2. American College of Sports Medicine. Joint position statement: Nutrition and athletic performance. *Med Sci Sports Exerc* 32:2130-2145, 2000.

3. American Heart Association. AHA Scientific Statement. American Heart Association Guide for Improving Cardiovascular Health at the Community Level, 2013 Update: A Scientific Statement for Public Health Practitioners, Healthcare Providers, and Health Policy Makers. 2013. www.heart.org/idc/groups/heart-public/@wcm/@adv/documents/downloadable/ucm_467504.pdf.

4. Ander, BP, Dupasquier, CM, Prociuk, MA, and Pierce, GN. Polyunsaturated fatty acids and their effects on cardiovascular disease. *Exp Clin Cardiol* 8:164-172, 2003.

5. Anderson, BM, and Ma, DW. Are all n-3 polyunsaturated fatty acids created equal? *Lipids Health Dis* 8:33, 2009.

6. Anderson, JW, Allgood, LD, Lawrence, A, Altringer, LA, Jerdack, GR, Hengehold, DA, and Morel, JG. Cholesterol-lowering effects of psyllium intake adjunctive to diet therapy in men and women with hypercholesterolemia: Meta-analysis of 8 controlled trials. *Am J Clin Nutr* 71:472-479, 2000.

7. Aro, A, Antoine, J, Pizzoferrato, L, Reykdala, O, and van Poppel, G. Trans fatty acids and dairy and meat products from 14 European countries: The TRANSFAIR study. *J Food Compost Anal* 11:150-160, 1998.

8. Aro, A, Jauhiainen, M, Partanen, R, Salminen, I, and Mutanen, M. Stearic acid, trans fatty acids, and dairy fat: Effects on serum and lipoprotein lipids, apolipoproteins, lipoprotein(a), and lipid transfer proteins in healthy subjects. *Am J Clin Nutr* 65:1419-1426, 1997.

9. Aronis, KN, Khan, SM, and Mantzoros, CS. Effects of trans fatty acids on glucose homeostasis: A meta-analysis of randomized, placebo-controlled clinical trials. *Am J Clin Nutr* 96:1093-1099, 2012.

10. Bendsen, NT, Chabanova, E, Thomsen, HS, Larsen, TM, Newman, JW, Stender, S, Dyerberg, J, Haugaard, SB, and Astrup, A. Effect of trans fatty acid intake on abdominal and liver fat deposition and blood lipids: A randomized trial in overweight postmenopausal women. *Nutr Diabetes* 1:e4, 2011.

11. Bendsen, NT, Stender, S, Szecsi, PB, Pedersen, SB, Basu, S, Hellgren, LI, Newman, JW, Larsen, TM, Haugaard, SB, and Astrup, A. Effect of industrially produced trans fat on markers of systemic inflammation: Evidence from a randomized trial in women. *J Lipid Res* 52:1821-1828, 2011.

12. Berry, SE. Triacylglycerol structure and interesterification of palmitic and stearic acid-rich fats: An overview and implications for cardiovascular disease. *Nutr Res Rev* 22:3-17, 2009.

13. Bettelheim, FA, Brown, WH, Campbell, MK, and Farrell, SO. *Introduction to General, Organic, and Biochemistry.* 9th ed. Boston, MA: Brooks/Cole, Cengage Learning.

14. Beynen, AC, Katan, MB, and Van Zutphen, LF. Hypo- and hyperresponders: Individual differences in the response of serum cholesterol concentration to changes in diet. *Adv Lipid Res* 22:115-171, 1987.

15. Biong, AS, Muller, H, Seljeflot, I, Veierod, MB, and Pedersen, JI. A comparison of the effects of cheese and butter on serum lipids, haemostatic variables and homocysteine. *Br J Nutr* 92:791-797, 2004.

16. Bosch, J, Gerstein, HC, Dagenais, GR, Diaz, R, Dyal, L, Jung, H, Maggiono, AP, Probstfield, J, Ramachandran, A, Riddle, MC, Ryden, LE, and Yusuf, S. N-3 fatty acids and cardiovascular outcomes in patients with dysglycemia. *N Engl J Med* 367:309-318, 2012.

17. Brown, L, Rosner, B, Willett, WW, and Sacks, FM. Cholesterol-lowering effects of dietary fiber: A meta-analysis. *Am J Clin Nutr* 69:30-42, 1999.

18. Burdge, GC, and Wootton, SA. Conversion of alpha-linolenic acid to eicosapentaenoic, docosapentaenoic and docosahexaenoic acids in young women. *Br J Nutr* 88:411-420, 2002.

19. Burke, LM. Fueling strategies to optimize performance: training high or training low? *Scand J Med Sci Sports* 20 Suppl 2:48-58, 2010.

20. Burr, ML, Fehily, AM, Gilbert, JF, Rogers, S, Holliday, RM, Sweetnam, PM, Elwood, PC, and Deadman, NM. Effects of changes in fat, fish, and fibre intakes on death and myocardial reinfarction: Diet and reinfarction trial (DART). *Lancet* 2:757-761, 1989.

21. de Oliveira Otto, MC, Mozaffarian, D, Kromhout, D, Bertoni, AG, Sibley, CT, Jacobs, DR, Jr., and Nettleton, JA. Dietary intake of saturated fat by food source and incident cardiovascular disease: The Multi-Ethnic Study of Atherosclerosis. *Am J Clin Nutr* 96:397-404, 2012.

22. Dhaka, V, Gulia, N, Ahlawat, KS, and Khatkar, BS. Trans fats—Sources, health risks and alternative approach: A review. *J Food Sci Technol* 48:534-541, 2011.

23. Dirlewanger, M, di Vetta, V, Guenat, E, Battilana, P, Seematter, G, Schneiter, P, Jequier, E, and Tappy, L. Effects of short-term carbohydrate or fat overfeeding on energy expenditure and plasma leptin concentrations in healthy female subjects. *Int J Obes Relat Metab Disord* 24:1413-1418, 2000.

24. Eslick, GD, Howe, PR, Smith, C, Priest, R, and Bensoussan, A. Benefits of fish oil supplementation in hyperlipidemia: A systematic review and meta-analysis. *Int J Cardiol* 136:4-16, 2009.

25. Ferrier, D. *Biochemistry*. 6th ed. Baltimore, MD: Lippinocott, Williams & Wilkins, 2014.

26. Field, CJ, Blewett, HH, Proctor, S, and Vine, D. Human health benefits of vaccenic acid. *Appl Physiol Nutr Metab* 34:979-991, 2009.

27. Filippou, A, Teng, KT, Berry, SE, and Sanders, TA. Palmitic acid in the sn-2 position of dietary triacylglycerols does not affect insulin secretion or glucose homeostasis in healthy men and women. *Eur J Clin Nutr* 68:1036-1041, 2014.

28. Fleming, JA, and Kris-Etherton, PM. The evidence for alpha-linolenic acid and cardiovascular disease benefits: Comparisons with eicosapentaenoic acid and docosahexaenoic acid. *Adv Nutr* 5:863S-876S, 2014.

29. Frost, E. Effect of Dietary Protein Intake on Diet-Induced Thermogenesis During Overfeeding. . Oral abstract presentation at The Obesity Society Annual Meeting, 2014.

30. Gebauer, SK, Chardigny, JM, Jakobsen, MU, Lamarche, B, Lock, AL, Proctor, SD, and Baer, DJ. Effects of ruminant trans fatty acids on cardiovascular disease and cancer: A comprehensive review of epidemiological, clinical, and mechanistic studies. *Adv Nutr* 2:332-354, 2011.

31. GISSI-Prevenzione Investigators. Dietary supplementation with n-3 polyunsaturated fatty acids and vitamin E after myocardial infarction: Results of the GISSI-Prevenzione trial. *Lancet* 354:447-455, 1999.

32. Goldberg, RJ, and Katz, J. A meta-analysis of the analgesic effects of omega-3 polyunsaturated fatty acid supplementation for inflammatory joint pain. *Pain* 129:210-223, 2007.

33. Hall, KD. What is the required energy deficit per unit weight loss? *Int J Obes (Lond)* 32:573-576, 2008.

34. Harris, WS. Are n-3 fatty acids still cardioprotective? *Curr Opin Clin Nutr Metab Care* 16:141-149, 2013.

35. Harris, WS, Lemke, SL, Hansen, SN, Goldstein, DA, DiRienzo, MA, Su, H, Nemeth, MA, Taylor, ML, Ahmed, G, and George, C. Stearidonic acid-enriched soybean oil increased the omega-3 index, an emerging cardiovascular risk marker. *Lipids* 43:805-811, 2008.

36. Hawley, JA, Schabort, EJ, Noakes, TD, and Dennis, SC. Carbohydrate-loading and exercise performance. An update. *Sports Med* 24:73-81, 1997.

37. Hayes, KC. Synthetic and modified glycerides: Effects on plasma lipids. *Curr Opin Lipidol* 12:55-60, 2001.

38. He, K, Song, Y, Daviglus, ML, Liu, K, Van Horn, L, Dyer, AR, and Greenland, P. Accumulated evidence on fish consumption and coronary heart disease mortality: A meta-analysis of cohort studies. *Circulation* 109:2705-2711, 2004.

39. Helge, JW, Watt, PW, Richter, EA, Rennie, MJ, and Kiens, B. Fat utilization during exercise: Adaptation to a fat-rich diet increases utilization of plasma fatty acids and very low density lipoprotein-triacylglycerol in humans. *J Physiol* 537:1009-1020, 2001.

40. Hjerpsted, J, Leedo, E, and Tholstrup, T. Cheese intake in large amounts lowers LDL-cholesterol concentrations compared with butter intake of equal fat content. *Am J Clin Nutr* 94:1479-1484, 2011.

41. Horton, TJ, Drougas, H, Brachey, A, Reed, GW, Peters, JC, and Hill, JO. Fat and carbohydrate overfeeding in humans: Different effects on energy storage. *Am J Clin Nutr* 62:19-29, 1995.

42. Hulston, CJ, Venables, MC, Mann, CH, Martin, C, Philp, A, Baar, K, and Jeukendrup, AE. Training with low muscle glycogen enhances fat metabolism in well-trained

cyclists. *Med Sci Sports Exerc* 42:2046-2055, 2010.

43. Hunter, JE. Studies on effects of dietary fatty acids as related to their position on triglycerides. *Lipids* 36:655-668, 2001.

44. Hunter, JE, Zhang, J, and Kris-Etherton, PM. Cardiovascular disease risk of dietary stearic acid compared with trans, other saturated, and unsaturated fatty acids: A systematic review. *Am J Clin Nutr* 91:46-63, 2010.

45. Hussain, MM. A proposed model for the assembly of chylomicrons. *Atherosclerosis* 148:1-15, 2000.

46. Igel, M, Giesa, U, Lutjohann, D, and von Bergmann, K. Comparison of the intestinal uptake of cholesterol, plant sterols, and stanols in mice. *J Lipid Res* 44:533-538, 2003.

47. IUPAC-IUB Commission on Biochemical Nomenclature. The nomenclature of lipids (Recommendations 1976) *Biochem J* 171:21-35, 1978.

48. James, MJ, Sullivan, TR, Metcalf, RG, and Cleland, LG. Pitfalls in the use of randomised controlled trials for fish oil studies with cardiac patients. *Br J Nutr* 112:812-820, 2014.

49. James, MJ, Ursin, VM, and Cleland, LG. Metabolism of stearidonic acid in human subjects: Comparison with the metabolism of other n-3 fatty acids. *Am J Clin Nutr* 77:1140-1145, 2003.

50. Jeukendrup, AE. Regulation of fat metabolism in skeletal muscle. *Ann N Y Acad Sci* 967:217-235, 2002.

51. Joint FAO/WHO Expert Consultation on Fats and Fatty Acids in Human Nutrition. *Interim Summary of Conclusions and Dietary Recommendations on Total Fat & Fatty Acids.* Geneva: WHO, 2008.

52. Judd, JT, Clevidence, BA, Muesing, RA, Wittes, J, Sunkin, ME, and Podczasy, JJ. Dietary trans fatty acids: Effects on plasma lipids and lipoproteins of healthy men and women. *Am J Clin Nutr* 59:861-868, 1994.

53. Katan, MB, van Gastel, AC, de Rover, CM, van Montfort, MA, and Knuiman, JT. Differences in individual responsiveness of serum cholesterol to fat-modified diets in man. *Eur J Clin Invest* 18:644-647, 1988.

54. Kiessling, G, Schneider, J, and Jahreis, G. Long-term consumption of fermented dairy products over 6 months increases HDL cholesterol. *Eur J Clin Nutr* 56:843-849, 2002.

55. Klonoff, DC. Replacements for trans fats—Will there be an oil shortage? *J Diabetes Sci Technol* 1:415-422, 2007.

56. Konig, A, Bouzan, C, Cohen, JT, Connor, WE, Kris-Etherton, PM, Gray, GM, Lawrence, RS, Savitz, DA, and Teutsch, SM. A quantitative analysis of fish consumption and coronary heart disease mortality. *Am J Prev Med* 29:335-346, 2005.

57. Kris-Etherton, PM. AHA science advisory: Monounsaturated fatty acids and risk of cardiovascular disease. *J Nutr* 129:2280-2284, 1999.

58. Kromhout, D, Giltay, EJ, and Geleijnse, JM. N-3 fatty acids and cardiovascular events after myocardial infarction. *N Engl J Med* 363:2015-2026, 2010.

59. Lands, B. Omega-3 PUFAs lower the propensity for arachidonic acid cascade overreactions. *Biomed Res Int* 2015:285135, 2015.

60. Lemke, SL, Maki, KC, Hughes, G, Taylor, ML, Krul, ES, Goldstein, DA, Su, H, Rains, TM, and Mukherjea, R. Consumption of stearidonic acid-rich oil in foods increases red blood cell eicosapentaenoic acid. *J Acad Nutr Diet* 113:1044-1056, 2013.

61. Lewis, EJ, Radonic, PW, Wolever, TM, and Wells, GD. 21 days of mammalian omega-3 fatty acid supplementation improves aspects of neuromuscular function and performance in male athletes compared to olive oil placebo. *J Int Soc Sports Nutr* 12:28, 2015.

62. Li, K, Huang, T, Zheng, J, Wu, K, and Li, D. Effect of marine-derived n-3 polyunsaturated fatty acids on C-reactive protein, interleukin 6 and tumor necrosis factor alpha: A meta-analysis. *PLoS One* 9:e88103, 2014.

63. Li, Y, Hruby, A, Bernstein, AM, Ley, SH, Wang, DD, Chiuve, SE, Sampson, L, Rexrode, KM, Rimm, EB, Willett, WC, and Hu, FB. Saturated fats compared with unsaturated fats and sources of carbohydrates in relation to risk of coronary heart disease: A prospective cohort study. *J Am Coll Cardiol* 66:1538-1548, 2015.

64. Lichtenstein, AH, Ausman, LM, Jalbert, SM, and Schaefer, EJ. Effects of different forms of dietary hydrogenated fats on serum lipoprotein cholesterol levels. *N Engl J Med* 340:1933-1940, 1999.

65. Liu, YM. Medium-chain triglyceride (MCT) ketogenic therapy. *Epilepsia* 49 Suppl 8:33-36, 2008.

66. Marchioli, R, and Levantesi, G. N-3 PUFAs in cardiovascular disease. *Int J Cardiol* 170:S33-38, 2013.

67. McNamara, DJ, Lowell, AE, and Sabb, JE. Effect of yogurt intake on plasma lipid and lipoprotein levels in normolipidemic males. *Atherosclerosis* 79:167-171, 1989.

68. Meier, TB, Bellgowan, PS, Singh, R, Kuplicki, R, Polanski, DW, and Mayer, AR. Recovery of cerebral blood flow following sports-related concussion. *JAMA Neurol* 72:530-538, 2015.

69. Meijer, GW, and Weststrate, JA. Interesterification of fats in margarine: Effect on blood lipids, blood enzymes, and hemostasis parameters. *Eur J Clin Nutr* 51:527-534, 1997.

70. Mensink, RP, Zock, PL, Kester, AD, and Katan, MB. Effects of dietary fatty acids and carbohydrates on the ratio of serum total to HDL cholesterol and on serum lipids and apolipoproteins: a meta-analysis of 60 controlled trials. *Am J Clin Nutr* 77:1146-1155, 2003.

71. Miles, EA, and Calder, PC. Influence of marine n-3 polyunsaturated fatty acids on immune function and a systematic review of their effects on clinical outcomes in rheumatoid arthritis. *Br J Nutr* 107 Suppl 2:S171-S184, 2012.

72. Miller, PE, Van Elswyk, M, and Alexander, DD. Long-chain omega-3 fatty acids eicosapentaenoic acid and docosahexaenoic acid and blood pressure: A meta-analysis of randomized controlled trials. *Am J Hypertens* 27:885-896, 2014.

73. Mills, JD, Bailes, JE, Sedney, CL, Hutchins, H, and Sears, B. Omega-3 fatty acid supplementation and reduction of traumatic axonal injury in a rodent head injury model. *J Neurosurg* 114:77-84, 2011.

74. Mills, JD, Hadley, K, and Bailes, JE. Dietary supplementation with the omega-3 fatty acid docosahexaenoic acid in traumatic brain injury. *Neurosurgery* 68:474-481, 2011.

75. Mosley, EE, McGuire, MK, Williams, JE, and McGuire, MA. Cis-9, trans-11 conjugated linoleic acid is synthesized from vaccenic acid in lactating women. *J Nutr* 136:2297-2301, 2006.

76. Motard-Belanger, A, Charest, A, Grenier, G, Paquin, P, Chouinard, Y, Lemieux, S, Couture, P, and Lamarche, B. Study of the effect of trans fatty acids from ruminants on blood lipids and other risk factors for cardiovascular disease. *Am J Clin Nutr* 87:593-599, 2008.

77. Mozaffarian, D. Does alpha-linolenic acid intake reduce the risk of coronary heart disease? A review of the evidence. *Altern Ther Health Med* 11:24-30, 2005.

78. Mozaffarian, D. Fish and n-3 fatty acids for the prevention of fatal coronary heart disease and sudden cardiac death. *Am J Clin Nutr* 87:1991S-1996S, 2008.

79. Mozaffarian, D, Aro, A, and Willett, WC. Health effects of trans-fatty acids: Experimental and observational evidence. *Eur J Clin Nutr* 63 Suppl 2:S5-S21, 2009.

80. Mozaffarian, D, Katan, MB, Ascherio, A, Stampfer, MJ, and Willett, WC. Trans fatty acids and cardiovascular disease. *N Engl J Med* 354:1601-1613, 2006.

81. Mozaffarian, D, Micha, R, and Wallace, S. Effects on coronary heart disease of increasing polyunsaturated fat in place of saturated fat: A systematic review and meta-analysis of randomized controlled trials. *PLoS Med* 7:e1000252, 2010.

82. Mozaffarian, D, and Rimm, EB. Fish intake, contaminants, and human health: Evaluating the risks and the benefits. *JAMA* 296:1885-1899, 2006.

83. National Cholesterol Education Program. *Third Report of the National Cholesterol Education Program (NCEP) Expert Panel on Detection, Evaluation, and Treatment of High Blood Cholesterol in Adults (Adult Treatment Panel III)*. Washington, DC: National Institutes of Health, 2002.

84. National Research Council. *Diet and Health: Implications for Reducing Chronic Disease Risk*. Washington, DC: National Academies Press, 1989.

85. Nestel, P, Shige, H, Pomeroy, S, Cehun, M, Abbey, M, and Raederstorff, D. The n-3 fatty acids eicosapentaenoic acid and docosahexaenoic acid increase systemic arterial compliance in humans. *Am J Clin Nutr* 76:326-330, 2002.

86. Nishida, C, and Uauy, R. WHO Scientific Update on health consequences of trans fatty acids: Introduction. *Eur J Clin Nutr* 63 Suppl 2:S1-S4, 2009.

87. Noakes, M, and Clifton, PM. Oil blends containing partially hydrogenated or interesterified fats: Differential effects on plasma lipids. *Am J Clin Nutr* 68:242-247, 1998.

88. O'Donnell-Megaro, AM, Barbano, DM, and Bauman, DE. Survey of the fatty acid composition of retail milk in the United States including regional and seasonal variations. *J Dairy Sci* 94:59-65, 2011.

89. Ordovas, JM. Nutrigenetics, plasma lipids, and cardiovascular risk. *J Am Diet Assoc* 106:1074-1081, 2006.

90. Otten, J, Hellwig, J, and Meyers, L. *Dietary Reference Intakes: The Essential Guide to Nutrient Requirements*. Washington, DC: National Academies Press, 2006.

91. Pendergast, DR, Horvath, PJ, Leddy, JJ, and Venkatraman, JT. The role of dietary fat on performance, metabolism, and health. *Am J Sports Med* 24:S53-58, 1996.

92. Pitsiladis, YP, Duignan, C, and Maughan, RJ. Effects of alterations in dietary carbohydrate intake on running performance during a 10 km treadmill time trial. *Br J Sports Med* 30:226-231, 1996.

93. Plourde, M, and Cunnane, SC. Extremely limited synthesis of long chain polyunsaturates in adults: Implications for their dietary essentiality and use as supplements. *Appl Physiol Nutr Metab* 32:619-634, 2007.

94. Precht, D. Variation of trans fatty acids in milk fats. *Z Ernahrungswiss* 34:27-29, 1995.

95. Rauch, B, Schiele, R, Schneider, S, Diller, F, Victor, N, Gohlke, H, Gottwik, M, Steinbeck, G, Del Castillo, U, Sack, R, Worth, H, Katus, H, Spitzer, W, Sabin, G, Senges, J, and Group, OS. OMEGA, a randomized, placebo-controlled trial to test the effect of highly purified omega-3 fatty acids on top of modern guideline-adjusted therapy after myocardial infarction. *Circulation* 122:2152-2159, 2010.

96. Richelle, M, Enslen, M, Hager, C, Groux, M, Tavazzi, I, Godin, JP, Berger, A, Metairon, S, Quaile, S, Piguet-Welsch, C, Sagalowicz, L, Green, H, and Fay, LB. Both free and esterified plant sterols reduce cholesterol absorption and the bioavailability of beta-carotene and alpha-tocopherol in normocholesterolemic humans. *Am J Clin Nutr* 80:171-177, 2004.

97. Robins, AL, Davies, DM, and Jones, GE. The effect of nutritional manipulation on ultra-endurance performance: A case study. *Res Sports Med* 13:199-215, 2005.

98. Robinson, DM, Martin, NC, Robinson, LE, Ahmadi, L, Marangoni, AG, and Wright, AJ. Influence of interesterification of a stearic acid-rich spreadable fat on acute metabolic risk factors. *Lipids* 44:17-26, 2009.

99. Rodriguez, N, DiMarco, N, and Langley, S. Position of the American Dietetic Association, Dietitians of Canada, and the American College of Sports Medicine: Nutrition and athletic performance. *J Am Diet Assoc* 100:1543-1556, 2000.

100. Romijn, JA, Coyle, EF, Sidossis, LS, Gastaldelli, A, Horowitz, JF, Endert, E, and Wolfe, RR. Regulation of endogenous fat and carbohydrate metabolism in relation to exercise intensity and duration. *Am J Physiol* 265:E380-391, 1993.

101. Rosqvist, F, Iggman, D, Kullberg, J, Cedernaes, J, Johansson, HE, Larsson, A, Johansson, L, Ahlstrom, H, Arner, P, Dahlman, I, and Riserus, U. Overfeeding polyunsaturated and saturated fat causes distinct effects on liver and visceral fat accumulation in humans. *Diabetes* 63:2356-2368, 2014.

102. Rowlands, DS, and Hopkins, WG. Effects of high-fat and high-carbohydrate diets on metabolism and performance in cycling. *Metabolism* 51:678-690, 2002.

103. Salem, N, Jr., Litman, B, Kim, HY, and Gawrisch, K. Mechanisms of action of docosahexaenoic acid in the nervous system. *Lipids* 36:945-959, 2001.

104. Sanclemente, T, Marques-Lopes, I, Puzo, J, and Garcia-Otin, AL. Role of naturally-occurring plant sterols on intestinal cholesterol absorption and plasmatic levels. *J Physiol Biochem* 65:87-98, 2009.

105. Schrauwen-Hinderling, VB, Hesselink, MK, Schrauwen, P, and Kooi, ME. Intramyocellular lipid content in human skeletal muscle. *Obesity (Silver Spring)* 14:357-367, 2006.

106. Schwingshackl, L, and Hoffmann, G. Monounsaturated fatty acids and risk of cardiovascular disease: Synopsis of the evidence available from systematic reviews and meta-analyses. *Nutrients* 4:1989-2007, 2012.

107. Siri-Tarino, PW, Sun, Q, Hu, FB, and Krauss, RM. Meta-analysis of prospective cohort studies evaluating the association of saturated fat with cardiovascular disease. *Am J Clin Nutr* 91:535-546, 2010.

108. Siri-Tarino, PW, Sun, Q, Hu, FB, and Krauss, RM. Saturated fat, carbohydrate, and cardiovascular disease. *Am J Clin Nutr* 91:502-509, 2010.

109. Smith, GI, Atherton, P, Reeds, DN, Mohammed, BS, Rankin, D, Rennie, MJ, and Mittendorfer, B. Dietary omega-3 fatty acid supplementation increases the rate of muscle protein synthesis in older adults: A randomized controlled trial. *Am J Clin Nutr* 93:402-412, 2011.

110. Smith, GI, Julliand, S, Reeds, DN, Sinacore, DR, Klein, S, and Mittendorfer, B. Fish oil-derived n-3 PUFA therapy increases muscle mass and function in healthy older adults. *Am J Clin Nutr* 102:115-122, 2015.

111. Soerensen, KV, Thorning, TK, Astrup, A, Kristensen, M, and Lorenzen, JK. Effect of dairy calcium from cheese and milk on fecal fat excretion, blood lipids, and appetite in young men. *Am J Clin Nutr* 99:984-991, 2014.

112. Summers, LK, Fielding, BA, Bradshaw, HA, Ilic, V, Beysen, C, Clark, ML, Moore, NR, and Frayn, KN. Substituting dietary saturated fat with polyunsaturated fat changes abdominal fat distribution and improves insulin sensitivity. *Diabetologia* 45:369-377, 2002.

113. Sundram, K, Karupaiah, T, and Hayes, KC. Stearic acid-rich interesterified fat and trans-rich fat raise the LDL/HDL ratio and plasma glucose relative to palm olein in humans. *Nutr Metab (Lond)* 4:3, 2007.

114. Tarrago-Trani, MT, Phillips, KM, Lemar, LE, and Holden, JM. New and existing oils and fats used in products with reduced trans-fatty acid content. *J Am Diet Assoc* 106:867-880, 2006.

115. Tartibian, B, Maleki, BH, and Abbasi, A. Omega-3 fatty acids supplementation attenuates inflammatory markers after eccentric exercise in untrained men. *Clin J Sport Med* 21:131-137, 2011.

116. Tavazzi, L, Maggioni, AP, Marchioli, R, Barlera, S, Franzosi, MG, Latini, R, Lucci, D, Nicolosi, GL, Porcu, M, Tognoni, G, and Gissi, HFI. Effect of n-3 polyunsaturated fatty acids in patients with chronic heart failure (the GISSI-HF trial): A randomised, double-blind, placebo-controlled trial. *Lancet* 372:1223-1230, 2008.

117. Tholstrup, T, Hoy, CE, Andersen, LN, Christensen, RD, and Sandstrom, B. Does fat in milk, butter and cheese affect blood lipids and cholesterol differently? *J Am Coll Nutr* 23:169-176, 2004.

118. Thompson, FE, Subar, AF, Loria, CM, Reedy, JL, and Baranowski, T. Need for technological innovation in dietary assessment. *J Am Diet Assoc* 110:48-51, 2010.

119. Tsuchiya, Y, Yanagimoto, K, Nakazato, K, Hayamizu, K, and Ochi, E. Eicosapentaenoic and docosahexaenoic acids-rich fish oil supplementation attenuates strength loss and limited joint range of motion after eccentric contractions: A randomized, double-blind, placebo-controlled, parallel-group trial. *Eur J Appl Physiol* 116:1179-1188, 2016.

120. Turpeinen, AM, Mutanen, M, Aro, A, Salminen, I, Basu, S, Palmquist, DL, and Griinari,

JM. Bioconversion of vaccenic acid to conjugated linoleic acid in humans. *Am J Clin Nutr* 76:504-510, 2002.

121. U.S. Department of Agriculture. Glycerin: Handling/Processing. https://www.ams. usda.gov/sites/default/files/media/Glycerin%20Petition%20to%20remove%20 TR%202013.pdf.

122. U.S. Department of Agriculture. Nutrient Intakes From Food: Mean Amounts Consumed per Individual, by Gender and Age: What We Eat in America, NHANES 2009-2010. 2012. www.ars.usda.gov/ba/bhnrc/fsrg.

123. U.S. Department of Agriculture. USDA National Nutrient Database for Standard Reference, Release 26. 2013. www.ars.usda.gov/ba/bhnrc/ndl.

124. U.S. Department of Agriculture. 2015-2020 Dietary Guidelines for Americans. 2015. http://health.gov/dietaryguidelines/2015/guidelines.

125. U.S. Food and Drug Administration. Title 21: Food and drugs—Part 184: Direct food substances affirmed as generally recognized as safe. *Code of Federal Regulations*, 1997.

126. U.S. Food and Drug Administration. GRAS notices: GRN No. 283. 2009. www.accessdata.fda.gov/scripts/fdcc/index.cfm?-set=GRASNotices&id=283.

127. U.S. Food and Drug Administration. Final determination regarding partially hydrogenated oils. *Federal Register* 116:34650-34670 2015. https://www.federalregister.gov/articles/2015/06/17/2015-14883/final-determination-regarding-partially-hydrogenated-oils. 116.

128. U.S. Food and Drug Administration. Title 21: Food and drugs—Subpart I: Multipurpose additives. *Code of Federal Regulations* 3, 2015.

129. U.S. Food and Drug Administration. What You Need to Know About Mercury in Fish and Shellfish. March 2004. www.fda.gov/food/resourcesforyou/consumers/ucm110591.htm.

130. U.S. Institute of Medicine. *Dietary Reference Intakes for Energy, Carbohydrate, Fiber, Fat, Fatty Acids, Cholesterol, Protein and Amino Acids*. Washington, DC: National Academies Press, 2002.

131. Vannice, G, and Rasmussen, H. Position of the Academy of Nutrition and Dietetics: Dietary fatty acids for healthy adults. *J Acad Nutr Diet* 114:136-153, 2014.

132. Verkijk, M, Vecht, J, Gielkens, HA, Lamers, CB, and Masclee, AA. Effects of medium-chain and long-chain triglycerides on antroduodenal motility and small bowel transit time in man. *Dig Dis Sci* 42:1933-1939, 1997.

133. von Schacky, C. Omega-3 fatty acids in cardiovascular disease—An uphill battle. *Prostaglandins Leukot Essent Fatty Acids* 92:41-47, 2015.

134. Wachira, JK, Larson, MK, and Harris, WS. N-3 Fatty acids affect haemostasis but do not increase the risk of bleeding: Clinical observations and mechanistic insights. *Br J Nutr* 111:1652-1662, 2014.

135. Walker, CG, Jebb, SA, and Calder, PC. Stearidonic acid as a supplemental source of omega-3 polyunsaturated fatty acids to enhance status for improved human health. *Nutrition* 29:363-369, 2013.

136. Wang, C, Chung, M, Lichtenstein, A, Balk, E, Kupelnick, B, DeVine, D, Lawrence, A, and Lau, J. *Effects of Omega-3 Fatty Acids on Cardiovascular Disease: Evidence Report/Technology Assessment No. 94*. Rockville, MD: Agency for Healthcare Research and Quality, 2004.

137. Wang, C, Harris, WS, Chung, M, Lichtenstein, AH, Balk, EM, Kupelnick, B, Jordan, HS, and Lau, J. N-3 fatty acids from fish or fish-oil supplements, but not alpha-linolenic acid, benefit cardiovascular disease outcomes in primary- and secondary-prevention studies: A systematic review. *Am J Clin Nutr* 84:5-17, 2006.

138. Wang, T, Van, KC, Gavitt, BJ, Grayson, JK, Lu, YC, Lyeth, BG, and Pichakron, KO. Effect of fish oil supplementation in a rat model of multiple mild traumatic brain injuries. *Restor Neurol Neurosci* 31:647-659, 2013.

139. Wang, TY, Liu, M, Portincasa, P, and Wang, DQ. New insights into the molecular mechanism of intestinal fatty acid absorption. *Eur J Clin Invest* 43:1203-1223, 2013.

140. Wu, A, Ying, Z, and Gomez-Pinilla, F. Dietary omega-3 fatty acids normalize BDNF levels, reduce oxidative damage, and counteract learning disability after traumatic brain injury in rats. *J Neurotrauma* 21:1457-1467, 2004.

141. Wu, A, Ying, Z, and Gomez-Pinilla, F. Omega-3 fatty acids supplementation restores mechanisms that maintain brain homeostasis in traumatic brain injury. *J Neurotrauma* 24:1587-1595, 2007.

142. Wu, A, Ying, Z, and Gomez-Pinilla, F. The salutary effects of DHA dietary supplementation on cognition, neuroplasticity, and membrane homeostasis after brain trauma. *J Neurotrauma* 28:2113-2122, 2011.

143. Wu, A, Ying, Z, and Gomez-Pinilla, F. Exercise facilitates the action of dietary DHA on functional recovery after brain trauma. *Neuroscience* 248:655-663, 2013.

144. Wu, JH, and Mozaffarian, D. Omega-3 fatty acids, atherosclerosis progression and cardiovascular outcomes in recent trials: New pieces in a complex puzzle. *Heart* 100:530-533, 2014.

145. Zevenbergen, H, de Bree, A, Zeelenberg, M, Laitinen, K, van Duijn, G, and Floter, E. Foods with a high fat quality are essential for healthy diets. *Ann Nutr Metab* 54 Suppl 1:15-24, 2009.

Chapter 5

1. Abbatecola, AM, Chiodini, P, Gallo, C, Lakatta, E, Sutton-Tyrrell, K, Tylavsky, FA, Goodpaster, B, de Rekeneire, N, Schwartz, AV, Paolisso, G, and Harris, T. Pulse wave velocity is associated with muscle mass decline: Health ABC study. *Age* 34:469-478, 2012.

2. Areta, JL, Burke, LM, Camera, DM, West, DW, Crawshay, S, Moore, DR, Stellingwerff, T, Phillips, SM, Hawley, JA, and Coffey, VG. Reduced resting skeletal muscle protein synthesis is rescued by resistance exercise and protein ingestion following short-term energy deficit. *Am J Physiol Endocrinol Metab* 306:E989-997, 2014.

3. Bonaldo, P, and Sandri, M. Cellular and molecular mechanisms of muscle atrophy. *Dis Model Mech* 6:25-39, 2013.

4. Brocchieri, L, and Karlin, S. Protein length in eukaryotic and prokaryotic proteomes. *Nucleic Acids Res* 33:3390-3400, 2005.

5. Center for Disease Control and Prevention. FastStats: Diet/Nutrition. 2016. https://www.cdc.gov/nchs/fastats/diet.htm.

6. Churchward-Venne, TA, Burd, NA, Mitchell, CJ, West, DW, Philp, A, Marcotte, GR, Baker, SK, Baar, K, and Phillips, SM. Supplementation of a suboptimal protein dose with leucine or essential amino acids: Effects on myofibrillar protein synthesis at rest and following resistance exercise in men. *J Physiol* 590:2751-2765, 2012.

7. Dai, Z, Wu, Z, Jia, S, and Wu, G. Analysis of amino acid composition in proteins of animal tissues and foods as pre-column o-phthaldialdehyde derivatives by HPLC with fluorescence detection. *J Chromatogr B Analyt Technol Biomed Life Sci* 964:116-127, 2014.

8. Escott-Stump, S. *Nutrition and Diagnosis-Related Care.* Philadelphia: Wolters Kluwer, 2015.

9. Hartman, JW, Tang, JE, Wilkinson, SB, Tarnopolsky, MA, Lawrence, RL, Fullerton, AV, and Phillips, SM. Consumption of fat-free fluid milk after resistance exercise promotes greater lean mass accretion than does consumption of soy or carbohydrate in young, novice, male weightlifters. *Am J Clin Nutr* 86:373-381, 2007.

10. Institute of Medicine. *Dietary Reference Intakes for Energy, Carbohydrate, Fiber, Fat, Fatty Acids, Cholesterol, Protein, and Amino Acids (Macronutrients).* Washington, DC: National Academies Press, 2005.

11. Josse, AR, Atkinson, SA, Tarnopolsky, MA, and Phillips, SM. Increased consumption of dairy foods and protein during diet- and exercise-induced weight loss promotes fat mass loss and lean mass gain in overweight

and obese premenopausal women. *J Nutr* 141:1626-1634, 2011.

12. Josse, AR, Tang, JE, Tarnopolsky, MA, and Phillips, SM. Body composition and strength changes in women with milk and resistance exercise. *Med Sci Sports Exerc* 42:1122-1130, 2010.

13. Kato, H, Suzuki, K, Bannai, M, and Moore, DR. Protein requirements are elevated in endurance athletes after exercise as determined by the indicator amino acid oxidation method. *PLoS One* 11:e0157406, 2016.

14. Layman, DK. Dietary Guidelines should reflect new understandings about adult protein needs. *Nutr Metab (Lond)* 6:12, 2009.

15. Manore, MM. Exercise and the Institute of Medicine recommendations for nutrition. *Curr Sports Med Rep* 4:193-198, 2005.

16. Matthews, DE. Proteins and amino acids. In *Modern Nutrition in Health and Disease.* Ross, AC, ed. Philadelphia: Wolters Kluwer Health/Lippincott Williams & Wilkins, 2014.

17. Mettler, S, Mitchell, N, and Tipton, KD. Increased protein intake reduces lean body mass loss during weight loss in athletes. *Med Sci Sports Exerc* 42:326-337, 2010.

18. Mitchell, HH, Hamilton, TS, Steggerda, FR, and Bean, HW. The chemical composition of the adult human body and its bearing on the biochemistry of growth. *J Biol Chem* 158:625-637, 1945.

19. Moore, DR, and Slater, G. Protein. In *Clinical Sports Nutrition.* Burke, L, Deakin, V, eds.: McGraw-Hill Education, 2015.

20. Morton, RW, McGlory, C, and Phillips, SM. Nutritional interventions to augment resistance training-induced skeletal muscle hypertrophy. *Front Physiol* 6:245, 2015.

21. National Center for Health Statistics. National Health and Nutrition Examination Survey Data. 2014. www.cdc.gov/nchs/nhanes/about_nhanes.htm.

22. Pennings, B, Boirie, Y, Senden, JM, Gijsen, AP, Kuipers, H, and van Loon, LJ. Whey protein stimulates postprandial muscle protein accretion more effectively than do casein and casein hydrolysate in older men. *Am J Clin Nutr* 93:997-1005, 2011.

23. Phillips, SM. Dietary protein requirements and adaptive advantages in athletes. *Br J Nutr* 108 Suppl 2:S158-S167, 2012.

24. Phillips, SM, Chevalier, S, and Leidy, HJ. Protein "requirements" beyond the RDA: Implications for optimizing health. *Appl Physiol Nutr Metab* 41:565-572, 2016.

25. Phillips, SM, and Van Loon, LJ. Dietary protein for athletes: From requirements to optimum adaptation. *J Sports Sci* 29 Suppl 1:S29-S38, 2011.

26. Rand, WM, Pellett, PL, and Young, VR. Meta-analysis of nitrogen balance studies for estimating protein requirements in healthy adults. *Am J Clin Nutr* 77:109-127, 2003.

27. Rodriguez, NR, Vislocky, LM, and Gaine, PC. Dietary protein, endurance exercise, and human skeletal-muscle protein turnover. *Curr Opin Clin Nutr Metab Care* 10:40-45, 2007.

28. Rosenbloom, CA, and Coleman, EJ. *Sports Nutrition: A Practice Manual for Professionals.* Academy of Nutrition and Dietetics, 2012.

29. Sarwar, G, and McDonough, FE. Evaluation of protein digestibility-corrected amino acid score method for assessing protein quality of foods. *J Assoc Off Anal Chem* 73:347-356, 1990.

30. Thomas, DT, Erdman, KA, and Burke, LM. American College of Sports Medicine joint position statement: Nutrition and athletic performance. *Med Sci Sports Exerc* 48:543-568, 2016.

31. Tipton, KD, Elliott, TA, Cree, MG, Aarsland, AA, Sanford, AP, and Wolfe, RR. Stimulation of net muscle protein synthesis by whey protein ingestion before and after exercise. *Am J Physiol Endocrinol Metab* 292:E71-E76, 2007.

32. U.S. Department of Agriculture and U.S. Department of Health & Human Services. Dietary Guidelines for Americans 2015-2020. 2015. https://health.gov/dietaryguidelines/2015/resources/2015-2020_Dietary_Guidelines.pdf.

33. U.S. Department of Agriculture and U.S. Department of Health & Human Services. *Dietary Guidelines for Americans, 2015-2020.* Wise Age Books, 2015.

34. U.S. Food and Drug Administration. Guidance for Industry: A Food Labeling Guide (Appendix B: Additional Requirements for Nutrient Content Claims). 2015. www.fda.gov/Food/GuidanceRegulation/GuidanceDocumentsRegulatoryInformation/LabelingNutrition/ucm064916.htm.

35. Wall, BT, Morton, JP, and van Loon, LJ. Strategies to maintain skeletal muscle mass in the injured athlete: Nutritional considerations and exercise mimetics. *Eur J Sport Sci* 15:53-62, 2015.

36. Wentz, L, Liu, PY, Ilich, JZ, and Haymes, EM. Dietary and training predictors of stress fractures in female runners. *Int J Sport Nutr Exerc Metab* 22:374-382, 2012.

37. World Health Organization. *Protein and Amino Acid Requirements in Human Nutrition.* Geneva: World Health Organization, 2007.

38. Zaheer, K, and Humayoun Akhtar, M. An updated review of dietary isoflavones: Nutrition, processing, bioavailability and impacts on human health. *Crit Rev Food Sci Nutr* 57:1280-1293, 2017.

Chapter 6

1. Akhtar, S, Ahmed, A, Randhawa, MA, Atukorala, S, Arlappa, N, Ismail, T, and Ali, Z. Prevalence of vitamin A deficiency in South Asia: Causes, outcomes, and possible remedies. *J Health Popul Nutr* 31:413-423, 2013.

2. Allen, L, de Benoist, B, Dary, O, and Hurrell, R. *Guidelines on Food Fortification with Micronutrients.* Geneva: World Health Organization and Food and Agricultural Organization of the United Nations, 2006.

3. Allen, LH. How common is vitamin B-12 deficiency? *Am J Clin Nutr* 89:693S-696S, 2009.

4. Ardestani, A, Parker, B, Mathur, S, Clarkson, P, Pescatello, LS, Hoffman, HJ, Polk, DM, and Thompson, PD. Relation of vitamin D level to maximal oxygen uptake in adults. *Am J Cardiol* 107:1246-1249, 2011.

5. Armas, L, Hollis, B, and Heaney, RP. Vitamin D2 is much less effective than vitamin D3 in humans. *J Clin Endocrinol Metab* 89:5387-5391, 2004.

6. Bailey, RL, Carmel, R, Green, R, Pfeiffer, CM, Cogswell, ME, Osterloh, JD, Sempos, CT, and Yetley, EA. Monitoring of vitamin B-12 nutritional status in the United States by using plasma methylmalonic acid and serum vitamin B-12. *Am J Clin Nutr* 94:552-561, 2011.

7. Bailey, RL, Dodd, KW, Gahche, JJ, Dwyer, JT, McDowell, MA, Yetley, EA, Sempos, CA, Burt, VL, Radimer, KL, and Picciano, MF. Total folate and folic acid intake from foods and dietary supplements in the United States: 2003-2006. *Am J Clin Nutr* 91:231-237, 2010.

8. Barker, T, Martins, T, Hill, H, Kjeldsberg, C, Trawick, R, Weaver, L, and Traber, M. Low vitamin D impairs strength recovery after anterior cruciate ligament surgery. *JEBCAM* 16:201-209, 2011.

9. Beals, KA, and Manore, MM. Nutritional status of female athletes with subclinical eating disorders. *J Am Diet Assoc* 98:419-425, 1998.

10. Beaudart, C, Buckinx, F, Rabenda, V, Gillain, S, Cavalier, E, Slomian, J, Petermans, J, Reginster, JY, and Bruyere, O. The effects of vitamin D on skeletal muscle strength, muscle mass, and muscle power: A systematic review and meta-analysis of randomized controlled trials. *J Clin Endocrinol Metab* 99:4336-4345, 2014.

11. Beer, TM, and Myrthue, A. Calcitriol in cancer treatment: from the lab to the clinic. *Mol Cancer Ther* 3:373-381, 2004.

12. Belko, AZ, Meredith, MP, Kalkwarf, HJ, Obarzanek, E, Weinberg, S, Roach, R, McKeon, G, and Roe, DA. Effects of exercise on riboflavin requirements: Biological validation in weight reducing women. *Am J Clin Nutr* 41:270-277, 1985.

13. Bendich, A, and Cohen, M. Vitamin B6 safety issues. *Ann N Y Acad Sci* 585:321-330, 1990.

14. Bergen-Cico, DK, and Short, SH. Dietary intakes, energy expenditures, and anthropo-

metric characteristics of adolescent female cross-country runners. *J Am Diet Assoc* 92:611-612, 1992.

15. Bergstrom, J, Hultman, E, Jorfeldt, L, Pernow, B, and Wahren, J. Effect of nicotinic acid on physical working capacity and on metabolism of muscle glycogen in man. *J Appl Physiol* 26:170-176, 1969.

16. Berry, DJ, Hesketh, K, Power, C, and Hypponen, E. Vitamin D status has a linear association with seasonal infections and lung function in British adults. *Br J Nutr* 106:1433-1440, 2011.

17. Bescos Garcia, R, and Rodriquez Guisado, F. Low levels of vitamin D in professional basketball players after wintertime: Relationship with dietary intake of vitamin D and calcium. *Nutr Hosp* 26:945-951, 2011.

18. Bikle, DD. Vitamin D metabolism, mechanism of action, and clinical applications. *Chem Biol* 21:319-329, 2014.

19. Birge, SJ, and Haddad, JG. 25-hydroxycholecalciferol stimulation of muscle metabolism. *J Clin Invest* 56:1100-1107, 1975.

20. Bischoff-Ferrari, HA. Vitamin D and fracture prevention. *Endocrinol Metab Clin North Am* 39:347-353, 2010.

21. Bischoff-Ferrari, HA, Dietrich, T, Orav, EJ, Hu, FB, Zhang, Y, Karlson, EW, and Dawson-Hughes, B. Higher 25-hydroxyvitamin D concentrations are associated with better lower-extremity function in both active and inactive persons aged > or =60 y. *Am J Clin Nutr* 80:752-758, 2004.

22. Bischoff-Ferrari, HA, Shao, A, Dawson-Hughes, B, Hathcock, J, Giovannucci, E, and Willett, WC. Benefit-risk assessment of vitamin D supplementation. *Osteoporos Int* 21:1121-1132, 2010.

23. Blumberg, J, and Block, G. The alpha-tocopherol, beta-carotene cancer prevention study in finland. *Nutr Rev* 52:242-245, 1994.

24. Boldorini, R, Vago, L, Lechi, A, Tedeschi, F, and Trabattoni, GR. Wernicke's encephalopathy: occurrence and pathological aspects in a series of 400 AIDS patients. *Acta Biomed Ateneo Parmense* 63:43-49, 1992.

25. Boniol, M, Autier, P, Boyle, P, and Gandini, S. Cutaneous melanoma attributable to sunbed use: Systematic review and meta-analysis. *BMJ* 345:e4757, 2012.

26. Borowitz, D, Baker, RD, and Stallings, V. Consensus report on nutrition for pediatric patients with cystic fibrosis. *J Pediatr Gastroenterol Nutr* 35:246-259, 2002.

27. Braakhuis, AJ. Effect of vitamin C supplements on physical performance. *Curr Sports Med Rep* 11:180-184, 2012.

28. Braakhuis, AJ, and Hopkins, WG. Impact of dietary antioxidants on sport performance: A review. *Sports Med* 45:939-955, 2015.

29. Cantorna, MT, and Mahon, BD. D-hormone and the immune system. *J Rheumatol Suppl* 76:11-20, 2005.

30. Carmel, R. Malabsorption of food cobalamin. *Baillieres Clin Haematol* 8:639-655, 1995.

31. Carr, AC, and Frei, B. Toward a new recommended dietary allowance for vitamin C based on antioxidant and health effects in humans. *Am J Clin Nutr* 69:1086-1107, 1999.

32. Carrillo, AE, Murphy, RJ, and Cheung, SS. Vitamin C supplementation and salivary immune function following exercise-heat stress. *Int J Sports Physiol Perform* 3:516-530, 2008.

33. Centers for Disease Control and Prevention. Indoor Tanning Is Not Safe. 2016. www.cdc.gov/cancer/skin/basic_info/indoor_tanning.htm. Accessed July 12, 2016.

34. Chester, D, Goldman, J, Ahuja, J, and Moshfegh, A. *Dietary Intakes of Choline: What We Eat in America, NHANES 2007-2008.* 2011.

35. Ciocoiu, M, Badescu, M, and Paduraru, I. Protecting antioxidative effects of vitamins E and C in experimental physical stress. *J Physiol Biochem* 63:187-194, 2007.

36. Clark, M, Reed, DB, Crouse, SF, and Armstrong, RB. Pre- and post-season dietary intake, body composition, and performance indices of NCAA division I female soccer players. *Int J Sport Nutr Exerc Metab* 13:303-319, 2003.

37. Close, GL, Russell, J, Cobley, JN, Owens, DJ, Wilson, G, Gregson, W, Fraser, WD, and Morton, JP. Assessment of vitamin D concentration in non-supplemented professional athletes and healthy adults during the winter months in the UK: Implications for skeletal muscle function. *J Sports Sci* 31:344-353, 2013.

38. Colantonio, S, Bracken, MB, and Beecker, J. The association of indoor tanning and melanoma in adults: Systematic review and meta-analysis. *J Am Acad Dermatol* 70:847-857, 2014.

39. Dawson-Hughes, B, Harris, SS, Lichtenstein, AH, Dolnikowski, G, Palermo, NJ, and Rasmussen, H. Dietary fat increases vitamin D-3 absorption. *J Acad Nutr Diet* 115:225-230, 2015.

40. De Roos, AJ, Arab, L, Renner, JB, Craft, N, Luta, G, Helmick, CG, Hochberg, MC, and Jordan, JM. Serum carotenoids and radiographic knee osteoarthritis: The Johnston County Osteoarthritis Project. *Public Health Nutr* 4:935-942, 2001.

41. DeLuca, HF. The transformation of a vitamin into a hormone: The vitamin D story. *Harvey Lect* 75:333-379, 1979.

42. Deluca, HF, and Cantorna, MT. Vitamin D: Its role and uses in immunology. *FASEB J* 15:2579-2585, 2001.

43. Deuster, PA, Kyle, SB, Moser, PB, Vigersky, RA, Singh, A, and Schoomaker, EB. Nutritional survey of highly trained women runners. *Am J Clin Nutr* 44:954-962, 1986.

44. Dijkhuizen, MA, Wieringa, FT, West, CE, Muherdiyantiningsih, and Muhilal. Concurrent micronutrient deficiencies in lactating mothers and their infants in Indonesia. *Am J Clin Nutr* 73:786-791, 2001.

45. Doyle, MR, Webster, MJ, and Erdmann, LD. Allithiamine ingestion does not enhance isokinetic parameters of muscle performance. *Int J Sport Nutr* 7:39-47, 1997.

46. Economos, CD, Bortz, SS, and Nelson, ME. Nutritional practices of elite athletes: Practical recommendations. *Sports Med* 16:381-399, 1993.

47. Faber, M, and Benade, AJ. Mineral and vitamin intake in field athletes (discus-, hammer-, javelin-throwers and shotputters). *Int J Sports Med* 12:324-327, 1991.

48. Feldmeyer, L, Shojaati, G, Spanaus, KS, Navarini, A, Theler, B, Donghi, D, Urosevic-Maiwald, M, Glatz, M, Imhof, L, Barysch, MJ, Dummer, R, Roos, M, French, LE, Surber, C, and Hofbauer, GF. Phototherapy with UVB narrowband, UVA/UVBnb, and UVA1 differentially impacts serum 25-hydroxyvitamin-D3. *J Am Acad Dermatol* 69:530-536, 2013.

49. Fischer, LM, daCosta, KA, Kwock, L, Stewart, PW, Lu, TS, Stabler, SP, Allen, RH, and Zeisel, SH. Sex and menopausal status influence human dietary requirements for the nutrient choline. *Am J Clin Nutr* 85:1275-1285, 2007.

50. Fogelholm, M, Ruokonen, I, Laakso, JT, Vuorimaa, T, and Himberg, JJ. Lack of association between indices of vitamin B1, B2, and B6 status and exercise-induced blood lactate in young adults. *Int J Sport Nutr* 3:165-176, 1993.

51. Forrest, KY, and Stuhldreher, WL. Prevalence and correlates of vitamin D deficiency in US adults. *Nutr Res* 31:48-54, 2011.

52. Fulgoni, VL, 3rd, Keast, DR, Bailey, RL, and Dwyer, J. Foods, fortificants, and supplements: Where do Americans get their nutrients? *J Nutr* 141:1847-1854, 2011.

53. Gaeini, AA, Rahnama, N, and Hamedinia, MR. Effects of vitamin E supplementation on oxidative stress at rest and after exercise to exhaustion in athletic students. *J Sports Med Phys Fitness* 46:458-461, 2006.

54. Gdynia, HJ, Muller, T, Sperfeld, AD, Kuhnlein, P, Otto, M, Kassubek, J, and Ludolph, AC. Severe sensorimotor neuropathy after intake of highest dosages of vitamin B6. *Neuromuscul Disord* 18:156-158, 2008.

55. Gerster, H. The role of vitamin C in athletic performance. *J Am Coll Nutr* 8:636-643, 1989.

56. Ginde, AA, Mansbach, JM, and Camargo, CA, Jr. Association between serum

25-hydroxyvitamin D level and upper respiratory tract infection in the Third National Health and Nutrition Examination Survey. *Arch Intern Med* 169:384-390, 2009.

57. Ginter, E, Simko, V, and Panakova, V. Antioxidants in health and disease. *Bratisl Lek Listy* 115:603-606, 2014.

58. Girgis, CM, Clifton-Bligh, RJ, Hamrick, MW, Holick, MF, and Gunton, JE. The roles of vitamin D in skeletal muscle: form, function, and metabolism. *Endocr Rev* 34:33-83, 2013.

59. Gomez-Cabrera, MC, Salvador-Pascual, A, Cabo, H, Ferrando, B, and Vina, J. Redox modulation of mitochondriogenesis in exercise: Does antioxidant supplementation blunt the benefits of exercise training? *Free Radic Biol Med* 86:37-46, 2015.

60. Goodman, GE, Thornquist, MD, Balmes, J, Cullen, MR, Meyskens, FL, Jr., Omenn, GS, Valanis, B, and Williams, JH, Jr. The Beta-Carotene and Retinol Efficacy Trial: Incidence of lung cancer and cardiovascular disease mortality during 6-year follow-up after stopping beta-carotene and retinol supplements. *J Natl Cancer Inst* 96:1743-1750, 2004.

61. Grober, U, and Kisters, K. Influence of drugs on vitamin D and calcium metabolism. *Dermatoendocrinol* 4:158-166, 2012.

62. Gueant, JL, Safi, A, Aimone-Gastin, I, Rabesona, H, Bronowicki, JP, Plenat, F, Bigard, MA, and Haertle, T. Autoantibodies in pernicious anemia type I patients recognize sequence 251-256 in human intrinsic factor. *Proc Assoc Am Physicians* 109:462-469, 1997.

63. Halliday, TM, Peterson, NJ, Thomas, JJ, Kleppinger, K, Hollis, BW, and Larson-Meyer, DE. Vitamin D status relative to diet, lifestyle, injury, and illness in college athletes. *Med Sci Sports Exerc* 43:335-343, 2011.

64. Hamilton, B. Vitamin D and athletic performance: The potential role of muscle. *Asian J Sports Med* 2:211-219, 2011.

65. Hamilton, B, Grantham, J, Racinais, S, and Chalabi, H. Vitamin D deficiency is endemic in Middle Eastern sportsmen. *Public Health Nutr* 13:1528-1534, 2010.

66. Hartley, L, Clar, C, Ghannam, O, Flowers, N, Stranges, S, and Rees, K. Vitamin K for the primary prevention of cardiovascular disease. *Cochrane Database Syst Rev*:CD011148, 2015.

67. He, CS, Handzlik, M, Fraser, WD, Muhamad, A, Preston, H, Richardson, A, and Gleeson, M. Influence of vitamin D status on respiratory infection incidence and immune function during 4 months of winter training in endurance sport athletes. *Exerc Immunol Rev* 19:86-101, 2013.

68. Heaney, RP, and Holick, MF. Why the IOM recommendations for vitamin D are deficient. *J Bone Miner Res* 26:455-457, 2011.

69. Hickson, JF, Jr., Schrader, J, and Trischler, LC. Dietary intakes of female basketball and gymnastics athletes. *J Am Diet Assoc* 86:251-253, 1986.

70. Holick, MF. Environmental factors that influence the cutaneous production of vitamin D. *Am J Clin Nutr* 61:638S-645S, 1995.

71. Holick, MF. Vitamin D deficiency. *N Engl J Med* 357:266-281, 2007.

72. Holick, MF. Vitamin D status: Measurement, interpretation, and clinical application. *Ann Epidemiol* 19:73-78, 2009.

73. Holick, MF, Biancuzzo, R, Chen, T, Klein, E, Young, A, Bibuld, D, Reitz, R, Salameh, W, Ameri, A, and Tannenbaum, A. Vitamin D2 is as effective as vitamin D3 in maintaining circulating concentrations of 25-hydroxyvitamin D. *J Clin Endocrinol Metab* 93:677-681, 2008.

74. Holick, MF, Binkley, NC, Bischoff-Ferrari, HA, Gordon, CM, Hanley, DA, Heaney, RP, Murad, MH, Weaver, CM, and Endocrine, S. Evaluation, treatment, and prevention of vitamin D deficiency: An Endocrine Society clinical practice guideline. *J Clin Endocrinol Metab* 96:1911-1930, 2011.

75. Hoyumpa, AM, Jr. Mechanisms of thiamin deficiency in chronic alcoholism. *Am J Clin Nutr* 33:2750-2761, 1980.

76. Jermendy, G. Evaluating thiamine deficiency in patients with diabetes. *Diab Vasc Dis Res* 3:120-121, 2006.

77. Johnston, CS, Swan, PD, and Corte, C. Substrate utilization and work efficiency during submaximal exercise in vitamin C depleted-repleted adults. *Int J Vitam Nutr Res* 69:41-44, 1999.

78. Khan, MA, Gilbert, C, Khan, MD, Qureshi, MB, and Ahmad, K. Incidence of blinding vitamin A deficiency in North West Frontier Province and its adjoining Federally Administered Tribal Areas, Pakistan. *Ophthalmic Epidemiol* 16:2-7, 2009.

79. Kim, J, and Lee, J. A review of nutritional intervention on delayed onset muscle soreness. Part I. *J Exerc Rehabil* 10:349-356, 2014.

80. Kimura, M, Itokawa, Y, and Fujiwara, M. Cooking losses of thiamin in food and its nutritional significance. *J Nutr Sci Vitaminol (Tokyo)* 36 Suppl 1:S17-S24, 1990.

81. Klein, EA, Thompson, IM, Jr., Tangen, CM, Crowley, JJ, Lucia, MS, Goodman, PJ, Minasian, LM, Ford, LG, Parnes, HL, Gaziano, JM, Karp, DD, Lieber, MM, Walther, PJ, Klotz, L, Parsons, JK, Chin, JL, Darke, AK, Lippman, SM, Goodman, GE, Meyskens, FL, Jr., and Baker, LH. Vitamin E and the risk of prostate cancer: The Selenium and Vitamin E Cancer Prevention Trial (SELECT). *JAMA* 306:1549-1556, 2011.

82. Koundourakis, NE, Androulakis, NE, Malliaraki, N, and Margioris, AN. Vitamin D and exercise performance in professional soccer players. *PLoS One* 9:e101659, 2014.

83. Krause, R, Patruta, S, Daxbock, F, Fladerer, P, Biegelmayer, C, and Wenisch, C. Effect of vitamin C on neutrophil function after high-intensity exercise. *Eur J Clin Invest* 31:258-263, 2001.

84. Kukreja, RC, and Hess, ML. The oxygen free radical system: from equations through membrane-protein interactions to cardiovascular injury and protection. *Cardiovasc Res* 26:641-655, 1992.

85. LeBlanc, ES, Zakher, B, Daeges, M, Pappas, M, and Chou, R. Screening for vitamin D deficiency: A systematic review for the U.S. Preventive Services Task Force. *Ann Intern Med* 162:109-122, 2015.

86. Leonard, SW, and Leklem, JE. Plasma B-6 vitamer changes following a 50-km ultra-marathon. *Int J Sport Nutr Exerc Metab* 10:302-314, 2000.

87. Leppala, JM, Virtamo, J, Fogelholm, R, Huttunen, JK, Albanes, D, Taylor, PR, and Heinonen, OP. Controlled trial of alpha-tocopherol and beta-carotene supplements on stroke incidence and mortality in male smokers. *Arterioscler Thromb Vasc Biol* 20:230-235, 2000.

88. Lindenbaum, J, Rosenberg, IH, Wilson, PW, Stabler, SP, and Allen, RH. Prevalence of cobalamin deficiency in the Framingham elderly population. *Am J Clin Nutr* 60:2-11, 1994.

89. Lo, CW, Paris, PW, Clemens, TL, Nolan, J, and Holick, MF. Vitamin D absorption in healthy subjects and in patients with intestinal malabsorption syndromes. *Am J Clin Nutr* 42:644-649, 1985.

90. Lobo, GP, Amengual, J, Baus, D, Shivdasani, RA, Taylor, D, and von Lintig, J. Genetics and diet regulate vitamin A production via the homeobox transcription factor ISX. *J Biol Chem* 288:9017-9027, 2013.

91. Lobo, V, Patil, A, Phatak, A, and Chandra, N. Free radicals, antioxidants and functional foods: Impact on human health. *Pharmacogn Rev* 4:118-126, 2010.

92. Loosli, AR, and Benson, J. Nutritional intake in adolescent athletes. *Pediatr Clin North Am* 37:1143-1152, 1990.

93. Lotfi, A, Abdel-Nasser, AM, Hamdy, A, Omran, AA, and El-Rehany, MA. Hypovitaminosis D in female patients with chronic low back pain. *Clin Rheumatol* 26:1895-1901, 2007.

94. Lukaski, HC. Vitamin and mineral status: Effects on physical performance. *Nutrition* 20:632-644, 2004.

95. Mangin, M, Sinha, R, and Fincher, K. Inflammation and vitamin D: The infection connection. *Inflamm Res* 63:803-819, 2014.

96. Manore, MM. Effect of physical activity on thiamine, riboflavin, and vitamin B-6 requirements. *Am J Clin Nutr* 72:598S-606S, 2000.

97. Manore, MN, Leklem, JE, and Walter, MC. Vitamin B-6 metabolism as affected by exercise in trained and untrained women fed diets differing in carbohydrate and vitamin B-6 content. *Am J Clin Nutr* 46:995-1004, 1987.

98. Maroon, JC, Mathyssek, CM, Bost, JW, Amos, A, Winkelman, R, Yates, AP, Duca, MA, and Norwig, JA. Vitamin D profile in National Football League players. *Am J Sports Med* 43:1241-1245, 2015.

99. Matsuoka, LY, Ide, L, Wortsman, J, MacLaughlin, JA, and Holick, MF. Sunscreens suppress cutaneous vitamin D3 synthesis. *J Clin Endocrinol Metab* 64:1165-1168, 1987.

100. Matter, M, Stittfall, T, Graves, J, Myburgh, K, Adams, B, Jacobs, P, and Noakes, TD. The effect of iron and folate therapy on maximal exercise performance in female marathon runners with iron and folate deficiency. *Clin Sci (Lond)* 72:415-422, 1987.

101. McAlindon, T, LaValley, M, Schneider, E, Nuite, M, Lee, JY, Price, LL, Lo, G, and Dawson-Hughes, B. Effect of vitamin D supplementation on progression of knee pain and cartilage volume loss in patients with symptomatic osteoarthritis: A randomized controlled trial. *JAMA* 309:155-162, 2013.

102. McAlindon, TE, Jacques, P, Zhang, Y, Hannan, MT, Aliabadi, P, Weissman, B, Rush, D, Levy, D, and Felson, DT. Do antioxidant micronutrients protect against the development and progression of knee osteoarthritis? *Arthritis Rheum* 39:648-656, 1996.

103. McCormick, DB. Vitamin/mineral supplements: of questionable benefit for the general population. *Nutr Rev* 68:207-213, 2010.

104. Miller, JR, Dunn, KW, Ciliberti, LJ, Jr., Patel, RD, and Swanson, BA. Association of vitamin D with stress fractures: A retrospective cohort study. *J Foot Ankle Surg*, 2015.

105. Moran, DS, McClung, JP, Kohen, T, and Lieberman, HR. Vitamin D and physical performance. *Sports Med* 43:601-611, 2013.

106. Morrison, D, Hughes, J, Della Gatta, PA, Mason, S, Lamon, S, Russell, AP, and Wadley, GD. Vitamin C and E supplementation prevents some of the cellular adaptations to endurance-training in humans. *Free Radic Biol Med* 89:852-862, 2015.

107. Moshfegh, A, Goldman, J, and Cleveland, L. *Usual Intakes From Food and Water Compared to 1997 Dietary Reference Intakes: What We Eat in America, NHANES 2005-2006.* U.S. Department of Agriculture, Agricultural Research Service, 2005.

108. National Institutes of Health. *Your Guide to Anemia.* Washington, DC.

109. Nieman, DC, Henson, DA, Butterworth, DE, Warren, BJ, Davis, JM, Fagoaga, OR, and Nehlsen-Cannarella, SL. Vitamin C supplementation does not alter the immune response to 2.5 hours of running. *Int J Sport Nutr* 7:173-184, 1997.

110. Nieman, DC, Henson, DA, McAnulty, SR, McAnulty, L, Swick, NS, Utter, AC, Vinci, DM, Opiela, SJ, and Morrow, JD. Influence of vitamin C supplementation on oxidative and immune changes after an ultramarathon. *J Appl Physiol (1985)* 92:1970-1977, 2002.

111. Nikolaidis, MG, Kerksick, CM, Lamprecht, M, and McAnulty, SR. Does vitamin C and E supplementation impair the favorable adaptations of regular exercise? *Oxid Med Cell Longev* 2012:707941, 2012.

112. Oliveira-Menegozzo, JM, Bergamaschi, DP, Middleton, P, and East, CE. Vitamin A supplementation for postpartum women. *Cochrane Database Syst Rev*:CD005944, 2010.

113. Olson, JA. Adverse effects of large doses of vitamin A and retinoids. *Semin Oncol* 10:290-293, 1983.

114. Olson, JE, Hamilton, GC, Angelos, MG, Singer, JI, Eilers, ME, and Gaddis, M. Objectives to direct the training of emergency medicine residents on off-service rotations: research. *J Emerg Med* 10:631-636, 1992.

115. Paulsen, G, Cumming, KT, Hamarsland, H, Borsheim, E, Berntsen, S, and Raastad, T. Can supplementation with vitamin C and E alter physiological adaptations to strength training? *BMC Sports Sci Med Rehabil* 6:28, 2014.

116. Paulsen, G, Cumming, KT, Holden, G, Hallen, J, Ronnestad, BR, Sveen, O, Skaug, A, Paur, I, Bastani, NE, Ostgaard, HN, Buer, C, Midttun, M, Freuchen, F, Wiig, H, Ulseth, ET, Garthe, I, Blomhoff, R, Benestad, HB, and Raastad, T. Vitamin C and E supplementation hampers cellular adaptation to endurance training in humans: A double-blind, randomised, controlled trial. *J Physiol* 592:1887-1901, 2014.

117. Pawlak, R, Lester, SE, and Babatunde, T. The prevalence of cobalamin deficiency among vegetarians assessed by serum vitamin B12: A review of literature. *Eur J Clin Nutr* 68:541-548, 2014.

118. Pellegrini, N, Serafini, M, Colombi, B, Del Rio, D, Salvatore, S, Bianchi, M, and Brighenti, F. Total antioxidant capacity of plant foods, beverages and oils consumed in Italy assessed by three different in vitro assays. *J Nutr* 133:2812-2819, 2003.

119. Peters, EM, Goetzsche, JM, Grobbelaar, B, and Noakes, TD. Vitamin C supplementation reduces the incidence of postrace symptoms of upper-respiratory-tract infection in ultramarathon runners. *Am J Clin Nutr* 57:170-174, 1993.

120. Pfeifer, M, Begerow, B, and Minne, HW. Vitamin D and muscle function. *Osteoporos Int* 13:187-194, 2002.

121. Phillips, KM, Ruggio, DM, Horst, RL, Minor, B, Simon, RR, Feeney, MJ, Byrdwell, WC, and Haytowitz, DB. Vitamin D and sterol composition of 10 types of mushrooms from retail suppliers in the United States. *J Agric Food Chem* 59:7841-7853, 2011.

122. Powers, SK, and Jackson, MJ. Exercise-induced oxidative stress: cellular mechanisms and impact on muscle force production. *Physiol Rev* 88:1243-1276, 2008.

123. Read, MH, and McGuffin, SL. The effect of B-complex supplementation on endurance performance. *J Sports Med Phys Fitness* 23:178-184, 1983.

124. Reginato, AJ, and Coquia, JA. Musculoskeletal manifestations of osteomalacia and rickets. *Best Pract Res Clin Rheumatol* 17:1063-1080, 2003.

125. Ring, SM, Dannecker, EA, and Peterson, CA. Vitamin D status is not associated with outcomes of experimentally-induced muscle weakness and pain in young, healthy volunteers. *J Nutr Metab* 2010:674240, 2010.

126. Rkain, H, Bouaddi, I, Ibrahimi, A, Lakhdar, T, Abouqal, R, Allali, F, and Hajjaj-Hassouni, N. Relationship between vitamin D deficiency and chronic low back pain in postmenopausal women. *Curr Rheumatol Rev* 9:63-67, 2013.

127. Rokitzki, L, Sagredos, AN, Reuss, F, Buchner, M, and Keul, J. Acute changes in vitamin B6 status in endurance athletes before and after a marathon. *Int J Sport Nutr* 4:154-165, 1994.

128. Ross, AC, Manson, JE, Abrams, SA, Aloia, JF, Brannon, PM, Clinton, SK, Durazo-Arvizu, RA, Gallagher, JC, Gallo, RL, Jones, G, Kovacs, CS, Mayne, ST, Rosen, CJ, and Shapses, SA. The 2011 report on Dietary Reference Intakes for calcium and vitamin D from the Institute of Medicine: What clinicians need to know. *J Clin Endocrinol Metab* 96:53-58, 2011.

129. Sabetta, JR, DePetrillo, P, Cipriani, RJ, Smardin, J, Burns, LA, and Landry, ML. Serum 25-hydroxyvitamin d and the incidence of acute viral respiratory tract infections in healthy adults. *PLoS One* 5:e11088, 2010.

130. Saito, N, Kimura, M, Kuchiba, A, and Itokawa, Y. Blood thiamine levels in outpatients with diabetes mellitus. *J Nutr Sci Vitaminol (Tokyo)* 33:421-430, 1987.

131. Sallander, E, Wester, U, Bengtsson, E, and Wiegleb Edstrom, D. Vitamin D levels after UVB radiation: effects by UVA additions in a randomized controlled trial. *Photodermatol Photoimmunol Photomed* 29:323-329, 2013.

132. Sanders, LM, and Zeisel, SH. Choline: Dietary requirements and role in brain development. *Nutr Today* 42:181-186, 2007.

133. Sanjoaquin, MA, and Molyneux, ME. Malaria and vitamin A deficiency in African children: A vicious circle? *Malar J* 8:134, 2009.

134. Sato, Y, Iwamoto, J, Kanoko, T, and Satoh, K. Low-dose vitamin D prevents muscular atrophy and reduces falls and hip fractures in women after stroke: A randomized controlled trial. *Cerebrovasc Dis* 20:187-192, 2005.

135. Schurgers, LJ. Vitamin K: Key vitamin in controlling vascular calcification in chronic kidney disease. *Kidney Int* 83:782-784, 2013.

136. Schwalfenberg, G. Improvement of chronic back pain or failed back surgery with vitamin D repletion: A case series. *J Am Board Fam Med* 22:69-74, 2009.

137. Sharman, IM, Down, MG, and Norgan, NG. The effects of vitamin E on physiological function and athletic performance of trained swimmers. *J Sports Med Phys Fitness* 16:215-225, 1976.

138. Shindle, M, Voos, J, Gulotta, L, Weiss, L, Rodeo, S, Kelly, B, Land, J, Barnes, R, and Warren, R. Vitamin D status in a professional American football team. Presented at American Orthopaedic Society of Sports Medicine 2011 annual meeting, San Diego, CA, July 2011.

139. Short, SH, and Short, WR. Four-year study of university athletes' dietary intake. *J Am Diet Assoc* 82:632-645, 1983.

140. Simpson, JL, Bailey, LB, Pietrzik, K, Shane, B, and Holzgreve, W. Micronutrients and women of reproductive potential: Required dietary intake and consequences of dietary deficiency or excess. Part I—Folate, vitamin B12, vitamin B6. *J Matern Fetal Neonatal Med* 23:1323-1343, 2010.

141. Sommer, A. Vitamin a deficiency and clinical disease: An historical overview. *J Nutr* 138:1835-1839, 2008.

142. Spector, SA, Jackman, MR, Sabounjian, LA, Sakkas, C, Landers, DM, and Willis, WT. Effect of choline supplementation on fatigue in trained cyclists. *Med Sci Sports Exerc* 27:668-673, 1995.

143. Suboticanec, K, Stavljenic, A, Schalch, W, and Buzina, R. Effects of pyridoxine and riboflavin supplementation on physical fitness in young adolescents. *Int J Vitam Nutr Res* 60:81-88, 1990.

144. Sullivan, G, Wells, KB, and Leake, B. Clinical factors associated with better quality of life in a seriously mentally ill population. *Hosp Community Psychiatry* 43:794-798, 1992.

145. Taghiyar, M, Ghiasvand, R, Askari, G, Feizi, A, Hariri, M, Mashhadi, NS, and Darvishi, L. The effect of vitamins C and E supplementation on muscle damage, performance, and body composition in athlete women: A clinical trial. *Int J Prev Med* 4:S24-S30, 2013.

146. Tang, G. Bioconversion of dietary provitamin A carotenoids to vitamin A in humans. *Am J Clin Nutr* 91:1468S-1473S, 2010.

147. Traber, MG. Vitamin E and K interactions—A 50-year-old problem. *Nutr Rev* 66:624-629, 2008.

148. Trang, H, Cole, D, Rubin, L, Pierratos, A, Siu, S, and Vieth, R. Evidence that vitamin D3 increases serum 25-hydroxyvitamin D more efficiently than does vitamin D2. *Am J Clin Nutr* 68:854-858, 1998.

149. Trivedi, DP, Doll, R, and Khaw, KT. Effect of four monthly oral vitamin D3 (cholecalciferol) supplementation on fractures and mortality in men and women living in the community: Randomised double blind controlled trial. *BMJ* 326:469, 2003.

150. U.S. Department of Agriculture. Nutrient Intakes From Food: Mean Amounts Consumed per Individual, by Gender and Age: What We Eat in America, NHANES 2009-2010. 2012. www.ars.usda.gov/ba/bhnrc/fsrg.

151. U.S. Department of Agriculture. USDA National Nutrient Database for Standard Reference, Release 26. 2013. www.ars.usda.gov/ba/bhnrc/ndl.

152. U.S. Food and Drug Administration. Title 21: Food and drugs—Chapter 1: Food and Drug Administration—Subchapter B: Food for human consumption—Part 101: Food labeling. *Code of Federal Regulations*.

153. U.S. Food and Drug Administration. How to Understand and Use the Nutrition Facts Label. 2015. www.fda.gov/Food/IngredientsPackagingLabeling/LabelingNutrition/ucm274593.htm#percent_daily_value. Accessed March 23, 2016.

154. U.S. Food and Drug Administration. Tanning Products. 2015. www.fda.gov/Radiation-EmittingProducts/RadiationEmitting ProductsandProcedures/Tanning/ ucm116434.htm. July 12, 2016.

155. U.S. Food and Drug Administration. Title 21: Food and drugs. *Code of Federal Regulations*, 2015.

156. U.S. Institute of Medicine. *Dietary Reference Intakes for Thiamin, Riboflavin, Niacin, Vitamin B6, Folate, Vitamin B12, Pantothenic Acid, Biotin, and Choline*. Washington, DC: National Academies Press, 1998.

157. U.S. Institute of Medicine. *Dietary Reference Intakes for Vitamin C, Vitamin E, Selenium, and Carotenoids*. Washington, DC: National Academies Press, 2000.

158. U.S. Institute of Medicine. *Dietary Reference Intakes for Vitamin A, Vitamin K, Arsenic, Boron, Chromium, Copper, Iodine, Iron, Manganese, Molybdenum, Nickel, Silicon, Vanadium, and Zinc*. Washington, DC: National Academies Press, 2001.

159. U.S. Institute of Medicine. *Dietary Reference Intakes: Guiding Principles for Nutrition Labeling and Fortification*. Washington, DC: National Academies Press, 2003.

160. U.S. Institute of Medicine. *Dietary Reference Intakes for Calcium and Vitamin D*. Washington, DC: National Academies Press, 2011.

161. Valko, M, Rhodes, CJ, Moncol, J, Izakovic, M, and Mazur, M. Free radicals, metals and antioxidants in oxidative stress-induced cancer. *Chem Biol Interact* 160:1-40, 2006.

162. van der Beek, EJ, van Dokkum, W, Wedel, M, Schrijver, J, and van den Berg, H. Thiamin, riboflavin and vitamin B6: Impact of restricted intake on physical performance in man. *J Am Coll Nutr* 13:629-640, 1994.

163. van Etten, E, and Mathieu, C. Immunoregulation by 1,25-dihydroxyvitamin D3: Basic concepts. *J Steroid Biochem Mol Biol* 97:93-101, 2005.

164. Veugelers, PJ, and Ekwaru, JP. A statistical error in the estimation of the recommended dietary allowance for vitamin D. *Nutrients* 6:4472-4475, 2014.

165. Vieth, R. Vitamin D supplementation, 25-hydroxyvitamin D concentrations, and safety. *Am J Clin Nutr* 69:842-856, 1999.

166. Virtamo, J, Pietinen, P, Huttunen, JK, Korhonen, P, Malila, N, Virtanen, MJ, Albanes, D, Taylor, PR, Albert, P, and Group, AS. Incidence of cancer and mortality following alpha-tocopherol and beta-carotene supplementation: A postintervention follow-up. *JAMA* 290:476-485, 2003.

167. Vognar, L, and Stoukides, J. The role of low plasma thiamin levels in cognitively impaired elderly patients presenting with acute behavioral disturbances. *J Am Geriatr Soc* 57:2166-2168, 2009.

168. Walsh, NP, Gleeson, M, Pyne, DB, Nieman, DC, Dhabhar, FS, Shephard, RJ, Oliver, SJ, Bermon, S, and Kajeniene, A. Position statement. Part two: Maintaining immune health. *Exerc Immunol Rev* 17:64-103, 2011.

169. Wang, Y, Hodge, AM, Wluka, AE, English, DR, Giles, GG, O'Sullivan, R, Forbes, A, and Cicuttini, FM. Effect of antioxidants on knee cartilage and bone in healthy, middle-aged subjects: A cross-sectional study. *Arthritis Res Ther* 9:R66, 2007.

170. War, AR, Paulraj, MG, Ahmad, T, Buhroo, AA, Hussain, B, Ignacimuthu, S, and Sharma, HC. Mechanisms of plant defense against insect herbivores. *Plant Signal Behav* 7:1306-1320, 2012.

171. Ward, KA, Das, G, Berry, JL, Roberts, SA, Rawer, R, Adams, JE, and Mughal, Z. Vitamin D status and muscle function in post-menarchal adolescent girls. *J Clin Endocrinol Metab* 94:559-563, 2009.

172. Webster, MJ. Physiological and performance responses to supplementation with thiamin and pantothenic acid derivatives. *Eur J Appl Physiol Occup Physiol* 77:486-491, 1998.

173. Wharton, B, and Bishop, N. Rickets. *Lancet* 362:1389-1400, 2003.

174. Wilkinson, TJ, Hanger, HC, George, PM, and Sainsbury, R. Is thiamine deficiency in elderly people related to age or co-morbidity? *Age Ageing* 29:111-116, 2000.

175. Williamson, JD, and Scandalios, JG. Plant antioxidant gene responses to fungal pathogens. *Trends Microbiol* 1:239-245, 1993.

176. Willis, KS, Smith, DT, Broughton, KS, and Larson-Meyer, DE. Vitamin D status and biomarkers of inflammation in runners. *Open Access J Sports Med* 3:35-42, 2012.

177. Wood, B, Gijsbers, A, Goode, A, Davis, S, Mulholland, J, and Breen, K. A study of partial thiamin restriction in human volunteers. *Am J Clin Nutr* 33:848-861, 1980.

178. Woolf, K, and Manore, MM. B-vitamins and exercise: Does exercise alter requirements? *Int J Sport Nutr Exerc Metab* 16:453-484, 2006.

179. World Health Organization. *Global Prevalence of Vitamin A Deficiency in Populations at Risk 1995-2005: WHO Global Database on Vitamin A Deficiency.* Geneva: World Health Organization, 2009.

180. Xanthakos, SA. Nutritional deficiencies in obesity and after bariatric surgery. *Pediatr Clin North Am* 56:1105-1121, 2009.

181. Yamaguchi, M. Role of carotenoid beta-cryptoxanthin in bone homeostasis. *J Biomed Sci* 19:36, 2012.

182. Yao, Y, Zhu, L, He, L, Duan, Y, Liang, W, Nie, Z, Jin, Y, Wu, X, and Fang, Y. A meta-analysis of the relationship between vitamin D deficiency and obesity. *Int J Clin Exp Med* 8:14977-14984, 2015.

183. Zeisel, SH, Da Costa, KA, Franklin, PD, Alexander, EA, Lamont, JT, Sheard, NF, and Beiser, A. Choline, an essential nutrient for humans. *FASEB J* 5:2093-2098, 1991.

184. Zempleni, J, Hassan, YI, and Wijeratne, SS. Biotin and biotinidase deficiency. *Expert Rev Endocrinol Metab* 3:715-724, 2008.

185. Zhang, FF, Driban, JB, Lo, GH, Price, LL, Booth, S, Eaton, CB, Lu, B, Nevitt, M, Jackson, B, Garganta, C, Hochberg, MC, Kwoh, K, and McAlindon, TE. Vitamin D deficiency is associated with progression of knee osteoarthritis. *J Nutr* 144:2002-2008, 2014.

186. Ziegler, PJ, Nelson, JA, and Jonnalagadda, SS. Nutritional and physiological status of U.S. national figure skaters. *Int J Sport Nutr* 9:345-360, 1999.

187. Zimmerman, H. Vitamin A (retinol): Drugs used in dermatotherapy. In *Hepatotoxicity: The Adverse Effects of Drugs and Other Chemicals on the Liver.* Zimmerman, H, ed. Philadelphia, PA: Lippincott, 1999, pp. 727-729.

Chapter 7

1. Allen, L, de Benoist, B, Dary, O, and Hurrell, R. *Guidelines on Food Fortification with Micronutrients.* Geneva: World Health Organization and Food and Agricultural Organization of the United Nations, 2006.

2. Allison, MC, Howatson, AG, Torrance, CJ, Lee, FD, and Russell, RI. Gastrointestinal damage associated with the use of nonsteroidal antiinflammatory drugs. *N Engl J Med* 327:749-754, 1992.

3. Althuis, MD, Jordan, NE, Ludington, EA, and Wittes, JT. Glucose and insulin responses to dietary chromium supplements: A meta-analysis. *Am J Clin Nutr* 76:148-155, 2002.

4. Anderson, RA, Bryden, NA, and Polansky, MM. Dietary chromium intake: Freely chosen diets, institutional diet, and individual foods. *Biol Trace Elem Res* 32:117-121, 1992.

5. Aoi, W, Ogaya, Y, Takami, M, Konishi, T, Sauchi, Y, Park, EY, Wada, S, Sato, K, and Higashi, A. Glutathione supplementation suppresses muscle fatigue induced by prolonged exercise via improved aerobic metabolism. *J Int Soc Sports Nutr* 12:7, 2015.

6. Bailey, RL, Fulgoni, VL, 3rd, Keast, DR, and Dwyer, JT. Dietary supplement use is associated with higher intakes of minerals from food sources. *Am J Clin Nutr* 94:1376-1381, 2011.

7. Barbagallo, M, Belvedere, M, and Dominguez, LJ. Magnesium homeostasis and aging. *Magnes Res* 22:235-246, 2009.

8. Barrett-Connor, E, Chang, JC, and Edelstein, SL. Coffee-associated osteoporosis offset by daily milk consumption: The Rancho Bernardo Study. *JAMA* 271:280-283, 1994.

9. Beard, JL. Iron biology in immune function, muscle metabolism and neuronal functioning. *J Nutr* 131:568S-579S, 2001.

10. Behrens, SB, Deren, ME, Matson, A, Fadale, PD, and Monchik, KO. Stress fractures of the pelvis and legs in athletes: A review. *Sports Health* 5:165-174, 2013.

11. Bermejo, F, and Garcia-Lopez, S. A guide to diagnosis of iron deficiency and iron deficiency anemia in digestive diseases. *World J Gastroenterol* 15:4638-4643, 2009.

12. Betteridge, DJ. What is oxidative stress? *Metabolism* 49:3-8, 2000.

13. Bolland, MJ, Grey, A, Avenell, A, Gamble, GD, and Reid, IR. Calcium supplements with or without vitamin D and risk of cardiovascular events: Reanalysis of the Women's Health Initiative limited access dataset and meta-analysis. *BMJ* 342:d2040, 2011.

14. Brilla, LR, and Haley, TF. Effect of magnesium supplementation on strength training in humans. *J Am Coll Nutr* 11:326-329, 1992.

15. Brownlie, T, Utermohlen, V, Hinton, PS, Giordano, C, and Haas, JD. Marginal iron deficiency without anemia impairs aerobic adaptation among previously untrained women. *Am J Clin Nutr* 75:734-742, 2002.

16. Brownlie, T, Utermohlen, V, Hinton, PS, and Haas, JD. Tissue iron deficiency without anemia impairs adaptation in endurance capacity after aerobic training in previously untrained women. *Am J Clin Nutr* 79:437-443, 2004.

17. Brun, JF, Dieu-Cambrezy, C, Charpiat, A, Fons, C, Fedou, C, Micallef, JP, Fussellier, M, Bardet, L, and Orsetti, A. Serum zinc in highly trained adolescent gymnasts. *Biol Trace Elem Res* 47:273-278, 1995.

18. Calton, JB. Prevalence of micronutrient deficiency in popular diet plans. *J Int Soc Sports Nutr* 7:24, 2010.

19. Caruso, TJ, Prober, CG, and Gwaltney, JM, Jr. Treatment of naturally acquired common colds with zinc: a structured review. *Clin Infect Dis* 45:569-574, 2007.

20. Carvil, P, and Cronin, J. Magnesium and implications on muscle function. *Strength Cond J* 32:48-54, 2010.

21. Chaudhary, DP, Sharma, R, and Bansal, DD. Implications of magnesium deficiency in type 2 diabetes: a review. *Biol Trace Elem Res* 134:119-129, 2010.

22. Chen, HY, Cheng, FC, Pan, HC, Hsu, JC, and Wang, MF. Magnesium enhances exercise performance via increasing glucose availability in the blood, muscle, and brain during exercise. *PLoS One* 9:e85486, 2014.

23. Chen, J, Gu, D, Huang, J, Rao, DC, Jaquish, CE, Hixson, JE, Chen, CS, Chen, J, Lu, F, Hu, D, Rice, T, Kelly, TN, Hamm, LL, Whelton, PK, and He, J. Metabolic syndrome and salt sensitivity of blood pressure in non-diabetic people in China: A dietary intervention study. *Lancet* 373:829-835, 2009.

24. Choi, HY, Park, HC, and Ha, SK. Salt Sensitivity and Hypertension: A Paradigm Shift from Kidney Malfunction to Vascular Endothelial Dysfunction. *Electrolyte Blood Press* 13:7-16, 2015.

25. Coris, EE, Ramirez, AM, and Van Durme, DJ. Heat illness in athletes: The dangerous combination of heat, humidity and exercise. *Sports Med* 34:9-16, 2004.

26. Dawson-Hughes, B, Harris, SS, Rasmussen, H, Song, L, and Dallal, GE. Effect of dietary protein supplements on calcium excretion in healthy older men and women. *J Clin Endocrinol Metab* 89:1169-1173, 2004.

27. de Lordes Lima, M, Cruz, T, Pousada, JC, Rodrigues, LE, Barbosa, K, and Cangucu, V. The effect of magnesium supplementation in increasing doses on the control of type 2 diabetes. *Diabetes Care* 21:682-686, 1998.

28. de Sousa, EF, Da Costa, TH, Nogueira, JA, and Vivaldi, LJ. Assessment of nutrient and water intake among adolescents from sports federations in the Federal District, Brazil. *Br J Nutr* 99:1275-1283, 2008.

29. De Souza, MJ, Williams, NI, Nattiv, A, Joy, E, Misra, M, Loucks, AB, Matheson, G, Olmsted, MP, Barrack, M, Mallinson, RJ, Gibbs, JC, Goolsby, M, Nichols, JF, Drinkwater, B, Sanborn, C, Agostini, R, Otis, CL, Johnson, MD, Hoch, AZ, Alleyne, JM, Wadsworth, LT, Koehler, K, VanHeest, J, Harvey, P, Kelly, AK, Fredericson, M, Brooks, GA, O'Donnell, E, Callahan, LR, Putukian, M, Costello, L, Hecht, S, Rauh, MJ, and McComb, J.

Misunderstanding the female athlete triad: Refuting the IOC consensus statement on Relative Energy Deficiency in Sport (RED-S). *Br J Sports Med* 48:1461-1465, 2014.

30. de Valk, HW, Verkaaik, R, van Rijn, HJ, Geerdink, RA, and Struyvenberg, A. Oral magnesium supplementation in insulin-requiring type 2 diabetic patients. *Diabet Med* 15:503-507, 1998.

31. DellaValle, DM, and Haas, JD. Impact of iron depletion without anemia on performance in trained endurance athletes at the beginning of a training season: A study of female collegiate rowers. *Int J Sport Nutr Exerc Metab* 21:501-506, 2011.

32. Dickens, BF, Weglicki, WB, Li, YS, and Mak, IT. Magnesium deficiency in vitro enhances free radical-induced intracellular oxidation and cytotoxicity in endothelial cells. *FEBS Lett* 311:187-191, 1992.

33. Dickinson, KM, Clifton, PM, and Keogh, JB. Endothelial function is impaired after a high-salt meal in healthy subjects. *Am J Clin Nutr* 93:500-505, 2011.

34. Dickinson, KM, Keogh, JB, and Clifton, PM. Effects of a low-salt diet on flow-mediated dilatation in humans. *Am J Clin Nutr* 89:485-490, 2009.

35. Eby, GA, and Halcomb, WW. Ineffectiveness of zinc gluconate nasal spray and zinc orotate lozenges in common-cold treatment: A double-blind, placebo-controlled clinical trial. *Altern Ther Health Med* 12:34-38, 2006.

36. Eftekhari, MH, Keshavarz, SA, Jalali, M, Elguero, E, Eshraghian, MR, and Simondon, KB. The relationship between iron status and thyroid hormone concentration in iron-deficient adolescent Iranian girls. *Asia Pac J Clin Nutr* 15:50-55, 2006.

37. Elin, RJ, Hosseini, JM, and Gill, JR, Jr. Erythrocyte and mononuclear blood cell magnesium concentrations are normal in hypomagnesemic patients with chronic renal magnesium wasting. *J Am Coll Nutr* 13:463-466, 1994.

38. Farquhar, WB, Edwards, DG, Jurkovitz, CT, and Weintraub, WS. Dietary sodium and health: More than just blood pressure. *J Am Coll Cardiol* 65:1042-1050, 2015.

39. Fenton, TR, Lyon, AW, Eliasziw, M, Tough, SC, and Hanley, DA. Meta-analysis of the effect of the acid-ash hypothesis of osteoporosis on calcium balance. *J Bone Miner Res* 24:1835-1840, 2009.

40. Finley, J, and Davis, C. Manganese deficiency and toxicity: Are high or low dietary amounts of manganese cause for concern? *BioFactors* 10:15-24, 1999.

41. Firoz, M, and Graber, M. Bioavailability of US commercial magnesium preparations. *Magnes Res* 14:257-262, 2001.

42. Ford, ES, and Mokdad, AH. Dietary magnesium intake in a national sample of US adults. *J Nutr* 133:2879-2882, 2003.

43. Freedman, AM, Mak, IT, Stafford, RE, Dickens, BF, Cassidy, MM, Muesing, RA, and Weglicki, WB. Erythrocytes from magnesium-deficient hamsters display an enhanced susceptibility to oxidative stress. *Am J Physiol* 262:C1371-1375, 1992.

44. Fujimura, R, Ashizawa, N, Watanabe, M, Mukai, N, Amagai, H, Fukubayashi, T, Hayashi, K, Tokuyama, K, and Suzuki, M. Effect of resistance exercise training on bone formation and resorption in young male subjects assessed by biomarkers of bone metabolism. *J Bone Miner Res* 12:656-662, 1997.

45. Fulgoni, VL, 3rd, Keast, DR, Auestad, N, and Quann, EE. Nutrients from dairy foods are difficult to replace in diets of Americans: Food pattern modeling and an analyses of the National Health and Nutrition Examination Survey 2003-2006. *Nutr Res* 31:759-765, 2011.

46. Fulgoni, VL, 3rd, Keast, DR, Bailey, RL, and Dwyer, J. Foods, fortificants, and supplements: Where do Americans get their nutrients? *J Nutr* 141:1847-1854, 2011.

47. Fung, TT, Manson, JE, Solomon, CG, Liu, S, Willett, WC, and Hu, FB. The association between magnesium intake and fasting insulin concentration in healthy middle-aged women. *J Am Coll Nutr* 22:533-538, 2003.

48. Galan, P, Preziosi, P, Durlach, V, Valeix, P, Ribas, L, Bouzid, D, Favier, A, and Hercberg, S. Dietary magnesium intake in a French adult population. *Magnes Res* 10:321-328, 1997.

49. Galy, B, Ferring-Appel, D, Kaden, S, Grone, HJ, and Hentze, MW. Iron regulatory proteins are essential for intestinal function and control key iron absorption molecules in the duodenum. *Cell Metab* 7:79-85, 2008.

50. Garfinkel, D, and Garfinkel, L. Magnesium and regulation of carbohydrate metabolism at the molecular level. *Magnesium* 7:249-261, 1988.

51. Giolo De Carvalho, F, Rosa, FT, Marques Miguel Suen, V, Freitas, EC, Padovan, GJ, and Marchini, JS. Evidence of zinc deficiency in competitive swimmers. *Nutrition* 28:1127-1131, 2012.

52. Gu, D, Rice, T, Wang, S, Yang, W, Gu, C, Chen, CS, Hixson, JE, Jaquish, CE, Yao, ZJ, Liu, DP, Rao, DC, and He, J. Heritability of blood pressure responses to dietary sodium and potassium intake in a Chinese population. *Hypertension* 50:116-122, 2007.

53. Guerrera, MP, Volpe, SL, and Mao, JJ. Therapeutic uses of magnesium. *Am Fam Physician* 80:157-162, 2009.

54. Guerrero-Romero, F, Tamez-Perez, HE, Gonzalez-Gonzalez, G, Salinas-Martinez, AM, Montes-Villarreal, J, Trevino-Ortiz, JH, and Rodriguez-Moran, M. Oral magnesium supplementation improves insulin sensitivity in non-diabetic subjects with insulin resistance: A double-blind placebo-controlled randomized trial. *Diabetes Metab* 30:253-258, 2004.

55. Haase, H, and Rink, L. Multiple impacts of zinc on immune function. *Metallomics* 6:1175-1180, 2014.

56. Haddy, FJ, Vanhoutte, PM, and Feletou, M. Role of potassium in regulating blood flow and blood pressure. *Am J Physiol Regul Integr Comp Physiol* 290:R546-R552, 2006.

57. Hagler, L, Askew, EW, Neville, JR, Mellick, PW, Coppes, RI, Jr., and Lowder, JF, Jr. Influence of dietary iron deficiency on hemoglobin, myoglobin, their respective reductases, and skeletal muscle mitochondrial respiration. *Am J Clin Nutr* 34:2169-2177, 1981.

58. Hajjar, IM, Grim, CE, George, V, and Kotchen, TA. Impact of diet on blood pressure and age-related changes in blood pressure in the US population: Analysis of NHANES III. *Arch Intern Med* 161:589-593, 2001.

59. Hallberg, L, Brune, M, and Rossander, L. Iron absorption in man: ascorbic acid and dose-dependent inhibition by phytate. *Am J Clin Nutr* 49:140-144, 1989.

60. Hawley, JA, Dennis, SC, Lindsay, FH, and Noakes, TD. Nutritional practices of athletes: Are they sub-optimal? *J Sports Sci* 13 Spec No:S75-S81, 1995.

61. He, J, Gu, D, Chen, J, Jaquish, CE, Rao, DC, Hixson, JE, Chen, JC, Duan, X, Huang, JF, Chen, CS, Kelly, TN, Bazzano, LA, and Whelton, PK. Gender difference in blood pressure responses to dietary sodium intervention in the GenSalt study. *J Hypertens* 27:48-54, 2009.

62. Heaney, RP, Kopecky, S, Maki, KC, Hathcock, J, Mackay, D, and Wallace, TC. A review of calcium supplements and cardiovascular disease risk. *Adv Nutr* 3:763-771, 2012.

63. Heaney, RP, and Layman, DK. Amount and type of protein influences bone health. *Am J Clin Nutr* 87:1567S-1570S, 2008.

64. Heaney, RP, and Rafferty, K. Carbonated beverages and urinary calcium excretion. *Am J Clin Nutr* 74:343-347, 2001.

65. Heaney, S, O'Connor, H, Gifford, J, and Naughton, G. Comparison of strategies for assessing nutritional adequacy in elite female athletes' dietary intake. *Int J Sport Nutr Exerc Metab* 20:245-256, 2010.

66. Henry, YM, Fatayerji, D, and Eastell, R. Attainment of peak bone mass at the lumbar spine, femoral neck and radius in men and women: Relative contributions of bone size and volumetric bone mineral density. *Osteoporos Int* 15:263-273, 2004.

67. Hinton, PS. Iron and the endurance athlete. *Appl Physiol Nutr Metab*:1-7, 2014.

68. Hinton, PS, Giordano, C, Brownlie, T, and Haas, JD. Iron supplementation improves endurance after training in iron-depleted, nonanemic women. *J Appl Physiol* 88:1103-1111, 2000.

69. Hoy, M, and Goldman, J. *Potassium Intake of the U.S. Population: What We Eat in America, NHANES 2009-2010.* U.S. Department of Agriculture, 2012.

70. Hoy, M, and Goldman, J. *Calcium Intake of the U.S. Population: What We Eat in America, NHANES 2009-2010.* U.S. Department of Agriculture, 2014.

71. Huerta, MG, Roemmich, JN, Kington, ML, Bovbjerg, VE, Weltman, AL, Holmes, VF, Patrie, JT, Rogol, AD, and Nadler, JL. Magnesium deficiency is associated with insulin resistance in obese children. *Diabetes Care* 28:1175-1181, 2005.

72. Imamura, H, Iide, K, Yoshimura, Y, Kumagai, K, Oshikata, R, Miyahara, K, Oda, K, Miyamoto, N, and Nakazawa, A. Nutrient intake, serum lipids and iron status of colligiate rugby players. *J Int Soc Sports Nutr* 10:9, 2013.

73. Jackson, S, Coleman King, S, Zhao, L, and Cogswell, M. Prevalence of excess sodium intake in the United States—NHANES, 2009-2012. *Morbidity and Mortality Weekly Report*, 2016. https://www.cdc.gov/mmwr/preview/mmwrhtml/mm6452a1.htm#tabl.

74. Jeejeebhoy, KN, Chu, RC, Marliss, EB, Greenberg, GR, and Bruce-Robertson, A. Chromium deficiency, glucose intolerance, and neuropathy reversed by chromium supplementation, in a patient receiving long-term total parenteral nutrition. *Am J Clin Nutr* 30:531-538, 1977.

75. Juzwiak, CR, Amancio, OM, Vitalle, MS, Pinheiro, MM, and Szejnfeld, VL. Body composition and nutritional profile of male adolescent tennis players. *J Sports Sci* 26:1209-1217, 2008.

76. Kamel, K, Lin, S, Yang, S, and Halperin, M. Clinical disorders of hyperkalemia. In *Seldin and Giebisch's The Kidney*. 5th ed. Alpern, R, Moe, O, Caplan, M, eds. Philadelphia PA: Elsevier, 2013.

77. Kass, L, Weekes, J, and Carpenter, L. Effect of magnesium supplementation on blood pressure: A meta-analysis. *Eur J Clin Nutr* 66:411-418, 2012.

78. Keith, RE, O'Keeffe, KA, Alt, LA, and Young, KL. Dietary status of trained female cyclists. *J Am Diet Assoc* 89:1620-1623, 1989.

79. Kerstetter, JE, O'Brien, KO, Caseria, DM, Wall, DE, and Insogna, KL. The impact of dietary protein on calcium absorption and kinetic measures of bone turnover in women. *J Clin Endocrinol Metab* 90:26-31, 2005.

80. Kim, SK, Kang, HS, Kim, CS, and Kim, YT. The prevalence of anemia and iron depletion in the population aged 10 years or older. *Korean J Hematol* 46:196-199, 2011.

81. Kramer, JH, Mak, IT, Phillips, TM, and Weglicki, WB. Dietary magnesium intake influences circulating pro-inflammatory neuropeptide levels and loss of myocardial tolerance to postischemic stress. *Exp Biol Med (Maywood)* 228:665-673, 2003.

82. Krebs, NF. Dietary zinc and iron sources, physical growth and cognitive development of breastfed infants. *J Nutr* 130:358S-360S, 2000.

83. Krotkiewski, M, Gudmundsson, M, Backstrom, P, and Mandroukas, K. Zinc and muscle strength and endurance. *Acta Physiol Scand* 116:309-311, 1982.

84. Leone, K. Calcium, magnesium, and phosphorus. In *Emergency Medicine: Clinical Essentials*. 2nd ed. Adams, J, ed. Philadelphia, PA: Elsevier Saunders, 2013.

85. Levenhagen, DK, Gresham, JD, Carlson, MG, Maron, DJ, Borel, MJ, and Flakoll, PJ. Postexercise nutrient intake timing in humans is critical to recovery of leg glucose and protein homeostasis. *Am J Physiol Endocrinol Metab* 280:E982-993, 2001.

86. Lewis, JR, Radavelli-Bagatini, S, Rejnmark, L, Chen, JS, Simpson, JM, Lappe, JM, Mosekilde, L, Prentice, RL, and Prince, RL. The effects of calcium supplementation on verified coronary heart disease hospitalization and death in postmenopausal women: A collaborative meta-analysis of randomized controlled trials. *J Bone Miner Res* 30:165-175, 2015.

87. Lindberg, JS, Zobitz, MM, Poindexter, JR, and Pak, CY. Magnesium bioavailability from magnesium citrate and magnesium oxide. *J Am Coll Nutr* 9:48-55, 1990.

88. Linder, MC, and Hazegh-Azam, M. Copper biochemistry and molecular biology. *Am J Clin Nutr* 63:797S-811S, 1996.

89. Lopez-Ridaura, R, Willett, WC, Rimm, EB, Liu, S, Stampfer, MJ, Manson, JE, and Hu, FB. Magnesium intake and risk of type 2 diabetes in men and women. *Diabetes Care* 27:134-140, 2004.

90. Luft, FC, Weinberger, MH, and Grim, CE. Sodium sensitivity and resistance in normotensive humans. *Am J Med* 72:726-736, 1982.

91. Lukaski, HC. Vitamin and mineral status: Effects on physical performance. *Nutrition* 20:632-644, 2004.

92. Lukaski, HC. Low dietary zinc decreases erythrocyte carbonic anhydrase activities and impairs cardiorespiratory function in men during exercise. *Am J Clin Nutr* 81:1045-1051, 2005.

93. Lukaski, HC, and Nielsen, FH. Dietary magnesium depletion affects metabolic responses during submaximal exercise in postmenopausal women. *J Nutr* 132:930-935, 2002.

94. Malczewska, J, Raczynski, G, and Stupnicki, R. Iron status in female endurance athletes and in non-athletes. *Int J Sport Nutr Exerc Metab* 10:260-276, 2000.

95. Mandal, AK. Hypokalemia and hyperkalemia. *Med Clin North Am* 81:611-639, 1997.

96. Manoguerra, AS, Erdman, AR, Booze, LL, Christianson, G, Wax, PM, Scharman, EJ, Woolf, AD, Chyka, PA, Keyes, DC, Olson, KR, Caravati, EM, and Troutman, WG. Iron ingestion: An evidence-based consensus guideline for out-of-hospital management. *Clin Toxicol (Phila)* 43:553-570, 2005.

97. Massey, LK, and Whiting, SJ. Caffeine, urinary calcium, calcium metabolism and bone. *J Nutr* 123:1611-1614, 1993.

98. Maughan, RJ, and Leiper, JB. Sodium intake and post-exercise rehydration in man. *Eur J Appl Physiol Occup Physiol* 71:311-319, 1995.

99. McCarty, MF. Magnesium may mediate the favorable impact of whole grains on insulin sensitivity by acting as a mild calcium antagonist. *Med Hypotheses* 64:619-627, 2005.

100. Michaelsson, K, Melhus, H, Warensjo Lemming, E, Wolk, A, and Byberg, L. Long term calcium intake and rates of all cause and cardiovascular mortality: Community based prospective longitudinal cohort study. *BMJ* 346:f228, 2013.

101. Micheletti, A, Rossi, R, and Rufini, S. Zinc status in athletes: Relation to diet and exercise. *Sports Med* 31:577-582, 2001.

102. Mishell, DR, Jr. Pharmacokinetics of depot medroxyprogesterone acetate contraception. *J Reprod Med* 41:381-390, 1996.

103. Misner, B. Food alone may not provide sufficient micronutrients for preventing deficiency. *J Int Soc Sports Nutr* 3:51-55, 2006.

104. Monsen, ER. Iron nutrition and absorption: Dietary factors which impact iron bioavailability. *J Am Diet Assoc* 88:786-790, 1988.

105. Morris, RC, Jr., Sebastian, A, Forman, A, Tanaka, M, and Schmidlin, O. Normotensive salt sensitivity: Effects of race and dietary potassium. *Hypertension* 33:18-23, 1999.

106. Moshfegh, A, Goldman, J, Ahuja, J, Rhodes, D, and LaComb, R. *What We Eat in America, NHANES 2005-2006: Usual Nutrient Intakes from Food and Water Compared to 1997 Dietary Reference Intakes for Vitamin D, Calcium, Phosphorus, and Magnesium.* U.S. Department of Agriculture, Agricultural Research Service, 2009.

107. Muhlbauer, B, Schwenk, M, Coram, WM, Antonin, KH, Etienne, P, Bieck, PR, and Douglas, FL. Magnesium-L-aspartate-HCl and magnesium-oxide: Bioavailability in healthy volunteers. *Eur J Clin Pharmacol* 40:437-438, 1991.

108. Muller, MJ, Bosy-Westphal, A, Klaus, S, Kreymann, G, Luhrmann, PM, Neuhauser-Berthold, M, Noack, R, Pirke, KM, Platte, P, Selberg, O, and Steiniger, J. World Health Organization equations have shortcomings for predicting resting energy expenditure in persons from a modern, affluent population: Generation of a new reference standard

from a retrospective analysis of a German database of resting energy expenditure. *Am J Clin Nutr* 80:1379-1390, 2004.

109. Musso, CG. Magnesium metabolism in health and disease. *Int Urol Nephrol* 41:357-362, 2009.

110. Naghii, MR, and Fouladi, AI. Correct assessment of iron depletion and iron deficiency anemia. *Nutr Health* 18:133-139, 2006.

111. National Insitutes of Health. Osteoporosis: Peak Bone Mass in Women. 2015. www.niams.nih.gov/health_info/bone/osteoporosis/bone_mass.asp.

112. National Institutes of Health. Multivitamin/Mineral Supplements. 2016. https://ods.od.nih.gov/factsheets/MVMS-Consumer.

113. Newhouse, IJ, and Finstad, EW. The effects of magnesium supplementation on exercise performance. *Clin J Sport Med* 10:195-200, 2000.

114. Nielsen, FH, and Lukaski, HC. Update on the relationship between magnesium and exercise. *Magnes Res* 19:180-189, 2006.

115. Nishiyama, S, Irisa, K, Matsubasa, T, Higashi, A, and Matsuda, I. Zinc status relates to hematological deficits in middle-aged women. *J Am Coll Nutr* 17:291-295, 1998.

116. Nishlyama, S, Inomoto, T, Nakamura, T, Higashi, A, and Matsuda, I. Zinc status relates to hematological deficits in women endurance runners. *J Am Coll Nutr* 15:359-363, 1996.

117. Noda, Y, Iide, K, Masuda, R, Kishida, R, Nagata, A, Hirakawa, F, Yoshimura, Y, and Imamura, H. Nutrient intake and blood iron status of male collegiate soccer players. *Asia Pac J Clin Nutr* 18:344-350, 2009.

118. O'Donnell, M, Mente, A, Rangarajan, S, McQueen, MJ, Wang, X, Liu, L, Yan, H, Lee, SF, Mony, P, Devanath, A, Rosengren, A, Lopez-Jaramillo, P, Diaz, R, Avezum, A, Lanas, F, Yusoff, K, Iqbal, R, Ilow, R, Mohammadifard, N, Gulec, S, Yusufali, AH, Kruger, L, Yusuf, R, Chifamba, J, Kabali, C, Dagenais, G, Lear, SA, Teo, K, and Yusuf, S. Urinary sodium and potassium excretion, mortality, and cardiovascular events. *N Engl J Med* 371:612-623, 2014.

119. O'Neal, SL, and Zheng, W. Manganese toxicity upon overexposure: A decade in review. *Curr Environ Health Rep* 2:315-328, 2015.

120. Oh, YS, Appel, LJ, Galis, ZS, Hafler, DA, He, J, Hernandez, AL, Joe, B, Karumanchi, SA, Maric-Bilkan, C, Mattson, D, Mehta, NN, Randolph, G, Ryan, M, Sandberg, K, Titze, J, Tolunay, E, Toney, GM, and Harrison, DG. National Heart, Lung, and Blood Institute Working Group Report on Salt in Human Health and Sickness: Building on the Current Scientific Evidence. *Hypertension* 68:281-288, 2016.

121. Otten, J, Hellwig, J, and Meyers, L. *Dietary Reference Intakes: The Essential Guide to Nutrient Requirements.* Washington, DC: National Academies Press, 2006.

122. Paolisso, G, Scheen, A, Cozzolino, D, Di Maro, G, Varricchio, M, D'Onofrio, F, and Lefebvre, PJ. Changes in glucose turnover parameters and improvement of glucose oxidation after 4-week magnesium administration in elderly noninsulin-dependent (type II) diabetic patients. *J Clin Endocrinol Metab* 78:1510-1514, 1994.

123. Paolisso, G, Sgambato, S, Gambardella, A, Pizza, G, Tesauro, P, Varricchio, M, and D'Onofrio, F. Daily magnesium supplements improve glucose handling in elderly subjects. *Am J Clin Nutr* 55:1161-1167, 1992.

124. Park, SC, Chun, HJ, Kang, CD, and Sul, D. Prevention and management of nonsteroidal anti-inflammatory drugs-induced small intestinal injury. *World J Gastroenterol* 17:4647-4653, 2011.

125. Peake, JM, Gerrard, DF, and Griffin, JF. Plasma zinc and immune markers in runners in response to a moderate increase in training volume. *Int J Sports Med* 24:212-216, 2003.

126. Petry, N, Egli, I, Gahutu, JB, Tugirimana, PL, Boy, E, and Hurrell, R. Phytic acid concentration influences iron bioavailability from biofortified beans in Rwandese women with low iron status. *J Nutr* 144:1681-1687, 2014.

127. Prasad, AS, Beck, FW, Bao, B, Snell, D, and Fitzgerald, JT. Duration and severity of symptoms and levels of plasma interleukin-1 receptor antagonist, soluble tumor necrosis factor receptor, and adhesion molecules in patients with common cold treated with zinc acetate. *J Infect Dis* 197:795-802, 2008.

128. Ranade, VV, and Somberg, JC. Bioavailability and pharmacokinetics of magnesium after administration of magnesium salts to humans. *Am J Ther* 8:345-357, 2001.

129. Rink, L, and Gabriel, P. Zinc and the immune system. *Proc Nutr Soc* 59:541-552, 2000.

130. Risser, WL, Lee, EJ, Poindexter, HB, West, MS, Pivarnik, JM, Risser, JM, and Hickson, JF. Iron deficiency in female athletes: Its prevalence and impact on performance. *Med Sci Sports Exerc* 20:116-121, 1988.

131. Rivlin, RS. Magnesium deficiency and alcohol intake: Mechanisms, clinical significance and possible relation to cancer development (a review). *J Am Coll Nutr* 13:416-423, 1994.

132. Rodriguez-Moran, M, and Guerrero-Romero, F. Oral magnesium supplementation improves insulin sensitivity and metabolic control in type 2 diabetic subjects: A randomized double-blind controlled trial. *Diabetes Care* 26:1147-1152, 2003.

133. Rodriguez, NR, DiMarco, NM, Langley, S, American Dietetic, A, Dietitians of, C, American College of Sports Medicine, N, and Athletic, P. Position of the American Dietetic Association, Dietitians of Canada, and the American College of Sports Medicine: Nutrition and athletic performance. *J Am Diet Assoc* 109:509-527, 2009.

134. Ross, AC, Manson, JE, Abrams, SA, Aloia, JF, Brannon, PM, Clinton, SK, Durazo-Arvizu, RA, Gallagher, JC, Gallo, RL, Jones, G, Kovacs, CS, Mayne, ST, Rosen, CJ, and Shapses, SA. The 2011 report on Dietary Reference Intakes for calcium and vitamin D from the Institute of Medicine: What clinicians need to know. *J Clin Endocrinol Metab* 96:53-58, 2011.

135. Ross, AC, Manson, JE, Abrams, SA, Aloia, JF, Brannon, PM, Clinton, SK, Durazo-Arvizu, RA, Gallagher, JC, Gallo, RL, Jones, G, Kovacs, CS, Mayne, ST, Rosen, CJ, and Shapses, SA. Clarification of DRIs for calcium and vitamin D across age groups. *J Am Diet Assoc* 111:1467, 2011.

136. Rossi, L, Migliaccio, S, Corsi, A, Marzia, M, Bianco, P, Teti, A, Gambelli, L, Cianfarani, S, Paoletti, F, and Branca, F. Reduced growth and skeletal changes in zinc-deficient growing rats are due to impaired growth plate activity and inanition. *J Nutr* 131:1142-1146, 2001.

137. Sacks, FM, Svetkey, LP, Vollmer, WM, Appel, LJ, Bray, GA, Harsha, D, Obarzanek, E, Conlin, PR, Miller, ER, 3rd, Simons-Morton, DG, Karanja, N, and Lin, PH. Effects on blood pressure of reduced dietary sodium and the Dietary Approaches to Stop Hypertension (DASH) diet. *N Engl J Med* 344:3-10, 2001.

138. Sandstead, HH. Requirements and toxicity of essential trace elements, illustrated by zinc and copper. *Am J Clin Nutr* 61:621S-624S, 1995.

139. Santos, DA, Matias, CN, Monteiro, CP, Silva, AM, Rocha, PM, Minderico, CS, Bettencourt Sardinha, L, and Laires, MJ. Magnesium intake is associated with strength performance in elite basketball, handball and volleyball players. *Magnes Res* 24:215-219, 2011.

140. Sawka, MN, Burke, LM, Eichner, ER, Maughan, RJ, Montain, SJ, and Stachenfeld, NS. American College of Sports Medicine position stand: Exercise and fluid replacement. *Med Sci Sports Exerc* 39:377-390, 2007.

141. Schmidlin, O, Forman, A, Sebastian, A, and Morris, RC, Jr. Sodium-selective salt sensitivity: Its occurrence in blacks. *Hypertension* 50:1085-1092, 2007.

142. Scott, SP, and Murray-Kolb, LE. Iron status is associated with performance on executive functioning tasks in nonanemic young women. *J Nutr* 146:30-37, 2016.

143. Seifter, J. Potassium disorders. In *Goldman's Cecil Medicine*. Goldman, L, Schafer, A, eds. Philadelphia, PA: Elsevier Saunders, 2016.

144. Setaro, L, Santos-Silva, PR, Nakano, EY, Sales, CH, Nunes, N, Greve, JM, and Colli, C. Magnesium status and the physical performance of volleyball players: Effects of magnesium supplementation. *J Sports Sci* 32:438-445, 2014.

145. Silva, MR, and Paiva, T. Low energy availability and low body fat of female gymnasts before an international competition. *Eur J Sport Sci* 15:591-599, 2015.

146. Singh, M, and Das, RR. Zinc for the common cold. *Cochrane Database Syst Rev*:CD001364, 2011.

147. Smith, SM, Heer, MA, Shackelford, LC, Sibonga, JD, Ploutz-Snyder, L, and Zwart, SR. Benefits for bone from resistance exercise and nutrition in long-duration spaceflight: Evidence from biochemistry and densitometry. *J Bone Miner Res* 27:1896-1906, 2012.

148. Song, Y, Manson, JE, Buring, JE, and Liu, S. Dietary magnesium intake in relation to plasma insulin levels and risk of type 2 diabetes in women. *Diabetes Care* 27:59-65, 2004.

149. Spencer, H, Norris, C, and Williams, D. Inhibitory effects of zinc on magnesium balance and magnesium absorption in man. *J Am Coll Nutr* 13:479-484, 1994.

150. Straub, DA. Calcium supplementation in clinical practice: A review of forms, doses, and indications. *Nutr Clin Pract* 22:286-296, 2007.

151. Tapiero, H, Gate, L, and Tew, KD. Iron: Deficiencies and requirements. *Biomed Pharmacother* 55:324-332, 2001.

152. Testa, G, Pavone, V, Mangano, S, Riccioli, M, Arancio, A, Evola, FR, Avonda, S, and Sessa, G. Normal nutritional components and effects on bone metabolism in prevention of osteoporosis. *J Biol Regul Homeost Agents* 29:729-736, 2015.

153. Toh, SY, Zarshenas, N, and Jorgensen, J. Prevalence of nutrient deficiencies in bariatric patients. *Nutrition* 25:1150-1156, 2009.

154. Tosiello, L. Hypomagnesemia and diabetes mellitus. A review of clinical implications. *Arch Intern Med* 156:1143-1148, 1996.

155. Turner, RB, and Cetnarowski, WE. Effect of treatment with zinc gluconate or zinc acetate on experimental and natural colds. *Clin Infect Dis* 31:1202-1208, 2000.

156. Tzemos, N, Lim, PO, Wong, S, Struthers, AD, and MacDonald, TM. Adverse cardiovascular effects of acute salt loading in young normotensive individuals. *Hypertension* 51:1525-1530, 2008.

157. U.S. Department of Agriculture. USDA National Nutrient Database for Standard Reference, Release 26. 2013. www.ars.usda.gov/ba/bhnrc/ndl.

158. U.S. Department of Agriculture. 2015-2020 Dietary Guidelines for Americans. 2015. http://health.gov/dietaryguidelines/2015/guidelines.

159. U.S. Department of Health and Human Services. *Bone Health and Osteoporosis: A Report of the Surgeon General.* Rockville, MD: U.S. Department of Health and Human Services,, 2004.

160. U.S. Food and Drug Administration. Title 21: Food and drugs—Chapter 1: Food and Drug Administration—Subchapter B: Food for human consumption—Part 101: Food labeling. *Code of Federal Regulations.*

161. U.S. Food and Drug Administration. Guidance for Industry: A Food Labeling Guide (Appendix F: Calculate the Percent Daily Value for the Appropriate Nutrients). 2013. www.fda.gov/Food/GuidanceRegulation/GuidanceDocumentsRegulatoryInformation/LabelingNutrition/ucm064928.htm. Accessed March 25, 2016.

162. U.S. House of Representatives. Title 21: Food and drugs—Subchapter II: Definitions—Chapter 9: Federal Food, Drug, and Cosmetic Act. *United States Code*, 2010. http://uscode.house.gov/view.xhtml?path=/prelim@title21/chapter9/subchapter2&edition=prelim.

163. U.S. Institute of Medicine. *Dietary Reference Intakes for Calcium, Phosphorus, Magnesium, Vitamin D, and Fluoride.* Washington, DC: National Academies Press, 1997.

164. U.S. Institute of Medicine. *Dietary Reference Intakes for Thiamin, Riboflavin, Niacin, Vitamin B6, Folate, Vitamin B12, Pantothenic Acid, Biotin, and Choline.* Washington, DC: National Academies Press, 1998.

165. U.S. Institute of Medicine. *Dietary Reference Intakes for Vitamin A, Vitamin K, Arsenic, Boron, Chromium, Copper, Iodine, Iron, Manganese, Molybdenum, Nickel, Silicon, Vanadium, and Zinc.* Washington, DC: National Academies Press, 2001.

166. U.S. Institute of Medicine. *Dietary Reference Intakes for Water, Potassium, Sodium, Chloride, and Sulfate.* Washington, DC: National Academies Press, 2005.

167. U.S. Institute of Medicine. *Dietary Reference Intakes for Calcium and Vitamin D.* Washington, DC: National Academies Press, 2011.

168. U.S. Institute of Medicine, Strom, BL, Yaktine, AL, and Oria, M. *Sodium Intake in Populations: Assessment of Evidence.* Washington, DC: National Academies Press, 2013.

169. U.S. Preventive Services Task Force. Final Recommendation Statement: Vitamin D and Calcium to Prevent Fractures: Preventive Medication. 2015. www.uspreventiveservicestaskforce.org/Page/Document/RecommendationStatementFinal/vitamin-d-and-calcium-to-prevent-fractures-preventive-medication.

170. Vaquero, MP. Magnesium and trace elements in the elderly: Intake, status and recommendations. *J Nutr Health Aging* 6:147-153, 2002.

171. Veronese, N, Berton, L, Carraro, S, Bolzetta, F, De Rui, M, Perissinotto, E, Toffanello, ED, Bano, G, Pizzato, S, Miotto, F, Coin, A, Manzato, E, and Sergi, G. Effect of oral magnesium supplementation on physical performance in healthy elderly women involved in a weekly exercise program: a randomized controlled trial. *Am J Clin Nutr* 100:974-981, 2014.

172. Volpe, SL. Magnesium and the athlete. *Curr Sports Med Rep* 14:279-283, 2015.

173. Walker, AF, Marakis, G, Christie, S, and Byng, M. Mg citrate found more bioavailable than other Mg preparations in a randomised, double-blind study. *Magnes Res* 16:183-191, 2003.

174. Wallace, KL, Curry, SC, LoVecchio, F, and Raschke, RA. Effect of magnesium hydroxide on iron absorption after ferrous sulfate. *Ann Emerg Med* 34:685-687, 1999.

175. Weaver, CM, Gordon, CM, Janz, KF, Kalkwarf, HJ, Lappe, JM, Lewis, R, O'Karma, M, Wallace, TC, and Zemel, BS. The National Osteoporosis Foundation's position statement on peak bone mass development and lifestyle factors: A systematic review and implementation recommendations. *Osteoporos Int* 27:1281-1386, 2016.

176. Weglicki, WB, Dickens, BF, Wagner, TL, Chmielinska, JJ, and Phillips, TM. Immunoregulation by neuropeptides in magnesium deficiency: Ex vivo effect of enhanced substance P production on circulating T lymphocytes from magnesium-deficient mice. *Magnes Res* 9:3-11, 1996.

177. Whelton, PK, He, J, Cutler, JA, Brancati, FL, Appel, LJ, Follmann, D, and Klag, MJ. Effects of oral potassium on blood pressure: Meta-analysis of randomized controlled clinical trials. *JAMA* 277:1624-1632, 1997.

178. Wierniuk, A, and Wlodarek, D. Estimation of energy and nutritional intake of young men practicing aerobic sports. *Rocz Panstw Zakl Hig* 64:143-148, 2013.

179. Wierzejska, R. Tea and health—A review of the current state of knowledge. *Przegl Epidemiol* 68:501-506, 595-509, 2014.

180. Yang, J, Punshon, T, Guerinot, ML, and Hirschi, KD. Plant calcium content: Ready to remodel. *Nutrients* 4:1120-1136, 2012.

181. Yokota, K, Kato, M, Lister, F, Ii, H, Hayakawa, T, Kikuta, T, Kageyama, S, and Tajima, N. Clinical efficacy of magnesium supplementation in patients with type 2 diabetes. *J Am Coll Nutr* 23:506S-509S, 2004.

182. Zalcman, I, Guarita, HV, Juzwiak, CR, Crispim, CA, Antunes, HK, Edwards, B, Tufik, S, and de Mello, MT. Nutritional status of adventure racers. *Nutrition* 23:404-411, 2007.

183. Zhang, X, Li, Y, Del Gobbo, LC, Rosanoff, A, Wang, J, Zhang, W, and Song, Y. Effects of magnesium supplementation on blood pressure: A meta-analysis of randomized

double-blind placebo-controlled trials. *Hypertension* 68:324-333, 2016.

184. Ziegler, PJ, Nelson, JA, and Jonnalagadda, SS. Nutritional and physiological status of U.S. national figure skaters. *Int J Sport Nutr* 9:345-360, 1999.

Chapter 8

1. Adan, A. Cognitive performance and dehydration. *J Am Coll Nutr* 31:71-78, 2012.

2. Adeleye, O, Faulkner, M, Adeola, T, and ShuTangyie, G. Hypernatremia in the elderly. *J Natl Med Assoc* 94:701-705, 2002.

3. Almond, CS, Shin, AY, Fortescue, EB, Mannix, RC, Wypij, D, Binstadt, BA, Duncan, CN, Olson, DP, Salerno, AE, Newburger, JW, and Greenes, DS. Hyponatremia among runners in the Boston Marathon. *N Engl J Med* 352:1550-1556, 2005.

4. American Academy of Pediatrics. Climatic heat stress and the exercising child and adolescent. *Pediatrics* 106:158-159, 2000.

5. Arieff, AI, Llach, F, and Massry, SG. Neurological manifestations and morbidity of hyponatremia: Correlation with brain water and electrolytes. *Medicine (Baltimore)* 55:121-129, 1976.

6. Armstrong, LE. Assessing hydration status: The elusive gold standard. *J Am Coll Nutr* 26:575S-584S, 2007.

7. Armstrong, LE, Ganio, MS, Casa, DJ, Lee, EC, McDermott, BP, Klau, JF, Jimenez, L, Le Bellego, L, Chevillotte, E, and Lieberman, HR. Mild dehydration affects mood in healthy young women. *J Nutr* 142:382-388, 2012.

8. Armstrong, LE, Maresh, CM, Castellani, JW, Bergeron, MF, Kenefick, RW, LaGasse, KE, and Riebe, D. Urinary indices of hydration status. *Int J Sport Nutr* 4:265-279, 1994.

9. Baker, LB, Dougherty, KA, Chow, M, and Kenney, WL. Progressive dehydration causes a progressive decline in basketball skill performance. *Med Sci Sports Exerc* 39:1114-1123, 2007.

10. Bar-Or, O, Blimkie, CJ, Hay, JA, MacDougall, JD, Ward, DS, and Wilson, WM. Voluntary dehydration and heat intolerance in cystic fibrosis. *Lancet* 339:696-699, 1992.

11. Bar-Or, O, Dotan, R, Inbar, O, Rotshtein, A, and Zonder, H. Voluntary hypohydration in 10- to 12-year-old boys. *J Appl Physiol Respir Environ Exerc Physiol* 48:104-108, 1980.

12. Bardis, CN, Kavouras, SA, Kosti, L, Markousi, M, and Sidossis, LS. Mild hypohydration decreases cycling performance in the heat. *Med Sci Sports Exerc* 45:1782-1789, 2013.

13. Batchelder, BC, Krause, BA, Seegmiller, JG, and Starkey, CA. Gastrointestinal temperature increases and hypohydration exists after collegiate men's ice hockey participation. *J Strength Cond Res* 24:68-73, 2010.

14. Bergeron, MF. Heat cramps: Fluid and electrolyte challenges during tennis in the heat. *J Sci Med Sport* 6:19-27, 2003.

15. Bergeron, MF, Devore, CD, and Rice, SG. Climatic heat stress and exercising children and adolescents. *Pediatrics* 128:e741-e747, 2011.

16. Bergeron, MF, McLeod, KS, and Coyle, JF. Core body temperature during competition in the heat: National Boys' 14s Junior Championships. *Br J Sports Med* 41:779-783, 2007.

17. Bergeron, MF, Waller, JL, and Marinik, EL. Voluntary fluid intake and core temperature responses in adolescent tennis players: Sports beverage versus water. *Br J Sports Med* 40:406-410, 2006.

18. Binkley, HM, Beckett, J, Casa, DJ, Kleiner, DM, and Plummer, PE. National Athletic Trainers' Association position statement: Exertional heat illnesses. *J Athl Train* 37:329-343, 2002.

19. Casa, DJ, Armstrong, LE, Hillman, SK, Montain, SJ, Reiff, RV, Rich, BS, Roberts, WO, and Stone, JA. National Athletic Trainers' Association position statement: Fluid replacement for athletes. *J Athl Train* 35:212-224, 2000.

20. Cheuvront, SN, Carter, R, 3rd, Castellani, JW, and Sawka, MN. Hypohydration impairs endurance exercise performance in temperate but not cold air. *J Appl Physiol* 99:1972-1976, 2005.

21. Conley, SB. Hypernatremia. *Pediatr Clin North Am* 37:365-372, 1990.

22. Coris, EE, Ramirez, AM, and Van Durme, DJ. Heat illness in athletes: The dangerous combination of heat, humidity and exercise. *Sports Med* 34:9-16, 2004.

23. Dalbo, VJ, Roberts, MD, Stout, JR, and Kerksick, CM. Putting to rest the myth of creatine supplementation leading to muscle cramps and dehydration. *Br J Sports Med* 42:567-573, 2008.

24. Davies, CT. Thermal responses to exercise in children. *Ergonomics* 24:55-61, 1981.

25. Davis, JK, Laurent, CM, Allen, KE, Green, JM, Stolworthy, NI, Welch, TR, and Nevett, ME. Influence of dehydration on intermittent sprint performance. *J Strength Cond Res* 29:2586-2593, 2015.

26. Distefano, LJ, Casa, DJ, Vansumeren, MM, Karslo, RM, Huggins, RA, Demartini, JK, Stearns, RL, Armstrong, LE, and Maresh, CM. Hypohydration and hyperthermia impair neuromuscular control after exercise. *Med Sci Sports Exerc* 45:1166-1173, 2013.

27. Docherty, D, Eckerson, JD, and Hayward, JS. Physique and thermoregulation in prepubertal males during exercise in a warm, humid environment. *Am J Phys Anthropol* 70:19-23, 1986.

28. Draper, SB, Mori, KJ, Lloyd-Owen, S, and Noakes, T. Overdrinking-induced hyponatraemia in the 2007 London Marathon. *BMJ Case Rep*, 2009.

29. Duffield, R, McCall, A, Coutts, AJ, and Peiffer, JJ. Hydration, sweat and thermoregulatory responses to professional football training in the heat. *J Sports Sci* 30:957-965, 2012.

30. Engell, DB, Maller, O, Sawka, MN, Francesconi, RN, Drolet, L, and Young, AJ. Thirst and fluid intake following graded hypohydration levels in humans. *Physiol Behav* 40:229-236, 1987.

31. Fletcher, GO, Dawes, J, and Spano, M. The potential dangers of using rapid weight loss techniques. *Strength Cond J* 36:45-48, 2014.

32. Ganio, MS, Armstrong, LE, Casa, DJ, McDermott, BP, Lee, EC, Yamamoto, LM, Marzano, S, Lopez, RM, Jimenez, L, Le Bellego, L, Chevillotte, E, and Lieberman, HR. Mild dehydration impairs cognitive performance and mood of men. *Br J Nutr* 106:1535-1543, 2011.

33. Gerber, G, and Brendler, C. Evaluation of the urologic patient: History, physical examination, and the urinalysis. In *Campbell-Walsh Urology*. 10th ed. AJ, W, ed. Philadelphia, PA: Saunders Elsevier, 2011, pp. 1-25.

34. Gibson, JC, Stuart-Hill, LA, Pethick, W, and Gaul, CA. Hydration status and fluid and sodium balance in elite Canadian junior women's soccer players in a cool environment. *Appl Physiol Nutr Metab* 37:931-937, 2012.

35. Godek, SF, Peduzzi, C, Burkholder, R, Condon, S, Dorshimer, G, and Bartolozzi, AR. Sweat rates, sweat sodium concentrations, and sodium losses in 3 groups of professional football players. *J Athl Train* 45:364-371, 2010.

36. Gonzalez-Alonso, J, Calbet, JA, and Nielsen, B. Muscle blood flow is reduced with dehydration during prolonged exercise in humans. *J Physiol* 513:895-905, 1998.

37. Greenleaf, JE. Problem: Thirst, drinking behavior, and involuntary dehydration. *Med Sci Sports Exerc* 24:645-656, 1992.

38. Greenwood, M, Kreider, RB, Melton, C, Rasmussen, C, Lancaster, S, Cantler, E, Milnor, P, and Almada, A. Creatine supplementation during college football training does not increase the incidence of cramping or injury. *Mol Cell Biochem* 244:83-88, 2003.

39. Hayes, LD, and Morse, CI. The effects of progressive dehydration on strength and power: Is there a dose response? *Eur J Appl Physiol* 108:701-707, 2010.

40. Jentjens, RL, Achten, J, and Jeukendrup, AE. High oxidation rates from combined carbohydrates ingested during exercise. *Med Sci Sports Exerc* 36:1551-1558, 2004.

41. Jequier, E, and Constant, F. Water as an essential nutrient: The physiological basis of hydration. *Eur J Clin Nutr* 64:115-123, 2010.

42. Jones, LC, Cleary, MA, Lopez, RM, Zuri, RE, and Lopez, R. Active dehydration impairs upper and lower body anaerobic muscular power. *J Strength Cond Res* 22:455-463, 2008.

43. Judelson, DA, Maresh, CM, Farrell, MJ, Yamamoto, LM, Armstrong, LE, Kraemer, WJ, Volek, JS, Spiering, BA, Casa, DJ, and Anderson, JM. Effect of hydration state on strength, power, and resistance exercise performance. *Med Sci Sports Exerc* 39:1817-1824, 2007.

44. Kavouras, SA. Assessing hydration status. *Curr Opin Clin Nutr Metab Care* 5:519-524, 2002.

45. Kavouras, SA, Arnaoutis, G, Makrillos, M, Garagouni, C, Nikolaou, E, Chira, O, Ellinikaki, E, and Sidossis, LS. Educational intervention on water intake improves hydration status and enhances exercise performance in athletic youth. *Scand J Med Sci Sports* 22:684-689, 2012.

46. Kovacs, EM, Senden, JM, and Brouns, F. Urine color, osmolality and specific electrical conductance are not accurate measures of hydration status during postexercise rehydration. *J Sports Med Phys Fitness* 39:47-53, 1999.

47. Kovacs, MS. A review of fluid and hydration in competitive tennis. *Int J Sports Physiol Perform* 3:413-423, 2008.

48. Matias, CN, Santos, DA, Judice, PB, Magalhaes, JP, Minderico, CS, Fields, DA, Lukaski, HC, Sardinha, LB, and Silva, AM. Estimation of total body water and extracellular water with bioimpedance in athletes: A need for athlete-specific prediction models. *Clin Nutr* 35:468-474, 2016.

49. Maughan, RJ, and Leiper, JB. Sodium intake and post-exercise rehydration in man. *Eur J Appl Physiol Occup Physiol* 71:311-319, 1995.

50. Maughan, RJ, Watson, P, and Shirreffs, SM. Heat and cold: What does the environment do to the marathon runner? *Sports Med* 37:396-399, 2007.

51. Meyer, F, Bar-Or, O, MacDougall, D, and Heigenhauser, GJ. Sweat electrolyte loss during exercise in the heat: effects of gender and maturation. *Med Sci Sports Exerc* 24:776-781, 1992.

52. Mitchell, JB, Costill, DL, Houmard, JA, Fink, WJ, Robergs, RA, and Davis, JA. Gastric emptying: Influence of prolonged exercise and carbohydrate concentration. *Med Sci Sports Exerc* 21:269-274, 1989.

53. Montain, SJ, and Coyle, EF. Influence of graded dehydration on hyperthermia and cardiovascular drift during exercise. *J Appl Physiol (1985)* 73:1340-1350, 1992.

54. Morris, DM, Huot, JR, Jetton, AM, Collier, SR, and Utter, AC. Acute sodium ingestion before exercise increases voluntary water consumption resulting in preexercise hyperrhydration and improvement in exercise performance in the heat. *Int J Sport Nutr Exerc Metab* 25:456-462, 2015.

55. Nadel, ER. Control of sweating rate while exercising in the heat. *Med Sci Sports* 11:31-35, 1979.

56. National Center for Complementary and Integrative Health. "Detoxes" and "Cleanses." https://nccih.nih.gov/health/detoxes-cleanses.

57. National Institute on Alcohol Abuse and Alcoholism. *Beyond Hangovers: Understanding Alcohol's Impact on Your Health.* National Institutes of Health, 2010. http://pubs.niaaa.nih.gov/publications/Hangovers/beyond-Hangovers.htm.

58. Nielsen, FH, and Lukaski, HC. Update on the relationship between magnesium and exercise. *Magnes Res* 19:180-189, 2006.

59. Noakes, TD, Sharwood, K, Speedy, D, Hew, T, Reid, S, Dugas, J, Almond, C, Wharam, P, and Weschler, L. Three independent biological mechanisms cause exercise-associated hyponatremia: Evidence from 2,135 weighed competitive athletic performances. *Proc Natl Acad Sci U S A* 102:18550-18555, 2005.

60. O'Brien, C, Young, AJ, and Sawka, MN. Bioelectrical impedance to estimate changes in hydration status. *Int J Sports Med* 23:361-366, 2002.

61. Oppliger, RA, Magnes, SA, Popowski, LA, and Gisolfi, CV. Accuracy of urine specific gravity and osmolality as indicators of hydration status. *Int J Sport Nutr Exerc Metab* 15:236-251, 2005.

62. Osterberg, KL, Horswill, CA, and Baker, LB. Pregame urine specific gravity and fluid intake by National Basketball Association players during competition. *J Athl Train* 44:53-57, 2009.

63. Palmer, MS, and Spriet, LL. Sweat rate, salt loss, and fluid intake during an intense on-ice practice in elite Canadian male junior hockey players. *Appl Physiol Nutr Metab* 33:263-271, 2008.

64. Penning, R, van Nuland, M, Fliervoet, LA, Olivier, B, and Verster, JC. The pathology of alcohol hangover. *Curr Drug Abuse Rev* 3:68-75, 2010.

65. Popkin, BM, D'Anci, KE, and Rosenberg, IH. Water, hydration, and health. *Nutr Rev* 68:439-458, 2010.

66. Popowski, LA, Oppliger, RA, Patrick Lambert, G, Johnson, RF, Kim Johnson, A, and Gisolf, CV. Blood and urinary measures of hydration status during progressive acute dehydration. *Med Sci Sports Exerc* 33:747-753, 2001.

67. Raymond, JR, and Yarger, WE. Abnormal urine color: Differential diagnosis. *South Med J* 81:837-841, 1988.

68. Riebl, SK, and Davy, BM. The hydration equation: Update on water balance and cognitive performance. *ACSMs Health Fit J* 17:21-28, 2013.

69. Rivera-Brown, AM, Gutierrez, R, Gutierrez, JC, Frontera, WR, and Bar-Or, O. Drink composition, voluntary drinking, and fluid balance in exercising, trained, heat-acclimatized boys. *J Appl Physiol* 86:78-84, 1999.

70. Rogers, PJ, Heatherley, SV, Mullings, EL, and Smith, JE. Faster but not smarter: Effects of caffeine and caffeine withdrawal on alertness and performance. *Psychopharmacology (Berl)* 226:229-240, 2013.

71. Rowland, T. Fluid replacement requirements for child athletes. *Sports Med* 41:279-288, 2011.

72. Rowland, T, Hagenbuch, S, Pober, D, and Garrison, A. Exercise tolerance and thermoregulatory responses during cycling in boys and men. *Med Sci Sports Exerc* 40:282-287, 2008.

73. Sawka, MN. Physiological consequences of hypohydration: Exercise performance and thermoregulation. *Med Sci Sports Exerc* 24:657-670, 1992.

74. Sawka, MN, Burke, LM, Eichner, ER, Maughan, RJ, Montain, SJ, and Stachenfeld, NS. American College of Sports Medicine position stand: Exercise and fluid replacement. *Med Sci Sports Exerc* 39:377-390, 2007.

75. Schoffstall, JE, Branch, JD, Leutholtz, BC, and Swain, DE. Effects of dehydration and rehydration on the one-repetition maximum bench press of weight-trained males. *J Strength Cond Res* 15:102-108, 2001.

76. Shanholtzer, BA, and Patterson, SM. Use of bioelectrical impedance in hydration status assessment: Reliability of a new tool in psychophysiology research. *Int J Psychophysiol* 49:217-226, 2003.

77. Sharma, S, and Hemal, A. Chyluria—An overview. *Int J Nephrol Urol* 1:14-26, 2009.

78. Shirreffs, SM, and Maughan, RJ. Urine osmolality and conductivity as indices of hydration status in athletes in the heat. *Med Sci Sports Exerc* 30:1598-1602, 1998.

79. Shirreffs, SM, and Maughan, RJ. Volume repletion after exercise-induced volume depletion in humans: Replacement of water and sodium losses. *Am J Physiol* 274:F868-F875, 1998.

80. Shirreffs, SM, Taylor, AJ, Leiper, JB, and Maughan, RJ. Post-exercise rehydration in man: Effects of volume consumed and drink sodium content. *Med Sci Sports Exerc* 28:1260-1271, 1996.

81. Simerville, JA, Maxted, WC, and Pahira, JJ. Urinalysis: A comprehensive review. *Am Fam Physician* 71:1153-1162, 2005.

82. Smith, MF, Newell, AJ, and Baker, MR. Effect of acute mild dehydration on cognitive-motor performance in golf. *J Strength Cond Res* 26:3075-3080, 2012.

83. Spaeth, AM, Goel, N, and Dinges, DF. Cumulative neurobehavioral and physiological effects of chronic caffeine intake: Individual differences and implications for the use of caffeinated energy products. *Nutr Rev* 72 Suppl 1:34-47, 2014.

84. Stofan, JR, Zachwieja, JJ, Horswill, CA, Murray, R, Anderson, SA, and Eichner, ER. Sweat and sodium losses in NCAA football players: A precursor to heat cramps? *Int J Sport Nutr Exerc Metab* 15:641-652, 2005.

85. Stover, EA, Petrie, HJ, Passe, D, Horswill, CA, Murray, B, and Wildman, R. Urine specific gravity in exercisers prior to physical training. *Appl Physiol Nutr Metab* 31:320-327, 2006.

86. Stover, EA, Zachwieja, J, Stofan, J, Murray, R, and Horswill, CA. Consistently high urine specific gravity in adolescent American football players and the impact of an acute drinking strategy. *Int J Sports Med* 27:330-335, 2006.

87. Taivainen, H, Laitinen, K, Tahtela, R, Kilanmaa, K, and Valimaki, MJ. Role of plasma vasopressin in changes of water balance accompanying acute alcohol intoxication. *Alcohol Clin Exp Res* 19:759-762, 1995.

88. Thomas, DT, Erdman, KA, and Burke, LM. Position of the Academy of Nutrition and Dietetics, Dietitians of Canada, and the American College of Sports Medicine: Nutrition and athletic performance. *J Acad Nutr Diet* 116:501-528, 2016.

89. Tilkian, S, Boudreau, C, and Tilkian, A. *Clinical & Nursing Implications of Laboratory Tests.* 5th ed. St. Louis, MO: Mosby, 1995.

90. Tripette, J, Loko, G, Samb, A, Gogh, BD, Sewade, E, Seck, D, Hue, O, Romana, M, Diop, S, Diaw, M, Brudey, K, Bogui, P, Cisse, F, Hardy-Dessources, MD, and Connes, P. Effects of hydration and dehydration on blood rheology in sickle cell trait carriers during exercise. *Am J Physiol Heart Circ Physiol* 299:H908-H914, 2010.

91. Tsuzuki-Hayakawa, K, Tochihara, Y, and Ohnaka, T. Thermoregulation during heat exposure of young children compared to their mothers. *Eur J Appl Physiol Occup Physiol* 72:12-17, 1995.

92. U.S. Department of Agriculture. USDA National Nutrient Database for Standard Reference, Release 26. 2013. www.ars.usda.gov/ba/bhnrc/ndl.

93. U.S. Institute of Medicine. *Caffeine for the Sustainment of Mental Task Performance: Formulations for Military Operations.* National Academies Press. www.nap.edu/catalog/10219/caffeine-for-the-sustainment-of-mental-task-performance-formulations-for.

94. U.S. Institute of Medicine. *Fluid Replacement and Heat Stress.* National Academies Press, 1994.

95. U.S. Institute of Medicine. *Dietary Reference Intakes for Calcium, Phosphorus, Magnesium, Vitamin D, and Fluoride.* Washington, DC: National Academies Press, 1997.

96. U.S. Institute of Medicine. *Dietary Reference Intakes for Water, Potassium, Sodium, Chloride, and Sulfate.* Washington, DC: National Academies Press, 2005.

97. Urso, C, Brucculeri, S, and Caimi, G. Physiopathological, epidemiological, clinical and therapeutic aspects of exercise-associated hyponatremia. *J Clin Med* 3:1258-1275, 2014.

98. Volpe, SL, Poule, KA, and Bland, EG. Estimation of prepractice hydration status of National Collegiate Athletic Association Division I athletes. *J Athl Train* 44:624-629, 2009.

99. Wenos, DL, and Amato, HK. Weight cycling alters muscular strength and endurance, ratings of perceived exertion, and total body water in college wrestlers. *Percept Mot Skills* 87:975-978, 1998.

100. Whitfield, AH. Too much of a good thing? The danger of water intoxication in endurance sports. *Br J Gen Pract* 56:542-545, 2006.

101. Wilk, B, and Bar-Or, O. Effect of drink flavor and NaCl on voluntary drinking and hydration in boys exercising in the heat. *J Appl Physiol (1985)* 80:1112-1117, 1996.

102. Wilson, PB. Multiple transportable carbohydrates during exercise: Current limitations and directions for future research. *J Strength Cond Res* 29:2056-2070, 2015.

103. Yang, A, Palmer, AA, and de Wit, H. Genetics of caffeine consumption and responses to caffeine. *Psychopharmacology (Berl)* 211:245-257, 2010.

104. Zhang, Y, Coca, A, Casa, DJ, Antonio, J, Green, JM, and Bishop, PA. Caffeine and diuresis during rest and exercise: A meta-analysis. *J Sci Med Sport* 18:569-574, 2015.

Chapter 9

1. Akabas, SR, Vannice, G, Atwater, JB, Cooperman, T, Cotter, R, and Thomas, L. Quality Certification Programs for Dietary Supplements. *J Acad Nutr Diet* 116:1378-1379, 2016.

2. Alhosin, M, Anselm, E, Rashid, S, Kim, JH, Madeira, SV, Bronner, C, and Schini-Kerth, VB. Redox-sensitive up-regulation of eNOS by purple grape juice in endothelial cells: role of PI3-kinase/Akt, p38 MAPK, JNK, FoxO1 and FoxO3a. *PLoS One* 8:e57883, 2013.

3. American Academy of Pediatrics. 2016. https://www.aap.org. Accessed August 4, 2016.

4. American College of Sports Medicine. ACSM Current Comment: Alcohol and Athletic Performance. 2016. https://www.acsm.org/public-information/search-by-topic/search-by-topic/fact-sheets. Accessed January 18, 2016.

5. Andersen, T, and Fogh, J. Weight loss and delayed gastric emptying following a South American herbal preparation in overweight patients. *J Hum Nutr Diet* 14:243-250, 2001.

6. Astell, KJ, Mathai, ML, and Su, XQ. Plant extracts with appetite suppressing properties for body weight control: A systematic review of double blind randomized controlled clinical trials. *Complement Ther Med* 21:407-416, 2013.

7. Astell, KJ, Mathai, ML, and Su, XQ. A review on botanical species and chemical compounds with appetite suppressing properties for body weight control. *Plant Foods Hum Nutr* 68:213-221, 2013.

8. Astorino, TA, and Roberson, DW. Efficacy of acute caffeine ingestion for short-term high-intensity exercise performance: A systematic review. *J Strength Cond Res* 24:257-265, 2010.

9. Baladia, E, Basulto, J, Manera, M, Martinez, R, and Calbet, D. Effect of green tea or green tea extract consumption on body weight and body composition: Systematic review and meta-analysis. *Nutr Hosp* 29:479-490, 2014.

10. Banned Substances Control Group. 2016. www.bscg.org. Accessed October 13, 2016.

11. Barnes, MJ. Alcohol: Impact on sports performance and recovery in male athletes. *Sports Med* 44:909-919, 2014.

12. Berti Zanella, P, Donner Alves, F, and Guerini, DESC. Effects of beta-alanine supplementation on performance and muscle fatigue in athletes and non-athletes of different sports: A systematic review. *J Sports Med Phys Fitness*, 2016.

13. Boozer, CN, Daly, PA, Homel, P, Solomon, JL, Blanchard, D, Nasser, JA, Strauss, R, and Meredith, T. Herbal ephedra/caffeine for weight loss: a 6-month randomized safety and efficacy trial. *Int J Obes Relat Metab Disord* 26:593-604, 2002.

14. Bryan, NS, and Ivy, JL. Inorganic nitrite and nitrate: Evidence to support consideration as dietary nutrients. *Nutr Res* 35:643-654, 2015.

15. Burke, LM. Practical considerations for bicarbonate loading and sports performance. *Nestle Nutr Inst Workshop Ser* 75:15-26, 2013.

16. Burke, LM, Collier, GR, Broad, EM, Davis, PG, Martin, DT, Sanigorski, AJ, and Hargreaves, M. Effect of alcohol intake on muscle glycogen storage after prolonged exercise. *J Appl Physiol (1985)* 95:983-990, 2003.

17. Chorley, JN, and Anding, RH. Performance-enhancing substances. *Adolesc Med State Art Rev* 26:174-188, 2015.

18. Clements, WT, Lee, SR, and Bloomer, RJ. Nitrate ingestion: A review of the health and physical performance effects. *Nutrients* 6:5224-5264, 2014.

19. Cohen, PA. Hazards of hindsight—Monitoring the safety of nutritional supplements. *N Engl J Med* 370:1277-1280, 2014.

20. Cohen, PA, Maller, G, DeSouza, R, and Neal-Kababick, J. Presence of banned drugs in dietary supplements following FDA recalls. *JAMA* 312:1691-1693, 2014.

21. Collomp, K, Buisson, C, Lasne, F, and Collomp, R. DHEA, physical exercise and doping. *J Steroid Biochem Mol Biol* 145:206-212, 2015.

22. DiMarco, NM, West, NP, Burke, LM, Stear, SJ, and Castell, LM. A-Z of nutritional supplements: Dietary supplements, sports nutrition foods and ergogenic aids for health and performance—Part 30. *Br J Sports Med* 46:299-300, 2012.

23. Esteghamati, A, Mazaheri, T, Vahidi Rad, M, and Noshad, S. Complementary and alternative medicine for the treatment of obesity: A critical review. *Int J Endocrinol Metab* 13:e19678, 2015.

24. Forstermann, U, and Munzel, T. Endothelial nitric oxide synthase in vascular disease: From marvel to menace. *Circulation* 113:1708-1714, 2006.

25. Gallagher, B, Tjoumakaris, FP, Harwood, MI, Good, RP, Ciccotti, MG, and Freedman, KB. Chondroprotection and the prevention of osteoarthritis progression of the knee: A systematic review of treatment agents. *Am J Sports Med* 43:734-744, 2015.

26. Gleeson, M, Siegler, JC, Burke, LM, Stear, SJ, and Castell, LM. A-Z of nutritional supplements: Dietary supplements, sports nutrition foods and ergogenic aids for health and performance—Part 31. *Br J Sports Med* 46:377-378, 2012.

27. Graham-Paulson, TS, Perret, C, Smith, B, Crosland, J, and Goosey-Tolfrey, VL. Nutritional supplement habits of athletes with an impairment and their sources of information. *Int J Sport Nutr Exerc Metab* 25:387-395, 2015.

28. Graham, T, and Spriet, L. Caffeine and exercise performance. *Gatorade Sports Science Exchange* 9, 1996.

29. Gurley, BJ, Steelman, SC, and Thomas, SL. Multi-ingredient, caffeine-containing dietary supplements: History, safety, and efficacy. *Clin Ther* 37:275-301, 2015.

30. Hatton, CK, Green, GA, and Ambrose, PJ. Performance-enhancing drugs: Understanding the risks. *Phys Med Rehabil Clin N Am* 25:897-913, 2014.

31. Hobson, RM, Saunders, B, Ball, G, Harris, RC, and Sale, C. Effects of beta-alanine supplementation on exercise performance: A meta-analysis. *Amino Acids* 43:25-37, 2012.

32. Hursel, R, Viechtbauer, W, and Westerterp-Plantenga, MS. The effects of green tea on weight loss and weight maintenance: A meta-analysis. *Int J Obes (Lond)* 33:956-961, 2009.

33. Hursel, R, and Westerterp-Plantenga, MS. Catechin- and caffeine-rich teas for control of body weight in humans. *Am J Clin Nutr* 98:1682s-1693s, 2013.

34. Informed Choice. 2016. www.informed-choice.org. Accessed January 7, 2016.

35. James, C-B, and Uhl, TL. A review of articular cartilage pathology and the use of glucosamine sulfate. *Journal of Athletic Training* 36:413-419, 2001.

36. Janssens, PL, Hursel, R, and Westerterp-Plantenga, MS. Nutraceuticals for body-weight management: The role of green tea catechins. *Physiol Behav* 162:83-87, 2016.

37. Jones, AM. Dietary nitrate supplementation and exercise performance. *Sports Med* 44:35-45, 2014.

38. Jull, AB, Ni Mhurchu, C, Bennett, DA, Dunshea-Mooij, CA, and Rodgers, A. Chitosan for overweight or obesity. *Cochrane Database Syst Rev*:Cd003892, 2008.

39. Kelley, DS, Vemuri, M, Adkins, Y, Gill, SH, Fedor, D, and Mackey, BE. Flaxseed oil prevents trans-10, cis-12-conjugated linoleic acid-induced insulin resistance in mice. *Br J Nutr* 101:701-708, 2009.

40. Kim, HJ, Kim, CK, Carpentier, A, and Poortmans, JR. Studies on the safety of creatine supplementation. *Amino Acids* 40:1409-1418, 2011.

41. Kim, J, Lee, J, Kim, S, Yoon, D, Kim, J, and Sung, DJ. Role of creatine supplementation in exercise-induced muscle damage: A mini review. *J Exerc Rehabil* 11:244-250, 2015.

42. King, DS, Baskerville, R, Hellsten, Y, Senchina, DS, Burke, LM, Stear, SJ, and Castell, LM. A-Z of nutritional supplements: Dietary supplements, sports nutrition foods and ergogenic aids for health and performance—Part 34. *Br J Sports Med* 46:689-690, 2012.

43. Kley, RA, Vorgerd, M, and Tarnopolsky, MA. Creatine for treating muscle disorders. *Cochrane Database Syst Rev*:Cd004760, 2007.

44. Knapik, JJ, Steelman, RA, Hoedebecke, SS, Austin, KG, Farina, EK, and Lieberman, HR. Prevalence of dietary supplement use by athletes: Systematic review and meta-analysis. *Sports Med* 46:103-123, 2016.

45. Koboziev, I, Karlsson, F, and Grisham, MB. Gut-associated lymphoid tissue, T cell trafficking, and chronic intestinal inflammation. *Ann N Y Acad Sci* 1207:E86-E93, 2010.

46. Lamis, DA, Ellis, JB, Chumney, FL, and Dula, CS. Reasons for living and alcohol use among college students. *Death Stud* 33:277-286, 2009.

47. Lanhers, C, Pereira, B, Naughton, G, Trousselard, M, Lesage, FX, and Dutheil, F. Creatine supplementation and upper limb strength performance: A systematic review and meta-analysis. *Sports Med* 47:163-173, 2016.

48. Lehnen, TE, da Silva, MR, Camacho, A, Marcadenti, A, and Lehnen, AM. A review on effects of conjugated linoleic fatty acid (CLA) upon body composition and energetic metabolism. *J Int Soc Sports Nutr* 12:36, 2015.

49. Lopez-Garcia, E, van Dam, RM, Rajpathak, S, Willett, WC, Manson, JE, and Hu, FB. Changes in caffeine intake and long-term weight change in men and women. *Am J Clin Nutr* 83:674-680, 2006.

50. Mayo Clinic. Caffeine Content for Coffee, Tea, Soda and More. 2016. www.mayoclinic.org/healthy-lifestyle/nutrition-and-healthy-eating/in-depth/caffeine/art-20049372. Accessed October 13, 2016.

51. Molfino, A, Gioia, G, Rossi Fanelli, F, and Muscaritoli, M. Beta-hydroxy-beta-methylbutyrate supplementation in health and disease: A systematic review of randomized trials. *Amino Acids* 45:1273-1292, 2013.

52. Moloney, F, Yeow, T-P, Mullen, A, Nolan, JJ, and Roche, HM. Conjugated linoleic acid supplementation, insulin sensitivity, and lipoprotein metabolism in patients with type 2 diabetes mellitus. *Am J Clin Nutr* 80:887-895, 2004.

53. Mora-Rodriguez, R, and Pallares, JG. Performance outcomes and unwanted side effects associated with energy drinks. *Nutr Rev* 72 Suppl 1:108-120, 2014.

54. National Center for Complementary and Integrative Health. Using Dietary Supplements Wisely: Safety Considerations. 2016. https://nccih.nih.gov/health/supplements/wiseuse.htm#hed6. Accessed October 6, 2016.

55. National Center for Drug Free Sport. Drug Free Sport. 2016. www.drugfreesport.com. Accessed January 7, 2016.

56. National Institutes of Health. College Drinking. 2015. http://pubs.niaaa.nih.gov/publications/CollegeFactSheet/CollegeFactSheet.pdf. Accessed October 28, 2016.

57. National Institutes of Health. Dietary Supplements for Weight Loss. 2016. https://ods.od.nih.gov/factsheets/WeightLoss-Health-Professional. Accessed October 26, 2016.

58. National Institutes of Health. Green Tea. 2016. https://nccih.nih.gov/health/greentea. Accessed October 28, 2016.

59. NSF International. 2016. www.nsf.org. Accessed January 7, 2016.

60. Onakpoya, I, Posadzki, P, and Ernst, E. Chromium supplementation in overweight and obesity: A systematic review and meta-analysis of randomized clinical trials. *Obes Rev* 14:496-507, 2013.

61. Onakpoya, I, Posadzki, P, and Ernst, E. The efficacy of glucomannan supplementation in overweight and obesity: a systematic review and meta-analysis of randomized clinical trials. *J Am Coll Nutr* 33:70-78, 2014.

62. Parr, EB, Camera, DM, Areta, JL, Burke, LM, Phillips, SM, Hawley, JA, and Coffey, VG. Alcohol ingestion impairs maximal post-exercise rates of myofibrillar protein synthesis following a single bout of concurrent training. *PLoS One* 9:e88384, 2014.

63. Persky, AM, and Rawson, ES. Safety of creatine supplementation. *Subcell Biochem* 46:275-289, 2007.

64. Pittler, MH, Abbot, NC, Harkness, EF, and Ernst, E. Randomized, double-blind trial of

chitosan for body weight reduction. *Eur J Clin Nutr* 53:379-381, 1999.

65. Pittler, MH, Stevinson, C, and Ernst, E. Chromium picolinate for reducing body weight: Meta-analysis of randomized trials. *Int J Obes Relat Metab Disord* 27:522-529, 2003.

66. Pronsky, Z, and Crowe, S. *Food Medication Interactions*. Birchrunville, PA: Food-Medication Interactions, 2015.

67. Pyne, DB, West, NP, Cox, AJ, and Cripps, AW. Probiotics supplementation for athletes—Clinical and physiological effects. *Eur J Sport Sci* 15:63-72, 2015.

68. Quesnele, JJ, Laframboise, MA, Wong, JJ, Kim, P, and Wells, GD. The effects of beta-alanine supplementation on performance: A systematic review of the literature. *Int J Sport Nutr Exerc Metab* 24:14-27, 2014.

69. Riserus, U, Vessby, B, Arnlov, J, and Basu, S. Effects of cis-9,trans-11 conjugated linoleic acid supplementation on insulin sensitivity, lipid peroxidation, and proinflammatory markers in obese men. *Am J Clin Nutr* 80:279-283, 2004.

70. Sahlin, K. Muscle energetics during explosive activities and potential effects of nutrition and training. *Sports Med* 44 Suppl 2:S167-173, 2014.

71. Sawka, MN, Burke, LM, Eichner, ER, Maughan, RJ, Montain, SJ, and Stachenfeld, NS. American College of Sports Medicine position stand. Exercise and fluid replacement. *Med Sci Sports Exerc* 39:377-390, 2007.

72. Semwal, RB, Semwal, DK, Vermaak, I, and Viljoen, A. A comprehensive scientific overview of Garcinia cambogia. *Fitoterapia* 102:134-148, 2015.

73. Sindelar, JJ, and Milkowski, AL. Human safety controversies surrounding nitrate and nitrite in the diet. *Nitric Oxide* 26:259-266, 2012.

74. Spriet, LL. Exercise and sport performance with low doses of caffeine. *Sports Med* 44 Suppl 2:S175-184, 2014.

75. Stohs, SJ, Preuss, HG, and Shara, M. The safety of Citrus aurantium (bitter orange) and its primary protoalkaloid p-synephrine. *Phytother Res* 25:1421-1428, 2011.

76. Stohs, SJ, Preuss, HG, and Shara, M. A review of the human clinical studies involving Citrus aurantium (bitter orange) extract and its primary protoalkaloid p-synephrine. *Int J Med Sci* 9:527-538, 2012.

77. Tarnopolsky, MA. Clinical use of creatine in neuromuscular and neurometabolic disorders. *Subcell Biochem* 46:183-204, 2007.

78. Tarnopolsky, MA. Caffeine and creatine use in sport. *Ann Nutr Metab* 57 Suppl 2:1-8, 2010.

79. Tarnopolsky, MA. Creatine as a therapeutic strategy for myopathies. *Amino Acids* 40:1397-1407, 2011.

80. Thomas, DT, Erdman, KA, and Burke, LM. Position of the Academy of Nutrition and Dietetics, Dietitians of Canada, and the American College of Sports Medicine: Nutrition and athletic performance. *J Acad Nutr Diet* 116:501-528, 2016.

81. Tian, H, Guo, X, Wang, X, He, Z, Sun, R, Ge, S, and Zhang, Z. Chromium picolinate supplementation for overweight or obese adults. *Cochrane Database Syst Rev* 11:Cd010063, 2013.

82. U.S. Anti-Doping Agency. 2016. www.usada.org. Accessed January 7, 2016.

83. U.S. Anti-Doping Agency. Supplement 411. 2016. www.usada.org/substances/supplement-411. Accessed January 7, 2016.

84. U.S. Food and Drug Administration. FDA to Investigate Added Caffeine. 2013. www.fda.gov/downloads/ForConsumers/ConsumerUpdates/UCM350740.pdf. Accessed October 28, 2016.

85. U.S. Food and Drug Administration. Dietary Supplements. 2016. www.fda.gov/Food/DietarySupplements/default.htm. Accessed January 5, 2016.

86. U.S. Food and Drug Administration. Food and Drug Administration Safety Alerts and Advisories. 2016. www.fda.gov/Food/RecallsOutbreaksEmergencies/SafetyAlertsAdvisories. Accessed August 3, 2016.

87. U.S. Food and Drug Administration. Guidance for Industry: A Food Labeling Guide (Appendix A: Definitions of Nutrient Content Claims). 2016. www.fda.gov/Food/GuidanceRegulation/GuidanceDocuments-RegulatoryInformation/LabelingNutrition/ucm064911.htm. Accessed Janaury 7, 2016.

88. U.S. Food and Drug Administration. Guidance for Industry: A Food Labeling Guide (Appendix B: Additional Requirements for Nutrient Content Claims). 2016. www.fda.gov/Food/GuidanceRegulation/GuidanceDocumentsRegulatoryInformation/LabelingNutrition/ucm064916.htm. Accessed Janaury 7, 2016.

89. U.S. Food and Drug Administration. Guidance for Industry: A Food Labeling Guide (Appendix C: Health Claims). 2016. www.fda.gov/Food/GuidanceRegulation/GuidanceDocumentsRegulatoryInformation/LabelingNutrition/ucm064919.htm. Accessed January 7, 2016.

90. U.S. Food and Drug Administration. Label Claims for Conventional Foods and Dietary Supplements. 2016. www.fda.gov/Food/IngredientsPackagingLabeling/LabelingNutrition/ucm111447.htm. Accessed January 5, 2016.

91. U.S. Food and Drug Administration. "Natural" on Food Labeling. 2016. www.fda.gov/Food/GuidanceRegulation/GuidanceDocumentsRegulatoryInformation/LabelingNutrition/ucm456090.htm. Accessed October 13, 2016.

92. U.S. Food and Drug Administration. Tainted Products Marketed as Dietary Supplements. 2016. www.accessdata.fda.gov/scripts/sda/sdNavigation.cfm?filter=&sortColumn=1d&sd=tainted_supplements_cder&page=1. Accessed January 7, 2016.

93. U.S. Food and Drug Administration. Why Isn't the Amount of Caffeine a Product Contains Required on a Food Label? 2016. www.fda.gov/AboutFDA/Transparency/Basics/ucm194317.htm. Accessed October 6, 2016.

94. U.S. Food and Drug Admistration. Food Labeling Guide. 2016. www.fda.gov/Food/GuidanceRegulation/GuidanceDocuments-RegulatoryInformation/LabelingNutrition/ucm2006828.htm. Accessed September 7, 2016.

95. U.S. Pharmacopeial Convention. 2016. www.usp.org. Accessed January 7, 2016.

96. United States Department of Agriculture. The Caffeine Content of Dietary Supplements Commonly Purchased in the U.S.: Analysis of 53 Products Having Caffeine-Containing Ingredients. 2007. https://www.ars.usda.gov/research/publications/publication/?seqNo115=213752. Accessed October 6, 2016.

97. van Rosendal, SP, and Coombes, JS. Glycerol use in hyperhydration and rehydration: Scientific update. *Med Sport Sci* 59:104-112, 2012.

98. van Rosendal, SP, Osborne, MA, Fassett, RG, and Coombes, JS. Physiological and performance effects of glycerol hyperhydration and rehydration. *Nutr Rev* 67:690-705, 2009.

99. Vemuri, M, Kelley, DS, Mackey, BE, Rasooly, R, and Bartolini, G. Docosahexaenoic acid (DHA) but not eicosapentaenoic acid (EPA) prevents trans-10, cis-12 conjugated linoleic acid (CLA)-induced insulin resistance in mice. *Metab Syndr Relat Disord* 5:315-322, 2007.

100. Web MD. NSAIDs (Nonsteroidal Anti-Inflammatory Drugs) and Arthritis. 2016. www.webmd.com/osteoarthritis/guide/anti-inflammatory-drugs#1. Accessed October 28, 2016.

101. Wruss, J, Waldenberger, G, Huemer, S, Uygun, P, Lanzerstorfer, P, Müller, U, Höglinger, O, and Weghuber, J. Compositional characteristics of commercial beetroot products and beetroot juice prepared from seven beetroot varieties grown in Upper Austria. *J Food Compost Anal* 42:46-55, 2015.

102. Wu, H, Xia, Y, Jiang, J, Du, H, Guo, X, Liu, X, Li, C, Huang, G, and Niu, K. Effect of beta-hydroxy-beta-methylbutyrate supplementation on muscle loss in older adults: A systematic review and meta-analysis. *Arch Gerontol Geriatr* 61:168-175, 2015.

103. Zalewski, BM, Chmielewska, A, and Szajewska, H. The effect of glucomannan on body weight in overweight or obese children and adults: A systematic review of randomized controlled trials. *Nutrition* 31:437-442, 2015.

104. Zalewski, BM, Chmielewska, A, Szajewska, H, Keithley, JK, Li, P, Goldsby, TU, and Allison, DB. Correction of data errors and reanalysis of "The effect of glucomannan on body weight in overweight or obese children and adults: A systematic review of randomized controlled trials". *Nutrition* 31:1056-1057, 2015.

105. Zanchi, NE, Gerlinger-Romero, F, Guimaraes-Ferreira, L, de Siqueira Filho, MA, Felitti, V, Lira, FS, Seelaender, M, and Lancha, AH, Jr. HMB supplementation: Clinical and athletic performance-related effects and mechanisms of action. *Amino Acids* 40:1015-1025, 2011.

106. Zhou, J, Heim, D, and Levy, A. Sports participation and alcohol use: Associations with sports-related identities and well-being. *J Stud Alcohol Drugs* 77:170-179, 2016.

Chapter 10

1. Aguilar-Valles, A, Inoue, W, Rummel, C, and Luheshi, GN. Obesity, adipokines and neuroinflammation. *Neuropharmacology* 96:124-134, 2015.

2. American College of Sports Medicine. *ACSM's Resource Manual for Guidelines for Exercise Testing and Prescritption.* Philadelphia: Wolters Kluwer-Lippincott, Williams, & Wilkins, 2014.

3. American Medical Association. Is Obesity a Disease? (Resolution 115-A-12). 2013. https://www.ama-assn.org/sites/default/files/media-browser/public/about-ama/councils/Council%20Reports/council-on-science-public-health/a13csaph3.pdf. Accessed February 20, 2017.

4. Centers for Disease Control and Prevention. About Adult BMI. www.cdc.gov/healthyweight/assessing/bmi/adult_bmi/index.html.

5. Centers for Disease Control and Prevention. Adult Obesity Causes and Consequences. www.cdc.gov/obesity/adult/causes.html.

6. Centers for Disease Control and Prevention. Assessing Your Weight. www.cdc.gov/healthyweight/assessing/index.html.

7. Durnin, JVGA, and Womersley, J. Body fat assessed from total body density and its estimation from skinfold thickness: Measurements of 481 men and women aged from 17-72 years. *Br J Nutr* 32:77-97, 1974.

8. Etchison, WC, Bloodgood, EA, Minton, CP, Thompson, NJ, Collins, MA, Hunter, SC, and Dai, H. Body mass index and percentage of body fat as indicators for obesity in an adolescent athletic population. *Sports Health* 3:249-252, 2011.

9. Freedman, DS, and Sherry, B. The validity of BMI as an indicator of body fatness and risk among children. *Pediatrics* 124 Suppl 1:S23-34, 2009.

10. Hall, DM, and Cole, TJ. What use is the BMI? *Arch Dis Child* 91:283-286, 2006.

11. Heyward, VH, and Wagner, DR. *Applied Body Composition Assessment.* Champaign, IL: Human Kinetics, 2004.

12. Hoffman, J. *Norms for Fitness, Performance, and Health.* Champaign, IL: Human Kinetics, 2006.

13. Howley, E, and Thompson, D. *Fitness Professional's Handbook.* Champaign, IL: Human Kinetics, 2017.

14. International Association for the Study of Obesity. Is Obesity a Disease? www.worldobesity.org/site_media/uploads/Is_obesity_a_disease.pdf. Accessed February 19, 2017.

15. Jackson, AS, and Pollock, ML. Practical assessment of body composition. *Phys Sportsmed* 13:76-90, 1985.

16. Jeukendrup, AE, and Gleeson, M. *Sport Nutrition.* Champaign, IL: Human Kinetics, 2010.

17. Jonnalagadda, SS, Skinner, R, and Moore, L. Overweight athlete: Fact or fiction? *Curr Sports Med Rep* 3:198-205, 2004.

18. Lohman, TG, and Going, SB. Multicompartment models in body composition research. *Basic Life Sci* 60:53-58, 1993.

19. Lohman, TG, Roche, AF, and Martorell, R. *Anthropometric Standardization Reference Manual.* Champaign, IL: Human Kinetics, 1988.

20. Manore, MM. Weight management for athletes and active individuals: A brief review. *Sports Med* 45 Suppl 1:83-92, 2015.

21. National Heart Lung and Blood Institute. Clinical Guidelines on the Identification, Evaluation, and Treatment of Overweight and Obesity in Adults: The Evidence Report. https://www.nhlbi.nih.gov/files/docs/guidelines/ob_gdlns.pdf. Accessed February 20, 2017.

22. Nattiv, A, Loucks, AB, Manore, MM, Sanborn, CF, Sundgot-Borgen, J, and Warren, MP. American College of Sports Medicine position stand. The female athlete triad. *Med Sci Sports Exerc* 39:1867-1882, 2007.

23. Radiological Society of North America. Bone Densitometry. 2017. www.radiologyinfo.org/en/info.cfm?pg=dexa.

24. Ross, CA, Caballero, B, Cousins, RJ, Tucker, KL, and Ziegler, TR. *Modern Nutrition in Health and Disease.* Baltimore, MD: Lippincott Williams & Wilkins, 2014.

25. Seidell, JC, Perusse, L, Despres, JP, and Bouchard, C. Waist and hip circumferences have independent and opposite effects on cardiovascular disease risk factors: The Quebec Family Study. *Am J Clin Nutr* 74:315-321, 2001.

26. Siri, WE. Body composition from fluid spaces and density: Analysis of methods. In *Techniques for Measuring Body Composition.* Brozek, J, Henschel, A, eds. Washington, DC: National Academy of Sciences, 1961, pp. 223-244.

27. Stoner, L, and Cornwall, J. Did the American Medical Association make the correct decision classifying obesity as a disease? *Australas Med J* 7:462-464, 2014.

28. Thomas, DT, Erdman, KA, and Burke, LM. Position of the Academy of Nutrition and Dietetics, Dietitians of Canada, and the American College of Sports Medicine: Nutrition and athletic performance. *J Acad Nutr Diet* 116:501-528, 2016.

29. Thompson, JL, Manore, MM, and Vaughan, LA. *The Science of Nutrition.* Upper Saddle River, NJ: Pearson Education, 2017.

30. U.S. Food and Drug Administration. Medications Target Long-Term Weight Control. www.fda.gov/downloads/ForConsumers/ConsumerUpdates/UCM312391.pdf.

31. Wallner-Liebmann, SJ, Kruschitz, R, Hubler, K, Hamlin, MJ, Schnedl, WJ, Moser, M, and Tafeit, E. A measure of obesity: BMI versus subcutaneous fat patterns in young athletes and nonathletes. *Coll Antropol* 37:351-357, 2013.

Chapter 11

1. Baar, K. Nutrition and the adaptation to endurance training. *Sports Med* 44 Suppl 1:S5-S12, 2014.

2. Bartlett, JD, Hawley, JA, and Morton, JP. Carbohydrate availability and exercise training adaptation: Too much of a good thing? *Eur J Sport Sci* 15:3-12, 2015.

3. Beelen, M, Burke, LM, Gibala, MJ, and van Loon, LJC. Nutritional strategies to promote postexercise recovery. *J Phys Act Health*:1-17, 2010.

4. Bergstrom, J, Hermanssen, L, and Saltin, B. Diet, muscle glycogen, andphysical performance. *Acta Physiol* 71:140-150, 1967.

5. Brooks, GA. Bioenergetics of exercising humans. *Compr Physiol* 2:537-562, 2012.

6. Brooks, GA, and Mercier, J. Balance of carbohydrate and lipid utilization during exercise: The "crossover" concept. *J Appl Physiol* 76:2253-2261, 1985.

7. Burke, LM. Nutrition strategies for the marathon: Fuel for training and racing. *Sports Med* 37:344-347, 2007.

8. Burke, LM. Fueling strategies to optimize performance: Training high or training low. *Scand J Med Sci Sports* 20:48-58, 2010.

9. Burke, LM. Re-examining high-fat diets for sports performance: Did we call the "nail in the coffin" too soon? *Sports Med* 45 Suppl 1:S33-49, 2015.

10. Burke, LM, Hawley, JA, Wong, SHS, and Jeukendrup, AE. Carbohydrates for training and competition. *J Sports Sci* 29:S17-S27, 2011.

11. Burke, LM, Kiens, B, and Ivy, JL. Carbohydrates and fat for training and recovery. *J Sports Sci* 22:15-30, 2004.

12. Burke, LM, Loucks, AB, and Broad, N. Energy and carbohydrates for training and recovery. *J Sports Sci* 24:675-685, 2006.

13. Cermak, NM, and van Loon, LJC. The use of carbohydrates during exercise as an ergogenic aid. *Sports Med* 43:1139-1155, 2013.

14. Coyle, EF. Timing and method of increased carbohydrate intake to cope with heavy training, competition and recovery. *J Sports Sci* 9:29-51, 1991.

15. Donaldson, C, Perry, T, and Rose, M. Glycemic index and endurance performance. *Int J Sport Nutr Exerc Metab* 20:154-165, 2010.

16. Hawley, JA, and Burke, LM. Carbohydrate availability and training adaptation: Effects on cell metabolism. *Exerc Sport Sci Rev* 38:152-160, 2010.

17. Ivy, JL. Muscle glycogen synthesis before and after exercise. *Sports Med* 11:6-19, 1991.

18. Jensen, J, Rustad, PI, Kolnes, AJ, and Lai, Y-C. The role of skeletal muscle glycogen breakdown for regulation of insulin sensitivity by exercise. *Front Physiol* 2:112, 2011.

19. Jeukendrup, AE. Nutrition for endurance sports: Marathon, triathlon, and road cycling. *J Sports Sci* 29:S91-S99, 2011.

20. Jeukendrup, AE. Performance and endurance in sport: Can it all be explained by metabolism and its manipulation? *Dialog Cardiovasc Med* 17:40-45, 2012.

21. Jeukendrup, AE. Multiple transportable carbohydrates and their benefits. *Gatorade Sports Science Exchange* 26:1-5, 2013.

22. Jeukendrup, AE. A step towards personalized sports nutrition: Carbohydrate intake during exercise. *Sports Med* 44:S25-S33, 2014.

23. Jeukendrup, AE, and Gleeson, M. *Sport Nutrition*. Champaign, IL: Human Kinetics, 2010.

24. Jeukendrup, AE, Rollo, I, and Carter, JM. Carbohydrate mouth rinse: Performance effects and mechanisms. *Gatorade Sports Science Exchange* 26:1-8, 2013.

25. Jozsi, AC, Trappe, TA, Starlling, RD, Goodpaster, B, Trappe, SW, Fink, WJ, and Costill, DL. The influence of starch structure on glycogen resynthesis and subsequent cycling performance. *Int J Sports Med* 17:373-378, 1996.

26. Karpinski, C, and Rosenbloom, C. *Sports Nutrition: A Handbook for Professionals*. Chicago, IL: Academy of Nutrition and Dietetics, 2017.

27. Kenny, WL, Wilmore, JH, and Costill, DL. *Physiology of Sport and Exercise*. Champaign, IL: Human Kinetics, 2015.

28. Kreher, JB, and Schwartz, JB. Overtraining syndrome: A practical guide. *Sports Health* 4:128-138, 2012.

29. Kreitzman, SN, Coxon, AY, and Szaz, KF. Glycogen storage: Illusions of easy weight loss, excessive weight regain, and distortions in estimates of body composition. *Am J Clin Nutr* 56:292s-293s, 1992.

30. Manore, MM. Weight management for athletes and active individuals: A brief review. *Sports Med* 45 Suppl 1:83-92, 2015.

31. Manore, MM, Brown, K, Houtkooper, L, Jakicic, JM, Peters, JC, Smith Edge, M, Steiber, A, Going, S, Guillermin Gable, L, and Krautheim, AM. Energy balance at a crossroads: Translating the science into action. *J Acad Nutr Diet* 114:1113-1119, 2014.

32. Meeusen, R, Duclos, M, Foster, C, Fry, A, Gleeson, M, Nieman, D, Raglin, J, Rietjens, G, Steinacker, J, and Urhausen, A. Prevention, diagnosis, and treatment of the overtraining syndrome: Joint consensus statement of the European College of Sports Medicine and the American College of Sports Medicine. *Med Sci Sports Exerc* 45:186-205, 2013.

33. Mountjoy, M, Sundgot-Borgen, J, Burke, L, Carter, S, Constantini, N, Lebrun, C, Meyer, N, Sherman, R, Steffen, K, Budgett, R, and Ljungqvist, A. The IOC consensus statement: Beyond the female athlete triad—Relative energy deficiency in sport (RED-S). *Br J Sports Med* 48:491-497, 2014.

34. National Academy of Sciences. Dietary Reference Intakes for Energy, Carbohydrate, Fiber, Fat, Fatty Acids, Cholesterol, Protein, and Amino Acids (Macronutrients). Washington, DC: National Academies Press, 2005.

35. O'Reilly, J, Wong, S, and Chen, Y. Glycaemic index, glycaemic load, and exercise performance. *Sports Med* 40:27-39, 2010.

36. Ormsbee, MJ, Bach, CW, and Baur, DA. Pre-exercise nutrition: The role of macronutrients, modified starches and supplements on metabolism and endurance performance. *Nutrients* 6:1782-1808, 2014.

37. Pfeiffer, B, Stellingwerf, T, Hodgson, AB, Randell, R, Pottgen, K, Res, P, and Jeukendrup, AE. Nutritional intake and gastrointestinal problems during competetive endurance events. *Med Sci Sports Exerc* 44:344-351, 2012.

38. Phillips, SM, and Van Loon, LJ. Dietary protein for athletes: From requirements to optimum adaptation. *J Sports Sci* 29 Suppl 1:S29-38, 2011.

39. Prado de Oliveira, E. Nutritional recommendations to avoid gastrointestinal complaints during exercise. *Gatorade Sports Science Exchange* 26:1-4, 2013.

40. Prado de Oliveira, E, Burini, RC, and Jeukendrup, AE. Gastrointestinal complaints during exercise: Prevalance, etiology, and nutritional recommendations. *Sports Med* 44:S79-S85, 2014.

41. Roberts, MD, Lockwood, C, Dalbo, VJ, Volek, J, and Kerksick, CM. Ingestion of a high-molecular-weight hydrothermally modified waxy maize starch alters metabolic responses to prolonged exercise in trained cyclists. *Nutrition* 27:659-665, 2011.

42. Romijn, JA, Coyle, EF, Sidossis, LS, Zhangm, XJ, and Wolfe, RR. Relationship between fatty acid delivery and fatty acid oxidation during strenuous exercise. *J Appl Physiol* 79:1939-1945, 1995.

43. Rong, Y, Sillick, M, and Gregson, CM. Determination of dextrose equivalent value and number average molecular weight of maltodextrin by osmometry. *J Food Sci* 74:C33-C40, 2009.

44. Sands, AL, Leidy, HJ, Hamaker, BR, Maguire, P, and Campbell, WW. Consumption of the slow-digesting waxy maize starch leads to blunted plasma glucose and insulin response but does not influence energy expenditure or appetite in humans. *Nutr Res* 29:383-390, 2009.

45. Shaw, CS, Clark, J, and Wagenmakers, AJ. The effect of exercise and nutrition on intramuscular fat metabolism and insulin sensitivity. *Annu Rev Nutr* 30:13-34, 2010.

46. Sherman, WM, Costill, DL, Fink, WJ, and Miller, JM. The effect of exercise and diet manipulation on muscle glycogen and its subsequent use during performance. *Int J Sports Med* 2:114-118, 1981.

47. Spriet, LL. New insights into the interaction of carbohydrate and fat metabolis, during exercise. *Sports Med* 44:S87-S96, 2014.

48. Stellingwerff, T, Maughan, RJ, and Burke, LM. Nutrition for power sports: Middle-distance running, track cycling, rowing, canoeing/kayaking, and swimming. *J Sports Sci* 29 Suppl 1:S79-89, 2011.

49. Stephens, FB, Roig, M, Armstrong, G, and Greenhaff, PL. Post-exercise ingestion of a unique, high molecular weight glucose polymer solution improves performance during a subsequent bout of cycling exercise. *J Sports Sci* 26:149-154, 2008.

50. Tarnopolsky, LJ, MacDougall, JD, Atkinson, SA, Tarnopolsky, MA, and Sutton, JR. Gender differences in substrate for endurance exercise. *J Appl Physiol* 68:302-308, 1990.

51. Tarnopolsky, MA, Bosman, M, Macdonald, JR, Vandeputte, D, Martin, J, and Roy, BD. Postexercise protein-carbohydrate and carbohydrate supplements increase muscle glycogen in men and women. *J Appl Physiol* 83:1877-1883, 1997.

52. Tarnopolsky, MA, Gibala, M, Jeukendrup, A, and Phillips, SM. Nutritional needs of elite endurance athletes. Part I: Carbohydrate and fluid requirements. *Eur J Sport Sci* 5:3 - 14, 2005.

53. Thomas, DT, Erdman, KA, and Burke, LM. Position of the Academy of Nutrition and Dietetics, Dietitians of Canada, and the American College of Sports Medicine: Nutrition and athletic performance. *J Acad Nutr Diet* 116:501-528, 2016.

54. U.S. Department of Health and Human Services and U.S. Department of Agricul-

ture. 2015–2020 Dietary Guidelines for Americans, The Dietary Guidelines for Americans: What It Is, What It Is Not. 2016. https://health.gov/dietaryguidelines/2015/guidelines/introduction/dietary-guidelines-for-americans. Accessed September 7, 2016.

55. U.S. Food and Drug Administration. Food Labeling Guide. Silver Spring, MD: U.S. Food and Drug Administration.

56. U.S. Food and Drug Administration. How Sweet It Is: All About Sugar Substitutes. 2014. www.fda.gov/ForConsumers/ConsumerUpdates/ucm397711.htm. Accessed Generic, May.

57. United States Department of Agriculture. National Agricultural Library Nutrient Data Lab. 2016. https://ndb.nal.usda.gov. Accessed July 30, 2016.

58. van Loon, LJ. Use of intramuscular triacylglycerol as a substrate source during exercise in humans. *J Appl Physiol* 97:1170-1187, 2004.

59. van Loon, LJ. Is there a need for protein ingestion during exercise? *Sports Med* 44 Suppl 1:S105-S111, 2014.

60. Walker, JL, Heigenhauser, GJ, Hultman, E, and Spriet, LL. Dietary carbohydrate, muscle glycogen content, and endurance performance in well-trained women. *J Appl Physiol* 88:2151-2158, 2000.

Chapter 12

1. Antonio, J, Peacock, CA, Ellerbroek, A, Fromhoff, B, and Silver, T. The effects of consuming a high protein diet (4.4 g/kg/d) on body composition in resistance-trained individuals. *J Int Soc Sports Nutr* 11:19, 2014.

2. Apro, W, Wang, L, Ponten, M, Blomstrand, E, and Sahlin, K. Resistance exercise induced mTORC1 signaling is not impaired by subsequent endurance exercise in human skeletal muscle. *Am J Physiol Endocrinol Metab* 305:E22-E32, 2013.

3. Areta, JL, Burke, LM, Camera, DM, West, DW, Crawshay, S, Moore, DR, Stellingwerff, T, Phillips, SM, Hawley, JA, and Coffey, VG. Reduced resting skeletal muscle protein synthesis is rescued by resistance exercise and protein ingestion following short-term energy deficit. *Am J Physiol Endocrinol Metab* 306:E989-E997, 2014.

4. Atherton, PJ, Etheridge, T, Watt, PW, Wilkinson, D, Selby, A, Rankin, D, Smith, K, and Rennie, MJ. Muscle full effect after oral protein: Time-dependent concordance and discordance between human muscle protein synthesis and mTORC1 signaling. *Am J Clin Nutr* 92:1080-1088, 2010.

5. Baar, K. Using molecular biology to maximize concurrent training. *Sports Med* 44 Suppl 2:S117-S125, 2014.

6. Babault, N, Paizis, C, Deley, G, Guerin-Deremaux, L, Saniez, MH, Lefranc-Millot, C, and Allaert, FA. Pea proteins oral supplementation promotes muscle thickness gains during resistance training: A double-blind, randomized, placebo-controlled clinical trial vs. whey protein. *J Int Soc Sports Nutr* 12:3, 2015.

7. Balon, TW, Horowitz, JF, and Fitzsimmons, KM. Effects of carbohydrate loading and weight-lifting on muscle girth. *Int J Sport Nutr* 2:328-334, 1992.

8. Beaudart, C, Buckinx, F, Rabenda, V, Gillain, S, Cavalier, E, Slomian, J, Petermans, J, Reginster, JY, and Bruyere, O. The effects of vitamin D on skeletal muscle strength, muscle mass, and muscle power: A systematic review and meta-analysis of randomized controlled trials. *J Clin Endocrinol Metab* 99:4336-4345, 2014.

9. Biolo, G, Maggi, SP, Williams, BD, Tipton, KD, and Wolfe, RR. Increased rates of muscle protein turnover and amino acid transport after resistance exercise in humans. *Am J Physiol* 268:E514-E520, 1995.

10. Bischoff-Ferrari, HA, Shao, A, Dawson-Hughes, B, Hathcock, J, Giovannucci, E, and Willett, WC. Benefit-risk assessment of vitamin D supplementation. *Osteoporos Int* 21:1121-1132, 2010.

11. Bohe, J, Low, JF, Wolfe, RR, and Rennie, MJ. Latency and duration of stimulation of human muscle protein synthesis during continuous infusion of amino acids. *J Physiol* 532:575-579, 2001.

12. Boisseau, N, and Delamarche, P. Metabolic and hormonal responses to exercise in children and adolescents. *Sports Med* 30:405-422, 2000.

13. Boisseau, N, Vermorel, M, Rance, M, Duche, P, and Patureau-Mirand, P. Protein requirements in male adolescent soccer players. *Eur J Appl Physiol* 100:27-33, 2007.

14. Borsheim, E, Cree, MG, Tipton, KD, Elliott, TA, Aarsland, A, and Wolfe, RR. Effect of carbohydrate intake on net muscle protein synthesis during recovery from resistance exercise. *J Appl Physiol (1985)* 96:674-678, 2004.

15. Bouillanne, O, Curis, E, Hamon-Vilcot, B, Nicolis, I, Chretien, P, Schauer, N, Vincent, JP, Cynober, L, and Aussel, C. Impact of protein pulse feeding on lean mass in malnourished and at-risk hospitalized elderly patients: A randomized controlled trial. *Clin Nutr* 32:186-192, 2013.

16. Brown, K, DeCoffe, D, Molcan, E, and Gibson, DL. Diet-induced dysbiosis of the intestinal microbiota and the effects on immunity and disease. *Nutrients* 4:1095-1119, 2012.

17. Brun, JF, Dieu-Cambrezy, C, Charpiat, A, Fons, C, Fedou, C, Micallef, JP, Fussellier, M, Bardet, L, and Orsetti, A. Serum zinc in highly trained adolescent gymnasts. *Biol Trace Elem Res* 47:273-278, 1995.

18. Burke, LM. Fueling strategies to optimize performance: Training high or training low? *Scand J Med Sci Sports* 20 Suppl 2:48-58, 2010.

19. Camera, DM, West, DW, Phillips, SM, Rerecich, T, Stellingwerff, T, Hawley, JA, and Coffey, VG. Protein ingestion increases myofibrillar protein synthesis after concurrent exercise. *Med Sci Sports Exerc* 47:82-91, 2015.

20. Campbell, B, Kreider, RB, Ziegenfuss, T, La Bounty, P, Roberts, M, Burke, D, Landis, J, Lopez, H, and Antonio, J. International Society of Sports Nutrition position stand: Protein and exercise. *J Int Soc Sports Nutr* 4:8, 2007.

21. Candow, DG, Burke, NC, Smith-Palmer, T, and Burke, DG. Effect of whey and soy protein supplementation combined with resistance training in young adults. *Int J Sport Nutr Exerc Metab* 16:233-244, 2006.

22. Casperson, SL, Sheffield-Moore, M, Hewlings, SJ, and Paddon-Jones, D. Leucine supplementation chronically improves muscle protein synthesis in older adults consuming the RDA for protein. *Clin Nutr* 31:512-519, 2012.

23. Cecelja, M, and Chowienczyk, P. Role of arterial stiffness in cardiovascular disease. *JRSM Cardiovasc Dis* 1, 2012.

24. Cermak, NM, Res, PT, de Groot, LC, Saris, WH, and van Loon, LJ. Protein supplementation augments the adaptive response of skeletal muscle to resistance-type exercise training: A meta-analysis. *Am J Clin Nutr* 96:1454-1464, 2012.

25. Charge, SB, and Rudnicki, MA. Cellular and molecular regulation of muscle regeneration. *Physiol Rev* 84:209-238, 2004.

26. Chen, HY, Cheng, FC, Pan, HC, Hsu, JC, and Wang, MF. Magnesium enhances exercise performance via increasing glucose availability in the blood, muscle, and brain during exercise. *PLoS One* 9:e85486, 2014.

27. Churchward-Venne, TA, Burd, NA, and Phillips, SM. Nutritional regulation of muscle protein synthesis with resistance exercise: Strategies to enhance anabolism. *Nutr Metab (Lond)* 9:40, 2012.

28. Coburn, JW, Housh, DJ, Housh, TJ, Malek, MH, Beck, TW, Cramer, JT, Johnson, GO, and Donlin, PE. Effects of leucine and whey protein supplementation during eight weeks of unilateral resistance training. *J Strength Cond Res* 20:284-291, 2006.

29. Coffey, VG, Jemiolo, B, Edge, J, Garnham, AP, Trappe, SW, and Hawley, JA. Effect of consecutive repeated sprint and resistance exercise bouts on acute adaptive responses in human skeletal muscle. *Am J Physiol Regul Integr Comp Physiol* 297:R1441-R1451, 2009.

30. Coppola, G, Natale, F, Torino, A, Capasso, R, D'Aniello, A, Pironti, E, Santoro, E, Calabro, R, and Verrotti, A. The impact of the ketogenic diet on arterial morphology and endothelial function in children and young adults with epilepsy: A case-control study. *Seizure* 23:260-265, 2014.

31. Cribb, PJ, Williams, AD, and Hayes, A. A creatine-protein-carbohydrate supplement enhances responses to resistance training. *Med Sci Sports Exerc* 39:1960-1968, 2007.

32. Deutz, NE, Pereira, SL, Hays, NP, Oliver, JS, Edens, NK, Evans, CM, and Wolfe, RR. Effect of beta-hydroxy-beta-methylbutyrate (HMB) on lean body mass during 10 days of bed rest in older adults. *Clin Nutr* 32:704-712, 2013.

33. Deutz, NE, and Wolfe, RR. Is there a maximal anabolic response to protein intake with a meal? *Clin Nutr* 32:309-313, 2013.

34. Devries, MC, and Phillips, SM. Creatine supplementation during resistance training in older adults: A meta-analysis. *Med Sci Sports Exerc* 46:1194-1203, 2014.

35. Donges, CE, Burd, NA, Duffield, R, Smith, GC, West, DW, Short, MJ, Mackenzie, R, Plank, LD, Shepherd, PR, Phillips, SM, and Edge, JA. Concurrent resistance and aerobic exercise stimulates both myofibrillar and mitochondrial protein synthesis in sedentary middle-aged men. *J Appl Physiol* 112:1992-2001, 2012.

36. Duplanty, AA, Budnar, RG, Luk, HY, Levitt, DE, Hill, DW, McFarlin, BK, Huggett, DB, and Vingren, JL. Effect of acute alcohol ingestion on resistance exercise induced mTORC1 signaling in human muscle. *J Strength Cond Res* 31, 2017.

37. Folland, JP, and Williams, AG. The adaptations to strength training: Morphological and neurological contributions to increased strength. *Sports Med* 37:145-168, 2007.

38. Frost, RA, and Lang, CH. Multifaceted role of insulin-like growth factors and mTOR in skeletal muscle. *Endocrinol Metab Clin North Am* 41:297-322, 2012.

39. Garfinkel, D, and Garfinkel, L. Magnesium and regulation of carbohydrate metabolism at the molecular level. *Magnesium* 7:249-261, 1988.

40. Gilani, GS, Cockell, KA, and Sepehr, E. Effects of antinutritional factors on protein digestibility and amino acid availability in foods. *J AOAC Int* 88:967-987, 2005.

41. Glynn, EL, Fry, CS, Drummond, MJ, Dreyer, HC, Dhanani, S, Volpi, E, and Rasmussen, BB. Muscle protein breakdown has a minor role in the protein anabolic response to essential amino acid and carbohydrate intake following resistance exercise. *Am J Physiol Regul Integr Comp Physiol* 299:R533-R540, 2010.

42. Gran, P, and Cameron-Smith, D. The actions of exogenous leucine on mTOR signalling and amino acid transporters in human myotubes. *BMC Physiol* 11:10, 2011.

43. Haff, GG, Koch, AJ, Potteiger, JA, Kuphal, KE, Magee, LM, Green, SB, and Jakicic, JJ. Carbohydrate supplementation attenuates muscle glycogen loss during acute bouts of resistance exercise. *Int J Sport Nutr Exerc Metab* 10:326-339, 2000.

44. Haff, GG, Lehmkuhl, MJ, McCoy, LB, and Stone, MH. Carbohydrate supplementation and resistance training. *J Strength Cond Res* 17:187-196, 2003.

45. Hall, KD, Chen, KY, Guo, J, Lam, YY, Leibel, RL, Mayer, LE, Reitman, ML, Rosenbaum, M, Smith, SR, Walsh, BT, and Ravussin, E. Energy expenditure and body composition changes after an isocaloric ketogenic diet in overweight and obese men. *Am J Clin Nutr* 104:324-333, 2016.

46. Hamada, K, Vannier, E, J.M., S, Witsell, AL, and Roubenoff, R. Senescence of human skeletal muscle impairs the local inflammatory cytokine response to acute eccentric exercise. *FASEB Journal* 19:264-266, 2005.

47. Hartman, JW, Tang, JE, Wilkinson, SB, Tarnopolsky, MA, Lawrence, RL, Fullerton, AV, and Phillips, SM. Consumption of fat-free fluid milk after resistance exercise promotes greater lean mass accretion than does consumption of soy or carbohydrate in young, novice, male weightlifters. *Am J Clin Nutr* 86:373-381, 2007.

48. Hatfield, DL, Kraemer, WJ, Volek, JS, Rubin, MR, Grebien, B, Gomez, AL, French, DN, Scheett, TP, Ratamess, NA, Sharman, MJ, McGuigan, MR, Newton, RU, and Hakkinen, K. The effects of carbohydrate loading on repetitive jump squat power performance. *J Strength Cond Res* 20:167-171, 2006.

49. Helge, JW, Watt, PW, Richter, EA, Rennie, MJ, and Kiens, B. Fat utilization during exercise: Adaptation to a fat-rich diet increases utilization of plasma fatty acids and very low density lipoprotein-triacylglycerol in humans. *J Physiol* 537:1009-1020, 2001.

50. Helms, ER, Aragon, AA, and Fitschen, PJ. Evidence-based recommendations for natural bodybuilding contest preparation: nutrition and supplementation. *J Int Soc Sports Nutr* 11:20, 2014.

51. Hubal, MJ, Gordish-Dressman, H, Thompson, PD, Price, TB, Hoffman, EP, Angelopoulos, TJ, Gordon, PM, Moyna, NM, Pescatello, LS, Visich, PS, Zoeller, RF, Seip, RL, and Clarkson, PM. Variability in muscle size and strength gain after unilateral resistance training. *Med Sci Sports Exerc* 37:964-972, 2005.

52. Hulmi, JJ, Laakso, M, Mero, AA, Hakkinen, K, Ahtiainen, JP, and Peltonen, H. The effects of whey protein with or without carbohydrates on resistance training adaptations. *J Int Soc Sports Nutr* 12:48, 2015.

53. Ivy, JL. Regulation of muscle glycogen repletion, muscle protein synthesis and repair following exercise. *J Sports Sci Med* 3:131-138, 2004.

54. Jacobs, I, Kaiser, P, and Tesch, P. Muscle strength and fatigue after selective glycogen depletion in human skeletal muscle fibers. *Eur J Appl Physiol Occup Physiol* 46:47-53, 1981.

55. Judelson, DA, Maresh, CM, Anderson, JM, Armstrong, LE, Casa, DJ, Kraemer, WJ, and Volek, JS. Hydration and muscular performance: Does fluid balance affect strength, power and high-intensity endurance? *Sports Med* 37:907-921, 2007.

56. Judelson, DA, Maresh, CM, Farrell, MJ, Yamamoto, LM, Armstrong, LE, Kraemer, WJ, Volek, JS, Spiering, BA, Casa, DJ, and Anderson, JM. Effect of hydration state on strength, power, and resistance exercise performance. *Med Sci Sports Exerc* 39:1817-1824, 2007.

57. Judelson, DA, Maresh, CM, Yamamoto, LM, Farrell, MJ, Armstrong, LE, Kraemer, WJ, Volek, JS, Spiering, BA, Casa, DJ, and Anderson, JM. Effect of hydration state on resistance exercise-induced endocrine markers of anabolism, catabolism, and metabolism. *J Appl Physiol (1985)* 105:816-824, 2008.

58. Kapetanakis, M, Liuba, P, Odermarsky, M, Lundgren, J, and Hallbook, T. Effects of ketogenic diet on vascular function. *Eur J Paediatr Neurol* 18:489-494, 2014.

59. Kerksick, C, Thomas, A, Campbell, B, Taylor, L, Wilborn, C, Marcello, B, Roberts, M, Pfau, E, Grimstvedt, M, Opusunju, J, Magrans-Courtney, T, Rasmussen, C, Wilson, R, and Kreider, RB. Effects of a popular exercise and weight loss program on weight loss, body composition, energy expenditure and health in obese women. *Nutr Metab (Lond)* 6:23, 2009.

60. Kerksick, CM, Wilborn, CD, Campbell, WI, Harvey, TM, Marcello, BM, Roberts, MD, Parker, AG, Byars, AG, Greenwood, LD, Almada, AL, Kreider, RB, and Greenwood, M. The effects of creatine monohydrate supplementation with and without D-pinitol on resistance training adaptations. *J Strength Cond Res* 23:2673-2682, 2009.

61. Kimball, SR, and Jefferson, LS. Regulation of protein synthesis by branched-chain amino acids. *Curr Opin Clin Nutr Metab Care* 4:39-43, 2001.

62. Koopman, R, Verdijk, L, Manders, RJ, Gijsen, AP, Gorselink, M, Pijpers, E, Wagenmakers, AJ, and van Loon, LJ. Co-ingestion of protein and leucine stimulates muscle protein synthesis rates to the same extent in young and elderly lean men. *Am J Clin Nutr* 84:623-632, 2006.

63. Krotkiewski, M, Gudmundsson, M, Backstrom, P, and Mandroukas, K. Zinc and muscle strength and endurance. *Acta Physiol Scand* 116:309-311, 1982.

64. Layman, DK. Dietary Guidelines should reflect new understandings about adult protein needs. *Nutr Metab (Lond)* 6:12, 2009.

65. LeBlanc, ES, Zakher, B, Daeges, M, Pappas, M, and Chou, R. Screening for vitamin D deficiency: A systematic review for the U.S. Preventive Services Task Force. *Ann Intern Med* 162:109-122, 2015.

66. Leenders, M, Verdijk, LB, van der Hoeven, L, van Kranenburg, J, Hartgens, F, Wodzig, WK, Saris, WH, and van Loon, LJ. Prolonged leucine supplementation does not augment muscle mass or affect glycemic control in elderly type 2 diabetic men. *J Nutr* 141:1070-1076, 2011.

67. Lemon, PW, and Mullin, JP. Effect of initial muscle glycogen levels on protein catabolism during exercise. *J Appl Physiol Respir Environ Exerc Physiol* 48:624-629, 1980.

68. Loenneke, JP, Loprinzi, PD, Murphy, CH, and Phillips, SM. Per meal dose and frequency of protein consumption is associated with lean mass and muscle performance. *Clin Nutr* 35:1506-1511, 2016.

69. Lundberg, TR, Fernandez-Gonzalo, R, Gustafsson, T, and Tesch, PA. Aerobic exercise alters skeletal muscle molecular responses to resistance exercise. *Med Sci Sports Exerc* 44:1680-1688, 2012.

70. Lundberg, TR, Fernandez-Gonzalo, R, Gustafsson, T, and Tesch, PA. Aerobic exercise does not compromise muscle hypertrophy response to short-term resistance training. *J Appl Physiol (1985)* 114:81-89, 2013.

71. MacDougall, JD, Ray, S, Sale, DG, McCartney, N, Lee, P, and Garner, S. Muscle substrate utilization and lactate production. *Can J Appl Physiol* 24:209-215, 1999.

72. MacDougall, JD, Ray, S, Sale, DG, McCartney, N, Lee, P, and Garner, S. Muscle substrate utilization and lactate production during weightlifting. *Can J Appl Physiol* 24:209-215, 1999.

73. Macnaughton, LS, Wardle, SL, Witard, OC, McGlory, C, Hamilton, DL, Jeromson, S, Lawrence, CE, Wallis, GA, and Tipton, KD. The response of muscle protein synthesis following whole-body resistance exercise is greater following 40 g than 20 g of ingested whey protein. *Physiol Rep* 4, 2016.

74. Mamerow, MM, Mettler, JA, English, KL, Casperson, SL, Arentson-Lantz, E, Sheffield-Moore, M, Layman, DK, and Paddon-Jones, D. Dietary protein distribution positively influences 24-h muscle protein synthesis in healthy adults. *J Nutr* 144:876-880, 2014.

75. Moore, DR, Churchward-Venne, TA, Witard, O, Breen, L, Burd, NA, Tipton, KD, and Phillips, SM. Protein ingestion to stimulate myofibrillar protein synthesis requires greater relative protein intakes in healthy older versus younger men. *J Gerontol A Biol Sci Med Sci* 70:57-62, 2015.

76. Moore, DR, Robinson, MJ, Fry, JL, Tang, JE, Glover, EI, Wilkinson, SB, Prior, T, Tarnopolsky, MA, and Phillips, SM. Ingested protein dose response of muscle and albumin protein synthesis after resistance exercise in young men. *Am J Clin Nutr* 89:161-168, 2009.

77. Mori, H. Effect of timing of protein and carbohydrate intake after resistance exercise on nitrogen balance in trained and untrained young men. *J Physiol Anthropol* 33:24, 2014.

78. Negro, M, Vandoni, M, Ottobrini, S, Codrons, E, Correale, L, Buonocore, D, and Marzatico, F. Protein supplementation with low fat meat after resistance training: effects on body composition and strength. *Nutrients* 6:3040-3049, 2014.

79. Norton, LE, Layman, DK, Bunpo, P, Anthony, TG, Brana, DV, and Garlick, PJ. The leucine content of a complete meal directs peak activation but not duration of skeletal muscle protein synthesis and mammalian target of rapamycin signaling in rats. *J Nutr* 139:1103-1109, 2009.

80. Paddon-Jones, D, and Leidy, H. Dietary protein and muscle in older persons. *Curr Opin Clin Nutr Metab Care* 17:5-11, 2014.

81. Paddon-Jones, D, and Rasmussen, BB. Dietary protein recommendations and the prevention of sarcopenia. *Curr Opin Clin Nutr Metab Care* 12:86-90, 2009.

82. Paddon-Jones, D, Sheffield-Moore, M, Zhang, XJ, Volpi, E, Wolf, SE, Aarsland, A, Ferrando, AA, and Wolfe, RR. Amino acid ingestion improves muscle protein synthesis in the young and elderly. *Am J Physiol Endocrinol Metab* 286:E321-E328, 2004.

83. Paoli, A, Grimaldi, K, D'Agostino, D, Cenci, L, Moro, T, Bianco, A, and Palma, A. Ketogenic diet does not affect strength performance in elite artistic gymnasts. *J Int Soc Sports Nutr* 9:34, 2012.

84. Parkin, JA, Carey, MF, Martin, IK, Stojanovska, L, and Febbraio, MA. Muscle glycogen storage following prolonged exercise: effect of timing of ingestion of high glycemic index food. *Med Sci Sports Exerc* 29:220-224, 1997.

85. Pascoe, DD, Costill, DL, Fink, WJ, Robergs, RA, and Zachwieja, JJ. Glycogen resynthesis in skeletal muscle following resistive exercise. *Med Sci Sports Exerc* 25:349-354, 1993.

86. Pasiakos, SM, Cao, JJ, Margolis, LM, Sauter, ER, Whigham, LD, McClung, JP, Rood, JC, Carbone, JW, Combs, GF, Jr., and Young, AJ. Effects of high-protein diets on fat-free mass and muscle protein synthesis following weight loss: A randomized controlled trial. *FASEB J* 27:3837-3847, 2013.

87. Pasiakos, SM, Vislocky, LM, Carbone, JW, Altieri, N, Konopelski, K, Freake, HC, Anderson, JM, Ferrando, AA, Wolfe, RR, and Rodriguez, NR. Acute energy deprivation affects skeletal muscle protein synthesis and associated intracellular signaling proteins in physically active adults. *J Nutr* 140:745-751, 2010.

88. Pennings, B, Boirie, Y, Senden, JM, Gijsen, AP, Kuipers, H, and van Loon, LJ. Whey protein stimulates postprandial muscle protein accretion more effectively than do casein and casein hydrolysate in older men. *Am J Clin Nutr* 93:997-1005, 2011.

89. Pennings, B, Groen, BB, van Dijk, JW, de Lange, A, Kiskini, A, Kuklinski, M, Senden, JM, and van Loon, LJ. Minced beef is more rapidly digested and absorbed than beef steak, resulting in greater postprandial protein retention in older men. *Am J Clin Nutr* 98:121-128, 2013.

90. Perez-Schindler, J, Hamilton, DL, Moore, DR, Baar, K, and Philp, A. Nutritional strategies to support concurrent training. *Eur J Sport Sci*:1-12, 2014.

91. Phillips, SM. A brief review of critical processes in exercise-induced muscular hypertrophy. *Sports Med* 44 Suppl 1:71-77, 2014.

92. Phillips, SM, Tipton, KD, Aarsland, A, Wolf, SE, and Wolfe, RR. Mixed muscle protein synthesis and breakdown after resistance exercise in humans. *Am J Physiol* 273:E99-E107, 1997.

93. Phinney, SD. Ketogenic diets and physical performance. *Nutr Metab (Lond)* 1:2, 2004.

94. Pugh, JK, Faulkner, SH, Jackson, AP, King, JA, and Nimmo, MA. Acute molecular responses to concurrent resistance and high-intensity interval exercise in untrained skeletal muscle. *Physiol Rep* 3, 2015.

95. Reidy, PT, Walker, DK, Dickinson, JM, Gundermann, DM, Drummond, MJ, Timmerman, KL, Fry, CS, Borack, MS, Cope, MB, Mukherjea, R, Jennings, K, Volpi, E, and Rasmussen, BB. Protein blend ingestion following resistance exercise promotes human muscle protein synthesis. *J Nutr* 143:410-416, 2013.

96. Rieu, I, Balage, M, Sornet, C, Giraudet, C, Pujos, E, Grizard, J, Mosoni, L, and Dardevet, D. Leucine supplementation improves muscle protein synthesis in elderly men independently of hyperaminoacidaemia. *J Physiol* 575:305-315, 2006.

97. Robinson, MJ, Burd, NA, Breen, L, Rerecich, T, Yang, Y, Hector, AJ, Baker, SK, and Phillips, SM. Dose-dependent responses of myofibrillar protein synthesis with beef ingestion are enhanced with resistance exercise in middle-aged men. *Appl Physiol Nutr Metab* 38:120-125, 2013.

98. Rodriguez, NR. Protein-centric meals for optimal protein utilization: Can it be that simple? *J Nutr* 144:797-798, 2014.

99. Rodriguez, NR. Introduction to Protein Summit 2.0: Continued exploration of the impact of high-quality protein on optimal health. *Am J Clin Nutr*, 2015.

100. Sarwar Gilani, G, Wu Xiao, C, and Cockell, KA. Impact of antinutritional factors in food proteins on the digestibility of protein and the bioavailability of amino acids and on protein quality. *Br J Nutr* 108 Suppl 2:S315-S332, 2012.

101. Schoenfeld, BJ, Aragon, AA, and Krieger, JW. The effect of protein timing on muscle strength and hypertrophy: A meta-analysis. *J Int Soc Sports Nutr* 10:53, 2013.

102. Schott, GD, and Wills, MR. Muscle weakness in osteomalacia. *Lancet* 1:626-629, 1976.

103. Stout, JR, Smith-Ryan, AE, Fukuda, DH, Kendall, KL, Moon, JR, Hoffman, JR, Wilson, JM, Oliver, JS, and Mustad, VA. Effect of calcium beta-hydroxy-beta-methylbutyrate (CaHMB) with and without resistance training in men and women 65+yrs: A randomized, double-blind pilot trial. *Exp Gerontol* 48:1303-1310, 2013.

104. Symons, TB, Sheffield-Moore, M, Wolfe, RR, and Paddon-Jones, D. A moderate serving of high-quality protein maximally stimulates skeletal muscle protein synthesis in young and elderly subjects. *J Am Diet Assoc* 109:1582-1586, 2009.

105. Tang, JE, Moore, DR, Kujbida, GW, Tarnopolsky, MA, and Phillips, SM. Ingestion of whey hydrolysate, casein, or soy protein isolate: Effects on mixed muscle protein synthesis at rest and following resistance exercise in young men. *J Appl Physiol* 107:987-992, 2009.

106. Tang, JE, Perco, JG, Moore, DR, Wilkinson, SB, and Phillips, SM. Resistance training alters the response of fed state mixed muscle protein synthesis in young men. *Am J Physiol Regul Integr Comp Physiol* 294:R172-R178, 2008.

107. Tarnopolsky, M. Caffeine and creatine use in sport. *Ann Nutr Metab* 57:1-8, 2010.

108. Tidball, JG. Inflammatory processes in muscle injury and repair. *Am J Physiol Regul Integr Comp Physiol* 288:R345-R353, 2005.

109. Tiidus, PM. *Skeletal Muscle Damage and Repair.* Champaign, IL: Human Kinetics, 2008.

110. Tipton, K, Gurkin, B, Matin, S, and Wolfe, R. Nonessential amino acids are not necessary to stimulate net muscle protein synthesis in healthy volunteers. *J Nutr Biochem* 10:89-95, 1999.

111. Tipton, KD, Elliott, TA, Cree, MG, Aarsland, AA, Sanford, AP, and Wolfe, RR. Stimulation of net muscle protein synthesis by whey protein ingestion before and after exercise. *Am J Physiol Endocrinol Metab* 292:E71-E76, 2007.

112. Tipton, KD, Ferrando, AA, Phillips, SM, Doyle, D, Jr., and Wolfe, RR. Postexercise net protein synthesis in human muscle from orally administered amino acids. *Am J Physiol* 276:E628-E634, 1999.

113. Tipton, KD, Rasmussen, BB, Miller, SL, Wolf, SE, Owens-Stovall, SK, Petrini, BE, and Wolfe, RR. Timing of amino acid-carbohydrate ingestion alters anabolic response of muscle to resistance exercise. *Am J Physiol Endocrinol Metab* 281:E197-E206, 2001.

114. U.S. Department of Agriculture. Nutrient Intakes From Food: Mean Amounts Consumed per Individual, by Gender and Age: What We Eat in America, NHANES 2009-2010. 2012. www.ars.usda.gov/ba/bhnrc/fsrg.

115. U.S. Department of Agriculture. USDA National Nutrient Database for Standard Reference, Release 26. 2013. www.ars.usda.gov/ba/bhnrc/ndl.

116. Van Koevering, M, and Nissen, S. Oxidation of leucine and alpha-ketoisocaproate to beta-hydroxy-beta-methylbutyrate in vivo. *Am J Physiol* 262:E27-E31, 1992.

117. Van Loan, MD, Sutherland, B, Lowe, NM, Turnlund, JR, and King, JC. The effects of zinc depletion on peak force and total work of knee and shoulder extensor and flexor muscles. *Int J Sport Nutr* 9:125-135, 1999.

118. Verdijk, L, Jonkers, R, Gleeson, B, Beelen, M, Meijer, K, Savelberg, H, Wodzig, W, Dendale, P, and van Loon, L. Protein supplementation before and after exercise does not further augment skeletal muscle hypertrophy after resistance training in elderly men. *Am J Clin Nutr* 89:608-616, 2009.

119. Verhoeven, S, Vanschoonbeek, K, Verdijk, LB, Koopman, R, Wodzig, WK, Dendale, P, and van Loon, LJ. Long-term leucine supplementation does not increase muscle mass or strength in healthy elderly men. *Am J Clin Nutr* 89:1468-1475, 2009.

120. Volek, JS, Noakes, T, and Phinney, SD. Rethinking fat as a fuel for endurance exercise. *Eur J Sport Sci* 15:13-20, 2015.

121. Vukovich, MD, Stubbs, NB, and Bohlken, RM. Body composition in 70-year-old adults responds to dietary beta-hydroxy-beta-methylbutyrate similarly to that of young adults. *J Nutr* 131:2049-2052, 2001.

122. Walsh, S, Kelsey, BK, Angelopoulos, TJ, Clarkson, PM, Gordon, PM, Moyna, NM, Visich, PS, Zoeller, RF, Seip, RL, Bilbie, S, Thompson, PD, Hoffman, EP, Price, TB, Devaney, JM, and Pescatello, LS. CNTF 1357 G --> A polymorphism and the muscle strength response to resistance training. *J Appl Physiol* 107:1235-1240, 2009.

123. Wax, B, Brown, SP, Webb, HE, and Kavazis, AN. Effects of carbohydrate supplementation on force output and time to exhaustion during static leg contractions superimposed with electromyostimulation. *J Strength Cond Res* 26:1717-1723, 2012.

124. West, DW, and Phillips, SM. Associations of exercise-induced hormone profiles and gains in strength and hypertrophy in a large cohort after weight training. *Eur J Appl Physiol* 112:2693-2702, 2012.

125. White, AM, Johnston, CS, Swan, PD, Tjonn, SL, and Sears, B. Blood ketones are directly related to fatigue and perceived effort during exercise in overweight adults adhering to low-carbohydrate diets for weight loss: A pilot study. *J Am Diet Assoc* 107:1792-1796, 2007.

126. Wilkinson, DJ, Hossain, T, Hill, DS, Phillips, BE, Crossland, H, Williams, J, Loughna, P, Churchward-Venne, TA, Breen, L, Phillips, SM, Etheridge, T, Rathmacher, JA, Smith, K, Szewczyk, NJ, and Atherton, PJ. Effects of leucine and its metabolite beta-hydroxy-beta-methylbutyrate on human skeletal muscle protein metabolism. *J Physiol* 591:2911-2923, 2013.

127. Wilkinson, S, Tarnopolsky, M, Macdonald, M, Macdonald, J, Armstrong, D, and Phillips, S. Consumption of fluid skim milk promotes greater muscle protein accretion after resistance exercise than does consumption of an isonitrogenous and isoenergetic soy-protein beverage. *Am J Clin Nutr* 85:1031-1040, 2007.

128. Wilson, JM, Marin, PJ, Rhea, MR, Wilson, SM, Loenneke, JP, and Anderson, JC. Concurrent training: A meta-analysis examining interference of aerobic and resistance exercises. *J Strength Cond Res* 26:2293-2307, 2012.

129. Witard, OC, Wardle, SL, Macnaughton, LS, Hodgson, AB, and Tipton, KD. Protein considerations for optimising skeletal muscle mass in healthy young and older adults. *Nutrients* 8:181, 2016.

130. Wolfe, RR. The underappreciated role of muscle in health and disease. *Am J Clin Nutr* 84:475-482, 2006.

Chapter 13

1. Ainsworth, BE, Haskell, WL, Herrmann, SD, Meckes, N, Bassett, DR, Jr., Tudor-Locke, C, Greer, JL, Vezina, J, Whitt-Glover, MC, and Leon, AS. 2011 compendium of physical activities: A second update of codes and MET values. *Med Sci Sports Exerc* 43:1575-1581, 2011.

2. Arabin, B, and Stupin, JH. Overweight and obesity before, during and after pregnancy: Part 2: Evidence-based risk factors and interventions. *Geburtshilfe Frauenheilkd* 74:646-655, 2014.

3. Areta, JL, Burke, LM, Camera, DM, West, DW, Crawshay, S, Moore, DR, Stellingwerff, T, Phillips, SM, Hawley, JA, and Coffey, VG. Reduced resting skeletal muscle protein synthesis is rescued by resistance exercise and protein ingestion following short-term energy deficit. *Am J Physiol Endocrinol Metab* 306:E989-E997, 2014.

4. Baer, DJ, Gebauer, SK, and Novotny, JA. Measured energy value of pistachios in the human diet. *Br J Nutr* 107:120-125, 2012.

5. Barr, SB, and Wright, JC. Postprandial energy expenditure in whole-food and processed-food meals: Implications for daily energy expenditure. *Food Nutr Res* 54, 2010.

6. Barry, VW, Baruth, M, Beets, MW, Durstine, JL, Liu, J, and Blair, SN. Fitness vs. fatness on all-cause mortality: A meta-analysis. *Prog Cardiovasc Dis* 56:382-390, 2014.

7. Berg, J, JL, T, and L, S. Fuel choice during exercise is determined by intensity and duration of activity. In *Biochemistr.* 5th ed. New York: W H Freeman, 2002.

8. Boisseau, N, Vermorel, M, Rance, M, Duche, P, and Patureau-Mirand, P. Protein requirements in male adolescent soccer players. *Eur J Appl Physiol* 100:27-33, 2007.

9. Borchers, JR, Clem, KL, Habash, DL, Nagaraja, HN, Stokley, LM, and Best, TM. Metabolic syndrome and insulin resistance in Division 1 collegiate football players. *Med Sci Sports Exerc* 41:2105-2110, 2009.

10. Bouchard, C, Tchernof, A, and Tremblay, A. Predictors of body composition and body energy changes in response to chronic overfeeding. *Int J Obes (Lond)* 38:236-242, 2014.

11. Boutcher, SH. High-intensity intermittent exercise and fat loss. *J Obes* 2011:868305, 2011.

12. Bray, GA, Smith, SR, de Jonge, L, Xie, H, Rood, J, Martin, CK, Most, M, Brock, C, Mancuso, S, and Redman, LM. Effect of dietary protein content on weight gain, energy expenditure, and body composition during overeating: A randomized controlled trial. *JAMA* 307:47-55, 2012.

13. Brunstrom, JM, Shakeshaft, NG, and Scott-Samuel, NE. Measuring "expected satiety" in a range of common foods using a method of constant stimuli. *Appetite* 51:604-614, 2008.

14. Byrne, NM, Wood, RE, Schutz, Y, and Hills, AP. Does metabolic compensation explain the majority of less-than-expected weight loss in obese adults during a short-term severe diet and exercise intervention? *Int J Obes (Lond)* 36:1472-1478, 2012.

15. Campbell, B, Kreider, RB, Ziegenfuss, T, La Bounty, P, Roberts, M, Burke, D, Landis, J, Lopez, H, and Antonio, J. International Society of Sports Nutrition position stand: Protein and exercise. *J Int Soc Sports Nutr* 4:8, 2007.

16. Caronia, LM, Martin, C, Welt, CK, Sykiotis, GP, Quinton, R, Thambundit, A, Avbelj, M, Dhruvakumar, S, Plummer, L, Hughes, VA, Seminara, SB, Boepple, PA, Sidis, Y, Crowley, WF, Jr., Martin, KA, Hall, JE, and Pitteloud, N. A genetic basis for functional hypothalamic amenorrhea. *N Engl J Med* 364:215-225, 2011.

17. Casperson, SL, Sheffield-Moore, M, Hewlings, SJ, and Paddon-Jones, D. Leucine supplementation chronically improves muscle protein synthesis in older adults consuming the RDA for protein. *Clin Nutr* 31:512-519, 2012.

18. Chaston, TB, Dixon, JB, and O'Brien, PE. Changes in fat-free mass during significant weight loss: A systematic review. *Int J Obes (Lond)* 31:743-750, 2007.

19. Churchward-Venne, TA, Burd, NA, and Phillips, SM. Nutritional regulation of muscle protein synthesis with resistance exercise: Strategies to enhance anabolism. *Nutr Metab (Lond)* 9:40, 2012.

20. Cribb, PJ, Williams, AD, and Hayes, A. A creatine-protein-carbohydrate supplement enhances responses to resistance training. *Med Sci Sports Exerc* 39:1960-1968, 2007.

21. Cummings, DE, and Overduin, J. Gastrointestinal regulation of food intake. *J Clin Invest* 117:13-23, 2007.

22. Curioni, CC, and Lourenco, PM. Long-term weight loss after diet and exercise: A systematic review. *Int J Obes (Lond)* 29:1168-1174, 2005.

23. de Graaf, C, Blom, WA, Smeets, PA, Stafleu, A, and Hendriks, HF. Biomarkers of satiation and satiety. *Am J Clin Nutr* 79:946-961, 2004.

24. Deurenberg, P, Weststrate, JA, and Hautvast, JG. Changes in fat-free mass during weight loss measured by bioelectrical impedance and by densitometry. *Am J Clin Nutr* 49:33-36, 1989.

25. Devries, MC, and Phillips, SM. Creatine supplementation during resistance training in older adults: A meta-analysis. *Med Sci Sports Exerc* 46:1194-1203, 2014.

26. Dhurandhar, EJ, Kaiser, KA, Dawson, JA, Alcorn, AS, Keating, KD, and Allison, DB. Predicting adult weight change in the real world: A systematic review and meta-analysis accounting for compensatory changes in energy intake or expenditure. *Int J Obes (Lond)* 39:1181-1187, 2015.

27. Diliberti, N, Bordi, PL, Conklin, MT, Roe, LS, and Rolls, BJ. Increased portion size leads to increased energy intake in a restaurant meal. *Obes Res* 12:562-568, 2004.

28. Djiogue, S, Nwabo Kamdje, AH, Vecchio, L, Kipanyula, MJ, Farahna, M, Aldebasi, Y, and Seke Etet, PF. Insulin resistance and cancer: The role of insulin and IGFs. *Endocr Relat Cancer* 20:R1-R17, 2013.

29. Duhamel, TA, Perco, JG, and Green, HJ. Manipulation of dietary carbohydrates after prolonged effort modifies muscle sarcoplasmic reticulum responses in exercising males. *Am J Physiol Regul Integr Comp Physiol* 291:R1100-R1110, 2006.

30. Duncan, GE. The "fit but fat" concept revisited: Population-based estimates using NHANES. *Int J Behav Nutr Phys Act* 7:47, 2010.

31. Elsayed, EF, Tighiouart, H, Weiner, DE, Griffith, J, Salem, D, Levey, AS, and Sarnak, MJ. Waist-to-hip ratio and body mass index as risk factors for cardiovascular events in CKD. *Am J Kidney Dis* 52:49-57, 2008.

32. Fox, CS. Cardiovascular disease risk factors, type 2 diabetes mellitus, and the Framingham Heart Study. *Trends Cardiovasc Med* 20:90-95, 2010.

33. Frost, E. Effect of Dietary Protein Intake on Diet-Induced Thermogenesis During Overfeeding. Oral abstract presentation at The Obesity Society Annual Meeting, 2014.

34. Garthe, I, Raastad, T, Refsnes, PE, Koivisto, A, and Sundgot-Borgen, J. Effect of two different weight-loss rates on body composition and strength and power-related performance in elite athletes. *Int J Sport Nutr Exerc Metab* 21:97-104, 2011.

35. Gastaldelli, A, Miyazaki, Y, Pettiti, M, Matsuda, M, Mahankali, S, Santini, E, DeFronzo, RA, and Ferrannini, E. Metabolic effects of visceral fat accumulation in type 2 diabetes. *J Clin Endocrinol Metab* 87:5098-5103, 2002.

36. Golan, R, Shelef, I, Rudich, A, Gepner, Y, Shemesh, E, Chassidim, Y, Harman-Boehm, I, Henkin, Y, Schwarzfuchs, D, Ben Avraham, S, Witkow, S, Liberty, IF, Tangi-Rosental, O, Sarusi, B, Stampfer, MJ, and Shai, I. Abdominal superficial subcutaneous fat: A putative distinct protective fat subdepot in type 2 diabetes. *Diabetes Care* 35:640-647, 2012.

37. Greer, BK, Sirithienthad, P, Moffatt, RJ, Marcello, RT, and Panton, LB. EPOC comparison between isocaloric bouts of steady-state aerobic, intermittent aerobic, and resistance training. *Res Q Exerc Sport* 86:190-195, 2015.

38. Gregor, MF, and Hotamisligil, GS. Inflammatory mechanisms in obesity. *Annu Rev Immunol* 29:415-445, 2011.

39. Guffey, CR, Fan, D, Singh, UP, and Murphy, EA. Linking obesity to colorectal cancer: Recent insights into plausible biological mechanisms. *Curr Opin Clin Nutr Metab Care* 16:595-600, 2013.

40. Hall, DM, and Cole, TJ. What use is the BMI? *Arch Dis Child* 91:283-286, 2006.

41. Hall, KD, Chen, KY, Guo, J, Lam, YY, Leibel, RL, Mayer, LE, Reitman, ML, Rosenbaum, M, Smith, SR, Walsh, BT, and Ravussin, E. Energy expenditure and body composition changes after an isocaloric ketogenic diet in overweight and obese men. *Am J Clin Nutr* 104:324-333, 2016.

42. Hall, KD, Heymsfield, SB, Kemnitz, JW, Klein, S, Schoeller, DA, and Speakman, JR. Energy balance and its components: Implications for body weight regulation. *Am J Clin Nutr* 95:989-994, 2012.

43. Hall, KD, Sacks, G, Chandramohan, D, Chow, CC, Wang, YC, Gortmaker, SL, and Swinburn, BA. Quantification of the effect of energy imbalance on bodyweight. *Lancet* 378:826-837, 2011.

44. Hardy, OT, Czech, MP, and Corvera, S. What causes the insulin resistance underlying obesity? *Curr Opin Endocrinol Diabetes Obes* 19:81-87, 2012.

45. Harnack, LJ, Jeffery, RW, and Boutelle, KN. Temporal trends in energy intake in the United States: An ecologic perspective. *Am J Clin Nutr* 71:1478-1484, 2000.

46. Harris, J, and Benedict, F. *A biometric study of basal metabolism in man.* Washington, DC: Carnegie Institution, 1919.

47. Hector, AJ, Marcotte, GR, Churchward-Venne, TA, Murphy, CH, Breen, L, von Allmen, M, Baker, SK, and Phillips, SM. Whey protein supplementation preserves postprandial myofibrillar protein synthesis during short-term energy restriction in overweight and obese adults. *J Nutr* 145:246-252, 2015.

48. Heydari, M, Freund, J, and Boutcher, SH. The effect of high-intensity intermittent exercise on body composition of overweight young males. *J Obes* 2012:480467, 2012.

49. Heymsfield, SB, Gonzalez, MC, Shen, W, Redman, L, and Thomas, D. Weight loss composition is one-fourth fat-free mass: A critical review and critique of this widely cited rule. *Obes Rev* 15:310-321, 2014.

50. Hill, JO, and Peters, JC. Environmental contributions to the obesity epidemic. *Science* 280:1371-1374, 1998.

51. Horton, TJ, Drougas, H, Brachey, A, Reed, GW, Peters, JC, and Hill, JO. Fat and carbohydrate overfeeding in humans: Different effects on energy storage. *Am J Clin Nutr* 62:19-29, 1995.

52. Institute, NHLaB. What Is Cholesterol? https://www.nhlbi.nih.gov/health/health-topics/topics/hbc/. Accessed May 1, 2016.

53. Jensen, MD, Ryan, DH, Apovian, CM, Ard, JD, Comuzzie, AG, Donato, KA, Hu, FB, Hubbard, VS, Jakicic, JM, Kushner, RF, Loria, CM, Millen, BE, Nonas, CA, Pi-Sunyer, FX, Stevens, J, Stevens, VJ, Wadden, TA, Wolfe, BM, Yanovski, SZ, Jordan, HS, Kendall, KA, Lux, LJ, Mentor-Marcel, R, Morgan, LC, Trisolini, MG, Wnek, J, Anderson, JL, Halperin, JL, Albert, NM, Bozkurt, B, Brindis, RG, Curtis, LH, DeMets, D, Hochman, JS, Kovacs, RJ, Ohman, EM, Pressler, SJ, Sellke, FW, Shen, WK, Smith, SC, Jr., and Tomaselli, GF. 2013 AHA/ACC/TOS guideline for the management of overweight and obesity in adults: A report of the American College of Cardiology/American Heart Association Task Force on Practice Guidelines and The Obesity Society. *Circulation* 129:S102-S138, 2014.

54. Johannsen, DL, Knuth, ND, Huizenga, R, Rood, JC, Ravussin, E, and Hall, KD. Metabolic slowing with massive weight loss despite preservation of fat-free mass. *J Clin Endocrinol Metab* 97:2489-2496, 2012.

55. Johnston, BC, Kanters, S, Bandayrel, K, Wu, P, Naji, F, Siemieniuk, RA, Ball, GD, Busse, JW, Thorlund, K, Guyatt, G, Jansen, JP, and Mills, EJ. Comparison of weight loss among named diet programs in overweight and obese adults: A meta-analysis. *JAMA* 312:923-933, 2014.

56. Jonnalagadda, SS, Skinner, R, and Moore, L. Overweight athlete: Fact or fiction? *Curr Sports Med Rep* 3:198-205, 2004.

57. Kelleher, AR, Hackney, KJ, Fairchild, TJ, Keslacy, S, and Ploutz-Snyder, LL. The metabolic costs of reciprocal supersets vs. traditional resistance exercise in young recreationally active adults. *J Strength Cond Res* 24:1043-1051, 2010.

58. Kelly, B, King, JA, Goerlach, J, and Nimmo, MA. The impact of high-intensity intermittent exercise on resting metabolic rate in healthy males. *Eur J Appl Physiol* 113:3039-3047, 2013.

59. Kerksick, CM, Wilborn, CD, Campbell, WI, Harvey, TM, Marcello, BM, Roberts, MD, Parker, AG, Byars, AG, Greenwood, LD, Almada, AL, Kreider, RB, and Greenwood, M. The effects of creatine monohydrate supplementation with and without D-pinitol on resistance training adaptations. *J Strength Cond Res* 23:2673-2682, 2009.

60. King, LK, March, L, and Anandacoomarasamy, A. Obesity & osteoarthritis. *Indian J Med Res* 138:185-193, 2013.

61. Knuth, ND, Johannsen, DL, Tamboli, RA, Marks-Shulman, PA, Huizenga, R, Chen, KY, Abumrad, NN, Ravussin, E, and Hall, KD. Metabolic adaptation following massive weight loss is related to the degree of energy imbalance and changes in circulating leptin. *Obesity (Silver Spring)* 22:2563-2569, 2014.

62. Kristeller, JL, and Wolever, RQ. Mindfulness-based eating awareness training for treating binge eating disorder: The conceptual foundation. *Eat Disord* 19:49-61, 2011.

63. Layman, DK. Dietary Guidelines should reflect new understandings about adult protein needs. *Nutr Metab (Lond)* 6:12, 2009.

64. Leidy, HJ, Bales-Voelker, LI, and Harris, CT. A protein-rich beverage consumed as a breakfast meal leads to weaker appetitive and dietary responses v. a protein-rich solid breakfast meal in adolescents. *Br J Nutr* 106:37-41, 2011.

65. Leidy, HJ, Bossingham, MJ, Mattes, RD, and Campbell, WW. Increased dietary protein consumed at breakfast leads to an initial and sustained feeling of fullness during energy restriction compared to other meal times. *Br J Nutr* 101:798-803, 2009.

66. Levine, JA. Non-exercise activity thermogenesis (NEAT). *Best Pract Res Clin Endocrinol Metab* 16:679-702, 2002.

67. Li, C, Ford, ES, Zhao, G, Balluz, LS, and Giles, WH. Estimates of body composition with dual-energy X-ray absorptiometry in adults. *Am J Clin Nutr* 90:1457-1465, 2009.

68. Lima, MM, Pareja, JC, Alegre, SM, Geloneze, SR, Kahn, SE, Astiarraga, BD, Chaim, EA, Baracat, J, and Geloneze, B. Visceral fat resection in humans: Effect on insulin sensitivity, beta-cell function, adipokines, and inflammatory markers. *Obesity (Silver Spring)* 21:E182-189, 2013.

69. Long, SJ, Jeffcoat, AR, and Millward, DJ. Effect of habitual dietary-protein intake on appetite and satiety. *Appetite* 35:79-88, 2000.

70. Longland, TM, Oikawa, SY, Mitchell, CJ, Devries, MC, and Phillips, SM. Higher compared with lower dietary protein during an energy deficit combined with intense exercise promotes greater lean mass gain and fat mass loss: A randomized trial. *Am J Clin Nutr* 103:738-746, 2016.

71. Lowery, LM. Dietary fat and sports nutrition: A primer. *J Sports Sci Med* 3:106-117, 2004.

72. MacDougall, JD, Ray, S, Sale, DG, McCartney, N, Lee, P, and Garner, S. Muscle substrate utilization and lactate production. *Can J Appl Physiol* 24:209-215, 1999.

73. Makris, A, and Foster, GD. Dietary approaches to the treatment of obesity. *Psychiatr Clin North Am* 34:813-827, 2011.

74. Mamerow, MM, Mettler, JA, English, KL, Casperson, SL, Arentson-Lantz, E, Sheffield-Moore, M, Layman, DK, and Paddon-Jones, D. Dietary protein distribution positively influences 24-h muscle protein synthesis in healthy adults. *J Nutr* 144:876-880, 2014.

75. Manore, MM. Weight management for athletes and active individuals: A brief review. *Sports Med* 45 Suppl 1:S83-S92, 2015.

76. Marshall, NE, and Spong, CY. Obesity, pregnancy complications, and birth outcomes. *Semin Reprod Med* 30:465-471, 2012.

77. Martin, CK, Heilbronn, LK, de Jonge, L, DeLany, JP, Volaufova, J, Anton, SD, Redman, LM, Smith, SR, and Ravussin, E. Effect of calorie restriction on resting metabolic rate and spontaneous physical activity. *Obesity (Silver Spring)* 15:2964-2973, 2007.

78. McArdle, W, Katch, F, and Katch, V. *Exercise Physiology, Energy, Nutrition, and Human Performance.* 6th ed. Baltimore, MD: Lippincott Williams & Wilkins, 2007.

79. McCrory, MA, Fuss, PJ, Hays, NP, Vinken, AG, Greenberg, AS, and Roberts, SB. Overeating in America: Association between restaurant food consumption and body fatness in healthy adult men and women ages 19 to 80. *Obes Res* 7:564-571, 1999.

80. Miller, M, Stone, NJ, Ballantyne, C, Bittner, V, Criqui, MH, Ginsberg, HN, Goldberg, AC, Howard, WJ, Jacobson, MS, Kris-Etherton, PM, Lennie, TA, Levi, M, Mazzone, T, and Pennathur, S. Triglycerides and cardiovascular disease: A scientific statement from the American Heart Association. *Circulation* 123:2292-2333, 2011.

81. Mojtahedi, MC, Thorpe, MP, Karampinos, DC, Johnson, CL, Layman, DK, Georgiadis, JG, and Evans, EM. The effects of a higher protein intake during energy restriction on changes in body composition and physical function in older women. *J Gerontol A Biol Sci Med Sci* 66:1218-1225, 2011.

82. Moore, DR, Robinson, MJ, Fry, JL, Tang, JE, Glover, EI, Wilkinson, SB, Prior, T, Tarnopolsky, MA, and Phillips, SM. Ingested protein dose response of muscle and albumin

protein synthesis after resistance exercise in young men. *Am J Clin Nutr* 89:161-168, 2009.

83. Mori, H. Effect of timing of protein and carbohydrate intake after resistance exercise on nitrogen balance in trained and untrained young men. *J Physiol Anthropol* 33:24, 2014.

84. Multhoff, G, Molls, M, and Radons, J. Chronic inflammation in cancer development. *Front Immunol* 2:98, 2011.

85. Murphy, CH, Churchward-Venne, TA, Mitchell, CJ, Kolar, NM, Kassis, A, Karagounis, LG, Burke, LM, Hawley, JA, and Phillips, SM. Hypoenergetic diet-induced reductions in myofibrillar protein synthesis are restored with resistance training and balanced daily protein ingestion in older men. *Am J Physiol Endocrinol Metab* 308:E734-E743, 2015.

86. Murphy, CH, Hector, AJ, and Phillips, SM. Considerations for protein intake in managing weight loss in athletes. *Eur J Sport Sci*:1-8, 2014.

87. National Heart Lung and Blood Institute. *Clinical Guidelines on the Identification, Evaluation, and Treatment of Overweight and Obesity in Adults.* Bethesda, MD: National Heart Lung and Blood Institute, 1998.

88. National Heart Lung and Blood Institute. Atherosclerosis. 2014. www.ncbi.nlm.nih.gov/pubmedhealth/PMH0062943/. Accessed April 16, 2016.

89. National Institute of Diabetes and Digestive and Kidney Diseases. *Insulin Resistance and Prediabetes.* Bethesda, MD: National Institutes of Health, 2014.

90. Nordestgaard, BG, and Varbo, A. Triglycerides and cardiovascular disease. *Lancet* 384:626-635, 2014.

91. Novotny, JA, Gebauer, SK, and Baer, DJ. Discrepancy between the Atwater factor predicted and empirically measured energy values of almonds in human diets. *Am J Clin Nutr* 96:296-301, 2012.

92. Ogden, CL, Carroll, MD, Kit, BK, and Flegal, KM. Prevalence of childhood and adult obesity in the United States, 2011-2012. *JAMA* 311:806-814, 2014.

93. Ortenblad, N, Nielsen, J, Saltin, B, and Holmberg, HC. Role of glycogen availability in sar-

coplasmic reticulum Ca2+ kinetics in human skeletal muscle. *J Physiol* 589:711-725, 2011.

94. Ortenblad, N, Westerblad, H, and Nielsen, J. Muscle glycogen stores and fatigue. *J Physiol* 591:4405-4413, 2013.

95. Paddon-Jones, D, and Leidy, H. Dietary protein and muscle in older persons. *Curr Opin Clin Nutr Metab Care* 17:5-11, 2014.

96. Paddon-Jones, D, and Rasmussen, BB. Dietary protein recommendations and the prevention of sarcopenia. *Curr Opin Clin Nutr Metab Care* 12:86-90, 2009.

97. Paschos, P, and Paletas, K. Non alcoholic fatty liver disease and metabolic syndrome. *Hippokratia* 13:9-19, 2009.

98. Pasiakos, SM, Cao, JJ, Margolis, LM, Sauter, ER, Whigham, LD, McClung, JP, Rood, JC, Carbone, JW, Combs, GF, Jr., and Young, AJ. Effects of high-protein diets on fat-free mass and muscle protein synthesis following weight loss: A randomized controlled trial. *FASEB J* 27:3837-3847, 2013.

99. Pasiakos, SM, Vislocky, LM, Carbone, JW, Altieri, N, Konopelski, K, Freake, HC, Anderson, JM, Ferrando, AA, Wolfe, RR, and Rodriguez, NR. Acute energy deprivation affects skeletal muscle protein synthesis and associated intracellular signaling proteins in physically active adults. *J Nutr* 140:745-751, 2010.

100. Peters, HP, Boers, HM, Haddeman, E, Melnikov, SM, and Qvyjt, F. No effect of added beta-glucan or of fructooligosaccharide on appetite or energy intake. *Am J Clin Nutr* 89:58-63, 2009.

101. Phillips, SM. A brief review of critical processes in exercise-induced muscular hypertrophy. *Sports Med* 44 Suppl 1:71-77, 2014.

102. Phillips, SM. A brief review of higher dietary protein diets in weight loss: A focus on athletes. *Sports Med* 44 Suppl 2:S149-S153, 2014.

103. Pi-Sunyer, X. The medical risks of obesity. *Postgrad Med* 121:21-33, 2009.

104. Polednak, AP. Estimating the number of U.S. incident cancers attributable to obesity and the impact on temporal trends in incidence rates for obesity-related cancers. *Cancer Detect Prev* 32:190-199, 2008.

105. Pouliot, MC, Despres, JP, Lemieux, S, Moorjani, S, Bouchard, C, Tremblay, A, Nadeau, A, and Lupien, PJ. Waist circumference and abdominal sagittal diameter: Best simple anthropometric indexes of abdominal visceral adipose tissue accumulation and related cardiovascular risk in men and women. *Am J Cardiol* 73:460-468, 1994.

106. Roberts, DL, Dive, C, and Renehan, AG. Biological mechanisms linking obesity and cancer risk: New perspectives. *Annu Rev Med* 61:301-316, 2010.

107. Rolls, BJ, Morris, EL, and Roe, LS. Portion size of food affects energy intake in normal-weight and overweight men and women. *Am J Clin Nutr* 76:1207-1213, 2002.

108. Rolls, BJ, Roe, LS, Kral, TV, Meengs, JS, and Wall, DE. Increasing the portion size of a packaged snack increases energy intake in men and women. *Appetite* 42:63-69, 2004.

109. Rolls, BJ, Roe, LS, Meengs, JS, and Wall, DE. Increasing the portion size of a sandwich increases energy intake. *J Am Diet Assoc* 104:367-372, 2004.

110. Ryan, DH, and Kushner, R. The state of obesity and obesity research. *JAMA* 304:1835-1836, 2010.

111. Schmieder, RE, and Messerli, FH. Does obesity influence early target organ damage in hypertensive patients? *Circulation* 87:1482-1488, 1993.

112. Schoenfeld, BJ, Aragon, AA, and Krieger, JW. The effect of protein timing on muscle strength and hypertrophy: A meta-analysis. *J Int Soc Sports Nutr* 10:53, 2013.

113. Schwab, RJ, Pasirstein, M, Pierson, R, Mackley, A, Hachadoorian, R, Arens, R, Maislin, G, and Pack, AI. Identification of upper airway anatomic risk factors for obstructive sleep apnea with volumetric magnetic resonance imaging. *Am J Respir Crit Care Med* 168:522-530, 2003.

114. Schwingshackl, L, Dias, S, and Hoffmann, G. Impact of long-term lifestyle programmes on weight loss and cardiovascular risk factors in overweight/obese participants: A systematic review and network meta-analysis. *Syst Rev* 3:130, 2014.

115. Seagle, HM, Strain, GW, Makris, A, Reeves, RS, and American Dietetic, A. Position of the American Dietetic Association: Weight management. *J Am Diet Assoc* 109:330-346, 2009.

116. Shaw, K, Gennat, H, O'Rourke, P, and Del Mar, C. Exercise for overweight or obesity. *Cochrane Database Syst Rev*:CD003817, 2006.

117. Spriet, LL. New insights into the interaction of carbohydrate and fat metabolism during exercise. *Sports Med* 44 Suppl 1:S87-S96, 2014.

118. Stark, M, Lukaszuk, J, Prawitz, A, and Salacinski, A. Protein timing and its effects on muscular hypertrophy and strength in individuals engaged in weight-training. *J Int Soc Sports Nutr* 9:54, 2012.

119. Stefan, N, Haring, HU, Hu, FB, and Schulze, MB. Metabolically healthy obesity: epidemiology, mechanisms, and clinical implications. *Lancet Diabetes Endocrinol* 1:152-162, 2013.

120. Stephens, AM, Dean, LL, Davis, JP, Osborne, JA, and Sanders, TH. Peanuts, peanut oil, and fat free peanut flour reduced cardiovascular disease risk factors and the development of atherosclerosis in Syrian golden hamsters. *J Food Sci* 75:H116-H122, 2010.

121. Stiegler, P, and Cunliffe, A. The role of diet and exercise for the maintenance of fat-free mass and resting metabolic rate during weight loss. *Sports Med* 36:239-262, 2006.

122. Sundgot-Borgen, J, and Garthe, I. Elite athletes in aesthetic and Olympic weight-class sports and the challenge of body weight and body compositions. *J Sports Sci* 29 Suppl 1:S101-S114, 2011.

123. Sundgot-Borgen, J, Meyer, NL, Lohman, TG, Ackland, TR, Maughan, RJ, Stewart, AD, and Muller, W. How to minimise the health risks to athletes who compete in weight-sensitive sports: Review and position statement on behalf of the Ad Hoc Research Working Group on Body Composition, Health and Performance, under the auspices of the IOC Medical Commission. *Br J Sports Med* 47:1012-1022, 2013.

124. Syrotuik, DG, and Bell, GJ. Acute creatine monohydrate supplementation: A descrip-

tive physiological profile of responders vs. nonresponders. *J Strength Cond Res* 18:610-617, 2004.

125. Thomas, DM, Bouchard, C, Church, T, Slentz, C, Kraus, WE, Redman, LM, Martin, CK, Silva, AM, Vossen, M, Westerterp, K, and Heymsfield, SB. Why do individuals not lose more weight from an exercise intervention at a defined dose? An energy balance analysis. *Obes Rev* 13:835-847, 2012.

126. Thomas, EL, Frost, G, Taylor-Robinson, SD, and Bell, JD. Excess body fat in obese and normal-weight subjects. *Nutr Res Rev* 25:150-161, 2012.

127. Thompson, J, and Manore, MM. Predicted and measured resting metabolic rate of male and female endurance athletes. *J Am Diet Assoc* 96:30-34, 1996.

128. Thompson, J, Manore, MM, and Skinner, JS. Resting metabolic rate and thermic effect of a meal in low- and adequate-energy intake male endurance athletes. *Int J Sport Nutr* 3:194-206, 1993.

129. Thompson, W. *ACSM's Guidelines for Exercise Testing and Prescription.* Philadelphia, PA: Lippincott Williams & Wilkins.

130. Traoret, CJ, Lokko, P, Cruz, AC, Oliveira, CG, Costa, NM, Bressan, J, Alfenas, RC, and Mattes, RD. Peanut digestion and energy balance. *Int J Obes (Lond)* 32:322-328, 2008.

131. Tsai, AG, and Wadden, TA. Systematic review: An evaluation of major commercial weight loss programs in the United States. *Ann Intern Med* 142:56-66, 2005.

132. Tsintzas, K, and Williams, C. Human muscle glycogen metabolism during exercise. Effect of carbohydrate supplementation. *Sports Med* 25:7-23, 1998.

133. Turocy, PS, DePalma, BF, Horswill, CA, Laquale, KM, Martin, TJ, Perry, AC, Somova, MJ, and Utter, AC. National Athletic Trainers' Association position statement: Safe weight loss and maintenance practices in sport and exercise. *J Athl Train* 46:322-336, 2011.

134. Urban, LE, McCrory, MA, Dallal, GE, Das, SK, Saltzman, E, Weber, JL, and Roberts, SB. Accuracy of stated energy contents of restaurant foods. *JAMA* 306:287-293, 2011.

135. Urban, LE, Weber, JL, Heyman, MB, Schichtl, RL, Verstraete, S, Lowery, NS, Das, SK, Schleicher, MM, Rogers, G, Economos, C, Masters, WA, and Roberts, SB. Energy contents of frequently ordered restaurant meals and comparison with human energy requirements and US Department of Agriculture database information: A multisite randomized study. *J Acad Nutr Diet* 116:590-598, 2016.

136. Valassi, E, Scacchi, M, and Cavagnini, F. Neuroendocrine control of food intake. *Nutr Metab Cardiovasc Dis* 18:158-168, 2008.

137. van Loon, LJ, Greenhaff, PL, Constantin-Teodosiu, D, Saris, WH, and Wagenmakers, AJ. The effects of increasing exercise intensity on muscle fuel utilisation in humans. *J Physiol* 536:295-304, 2001.

138. Vianna, JM, Werneck, FZ, Coelho, EF, Damasceno, VO, and Reis, VM. Oxygen uptake and heart rate kinetics after different types of resistance exercise. *J Hum Kinet* 42:235-244, 2014.

139. Wadei, HM, and Textor, SC. The role of the kidney in regulating arterial blood pressure. *Nat Rev Nephrol* 8:602-609, 2012.

140. Wang, SC, Bednarski, B, Patel, S, Yan, A, Kohoyda-Inglis, C, Kennedy, T, Link, E, Rowe, S, Sochor, M, and Arbabi, S. Increased depth of subcutaneous fat is protective against abdominal injuries in motor vehicle collisions. *Annu Proc Assoc Adv Automot Med* 47:545-559, 2003.

141. Wang, Z, Ying, Z, Bosy-Westphal, A, Zhang, J, Heller, M, Later, W, Heymsfield, SB, and Muller, MJ. Evaluation of specific metabolic rates of major organs and tissues: Comparison between men and women. *Am J Hum Biol* 23:333-338, 2011.

142. Weinheimer, EM, Sands, LP, and Campbell, WW. A systematic review of the separate and combined effects of energy restriction and exercise on fat-free mass in middle-aged and older adults: Implications for sarcopenic obesity. *Nutr Rev* 68:375-388, 2010.

143. Whitmore, C. Type 2 diabetes and obesity in adults. *Br J Nurs* 19:880, 882-886, 2010.

144. Williams, RL, Wood, LG, Collins, CE, and Callister, R. Effectiveness of weight loss interventions—Is there a difference between men and women: A systematic review. *Obes Rev* 16:171-186, 2015.

145. Wishnofsky, M. Caloric equivalents of gained or lost weight. *Am J Clin Nutr* 6:542-546, 1958.

146. Yerrakalva, D, Mullis, R, and Mant, J. The associations of "fatness," "fitness," and physical activity with all-cause mortality in older adults: A systematic review. *Obesity (Silver Spring)* 23:1944-1956, 2015.

147. Zanker, CL. Regulation of reproductive function in athletic women: An investigation of the roles of energy availability and body composition. *Br J Sports Med* 40:489-490; discussion 490, 2006.

148. Zhou, Y, and Rui, L. Leptin signaling and leptin resistance. *Front Med* 7:207-222, 2013.

Chapter 14

1. Adan, A. Cognitive performance and dehydration. *J Am Coll Nutr* 31:71-78, 2012.

2. American College of Obstetricians and Gynecologists. ACOG Committee opinion no. 548: Weight gain during pregnancy. *Obstet Gynecol* 121:210-212, 2013.

3. American College of Obstetricians and Gynecologists. ACOG Committee opinion no. 650: Physical activity and exercise during pregnancy and the postpartum period. *Obstet Gynecol* 126:e135-e142, 2015.

4. American Psychiatric Association. *Anxiety Disorders: DSM-5 Selections.* Arlington, VA: American Psychiatric Association Publishing, 2016.

5. Bennell, KL, Malcolm, SA, Wark, JD, and Brukner, PD. Skeletal effects of menstrual disturbances in athletes. *Sc and J Med Sci Sports* 7:261-273, 1997.

6. Bernhardt, IB, and Dorsey, DJ. Hypervitaminosis A and congenital renal anomalies in a human infant. *Obstet Gynecol* 43:750-755, 1974.

7. Bratland-Sanda, S, Martinsen, EW, and Sundgot-Borgen, J. Changes in physical fitness, bone mineral density and body composition during inpatient treatment of underweight and normal weight females with longstanding eating disorders. *Int J Environ Res Public Health* 9:315-330, 2012.

8. Bui, T, and Christin-Maitre, S. Vitamin D and pregnancy. *Ann Endocrinol (Paris)* 72 Suppl 1:S23-S28, 2011.

9. Burke, DG, Chilibeck, PD, Parise, G, Candow, DG, Mahoney, D, and Tarnopolsky, M. Effect of creatine and weight training on muscle creatine and performance in vegetarians. *Med Sci Sports Exerc* 35:1946-1955, 2003.

10. Cadore, EL, Rodriguez-Manas, L, Sinclair, A, and Izquierdo, M. Effects of different exercise interventions on risk of falls, gait ability, and balance in physically frail older adults: A systematic review. *Rejuvenation Res* 16:105-114, 2013.

11. Campbell, MK. *Biochemistry.* 3rd ed. Philadelphia: Saunders, 1999.

12. Churchward-Venne, TA, Burd, NA, Mitchell, CJ, West, DW, Philp, A, Marcotte, GR, Baker, SK, Baar, K, and Phillips, SM. Supplementation of a suboptimal protein dose with leucine or essential amino acids: Effects on myofibrillar protein synthesis at rest and following resistance exercise in men. *J Physiol* 590:2751-2765, 2012.

13. Churchward-Venne, TA, Tieland, M, Verdijk, LB, Leenders, M, Dirks, ML, de Groot, LC, and van Loon, LJ. There are no nonresponders to resistance-type exercise training in older men and women. *J Am Med Dir Assoc* 16:400-411, 2015.

14. Cowell, BS, Rosenbloom, CA, Skinner, R, and Summers, SH. Policies on screening female athletes for iron deficiency in NCAA Division I-A institutions. *Int J Sport Nutr Exerc Metab* 13:277-285, 2003.

15. Craig, WJ, and Mangels, AR. Position of the American Dietetic Association: Vegetarian diets. *J Am Diet Assoc* 109:1266-1282, 2009.

16. DeFronzo, RA. Dysfunctional fat cells, lipotoxicity and type 2 diabetes. *Int J Clin Pract Suppl*:9-21, 2004.

17. DellaValle, DM. Iron supplementation for female athletes: Effects on iron status and performance outcomes. *Curr Sports Med Rep* 12:234-239, 2013.

18. Desbrow, B, McCormack, J, Burke, LM, Cox, GR, Fallon, K, Hislop, M, Logan, R, Marino, N, Sawyer, SM, Shaw, G, Star, A, Vidgen, H, and Leveritt, M. Sports Dietitians Australia position statement: Sports nutrition for the adolescent athlete. *Int J Sport Nutr Exerc Metab* 24:570-584, 2014.

19. Donnelly, JE, Blair, SN, Jakicic, JM, Manore, MM, Rankin, JW, and Smith, BK. American College of Sports Medicine position stand: Appropriate physical activity intervention strategies for weight loss and prevention of weight regain for adults. *Med Sci Sports Exerc* 41:459-471, 2009.

20. Driskell, JA, and Wolinsky, I. *Sports Nutrition: Vitamins and Trace Elements.* 2nd ed. Boca Raton, FL: Taylor & Francis, 2005.

21. Durham, HA, Morey, MC, Lovelady, CA, Namenek Brouwer, RJ, Krause, KM, and Ostbye, T. Postpartum physical activity in overweight and obese women. *J Phys Act Health* 8:988-993, 2011.

22. Fink, HH, Burgoon, LA, and Mikesky, AE. *Practical Applications in Sports Nutrition.* 2nd ed. Sudbury, MA: Jones and Bartlett, 2009.

23. Fink, HH, Mikesky, AE, and Burgoon, LA. *Practical Applications in Sports Nutrition.* 3rd ed. Sudbury, MA: Jones and Bartlett, 2012.

24. Fuhrman, J, and Ferreri, DM. Fueling the vegetarian (vegan) athlete. *Curr Sports Med Rep* 9:233-241, 2010.

25. Gallen, I, Hume, C, and Lumb, A. Fueling the athlete with type 1 diabetes. *Diabetes Obes Metab* 13:130-136, 2011.

26. Garner, DM. *Eating Disorder Inventory-3: Professional Manual.* Lutz, FL: Psychological Assessment Resources, 2004.

27. Hanne, N, Dlin, R, and Rotstein, A. Physical fitness, anthropometric and metabolic parameters in vegetarian athletes. *J Sports Med Phys Fitness* 26:180-185, 1986.

28. Holick, MF, Binkley, NC, Bischoff-Ferrari, HA, Gordon, CM, Hanley, DA, Heaney, RP, Murad, MH, and Weaver, CM. Evaluation, treatment, and prevention of vitamin D deficiency: An Endocrine Society clinical practice guideline. *J Clin Endocrinol Metab* 96:1911-1930, 2011.

29. Hunt, JR. Bioavailability of iron, zinc, and other trace minerals from vegetarian diets. *Am J Clin Nutr* 78:633s-639s, 2003.

30. Institute of Medicine. *Dietary Reference Intakes for Vitamin A, Vitamin K, Arsenic, Boron, Chromium, Copper, Iodine, Iron, Manganese, Molybdenum, Nickel, Silicon, Vanadium, and Zinc.* Washington, DC: National Academies Press, 2001.

31. Institute of Medicine. *Dietary Reference Intakes for Energy, Carbohydrate, Fiber, Fat, Fatty Acids, Cholesterol, Protein, and Amino Acids (Macronutrients).* Washington, DC: National Academies Press, 2005.

32. Institute of Medicine and National Research Council Committee to Reexamine Institute of Medicine Pregnancy Weight Guidelines. The National Academies Collection: Reports funded by National Institutes of Health. In *Weight Gain During Pregnancy: Reexamining the Guidelines.* Rasmussen, KM, Yaktine, AL, eds. Washington, DC: National Academies Press, 2009.

33. Institute of Medicine Subcommittee on the Interpretation and Uses of Dietary Reference Intakes. *Dietary Reference Intakes: Applications in Dietary Planning.* Washington, DC: National Academies Press, 2003.

34. Jager, TE, Weiss, HB, Coben, JH, and Pepe, PE. Traumatic brain injuries evaluated in U.S. emergency departments, 1992-1994. *Acad Emerg Med* 7:134-140, 2000.

35. Jakicic, JM, and Otto, AD. Physical activity considerations for the treatment and prevention of obesity. *Am J Clin Nutr* 82:226s-229s, 2005.

36. Jensen, J. Nutritional concerns in the diabetic athlete. *Curr Sports Med Rep* 3:192-197, 2004.

37. Johnson, NF, Gold, BT, Bailey, AL, Clasey, JL, Hakun, JG, White, M, Long, DE, and Powell, DK. Cardiorespiratory fitness modifies the relationship between myocardial function and cerebral blood flow in older adults. *Neuroimage* 131:126-132, 2016.

38. Joy, E, De Souza, MJ, Nattiv, A, Misra, M, Williams, NI, Mallinson, RJ, Gibbs, JC, Olmsted, M, Goolsby, M, Matheson, G, Barrack, M, Burke, L, Drinkwater, B, Lebrun, C, Loucks, AB, Mountjoy, M, Nichols, J, and Borgen, JS. 2014 female athlete triad coalition consensus statement on treatment and return to play of the female athlete triad. *Curr Sports Med Rep* 13:219-232, 2014.

39. Kim, JS, Wilson, JM, and Lee, SR. Dietary implications on mechanisms of sarcopenia: roles of protein, amino acids and antioxidants. *J Nutr Biochem* 21:1-13, 2010.

40. Kushi, LH, Doyle, C, McCullough, M, Rock, CL, Demark-Wahnefried, W, Bandera, EV, Gapstur, S, Patel, AV, Andrews, K, and Gansler, T. American Cancer Society guidelines on nutrition and physical activity for cancer prevention: Reducing the risk of cancer with healthy food choices and physical activity. *CA Cancer J Clin* 62:30-67, 2012.

41. Landi, F, Liperoti, R, Russo, A, Giovannini, S, Tosato, M, Capoluongo, E, Bernabei, R, and Onder, G. Sarcopenia as a risk factor for falls in elderly individuals: Results from the ilSIRENTE study. *Clin Nutr* 31:652-658, 2012.

42. Leenders, M, Verdijk, LB, van der Hoeven, L, van Kranenburg, J, Nilwik, R, and van Loon, LJ. Elderly men and women benefit equally from prolonged resistance-type exercise training. *J Gerontol A Biol Sci Med Sci* 68:769-779, 2013.

43. Lukaski, HC. Vitamin and mineral status: Effects on physical performance. *Nutrition* 20:632-644, 2004.

44. Lukaszuk, JM, Robertson, RJ, Arch, JE, Moore, GE, Yaw, KM, Kelley, DE, Rubin, JT, and Moyna, NM. Effect of creatine supplementation and a lacto-ovo-vegetarian diet on muscle creatine concentration. *Int J Sport Nutr Exerc Metab* 12:336-348, 2002.

45. Lukaszuk, JM, Robertson, RJ, Arch, JE, and Moyna, NM. Effect of a defined lacto-ovo-vegetarian diet and oral creatine monohydrate supplementation on plasma creatine concentration. *J Strength Cond Res* 19:735-740, 2005.

46. Martinsen, M, and Sundgot-Borgen, J. Higher prevalence of eating disorders among adolescent elite athletes than controls. *Med Sci Sports Exerc* 45:1188-1197, 2013.

47. Maughan, RJ. *Sports Nutrition.* Wiley, 2013.

48. Mayo Clinic. Pregnancy Weight Gain: What's Healthy. 2017. www.mayoclinic.org/healthy-lifestyle/pregnancy-week-by-week/in-depth/pregnancy-weight-gain/art-20044360.

49. Melina, V, Craig, W, and Levin, S. Position of the Academy of Nutrition and Dietetics: Vegetarian diets. *J Acad Nutr Diet* 116:1970-1980, 2016.

50. Merkel, DL. Youth sport: Positive and negative impact on young athletes. *Open Access J Sports Med* 4:151-160, 2013.

51. Mountjoy, M, Sundgot-Borgen, J, Burke, L, Carter, S, Constantini, N, Lebrun, C, Meyer, N, Sherman, R, Steffen, K, Budgett, R, and Ljungqvist, A. The IOC consensus statement: Beyond the female athlete triad— Relative energy deficiency in sport (RED-S). *Br J Sports Med* 48:491-497, 2014.

52. National Heart Lung Blood Institute. Expert panel on integrated guidelines for cardiovascular health and risk reduction in children and adolescents: Summary report. *Pediatrics* 128 Suppl 5:S213-256, 2011.

53. National Institute of Arthritis and Musculoskeletal and Skin Diseases. Preventing Musculoskeletal Sports Injuries in Youth: A Guide for Parents. 2016. https://www.niams.nih.gov/Health_Info/Sports_Injuries/child_sports_injuries.asp.

54. National Institute of Diabetes and Digestive and Kidney Diseases. Helping Your Child Who Is Overweight. 2016. https://www.niddk.nih.gov/health-information/health-topics/weight-control/helping-overweight-child/Pages/helping-your-overweight-child.aspx. Accessed January 24, 2017.

55. Nattiv, A, Loucks, AB, Manore, MM, Sanborn, CF, Sundgot-Borgen, J, and Warren, MP. American College of Sports Medicine position stand: The female athlete triad. *Med Sci Sports Exerc* 39:1867-1882, 2007.

56. Ogden, CL, Carroll, MD, Fryar, CD, and Flegal, KM. Prevalence of obesity among adults and youth: United States, 2011-2014. *NCHS Data Brief*:1-8, 2015.

57. Paddon-Jones, D, and Leidy, H. Dietary protein and muscle in older persons. *Curr Opin Clin Nutr Metab Care* 17:5-11, 2014.

58. Peeling, P, Dawson, B, Goodman, C, Landers, G, and Trinder, D. Athletic induced iron deficiency: New insights into the role of inflammation, cytokines and hormones. *Eur J Appl Physiol* 103:381-391, 2008.

59. Peternelj, TT, and Coombes, JS. Antioxidant supplementation during exercise training: Beneficial or detrimental? *Sports Med* 41:1043-1069, 2011.

60. Praet, SF, Manders, RJ, Meex, RC, Lieverse, AG, Stehouwer, CD, Kuipers, H, Keizer, HA, and van Loon, LJ. Glycaemic instability is an underestimated problem in type II diabetes. *Clin Sci (Lond)* 111:119-126, 2006.

61. Praet, SF, and van Loon, LJ. Optimizing the therapeutic benefits of exercise in type 2 diabetes. *J Appl Physiol* 103:1113-1120, 2007.

62. Rizzoli, R, Reginster, JY, Arnal, JF, Bautmans, I, Beaudart, C, Bischoff-Ferrari, H, Biver, E, Boonen, S, Brandi, ML, Chines, A, Cooper, C, Epstein, S, Fielding, RA, Goodpaster, B, Kanis, JA, Kaufman, JM, Laslop, A, Malafarina, V, Manas, LR, Mitlak, BH, Oreffo, RO, Petermans, J, Reid, K, Rolland, Y, Sayer, AA, Tsouderos, Y, Visser, M, and Bruyere, O. Quality of life in sarcopenia and frailty. *Calcif Tissue Int* 93:101-120, 2013.

63. Rosenbloom, C, and Bahns, M. What can we learn about diet and physical activity from master athletes? *Holist Nurs Pract* 20:161-166, 2006.

64. Ross, AC, Manson, JE, Abrams, SA, Aloia, JF, Brannon, PM, Clinton, SK, Durazo-Arvizu, RA, Gallagher, JC, Gallo, RL, Jones, G, Kovacs, CS, Mayne, ST, Rosen, CJ, and Shapses, SA. The 2011 Dietary Reference Intakes for calcium and vitamin D: What dietetics practitioners need to know. *J Am Diet Assoc* 111:524-527, 2011.

65. Savoie, FA, Kenefick, RW, Ely, BR, Cheuvront, SN, and Goulet, ED. Effect of hypohydration on muscle endurance, strength, anaerobic power and capacity and vertical jumping ability: A meta-analysis. *Sports Med* 45:1207-1227, 2015.

66. Schneider, MB, and Benjamin, HJ. Sports drinks and energy drinks for children and adolescents: Are they appropriate? *Pediatrics* 127:1182-1189, 2011.

67. Stahler, C. How many vegetarians are there? *Vegetarian Journal*, 2009.

68. Sterling, DA, O'Connor, JA, and Bonadies, J. Geriatric falls: Injury severity is high and disproportionate to mechanism. *J Trauma* 50:116-119, 2001.

69. Stipanuk, MH. *Biochemical and Physiological Aspects of Human Nutrition*. Philadelphia: W.B. Saunders, 2000.

70. Sundgot-Borgen, J. Prevalence of eating disorders in elite female athletes. *Int J Sport Nutr* 3:29-40, 1993.

71. Sundgot-Borgen, J, Meyer, NL, Lohman, TG, Ackland, TR, Maughan, RJ, Stewart, AD, and Muller, W. How to minimise the health risks to athletes who compete in weight-sensitive sports: Review and position statement on behalf of the Ad Hoc Research Working Group on Body Composition, Health and Performance, under the auspices of the IOC Medical Commission. *Br J Sports Med* 47:1012-1022, 2013.

72. Sundgot-Borgen, J, and Torstveit, MK. Prevalence of eating disorders in elite athletes is higher than in the general population. *Clin J Sport Med* 14:25-32, 2004.

73. Sundgot-Borgen, J, and Torstveit, MK. Aspects of disordered eating continuum in elite high-intensity sports. *Scand J Med Sci Sports* 20 Suppl 2:112-121, 2010.

74. Szabo, AN, Washburn, RA, Sullivan, DK, Honas, JJ, Mayo, MS, Goetz, J, Lee, J, and Donnelly, JE. The Midwest exercise trial for the prevention of weight regain: MET POWeR. *Contemp Clin Trials* 36:470-478, 2013.

75. Tanaka, H, and Seals, DR. Endurance exercise performance in masters athletes: Age-associated changes and underlying physiological mechanisms. *The Journal of Physiology* 586:55-63, 2008.

76. Thomas, DT, Erdman, KA, and Burke, LM. American College of Sports Medicine joint position statement: Nutrition and athletic performance. *Med Sci Sports Exerc* 48:543-568, 2016.

77. Thompson, J, and Manore, MM. Predicted and measured resting metabolic rate of male and female endurance athletes. *J Am Diet Assoc* 96:30-34, 1996.

78. Tipton, KD, and Witard, OC. Protein requirements and recommendations for athletes: Relevance of ivory tower arguments for practical recommendations. *Clin Sports Med* 26:17-36, 2007.

79. Tseng, BY, Uh, J, Rossetti, HC, Cullum, CM, Diaz-Arrastia, RF, Levine, BD, Lu, H, and Zhang, R. Masters athletes exhibit larger regional brain volume and better cognitive performance than sedentary older adults. *J Magn Reson Imaging* 38:1169-1176, 2013.

80. U.S. Department of Agriculture and U.S. Department of Health & Human Services. Dietary Guidelines for Americans 2015-2020. 2015. https://health.gov/dietaryguidelines/2015/resources/2015-2020_Dietary_Guidelines.pdf.

81. United Nations Department of Economic and Social Affairs Population Division. Population Pyramids of the World from 1950 to 2100. 2015. https://populationpyramid.net/world/2040.

82. Velez, NF, Zhang, A, Stone, B, Perera, S, Miller, M, and Greenspan, SL. The effect of moderate impact exercise on skeletal integrity in master athletes. *Osteoporos Int* 19:1457-1464, 2008.

83. Venderley, AM, and Campbell, WW. Vegetarian diets: Nutritional considerations for athletes. *Sports Med* 36:293-305, 2006.

84. von Haehling, S, Morley, JE, and Anker, SD. An overview of sarcopenia: Facts and numbers on prevalence and clinical impact. *J Cachexia Sarcopenia Muscle* 1:129-133, 2010.

85. Wentz, L, Liu, PY, Ilich, JZ, and Haymes, EM. Dietary and training predictors of stress fractures in female runners. *Int J Sport Nutr Exerc Metab* 22:374-382, 2012.

86. Wicherts, IS, van Schoor, NM, Boeke, AJ, Visser, M, Deeg, DJ, Smit, J, Knol, DL, and Lips, P. Vitamin D status predicts physical performance and its decline in older persons. *J Clin Endocrinol Metab* 92:2058-2065, 2007.

87. Wilks, DC, Winwood, K, Gilliver, SF, Kwiet, A, Sun, LW, Gutwasser, C, Ferretti, JL, Sargeant, AJ, Felsenberg, D, and Rittweger, J. Age-dependency in bone mass and geometry: A pQCT study on male and female master sprinters, middle and long distance runners, race-walkers and sedentary people. *J Musculoskelet Neuronal Interact* 9:236-246, 2009.

88. Young, VR, and Pellett, PL. Plant proteins in relation to human protein and amino acid nutrition. *Am J Clin Nutr* 59:1203s-1212s, 1994.

Note: The italicized *f* and *t* following page numbers refer to figures and tables, respectively.

genetics and environment in 12-13

health impacts of 256, 312-315, 313*t*

high-fructose corn syrup and 87-88

inflammation and 256

insulin resistance in 344

metabolic syndrome and 344

muscle mass and 292

in older adults 341

in pregnancy 351

skinfold measurements and 267

sodium and blood pressure in 193

sugar intake and 87

vitamin D and 160, 163*t*

OGTT (oral glucose tolerance test) 73

oils 95, 97-98, 97*f*, 103, 107, 107*f*

older adults. *See also* aging

body weight in 341

bone resorption in 182-183

cardiovascular and metabolic health in 339-340

cognitive function in 341

dehydration in 210

energy needs of 341

fluid balance in 192

magnesium and 188, 189-190

muscle protein synthesis in 298-299, 300-301, 300*f*, 326

musculoskeletal health in 340-341

nutrition needs 341-342, 342*t*

omega-3 fatty acids and 105-106

protein needs of 6, 300–301, 326

sodium and blood pressure in 192-193

vitamin B$_{12}$ for 201

vitamin D and 160, 162, 163, 201

oleic acid 100, 101*t*

oligomenorrhea 365

oligosaccharides 67-68, 70

omega-3 fatty acids

food sources of 101*t*, 359

health effects of 101*t*, 102-106, 102*f*, 103*f*

structure of 95-96, 96*f*

omega-6 fatty acids 95-96, 96*f*, 100-102, 101*t*, 102*f*, 103*f*

ORAC (oxygen radical absorbance capacity) 167

oral glucose tolerance test (OGTT) 73

organelles 28, 29*f*

ornithine 117*t*, 240

OSFED (Other Specified Feeding or Eating Disorders) 364

osmolarity 208, 218, 222*t*

osteoarthritis 159, 168, 246, 315, 316

osteoporosis 182-183, 292, 340, 365, 365*f*

Other Specified Feeding or Eating Disorders (OSFED) 364

OTS (overtraining syndrome) 14-16, 15*f*, 289

overhydration 206, 210, 213. *See also* hydration status

overload principle 13

overreaching 15

overtraining syndrome (OTS) 14-16, 15*f*, 289

overweight

body fat patterns 260-261, 261*f*

in childhood and adolescence 336

definition of 256, 259*t*, 313*t*

genetics and environment in 12-13

health impacts of 256, 260

in older adults 341

pregnancy and 351

oxalates 146, 181, 183*f*, 216

oxaloacetate 40, 44-45, 50*f*

oxidative decarboxylation 28

oxidative phosphorylation 28, 29*f*, 32*f*, 41, 43*t*

oxidative stress 202

oxygen availability 33, 36, 38, 40, 45, 47

oxygen radical absorbance capacity (ORAC) 167

P

palm kernel oil 95, 101*t*

pancreas

diabetes and 314, 343-345, 343*f*, 344*f*

digestive enzymes from 70-71, 71*t*, 110, 129, 129*f*

in glucose transport into cells 73-74, 75*t*

insulin from 73-74, 75*t*, 282*f*, 343-344

pancreatic amylase 70-71, 71*t*

pantothenic acid (vitamin B$_5$) 40, 164*t*, 172-173

Parkinsonism, manganese-induced 199

Parkinson's disease 34

PDC (pyruvate dehydrogenase complex) 39-40

PDCAAS (protein digestibility corrected amino acid score) 137*t*, 139, 147

peak bone mass 182, 186*f*

peer-reviewed journals 231-232

pellagra 172

pepsin 128-129

pepsinogen 127-128

peptidases 130

peptide bonds 116, 121-122, 122*f*, 129*f*

peptide hormones 124-125, 125*f*

percent daily value (%DV) 82-83, 84*f*

periodization principle 14, 14*f*, 16

periodized training program 142-143, 353

pernicious anemia 174-175

personality, eating disorders and 362

perspiration, insensible 206

pH, blood 126-127

phenylalanine 116-118, 117*t*

phosphagen system 31, 32*f*, 32*t*, 33-34, 33*f*

phosphocreatine (PCr) 12, 13*f*, 31, 33-34, 33*f*, 240

phospholipids 97, 127*f*

phosphorus

bone health and 181-182, 183*f*, 184, 186*f*

intake recommendations 180*t*, 181*t*, 186, 197*t*

sources of 184-185, 196*t*

vitamin D and 161

photosynthesis 66, 66*f*

physical activity. *See* exercise

physical activity level 7, 347

physical fitness components 11-13, 13*f*

phytates 146, 194

phytic acid 183*f*, 194

pica 174-175

PINES (Professionals in Nutrition for Exercise and Sport) 20

plant-based diets 136, 146-147, 146*t*, 147*f*, 357, 358*f*. *See also* vegetarian diets

plant sterols 97

plaque in arteries 97, 110, 314-315, 314*f*

plasma osmolarity 208, 218, 222*t*

polydipsia 345, 345*f*, 346

polyols 86

polypeptides 122

polyphagia 345, 345*f*, 346

polyphenols 194, 238-239, 243

polysaccharides 70-71, 71*t*. *See also* fiber; glycogen; starch

polyunsaturated fatty acids (PUFA). *See also* omega-3 fatty acids; omega-6 fatty acids

food sources of 97*f*, 101*t*

health effects of 99-100, 101*t*, 102*f*

structure of 95-96, 96*f*

polyuria 345, 345*f*, 346

portal vein 129*f*, 130, 131*f*

portion sizes 8, 8*f*, 283, 283*f*, 285, 323*f*

postprandial hypoglycemia 78
potassium 180t, 181t, 190-191, 196t-197t, 214, 307
prebiotics 247
preformed vitamin A 154, 157
pregnancy 350-355
  carbohydrate needs in 79
  DEXA and 265
  diet recommendations in 350-354, 354t
  exercise in 350-351
  folate and 172, 201, 354
  gestational diabetes in 351, 352
  iron in 195, 198, 201, 355
  multiple babies 353
  vitamins in 354-355
  water intake in 207
  weight gain in 351-352, 352t, 355
primary protein structure 122, 122f
principle of detraining 14, 15, 48
principle of periodization 14, 14f, 16
principle of progressive overload 13
principle of specificity 13
probiotics 247
processed foods 202, 320-321, 323f
proenzymes 127-128
Professionals in Nutrition for Exercise and Sport (PINES) 20
prohormones 242
prolamins 85
proline 116, 117f, 118
proprietary blends 235
prostate cancer 167
protease activation cascade 129
protein 116-149
  absorption of 129-130, 130f, 131, 131f
  amino acids and 116-119, 116f, 117f, 119f. See also amino acids
  animal 121, 136, 146, 195, 299
  calcium and 182
  calories per gram 4
  catabolism of 118-121, 124, 132, 140-141, 141f, 346
  cell transporters 126-127, 127f, 128t
  chemical energy from 45-46
  for children and adolescents 337-338
  classification and function of 119-121, 120f, 121t
  collagen 118, 124
  deficiency and excess 147-148, 353-354
  denaturation 124
  diabetes and 348
  dietary recommendations 6, 133-135, 142-144, 143t, 302

digestion of 127-129, 129f
for endurance athletes 277, 283
as enzymes 123-124, 125f. See also enzymes
fluid maintenance 123, 125-126, 126f
as fuel in diabetes 346
functions 6, 123, 124f, 128f, 143
immunity and 125
leucine 304
maximum usable amount 304
metabolism and exercise 27f, 140-142, 141f
muscle mass and 325-326
muscle metabolic adaptation and 145, 145t
muscle protein synthesis 116, 144-145, 276, 295-299, 300f
nitrogen balance assessment 120, 132-133
older adult need for 298-299, 300-301, 300f, 342, 342t
overfeeding 111, 148, 325
oxidation of 141-142
peptide hormones 124-125, 125f
in pregnancy 353-354, 354t
protein synthesis 130-132, 131f, 132f, 144-145
quality of 135-140, 137t, 357, 358f
in resistance training 292, 293, 301-302
satiety and 320
sources of 121, 121t, 145-146
structure hierarchy in 121-123, 122f
timing of 142-144, 281, 299-300, 302-303, 302f
vegetarian and vegan sources 146-147, 146t, 147f, 357-359, 358f
in weight loss 305-307, 318-319, 327-328
protein digestibility corrected amino acid score (PDCAAS) 137t, 139, 147
protein efficiency ratio 137t, 139
proteinogenic, amino acids 116
protein powder 135
protein pumps 126-127, 127f
proton motive force 41
provitamin A carotenoids 154, 156f
pubertal age 335
PUFA. See polyunsaturated fatty acids
purging behavior 363
purging disorder 364. See also disordered eating
pyridoxine (vitamin B$_6$) 174
pyrophosphate 30

pyruvate
  in anaerobic system 35, 35f
  in carbohydrate breakdown 39-40, 41f, 42f, 43f
  in gluconeogenesis 50, 50f
  in glycolysis 39
  in protein catabolism 27, 29f, 132, 141
pyruvate dehydrogenase complex (PDC) 39-40

Q

quackery 17
quaternary protein structure 122, 122f

R

RAE (retinal activity equivalents) 154, 157
reactive hypoglycemia 78
recommended dietary allowance (RDA) 4-6, 5f, 79, 133-135, 162
REE (resting energy expenditure) 54, 58, 352
refined carbohydrate 86-87
registered dietitian nutritionist (RDN) 7, 19-20, 22, 85, 319, 348
relative energy deficiency in sport (RED-S) 60, 365, 366f, 367f
resistance training. See also resistance training, nutrition for
  concurrent training 301
  creatine and 240
  hydration during 292-293, 294
  for losing fat and gaining muscle 327-328
  muscle protein synthesis in 144, 295-299, 296f, 297f, 300f
  by older adults 300-301, 340-341
  overload principle in 13, 14
  protein oxidation in 140
  recommendations for adults 11
  sport supplements for 308
  strength training gains 300
  in weight loss 321-322
resistance training, nutrition for 292-308
  alcohol and 299
  carbohydrate in 293-294, 299, 305
  daily dietary intake 301-304, 302f, 303f
  glycogen replenishment 294-295
  hydration 292-293, 294
  ketogenic diets 305-307
  leucine in 295-299, 296f, 298f, 302
  low-carbohydrate diets 299, 305
  magnesium and 189-190
  protein and amino acids 145-146, 292-299, 301-304

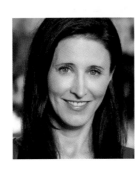

Marie A. Spano, MS, RD, CSCS, CSSD, is one of the country's leading sports nutritionists and the sports performance nutritionist for the Atlanta Hawks, Atlanta Braves, and Atlanta Falcons. She combines science with practical experience to help athletes implement customized nutrition plans to maximize athletic performance, recovery, and career longevity. Also a nutrition communications expert, Spano has appeared on CNN as well as on NBC, ABC, Fox, and CBS affiliates. She has authored hundreds of magazine and trade publication articles in addition to book chapters in *NSCA's Essentials of Strength Training and Conditioning* and *NSCA's Essentials of Personal Training.* She is coeditor of *NSCA's Guide to Exercise and Sport Nutrition.*

A three-sport collegiate athlete, Spano earned her master's degree in nutrition from the University of Georgia, where she worked in the athletic department as a graduate assistant running the sports nutrition program, and her bachelor's degree in exercise and sports science from the University of North Carolina at Greensboro, where she also ran Division I cross country. Her experiences as a college athlete provide her an effective perspective when working with athletes of all levels, especially student athletes, by giving her a firsthand understanding of how the demands of athletics, psychological aspects of injury, sleep, recovery, and nutrition can affect an athlete's overall well-being and performance.

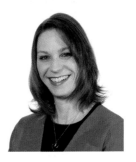

Laura J. Kruskall, PhD, RDN, CSSD, LD, FACSM, FAND, is an associate professor and director of nutrition sciences at University of Nevada, Las Vegas. She oversees the nutrition sciences academic degree programs and serves as program director for the ACEND-accredited dietetic internship. She has held numerous leadership positions at the local, state, and national levels, including serving on the board of trustees of the American College of Sports Medicine (ACSM) and as the cochair of the committee that authored "Standards of Practice and Standards of Professional Performance for Registered Dietitian Nutritionists (Competent, Proficient, and Expert) in Sports Nutrition and Dietetics," published in the *Journal of the Academy of Nutrition and Dietetics* in 2014. She is currently serving as the chair of the nutrition track for the ACSM Health and Fitness Summit and Exposition and is a member of the editorial board for *ACSM's Health & Fitness Journal.* Dr. Kruskall has been given fellow status by both ACSM and the Academy of Nutrition and Dietetics for her leadership and contributions to the profession.

Dr. Kruskall's areas of teaching and practice expertise are sports nutrition, weight management, and medical nutrition therapy. Her research interests include the effects of nutrition and exercise interventions on body composition and energy metabolism and the role of vitamin D in bone health and performance in collegiate athletes. In addition to her academic duties at the university, she is a nutrition consultant for Canyon Ranch SpaClub and Cirque du Soleil in Las Vegas.

Dr. Kruskall earned her PhD in nutrition from Penn State University. She also holds a certificate of training in Adult Weight Management Level 2 from the Commission on Dietetic Registration, is certified as an exercise physiologist by ACSM, holds the Exercise Is Medicine Credential II from ACSM, and is a Board Certified Specialist in Sports Dietetics (CSSD).

D. Travis Thomas, PhD, RDN, CSSD, LD, FAND, is an associate professor of clinical and sports nutrition in the College of Health Sciences and director of the undergraduate certificate program in nutrition for human performance at the University of Kentucky. Dr. Thomas is a Board Certified Specialist in Sports Dietetics (CSSD). He has held multiple national leadership positions for SCAN (a dietetic practice group of the Academy of Nutrition and Dietetics) and received honors as the lead author on the position statement "Nutrition for Athletic Performance" (March 2016, published in three journals).

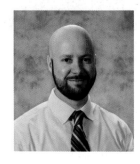

Dr. Thomas became a registered dietitian in 2001 and worked as a clinical dietitian in Greensboro, North Carolina, managing medical nutrition therapy for patients in general medicine, cardiac, rehabilitation, and intensive care units. Dr. Thomas then completed his PhD in nutrition at the University of North Carolina at Greensboro and a postdoctoral fellowship at the University of Kansas. Throughout his doctoral and postdoctoral studies, he expanded his clinical knowledge base to include aspects of exercise physiology, sports nutrition, body composition, and hormone physiology.

Dr. Thomas has more than nine years of experience conducting human studies involving nutrition and exercise interventions across the lifespan. Over the last six years, Dr. Thomas has served as an investigator on several research projects that focused on nutrition issues associated with the preservation and enhancement of skeletal muscle function and performance. These studies have included examining the relationship between vitamin D and muscle metabolic function, studies on nutrition and physical function in aging and athletic populations, nutrition interventions to reduce symptoms in patients with advanced heart failure, and investigating nutrition strategies to preserve physical performance and lean body mass in patients with head and neck cancer. Collectively, this work has resulted in multiple publications and has led to NIH funding to examine the contribution of vitamin D to muscle metabolic function.

Dr. Thomas is married and has two children, Averie and Collin. In his free time, he enjoys traveling, staying physically active, cooking, and gardening. He is an avid fan of collegiate sports.

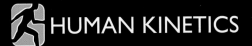
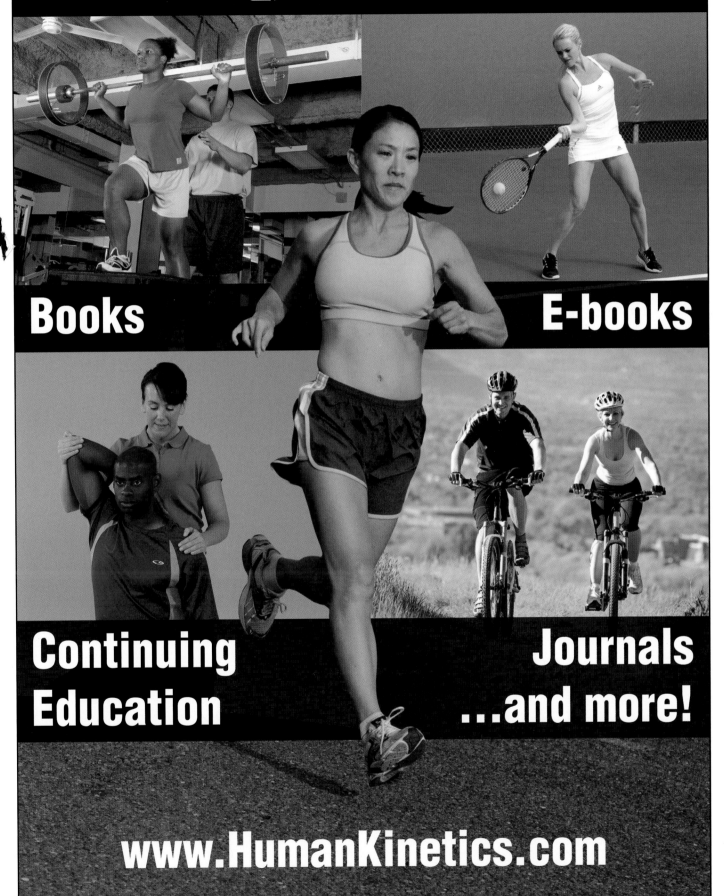